Cancer Disparities

Causes and Evidence-Based Solutions

Ronit Elk, PhD is Director of Cancer Control and Prevention Research and Director of the Priority Program in Health Disparities of the Extramural Research Grants at the American Cancer Society. Born in Israel, she grew up in Israel, Turkey, India, Uganda, Kenya, and South Africa. She received her PhD in Cape Town, South Africa, and shortly thereafter immigrated with her family to the United States. Prior to joining the American Cancer Society, Dr. Elk was an Associate Professor in the Department of Psychiatry and Behavioral Sciences at the University of Texas Health Sciences Center in Houston. She was Principal Investigator of two large National Institutes of Health (NIH) grants ($3 million); and co-investigator or consultant on 12 additional NIH grants. She has served on several research panels of the NIH, and published over 40 scientific papers in peer-reviewed journals. During her 10-year tenure with the American Cancer Society, she has spearheaded the Cancer Control and Prevention Research program, and led the targeted program in Disparities Research, resulting in a dramatic increase in applications and funded grants in these areas. She recently received the Society of Behavioral Medicine, Cancer Special Interest Group award, in recognition of her contribution to this field. Dr. Elk is the author, with Dr. Monica Morrow, of *Breast Cancer for Dummies*. She is also the author of two children's books, *A Surprise at Dancing Fields* and *It's the Elephant's Picnic*.

Hope Landrine, PhD is Director of the Center for Health Disparities Research and Professor of Psychology at East Carolina University. She received her PhD in Clinical Psychology at the University of Rhode Island, postdoctoral training in Social Psychology at Stanford University, and postdoctoral training in Cancer Prevention and Control as a National Cancer Institute Fellow at the University of Southern California Medical School. Her research focuses on sociocultural and contextual factors in cancer and other chronic disease disparities among African Americans. She has published numerous articles and books on this topic, and received six national awards for her research, including the American Psychological Association (APA) Dalmas Taylor Award for Lifetime, Distinguished Contributions to Research on Ethnic Minorities, and Fellow status in APA Divisions 35 (Women), 9 (Social Issues), 38 (Health), and 45 (Ethnic Minorities) for outstanding contributions to research. She is the former Director of Multicultural Health Behavior Research at the American Cancer Society, and continues to collaborate with American Cancer Society and National Cancer Institute scholars on studies of Black–White cancer disparities. Her current grants focus on improving quality of care for Black women breast cancer patients in oncology practices, and on novel strategies for providing cancer education to low-income, rural, minority communities.

Cancer Disparities

Causes and Evidence-Based Solutions

Ronit Elk, PhD
Hope Landrine, PhD
Editors

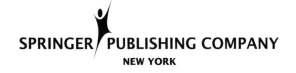

SPRINGER PUBLISHING COMPANY
NEW YORK

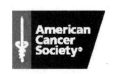
American Cancer Society®

Springer Publishing Company, LLC
11 West 42nd Street
New York, NY 10036
www.springerpub.com

Acquisitions Editor: Jennifer Perillo
Production Editor: Lindsay Claire
Composition: S4Carlisle Publishing Services

ISBN: 978-0-8261-0882-1
E-book ISBN: 978-0-8261-0883-8

10 11 12 13/ 5 4 3 2 1

The author and the publisher of this Work have made every effort to use sources believed to be reliable to provide information that is accurate and compatible with the standards generally accepted at the time of publication. Because medical science is continually advancing, our knowledge base continues to expand. Therefore, as new information becomes available, changes in procedures become necessary. We recommend that the reader always consult current research and specific institutional policies before performing any clinical procedure. The author and publisher shall not be liable for any special, consequential, or exemplary damages resulting, in whole or in part, from the readers' use of, or reliance on, the information contained in this book. The publisher has no responsibility for the persistence or accuracy of URLs for external or third-party Internet Web sites referred to in this publication and does not guarantee that any content on such Web sites is, or will remain, accurate or appropriate.

Library of Congress Cataloging-in-Publication Data

Cancer disparities : causes and evidence-based solutions / [edited by] Ronit Elk, Hope Landrine.
p. ; cm.
Includes bibliographical references.
ISBN 978-0-8261-0882-1 — ISBN 978-0-8261-0883-8 (e-book)
I. Elk, Ronit. II. Landrine, Hope, 1954-
[DNLM: 1. Neoplasms—epidemiology—United States. 2. African Americans—United States. 3. Health Status Disparities—United States. 4. Healthcare Disparities—United States. 5. Hispanic Americans—United States. 6. Socioeconomic Factors—United States. QZ 220 AA1]
LC-classification not assigned
614.5'9990973—dc23   2011028433

Printed in the United States of America by Bang Printing.

We owe a debt of gratitude to the many people—
researchers, clinicians, policy makers,
community advocates, and others—who have committed their
lives' work to reducing health disparities:
The leaders who paved the way;
Those who are currently engaged in the work, and
Future generations who will continue their commitment until
health equity is achieved.
To my father and grandfather
who instilled in me the value of
"tikkun olam" (fixing the world) through example.

Contents

Contributors

E. Kathleen Adams, PhD Professor, Department of Health Policy and Management, Emory University, Atlanta, Georgia

Elvira Aguirre Wendrell, BA Patient Navigator, Department of Health Behavior and Health Education, Fay W. Boozman College of Public Health, University of Arkansas for Medical Sciences, Little Rock, Arkansas

Karen O. Anderson, PhD, MPH Department of Symptom Research, Division of Internal Medicine, University of Texas M. D. Anderson Cancer Center, Houston, Texas

Elva Arredondo, PhD Institute for Behavioral and Community Health, San Diego State University, San Diego, California

Kimlin T. Ashing-Giwa, PhD Center of Community Alliance for Research and Education, City of Hope National Medical Center, Duarte, California

Guadalupe X. Ayala, PhD, MPH Institute for Behavioral and Community Health, San Diego State University, San Diego, California

David W. Baker, MD, MPH Division of General Internal Medicine, Department of Medicine, Northwestern University Feinberg School of Medicine, Chicago, Illinois

Priti Bandi, MS Epidemiologist, American Cancer Society, Atlanta, Georgia

Janice Baranowski, MPH, RD Assistant Professor of Pediatrics, USDA/ARS Children's Nutrition Research Center, Baylor College of Medicine, Houston, Texas

Tom Baranowski, PhD Professor of Pediatrics, USDA/ARS Children's Nutrition Research Center, Baylor College of Medicine, Houston, Texas

Linda G. Blount, MPH National Vice President, Health Disparities, American Cancer Society, Atlanta, Georgia

Ulrike Boehmer, PhD Department of Community Health Sciences, Boston University School of Public Health, Boston, Massachusetts

Morris Boswell, BA Director of Cosmetology, Guilford Technical Community College, BEAUTY Advisory Board Member, Jamestown, North Carolina

Deborah Bowen, PhD Department of Community Health Sciences, Boston University School of Public Health, Boston, Massachusetts

Otis W. Brawley, MD Chief Medical and Scientific Officer, American Cancer Society, Atlanta, Georgia

Richard Buday, FAIA President, Archimage, Inc., Houston, Texas

Zoran Bursac, PhD, MPH Associate Professor, Department of Biostatistic, College of Medicine and Fay W. Boozman College of Public Health, University of Arkansas for Medical Sciences, Bella Vista, Arkansas

Veronica Carlisle, MPH Project Manager, North Carolina BEAUTY and Health Project, University of North Carolina, Chapel Hill, North Carolina

Anabella G. Castillo, MPH Project Coordinator for *Esperanza y Vida*, Department of Oncological Sciences, Mount Sinai School of Medicine, New York, New York

Li-Nien Chien, PhD Post-Doctor at Taipei Medical University, Emory University, Atlanta, Georgia

Suzanne Christopher, PhD Professor, Department of Health and Human Development, Montana State University, Bozeman, Montana

Vilma Cokkinides, PhD Director, Risk Factors Research, American Cancer Society, Atlanta, Georgia

Jomary Colón Project Coordinator for *Esperanza y Vida*, Division of Cancer Control Prevention & Population Sciences, Roswell Park Cancer Institute, Buffalo, New York

Dexter Cooper, MPH Behavioral Research Center, American Cancer Society, Atlanta, Georgia

Irma Corral PhD, MPH Department of Psychiatric Medicine, Brody School of Medicine at East Carolina University, Greenville, North Carolina

Beldine Crooked Arm Pease, BS Program Assistant, Messengers for Health Program, Crow Agency, Montana

Karen W. Cullen, DrPH Associate Professor of Pediatrics, USDA/ARS Children's Nutrition Research Center, Baylor College of Medicine, Houston, Texas

Samuel Cykert, MD Professor, North Carolina Area Health Education Centers Program, AHEC Program and the Department of Internal Medicine and Clinical Epidemiology, University of North Carolina, Chapel Hill, North Carolina

John P. Elder, PhD, MPH Institute for Behavioral and Community Health, San Diego State University, San Diego, California

Moshe Engelberg, PhD, MPH Research Works, San Diego, California

Deborah O. Erwin, PhD Distinguished Member and Director, Office of Cancer Health Disparities Research, Division of Cancer Prevention and Population Sciences, Roswell Park Cancer Institute, Buffalo, New York

Kevin Fiscella, MD, MPH Department of Family Medicine, Community & Preventive Medicine and Oncology, University of Rochester Medical Center and Wilmot Cancer Center, Rochester, New York

Michael Fisch, MD, MPH Professor and Chair, Department of General Oncology, Division of Cancer Medicine, University of Texas M. D. Anderson Cancer Center, Houston, Texas

Julia C. Fondren, MA Professor, Center for Health Disparities Research, East Carolina University, Greenville, North Carolina

Pamela Ganschow, MD Co-Director, Breast Cancer Screening, Prevention and Treatment, Cook County Health and Hospitals System; Assistant Professor of Medicine, Rush Medical College, Chicago, Illinois

Araceli Garcia-Gonzalez, MD, DSc Department of Symptom Research, Division of Internal Medicine, University of Texas M. D. Anderson Cancer Center, Houston, Texas

Heather Honoré Goltz, PhD, LMSW Instructor, Department of Urology, Baylor College of Medicine, VA HSR & D Center of Excellence, Houston, Texas

Derek M. Griffith, PhD Center on Men's Health Disparities, School of Public Health, Department of Health Behavior & Health Education, University of Michigan, Ann Arbor, Michigan

Katie Gunter, MPH, MSW Center on Men's Health Disparities, School of Public Health, Department of Health Behavior & Health Education, University of Michigan, Ann Arbor, Michigan

Karin M. Hahn, MD, MPH Associate Professor, Department of General Oncology, Division of Cancer Medicine, University of Texas M. D. Anderson Cancer Center, Houston, Texas

María Hannigan, BS Northwestern Arkansas Patient Navigation Specialist for *Esperanza y Vida*, Department of Health Behavior and Health Education, Fay W. Boozman College of Public Health, University of Arkansas for Medical Sciences, Bella Vista, Arkansas

Yongping Hao, PhD National Center for Environmental Health, Centers for Disease Control and Prevention, Atlanta, Georgia

Cherise B. Harrington, PhD, MPH Cancer Health Disparities Postdoctoral Research Fellow, University of North Carolina at Chapel Hill, Lineberger Comprehensive Cancer Center, Chapel Hill, North Carolina

Kimala Harris, BA Clinical Research Assistant, Obstetrics and Gynecology & Women's Health, Division of Gynecologic Oncology, Montefiore Medical Center, Bronx, New York

Melanie Harris, PhD Lander College for Women, Touro College, New York, New York

Stacey L. Hart, PhD Associate Professor, Department of Psychology, Ryerson University, Toronto, Ontario

Samantha Hendren, MD, MPH Department of Surgery, Colorectal Surgery Division, University of Michigan School of Medicine, Ann Arbor, Michigan

Erika Hernandez, MA, MPH Institute for Behavioral and Community Health, San Diego, California

Dawn L. Hershmann, MD, MS   Associate Professor of Medicine and Epidemiology, Columbia University, New York, New York

Carol Horowitz, MD, MPH   Associate Professor, Department of Health Evidence and Policy, Mount Sinai School of Medicine, New York, New York

Lucy Horton, MSc, MPH   Institute for Behavioral and Community Health, San Diego, California

Carol Howe   Messengers for Health Executive Board, Lodge Grass, Montana

Sharon Humiston, MD, MPH   Department of Pediatrics, Division of Emergency and Urgent Care, Children's Mercy Hospitals and Clinics, Kansas City, Missouri

Leticia Ibarra, MPH   Director of Programs, Clinicas de Salud del Pueblo, Inc., Brawley, California

Russ Jago, PhD   Reader in Exercise, Nutrition & Health, University of Bristol, United Kingdom

Lina Jandorf, MA   Associate Professor, Department of Oncological Sciences, Mount Sinai School of Medicine, New York, New York

Lois Jefferson   Messengers for Health Executive Board, Crow Agency, Montana

Ahmedin Jemal, DVM, PhD   Surveillance Research, American Cancer Society, Atlanta, Georgia

Jung-won Lim, PhD   Mandel School of Applied Social Sciences, Case Western Reserve University, Cleveland, Ohio

Chiewkwei Kaw, MS   Behavioral Research Center, American Cancer Society, Atlanta, Georgia

Youngmee Kim, PhD   Department of Psychology, University of Miami, Coral Gables, Florida

Joy L. King, BA   Center for Health Disparities Research, East Carolina University, Greenville, North Carolina

Evelyn Kolidas, BA   Albert Einstein College of Medicine, Department of Epidemiology & Population Health, Bronx, New York

David M. Latini, PhD   Assistant Professor of Urology & Psychiatry, Baylor College of Medicine, VA HSR & D Center of Excellence, Houston, Texas

Deb LaVeaux, MS   Program Manager, Center for Native Health Partnerships, Montana State University, Bozeman, Montana

Myra Lefthand, MSW   Messengers for Health Executive Board, Crow Agency, Montana

Stephen J. Lepore, PhD   Professor and PhD Program Director, Temple University, Department of Public Health, Philadelphia, Pennsylvania

Eric Kai-Ping Liao, PhD   Department of Symptom Research, Division of Internal Medicine, University of Texas M. D. Anderson Cancer Center, Houston, Texas

Laura A. Linnan, ScD, CHES Professor, University of North Carolina at Chapel Hill; Member, Lineberger Comprehensive Cancer Center, Chapel Hill, North Carolina

Rochelle Lodgepole, BS Master's student, Montana State University, Bozeman, Montana

Wanda Lucas, MBA Cancer Control Program, Department of Oncology, Lombardi Comprehensive Cancer Center, Georgetown University Medical Center, Washington, District of Columbia

Jiemin Ma, PhD, MHS Surveillance Research, American Cancer Society, Atlanta, Georgia

Alma McCormick Project Coordinator, Messengers for Health Program, Crow Agency, Montana

Gregory Makoul, PhD Connecticut Institute for Primary Care Innovation, Saint Francis Care, Hartford, Connecticut; Department of Medicine, University of Connecticut School of Medicine, Farmington, Connecticut

Elsa Iris Mendez Patient Navigator, Department of Oncological Sciences, Mount Sinai School of Medicine, New York, New York

Tito R. Mendoza, PhD Department of Symptom Research, Division of Internal Medicine, University of Texas M. D. Anderson Cancer Center, Houston, Texas

Alyson B. Moadel, PhD Associate Professor, Albert Einstein College of Medicine, Department of Epidemiology & Population Health, Bronx, New York

Arden Morris, MD, MPH Associate Professor, Division of Colorectal Surgery, Department of Surgery, University of Michigan, Ann Arbor, Michigan

Arlene Nazario, MD Clinical Associate Professor, Department of General Oncology, Division of Cancer Medicine, University of Texas M. D. Anderson Cancer Center, Houston, Texas

Julie Ober Allen, MPH Center on Men's Health Disparities, School of Public Health, Department of Health Behavior & Health Education, University of Michigan, Ann Arbor, Michigan

Margaret K. Offermann, MD, PhD The Salutramed Group, Atlanta, Georgia

Larna Old Elk Bachelor student, Montana State University, Bozeman, Montana

Olufunmilayo I. Olopade, MD Division of Hematology and Oncology, Department of Medicine, University of Chicago Hospitals, Chicago, Illinois

Tracy L. Onega, PhD Department of Community and Family Medicine, Norris Cotton Cancer Center and the Dartmouth Institute for Health Policy and Clinical Practice, Dartmouth Medical School, Lebanon, New Hampshire

Eleanor Pretty On Top Messengers for Health Executive Board, Pryor, Montana

Guadalupe R. Palos, DrPH, LMSW, RN Manager, Clinical Protocol Research, Cancer Survivorship, University of Texas M. D. Anderson Cancer Center, Houston, Texas

Humberto Parada, MPH   Institute for Behavioral and Community Health, San Diego, California

Doru Paul, MD   Department of Medicine, Division of Hematology/Oncology, Lincoln Medical & Mental Health Center, Bronx, New York

Richard Payne, MD   Professor of Medicine and Divinity, Esther Colliflower Director, Duke Institute on Care at the End of Life, Duke University Divinity School, Durham, North Carolina

LeaVonne Pulley, PhD   Associate Professor, Department of Health Behavior and Health Education, Fay W. Boozman College of Public Health, University of Arkansas for Medical Sciences, Little Rock, Arkansas

Bruce D. Rapkin, PhD   Professor of Epidemiology and Population Health, Division of Community Collaboration & Implementation Science, Director, Marilyn & Stanley M. Katz Comprehensive Cancer Prevention & Control Research Program, Albert Einstein College of Medicine, Bronx, New York

Cheryl Rock, PhD   Department of Family and Preventive Medicine, and Cancer Prevention and Control Program, University of California, San Diego; Moores UCSD Cancer Center, La Jolla, California

John M. Rose, MA, PhD   Evaluation Coordinator, North Carolina BEAUTY and Health Project, Durham, North Carolina

Frances G. Saad-Harfouche, MSW   Research Assistant, Division of Cancer Prevention and Population Sciences, Roswell Park Cancer Institute, Buffalo, New York

Ruth Santizo, BA   Study Coordinator, Pediatric Hematology/Oncology, Montefiore Medical Center, Bronx, New York

Denise Scholtens, PhD   Department of Preventive Medicine and Robert H. Lurie Comprehensive Cancer Center, Northwestern University Feinberg School of Medicine, Chicago, Illinois

Leslie R. Schover, PhD   Professor of Behavioral Science, Department of Behavioral Science, University of Texas M. D. Anderson Cancer Center, Houston, Texas

Mayra Serrano, BA   Center of Community Alliance for Research and Education, City of Hope National Medical Center, Duarte, California

Vanessa B. Sheppard, PhD   Cancer Control Program, Department of Oncology, Lombardi Comprehensive Cancer Center, Georgetown University Medical Center, Washington, District of Columbia

Amy Shirong Lu, PhD   Assistant Professor of Media Arts and Science, Indiana University School of Informatics, Indianapolis, Indiana

Rebecca Siegel, MPH   Surveillance Research, American Cancer Society, Atlanta, Georgia

Colleen Simpson   Messengers for Health Executive Board, Billings, Montana

Donald Slymen, PhD   Institute for Behavioral and Community Health, San Diego State University, San Diego, California

Tenbroeck Smith, MA   Behavioral Research Center, American Cancer Society, Atlanta, Georgia

Kevin Stein, PhD   Behavioral Research Center, American Cancer Society, Atlanta, Georgia

Maudine Stewart   Messengers for Health Executive Board, Crow Agency, Montana

Brooke Sylvester, BS   Department of Medicine, University of Chicago, Chicago, Illinois

Linda D. Thélémaque, MPH   Data Manager, Department of Oncological Sciences, Mount Sinai School of Medicine, New York, New York

Debbe Thompson, PhD   Scientist Nutritionist, and Assistant Professor of Pediatrics, USDA/ARS Children's Nutrition Research Center, Baylor College of Medicine, Houston, Texas

Ann Trauscht, MD   Lake County Health Department and Community Health Center, Waukegan, Illinois

Michelle Treviño, MPH   Project Coordinator for *Esperanza y Vida*, Department of Health Behavior and Health Education, Fay W. Boozman College of Public Health, University of Arkansas for Medical Sciences, Little Rock, Arkansas

Vicente Valero, MD   Professor, Department of Breast Medical Oncology, Division of Cancer Medicine, University of Texas M. D. Anderson Cancer Center, Houston, Texas

Katherine Virgo PhD, MBA   Behavioral Research Center, American Cancer Society, Atlanta, Georgia

Sherri Flynt Wallington, PhD   Lombardi Comprehensive Cancer Center, Georgetown University Medical Center, Washington, District of Columbia

Elizabeth Ward, PhD   Vice President, Surveillance & Health Policy Research, American Cancer Society, Atlanta, Georgia

Vanessa Watts Simonds, ScD   Post-Doctoral Fellow, Robert Wood Johnson Foundation Center for Health Policy, MPH Program, Department of Family and Community Medicine, Albuquerque, New Mexico

J. Lee Westmaas, PhD   Director, Tobacco Research, American Cancer Society, Atlanta, Georgia

Chaplain Carol Whiteman   Messengers for Health Executive Board, Pryor, Montana

Karen Patricia Williams, PhD   Department of Obstetrics, Gynecology & Reproductive Biology, College of Human Medicine, Michigan State University, East Lansing, Michigan

Preface

American Cancer Society Strategies
for Reducing Cancer Disparities

Linda G. Blount

Significant progress has been made in the reduction of cancer incidence and mortality rates. Delay-adjusted incidence rates for all low-income, racial, and ethnic groups combined decreased by 0.7% per year from 1999 to 2007, after stabilizing from 1989 to 1999 and increasing by 1.2% per year from 1975 to 1989. The decline in overall mortality rates accelerated from 1.1% per year from 1993 to 2001 to 1.6% per year from 2001 to 2007 (Jemal et al., 2008). This is real progress. However, very real and widening gaps are masked by these statistics. In fact, cancer mortality rates are falling much faster for some populations than for others. And, in the case of breast cancer and colorectal cancer, the difference in mortality rates between African Americans and Caucasians, rich and poor, is greater now than 25 years ago.

There are many reasons why cancer disparities exist. These reasons have been analyzed and described in many books and peer-reviewed publications over the past 25 years. The role that social determinants of health, access to quality care, and culturally relevant health communications materials and delivery methods can play in cancer prevention and optimal cancer health outcomes is understood to a great degree. But where do researchers and practitioners turn for evidence-based interventions that have narrowed the disparities gap in cancer incidence and mortality? Unfortunately, very few scientific articles, and no book to date, explain these disparities in a language suitable for medical, public health, and social–behavioral scientists, and even fewer publications present concrete interventions that can be used to reduce or eliminate cancer disparities.

Cancer Disparities: Causes and Evidence-Based Solutions is the first book on cancer disparities that provides *evidence-based interventions proven to reduce cancer disparities*. This book constitutes a novel, long-overdue, comprehensive

approach to cancer disparities and their reduction. While cancer researchers, faculty, and graduate students in medical schools, cancer centers, and
schools of public health will find this book an important addition to the
academic syllabus, public health and cancer-control leaders in community
organizations will find this book a valuable resource for understanding cancer disparities and interventions efforts to end them. Eminently readable for
nonresearchers, this book will act as a guide to community-based studies
that have been evaluated and provide real-life examples of how barriers to
cancer care, prevention, and information can be reduced or even eliminated.

The research presented in this book reflects the commitment of the
American Cancer Society (ACS), the largest nongovernmental funder of cancer research, to reducing and eliminating cancer disparities. The Society has
a long history of funding research, programs, and services to help those facing a disproportionate cancer burden and inequities in cancer care. A decade
before Dr. David Satcher, Surgeon General of the United States, coined the
phrase "Elimination of Health Disparities," then ACS National President,
Dr. Harold Freeman, convened a Board-led Oversight Committee to study
cancer control in underserved communities. The 1989 report, *Cancer Control
and the Socioeconomically Disadvantaged*, was the first strategic plan by the
ACS to address cancer disparities, and was developed in response to ACS-
sponsored regional hearings on cancer in the poor. The report concluded
that reaching out to socioeconomically disadvantaged populations was "a
top priority" and that "all components of the Society should be involved"
(Freeman, 1989). The Committee's action strategies for the Society centered
around three areas: public policy (including calls for health reform); patient
advocacy and empowerment (working with community partners, adapting
the ACS direct response system to address the information needs of the poor,
and training staff and volunteers to address the cancer control needs of the
disadvantaged); and education and early detection (increasing behavioral
research on effective ways to reach culturally diverse subgroups, messaging and advertising campaigns to counteract the work of tobacco companies,
and funding community-level demonstration projects on cancer prevention,
detection, and education).

In 2002, a team of volunteers and staff reviewed progress toward
Dr. Freeman's plan and determined if new strategies were required. Their
recommendations largely supported those of the earlier initiative, including
implementing community outreach and partnerships with community-level
organizations, offering evidence-based interventions, providing education, disseminating information, focusing on government regulation and
legislative advocacy, and building more infrastructure and capacity at the
community level. Two years later, the Society adopted a strategic framework of information, prevention, detection, quality of life, and research that

represents the Society's optimal role in the fight against cancer. Because of its importance, strategies for reducing health care disparities were included in every aspect of that framework.

The formation of the Office of Health Disparities in 2007, working in collaboration with national and division departments, ensured the continuity of the strategic focus on health equity and the elimination of disparities, encompassing a broad spectrum of work, including: front-line advocacy for increased access to high-quality, affordable cancer care and work with state and local lawmakers to ensure that the needs of the underserved are met, particularly through adequate funding of the National Breast and Cervical Cancer Early Detection Program (NBCCEDP); linguistically and culturally appropriate awareness, prevention, and screening information; hip-hop artists targeting anti-tobacco messaging to youth and young adults; patient navigation programs in disproportionate share hospitals and *promotoras* serving low-income Hispanic patients; partnerships with minority media outlets, professional, and civic organizations; and scores of community-based programs that have provided patient support and increased understanding of cancer, prevention, and early detection among thousands of low-income and minority individuals.

The Society has both an intramural and an extramural research focus. Intramural research conducted by ACS scientists centers primarily on surveillance and analytic epidemiology and health services research. The Surveillance and Health Policy Research department plays a key role in promoting cancer control in the underserved population by compiling and disseminating information on disparities in cancer incidence, survival, mortality, and risk factors to cancer control advocates, the media, educators, and the general public. It does so through its annual *Facts and Figures* publications, the most widely cited cancer publications, and through its annual *Cancer Statistics* article in *CA: A Cancer Journal for Clinicians*, which reaches a wide clinical audience. The department's *Annual Report to the Nation* monitors the nation's progress in reducing cancer incidence and mortality overall, as well as by specific racial and ethnic populations. The Department of Analytic Epidemiology is responsible for the Society's largest intramural research study, Cancer Prevention Study III (CPS-III), which will eventually accrue up to 500,000 participants, 25% of whom will be racial and ethnic minorities (www.cancer.org). The research in this department also has, as a primary focus, studies on the impact of nutrition and physical activity on cancer risk, treatment, and outcomes. The findings of CPS-III should make a significant contribution to the understanding of cancer, its etiology, and the risk factors among racial and ethnic minorities. This department has conducted all of the Society's large cohort studies to provide insights about causes of cancer and prevention. The three main cohorts, Hammond-Horn and the CPS-I and

CPS-II, feature prominently in many Surgeon General Reports on tobacco (Thun, Calle, Rodriguez, & Wingo, 2000).

Over the past 60 years, the Society's Extramural Research Grants (ERG) Department has funded more than $3 billion in cancer research, primarily basic science, to help understand the etiology of cancer and to develop interventions to prevent and treat the disease. In 1999, in response to the Society's 2015 goals of eliminating disparities in cancer burdens, the ERG department designated poor and medically underserved populations as a high-priority area of focus, with set aside dollars. The goals of this focus area, called the Targeted Program, were to explore innovative research that would lead to the discovery of effective cancer treatments, prevention practices, and early detection measures for high-risk populations, and to increase the evidence base on which programmatic and public policy decisions were made. In recognition of the importance of this area of research, up to 10% of the total ERG budget, approximately $10 million per year, was set aside for this program. In the 10 years from 1999 to 2009, $99 million has been awarded to targeted research, constituting 10.9% of the $908 million awarded to nontargeted research over the same period.

In an effort to meet the goals of making ACS-funded research relevant to the policies and programs of the Society, and to enhance the implementation of evidence-based programs in the Divisions, the results of funded studies are shared through the Targeted Grants Program and the Office of Health Disparities on an ongoing basis with the National Department of Health Promotion and ACSCAN, and through partnerships formed with ACS-funded researchers and Divisions.

The Targeted Program of the Extramural Research Grants Department has been reviewed by several Advisory Boards over the years. In prior years, there were recommendations that the ERG Department continue with this special Targeted Program, due to its strong relevance to Society goals and its high potential to benefit the populations it is targeting. The 2009 evaluation recommended both expanding and broadening the scope of the program. On these recommendations, it has been made a high-priority area of funding in the Cancer Control and Prevention Research Program of the Extramural Grants Program.

Attracting new researchers into this field was another stated goal of the Targeted Program. This program has attracted researchers from racial and ethnic groups that are traditionally underrepresented in science (including researchers of African American, Hispanic, and Native American descent). While the majority of the applicants in both "Targeted" and "non-Targeted" extramural grants programs are Caucasian, significantly more applicants from populations underrepresented in science applied for research grants in the Targeted Program.

The Targeted Program has funded studies across the cancer continuum. By far the majority (86%) are those that focus on cancer control and prevention, quality of life, and health policy/health services research, with just a few in the clinical research or basic sciences. The majority of the funded studies focus on ethnic-minority populations in which health care disparities exist, with African Americans being the largest group studied. Ninety-three percent of funded studies examine an aspect of prevention, early detection, and screening. Prevention studies look at specific behaviors, with the largest number targeting diet and exercise modification, followed by smoking cessation. Screening and early detection primarily address breast, colorectal, and cervical cancer, with many examining the use of Lay Health Advisors to change screening behaviors.

A significant number of the studies used Community-Based Participatory Research (CBPR) methods, in which a partnership between the community of focus and the research team is formed in order to identify the questions of concern and the culturally appropriate methods for jointly finding solutions. Chapter 12 is an outstanding example of a true community-research partnership, in which Dr. Christopher and at least 20 women leaders from the Apsáalooke tribe worked hand in hand, at every step of the way, in designing and testing a program titled "Messengers for Health" that would enhance cervical cancer screening for women of the community.

Studies focusing on treatment include those describing treatment differences between various ethnic or other underserved groups, provider–patient interactions, and the effect of health care systems and policies on differential outcomes. In Chapter 16, Dr. Sheppard and colleagues describe a unique culturally based intervention, "Sisters Informing Sisters^{SM}," that is designed to help African American women understand and embrace the need to complete adjuvant treatment for breast cancer.

Health policy research is an important area of interest, particularly as health care reform implementation moves forward. In Chapter 11, Dr. Adams examines the effect of legislative change (extending Medicaid coverage to any uninsured woman under 65 in need of cancer treatment, with breast or cervical cancer or pre-cancerous cervical conditions) on outcome. Women got into the program more quickly, received the right treatment, and in the case of cervical cancer, extended treatment in some groups, in a timely manner.

This unique and highly competitive Targeted Program funds esteemed researchers across the nation to develop interventions to reduce cancer disparities and promote health equity. Fifteen of their studies, which highlight effective interventions across a broad range of underserved populations, were chosen for this book. They serve as evidence that, with the right culturally appropriate interventions, *change is possible.*

REFERENCES

Cancer Epidemiology, Biomarkers & Prevention September 2000 9; 861. http://www.cancer.org/Research/ResearchProgramsFunding/Epidemiology-Cancer PreventionStudies/CancerPreventionStudy-3/index.

Freeman, H. (1989). *Report of the Interdepartmental Oversight Committee on Cancer Control and the Socioeconomically Disadvantaged: Proposed plan of action.* Philadelphia, PA. 64 pp.

Jemal, A., Thun, M. J., Ward, E. E., Henley, S. J., Cokkinides, V. E., & Murray, T. E. (2008). Mortality from leading causes by education and race in the United States, 2001. *American Journal of Preventive Medicine, 34*(1), 1–8.

Thun, M. J., Calle, E. E., Rodriguez C., & Wingo, P. A. (2000). Epidemiological research at the American Cancer Society. Cancer Epidemiology, Biomarkers & Prevention, 9, 861–868.

Acknowledgments

We have been truly fortunate in collaborating with a group of outstanding American Cancer Society–funded researchers and colleagues. We chose your projects because of your outstanding research, and have been inspired by the effect of your interventions on reducing disparities. We look forward to watching the impact your work will have on future generations of researchers, clinicians, community workers, and, most importantly, the communities and patients we serve.

We are deeply grateful to the reviewers, national experts in their respective fields, who provided valuable critiques and constructive feedback on the initial chapter draft. [Listed in chapter order: Charles Saxe, PhD—American Cancer Society; Xiao-Cheng Wu, MD, MPH—Louisiana State University Health Science Center, Louisiana State University; Ted Gansler, MD, MBA—American Cancer Society; Jennifer Griggs, MD, MPH—University of Michigan; Deborah Bowen, PhD—Boston University School of Public Health; Latrice C. Pichon, PhD, MPH, CHES—The University of Memphis; Wendell Taylor, PhD, MPH—Univeristy of Texas, Houston; Janice Bowie, PhD, MPH—Johns Hopkins Bloomberg School of Public Health; Cheryl Holt, PhD—University of Maryland; Dianne S. Ward, PhD—University of North Carolina; Cathy Bradley, PhD—Virginia Commonwealth University; June Strickland, PhD, RN— University of Washington School of Nursing; Lisa Rey Thomas, PhD—University of Washington; Michael Pignone, MD, MPH—University of North Carolina; Richard G. Roetzheim, MD, MSPH—Moffitt Cancer Center; Roberta Baer, PhD—University of South Florida; Sandra Millon Underwood, RN, PhD, FAAN—University of Wisconsin Milwaukee; Suzanne K. Chambers, PhD—Cancer Council Queensland; April Vallerand, PhD, RN, FAAN—Wayne State College of Nursing; Mitch Golant, PhD—Cancer Support Community; Anna Maria Napoles, PhD, MPH—University of California San Francisco; Alicia Matthews, PhD—UIC College of Nursing.]

Warm thanks go to Kim A. Smith for her inestimable administrative help in sending out endless emails, collecting and compiling forms, creating spreadsheets, and making sure all the myriad pieces were in place. Teresa Aluku who volunteered to help with the bibliography and willingly jumped in during "crises," deserves a special thank you.

We owe a special debt of gratitude to our leaders, Drs. David Ringer and Otis Brawley, who believed in the importance of this project right from the beginning and supported our work on it throughout.

We also want to express our gratitude to Jennifer Perillo and Lindsay Claire, our acquisitions editor and senior production editor, respectively, at Springer Publishing, and Nandini Loganathan, our project manager at S4Carlisle, for their thoughtful feedback, enduring patience, and concerted efforts to keep the book on schedule.

Finally, we want to recognize the pioneers who have led the struggle for health equality. We are continuing the work, and hope to inspire future generations.

Introduction

Cancer Disparities: The Scope of the Problem and Possible Solutions

Otis W. Brawley

THE BIRTH OF A DISCIPLINE

In 1973, a landmark paper was published documenting the increasing disparities in cancer mortality between Black and White Americans (Henschke et al., 1973). In many ways, this paper was inspired by the U.S. Civil Rights Movement. It was the signal that the struggle for racial equality was broadening beyond social and economic equality to include equality in health care. The Henschke paper and similar papers related to other diseases would eventually be the start of the academic discipline known as "minority health." Over time, the field become known as "special populations" and later—in the mid-1990s, with the wisdom of then Surgeon General Dr. David Satcher—it became known as "health disparities" (Nkwa-Mullan et al., 2010). The name "health disparities" was descriptive of the field. The phrase was less open to criticism from politicians who did not support programs and research in minority health or special populations. It became difficult for a politician to stand up and speak up against programs intended to reduce disparities in health. Today, there is a movement toward calling the field "health equity." The documentation of disparities in race and the expansion of the discipline became a significant influence on the current health care debate.

The basic principle behind health disparities is the reality that there are populations that do not do as well as others in terms of health outcomes. Initially, those focusing on minority health were physicians who recognized racial differences in presentation of disease and mortality. As the academic field grew, it attracted the talents of professionals in diverse medical disciplines, epidemiologists, and social scientists. Anthropologists helped define populations, and nursing scientists and the palliative care movement helped expand the field further by better defining disparities and expanding the measures of disparities. Patient advocacy was equally important in the birthing of the field. In the 1980s, Congress legislated establishment of the National Institutes of Health (NIH) Office for Research on Minority Health and the Department of Health Education and Welfare (later the Department of Health and Human Services) Office of Minority Health. Eventually, almost every federal health agency opened an office for special populations and, later, an office for health disparities. Provisions within the NIH Revitalization Act of 1993 strengthened research into the field (Freedman et al., 1995) and in 2010, the Affordable Care Act transformed the NIH Office for Research on Minority Health into an institute, with the ability to fund grants and programs across the country. Cancer was one area where the disparities in screening and treatment were clearly documented (Greenberg, Weeks, & Stain, 2008). In an effort to address this, Congress passed legislation creating the Centers for Disease Control (CDC) Breast and Cervical Cancer Treatment Program, to give poor women access to breast and cervical cancer screening. (Later, this program was modified to pay for treatment for those diagnosed with those cancers, an evaluation of which appears in Chapter 11.)

HEALTH DISPARITIES BECOME MORE THAN BLACK AND WHITE

At one time, the only disparate outcomes discussed were differences in incidence and mortality among Blacks and Whites. Today, our concern for health disparities and achieving health equity has expanded beyond concern for the health of African Americans. During his tenure as volunteer president of the American Cancer Society in 1989, Harold Freeman brought tremendous focus on the fact that America's poor, be they Black, White, Hispanic, Asian, or Native American, have disparate cancer outcomes. In the early 1990s, National Cancer Institute director Sam Broder made a now famous statement that "poverty is a carcinogen." This led to studies of the effects of poverty and social deprivation on the cause and course of malignant disease. Health disparities research dramatically increased in the field of oncology (Freeman, 1998). Significant advances have been made in defining the scientific and political issues that cause disparities in health, and the interventions (public health, medical, and sociopolitical) that can alleviate such disparities and lead to health equity. Much can be learned through comparing and contrasting well-defined populations. Efforts to determine why one cohort has a low rate of a cancer can help us find interventions to lower that rate in other populations.

DATABASES ENHANCE THE MEASUREMENT OF DISPARITIES

The development of cancer databases and registries has increased the availability of data and helped to define disparities through assessment of other outcomes and in other populations. The CDC National Center for Health Statistics (NCHS), established in the early 1960s, began providing state-by-state mortality data. Eventually, NCHS began the National Health Interview Survey (NHIS) and the Behavioral Risk Factor Surveillance System (BRFSS) to provide additional data (Cyrus-David, King, Bevers, & Robinson, 2009). The NCI Surveillance, Epidemiology, and End Results (SEER) Program was launched in 1972 as part of the implementation of the National Cancer Act. It provided incidence and 5-year survival data. As its data matured, additional outcomes measures became available. Researchers began looking at practice patterns data and even geographic differences. In the early 1990s, the NCI SEER program went beyond publishing Black–White data and began publishing data for the five racial and ethnic categories as defined by the U.S. Office of Management and Budget (OMB). The National Cancer Data Base (NCDB) was launched in the late 1980s. It is run by the American College of Surgeons Commission on Cancer and supported by the American Cancer Society. The NCDB registry has grown to include hospitals that treat more than 70% of Americans with cancer. It gathers such demographic data as insurance status and time to treatment received, thereby allowing additional analysis of differences in quality of treatment. Questions addressed include the proportion with a specific disease not receiving standard care and differences in quality of treatment (Fry, Menck, & Winchester, 1996). Recently, quality of life for cancer patients and cancer survivors (pediatric and adult) has become a concern in the health disparities community. Focus areas include the availability of adequate pain control, as well as access to programs for physical and emotional rehabilitation (Lafleur, Said, McAdam-Marx, Jackson, & Mortazavi, 2007).

KEY ASPECTS TO CONSIDER IN CATEGORIZING POPULATIONS

If we are to truly attack disparities in health outcomes, we must be open minded, question the standard prejudices and paradigms, and carefully define the scientific and medical questions that need to be addressed. Key to defining the problem has been adequately categorizing populations, identifying the outcomes that are disparate, defining how to measure those outcomes, and defining the causes of disparities. Only then can we identify the interventions necessary to overcome the disparities (Brawley & Berger, 2008). Today, we recognize that there are numerous ways to define populations. Categories frequently used include race, ethnicity, and area of geographic origin or socioeconomic status. There are significant cautions that need to be taken when defining populations using these categories. These are words whose meaning and history are not well understood by the lay and medical public, and they are frequently used with differing meanings. Our race-based labels crudely predict for groups of people that are less likely to do well with cancer and other diseases, but we must realize the sociopolitical nature of these categories (Witzig, 1996). Race is not a biologic categorization. In the assessment of risk of cancer, a form of "benevolent racial profiling" is sometimes appropriate; however, overcommitment to this view without deep, careful thought can obscure the truth and actually impede science from benefiting disparate populations.

The concept of *race* originated in the eighteenth century. It has to do with superficial facial features and presumed geographic area of origin. It does not even deal with skin color, as dark-skinned people from the Indian subcontinent are considered Caucasian. There are no distinct races, and racial groups are overlapping populations (Brown, 2007). The one "drop rule" in which a person with just one known African ancestor is considered Black is still practiced in this country and is the ultimate example of how unscientific the concept of race is. Many who describe themselves as Black or African American are actually a mixture of European and African ancestries (Witzig, 1996). *Ethnicity* involves culture, habit, lifestyle, and behavioral patterns and other environmental influences that can cause disease or even lower the risk of disease (Faulkner and Merritt, 1998). Ethnicity defines foods consumed and how foods are prepared. Different ethnic groups often have different attitudes toward health and medical care. They interact differently with medical professionals. Appreciation of this is important to health care professionals who want to provide appropriate care. Ethnicity is appreciated as distinctly different from race. Both are important in cancer causation. Hispanic is an ethnicity. An individual can be categorized as Black race and Hispanic ethnicity or White race and Hispanic ethnicity. Ethnicity might be a bit more scientific than race, even though it is not necessarily static. Some people identify themselves as belonging to a particular ethnic group in one context, and to another in a different context (Corral & Landrine, 2008). The racial and ethnic categories used in most U.S. health care data are defined by the OMB. These definitions are used in the U.S. Census. The census data is then used to determine the size of the population in calculating rates of disease. In their directive defining race and ethnicity, OMB notes that the categories are sociopolitical in nature and not based in science.

Area of geographic origin is another way of categorizing populations. It can loosely correlate with ethnicity and race, but tends to be more specific than race. When asked about area of origin, Americans of Korean and African ancestry are more likely to identify as Korean and African, whereas racially they might consider themselves Black or African American.

Socioeconomic status (SES) is a category that often correlates with health status. Its definition has also evolved over time; SES was once defined by household income or education and occupation (Albano et al., 2007). Today, we recognize that insurance status and even degree of medical sophistication are important factors in outcomes. European social scientists have taken SES to a higher level, with deprivation indices that in some cases even take into account whether one has indoor plumbing or household help (Byers et al., 2008). SES can be highly correlated with differences in outcome and related to unknown environmental influences that cause cancer, cause a delay in diagnosis of cancer, or cause less than optimal treatment of cancer. Access to care and lack of convenient care are SES-based variables that play a tremendous role in disparities in the United States (Faggiano, Partanen, Kogevinas, & Boffetta, 1997). SES is also related to the quality and types of foods consumed, the neighborhood and environment one lives in, and the work one does (Faggiano et al., 1997). Numerous surveys suggest that poor Americans are more likely to have harmful health behaviors and less likely to practice healthy behaviors. The poor are more likely to consume higher-calorie diets and have diets higher in carbohydrates and fats. Poor Americans are also more likely to be overweight or obese, and less likely to consume diets high in fruits and vegetables, compared to middle- and upper-middle-class Americans (Satia-Abouta, Patterson, Neuhouser, & Elder, 2002).

Area of residence, too, can be a factor in cancer risk. In the United States, area of residence can be viewed as rural versus urban, with differing access to health care. It can include living in polluted areas with greater exposure to disease-causing chemicals, such as a landfill or an industrial area (Law & Morris, 1998). It can also include living in crime-ridden inner-city neighborhoods, where opportunities for healthful habits such as exercise are limited (Bennett et al., 2007; Gaskin, Price, Brandon, & Laveist, 2009).

These categories can overlap and make attribution of cause of disease difficult. For example, as discussed in Chapter 5, in the United States low SES can be associated with the Black race and living in an inner-city area. An outcome caused by low SES in a group of Blacks might be mistaken as being due to race or to area of residence. It could also be truly related to all three (Kaufman, Cooper, & McGee, 1997). A higher proportion of Americans of African heritage are poor compared to Whites. It is appropriate to ask what the effect of poverty is on our race-based health statistics. Indeed, socioeconomic status and its incumbent environmental influences may be the cause of many health disparities. It is possible that socioeconomic factors that act largely through and are associated with race are responsible for much of the disparity between Black and White (Ward et al., 2004).

RACE MEDICINE: DISPARITIES IN CANCER RISK AND INCIDENCE

Cancer is caused by an aberration of genetics. The aberration can be due to an inherent genetic mutation that can be passed on through generations. It can also be due to environmental influences on a gene or series of genes. Some cohorts have a higher prevalence of a specific genetic mutation or a series of genes that increase risk. Some cohorts have increased or decreased risk due to environmental exposures. An understanding of both cancer genetics *and* population genetics is critical for those who wish to approach disparities in health in a rational scientific way, in which pertinent questions are identified and clearly stated.

Over the years, American medicine has placed much interest on genetic differences among the races. The concept that phenotypic differences translate into biologic differences was the basis of "Race Medicine." This concept was commonly accepted in the America of the 19th and early 20th centuries. It was one of the reasons that the study commonly known as the "The Tuskegee Syphilis Study," which began in 1932, was thought reasonable and ethical. Syphilis was thought to be a very different disease in Blacks versus Whites. Many actually believed that syphilis rarely killed infected Blacks, but frequently killed infected Whites (Brawley, 1998). Race Medicine is still with us today. This belief in biologic differences among the races has crept into the discipline of health disparities (Goldson, Henschke, Leffall, & Schneider, 1981). It is unfortunate we do sometimes read that "breast cancer is a different disease in Blacks versus Whites" or that "prostate cancer is a different disease in Blacks versus Whites." Truth be told, as explained in chapter 1, there are highly aggressive, bad-prognosis cancers and there are less aggressive, good-prognosis cancers. No race has a monopoly on the good cancers or on the bad cancers. It is also true that a higher proportion of Black American women with breast cancer have the more aggressive types (Brawley, 2010; Lund et al., 2009).

A good scientific question is, "Why do a higher proportion of Black women with breast cancer have the poorer-prognosis disease compared to White women?" A second good question rarely discussed is, "Why do a higher proportion of White women have the good-prognosis breast cancers?" It is known that there are racial differences in a number of environmental factors that are correlated with breast cancer risk. Indeed, in the United States there are racial differences in the proportion beginning menstruation at an early age, birthing patterns, the proportion that is obese, and the use of postmenopausal hormones (Lund et al., 2008). Could race be a surrogate for SES status? Some data suggests that SES and social deprivation not only correlate with the risk of cancer, but also with pathologic factors (Gordon, 1995; Gordon, 2003). Several studies suggest that poor White women with breast cancer are more likely to be diagnosed with estrogen receptor negative tumors (Gordon, 1995; Thomson, Hole, Twelves, Brewster, & Black, 2001). It is unknown how poverty influences pathology of disease. It may be through lifelong diet, and birthing habits. Diets high in calories during childhood can affect age at menarche. Earlier age at menarche is known to be associated with increased breast cancer risk later in life. A higher proportion of the poor are overweight or obese. Increased body mass index has been correlated with increased risk of postmenopausal breast cancer. Similarly, increased body mass index, which is more common in African American males compared to White males, has been correlated with increased risk for more aggressive prostate cancer (Amling et al., 2004; Spangler et al., 2007).

While it is important to study race, it is also important not to overemphasize race. Even when a specific genetic difference is highly associated with a race or ethnicity, it might more appropriately be considered familial rather than racial or ethnic. A specific gene or series of genes can be conserved among families, and a closed society will conserve genetic traits within that society. Segregation on the basis of race, ethnicity, economics, or other factors can lead to increased prevalence of a specific gene or series of genes in the segregated population. This has been demonstrated in several diseases with a well-defined genetic basis, such as Tay Sachs disease, cystic fibrosis, and sickle cell disease. Each of these diseases has a higher prevalence in, but is not exclusive to, a specific racial/ethnic group. Even the mutation of BRCA common among Ashkenazi Jews has been linked to a small number of individuals having it about 1,000 years ago, and it is now preserved through ethnic segregation. As populations in Europe and America mix, these genetic differences will lessen (Offit et al., 1996).

There are genetic variations between human populations. A gene, or even a single nucleotide polymorphism (SNP) allele, that is common in one geographic, racial, or ethnic group may be rare in another. Some of these genetically based differences translate into a difference in disease risk among populations. Some of these differences have been associated with an environmental influence and can offer a survival advantage. Sickle cell disease, for example, is associated with area of geographic origin. People from Spain, Italy, Greece, and the Middle East, as well as northern and sub-Saharan Africa, have sickle cell trait and sickle cell anemia. While the prevalence of sickle cell trait and sickle cell anemia is higher in sub-Saharan Africa, there is also a prevalence in people originating from southern Europe and considered to be of White race. Sickle cell is not found among Black Africans originating from southern Africa. This genetic mutation is thought to be an example of genetic selection. Those who had sickle cell trait had some advantage during a massive malaria epidemic several thousand years ago. That advantage extends to those with sickle cell trait to this day (Brawley et al., 2008). Sickle cell disease is an excellent example of environmental influences on genetics. The fact that it parallels a geographic area where people are considered of White race and Black race is also a good lesson, as most Americans think of sickle cell disease solely as an affliction of Blacks.

There are other genetic markers that correspond with areas of geographic origin far better than with skin color or race (Fijumara & Rajagoplan, 2011). Glucose 6 phosphate dehydrogenase deficiency is common in, but not monopolized by, people originating in the Middle East and Mediterranean regions (Beutler, Lisker, & Kuhl, 1990). Alcohol dehydrogenase deficiency is common in persons from certain areas of Asia. There are differences in metabolism of some drugs by genetic markers that tend to parallel area of geographic origin. The drug irinotecan, or CPT 11, is used in the treatment of colon cancer. It is metabolized by the UDP-glucuronosyltransferase 1-1 gene (*UGT1A1*) gene in the liver. Certain polymorphisms of the gene metabolize the drug slower than others. The U.S. Food and Drug Administration recommends that patients with certain polymorphisms of *UGT1A1* receive reduced doses of the drug. It is one of the first cancer drugs dosed according to genotype. Asian populations tend to have a slower *UGT1A1* compared to populations originating in Europe (Beutler, Gelbart, & Demina, 1998). The word "tend" is important. It is best to do the laboratory tests necessary to assess *UGT1A1* in the specific patient than to do racial medical profiling and assume that all Asians should be dose reduced. Racial medical profiling can deprive a patient of a therapeutic dose of this drug. The movement toward personalized medicine, with its emphasis on the genetics of the individual, may be one way that we stop racial medical profiling.

RACE MEDICINE: SCREENING, DIAGNOSIS, AND TREATMENT OF CANCER

Much cancer research shows that equal treatment yields equal outcomes, among equal patients (Bach, Cramer, Warren, & Begg, 1999). Race in and of itself need not be a factor in the outcomes of cancer treatment. Unfortunately, as is clearly documented in Chapter 6, numerous patterns of care studies show that there is not equal treatment; race *is* a factor in treatment (Shavers & Brown, 2002). There are Black–White disparities in both the availability and use of care and in the quality of care received. In the field of oncology, these studies overwhelmingly show that the proportion of Blacks getting adequate screening, diagnostics, and treatment is less than the proportion of Whites. Some studies show that Blacks in the southern United States are more likely to get less than optimal cancer care compared to Blacks in the northeast, who are less likely to get optimal care compared to Blacks in the west (Harlan, Brawley, Pommerenke, Wali, & Kramer, 1995).

As suggested earlier, while race is a correlative factor in these disparities, the driver of the disparities may be due to socioeconomic differences, and not racial. Studies suggest that some disparities in treatment are due to racism and some are due to SES discrimination. Other important factors are lack of access to good therapy or lack of convenient access to needed therapy. Comorbid diseases (including obesity) can also make aggressive cancer therapy inappropriate. Some disparities in cancer treatment may be due to comorbid diseases and may be appropriate (Griggs et al., 2007). Unfortunately, very few studies have looked at disparities by socioeconomic status, and even fewer have looked at practice pattern disparities in other racial/ethnic groups such as Hispanics, Asians, or Native Americans. Little effort has been put into assessing outcomes in other disenfranchised communities, such as refugee communities, or the lesbian, gay, bisexual, and transgender communities (Mayer et al., 2008). Chapter 21 discusses one of the few studies focusing on sexual-minority women with breast cancer.

Cultural differences in acceptance of therapy and lack of education about the disease are huge drivers in the disparate receipt of health care. Some cultures have fatalistic views toward cancer and a cancer diagnosis. This causes them to run away from good care when it is available. Culturally sensitive interventions to educate and create understanding about disease can help bring about health equity. Experience tells us that a successful intervention is created by someone who understands and cares about the population with the disparity. All interventions should be carefully and rigorously assessed for effectiveness before full implementation. These interventions must be implemented with sensitivity and by a trusted source. For example, as described in chapter 9, research has found that in some situations a beautician can be a highly trusted source and a very effective teacher. At the same time, a highly degreed health care expert may be unsuccessful. The concept of community-based participatory research is based on this finding (Ford et al., 2009).

CONCLUSION

Health equity can only be achieved through open-mindedness and a committed interest on the part of health care providers, social scientists, health consumers, and health advocates. In some instances, the medical and medical–social professions have to change their preconceived notions. In order to achieve health equity, it is imperative that we:

- Realize the meaning of race, ethnicity, area of geographic origin, and socio-economic status, and appreciate the limitations of those categories.
- Understand the role of cancer genetics, population genetics, and the role of environmental interactions with genes.
- Value the scientific method as we rigorously assess culturally sensitive interventions to reduce health disparities and bring about health equity.
- Care about the fact that there are disparities, and care about and respect the uniqueness of the patients we serve.

Each of the researchers whose works are presented in this book has taken steps along this journey. If we all follow these principles, think of the major impact we can have on the lives of future generations.

REFERENCES

Albano, J. D., Ward, E., Jemal, A., Anderson, R., Cokkinides, V. E., Murray, T., . . . Thun, M. J. (2007). Cancer mortality in the United States by education level and race. *Journal of the National Cancer Institute, 99*, 1384–1394.

Amling, C. L., Riffenburgh, R. H., Sun, L., Moul, J. W., Lance, R. S., Kusuda, L., . . . McLeod, D. G. (2004). Pathologic variables and recurrence rates as related to obesity and race in men with prostate cancer undergoing radical prostatectomy. *Journal of Clinical Oncology, 22*, 439–445.

Bach, P. B., Cramer, L. D., Warren, J. L., & Begg, C. B. (1999). Racial differences in the treatment of early-stage lung cancer. *New England Journal of Medicine, 341*, 1198–1205.

Bennett, G. G., McNeill, L. H., Wolin, K. Y., Duncan, D. T., Puleo, E., & Emmons, K. M. (2007). Safe to walk? Neighborhood safety and physical activity among public housing residents. *PLoS Medicine, 4*, 1599–1606.

Beutler, E., Gelbart, T., & Demina, A. (1998). Racial variability in the UDP-glucuronosyltransferase 1 (UGT1A1) promoter: A balanced polymorphism for regulation of bilirubin metabolism? *Proceedings of the National Academy of Sciences of the United States of America, 95*(14), 8170–8174.

Beutler, E., Lisker, R., & Kuhl, W. (1990). Molecular biology of G 6 PD variants. *Biomedica Biochimica Acta, 49*, S236–S241.

Brawley, O. W. (1998). The study of untreated syphilis in the negro male. *International Journal of Radiation Oncology, Biology, Physics, 40*, 5–8.

Brawley, O. W. & Berger, M. Z. (2008). Cancer and disparities in health: Perspectives on health Statistics and research questions. *Cancer, 113*, 1744–1754.

Brawley, O. W. (2010). Towards a better understanding of race and cancer. *Clinical Cancer Research, 16*(24), 5920–5922.

Brawley, O. W., Cornelius, L. J., Edwards, L. R., Gamble, V. N., Green, B. L., Inturrisi, C., . . . Schori, M. (2008). National Institutes of Health Consensus Development Conference statement: Hydroxyurea treatment for sickle cell disease. *Annals of Internal Medicine, 148*, 932–938.

Brown, M. (2007). Defining human differences in biomedicine. *PLoS Medicine, 4*, e288.

Byers, T. E., Wolf, H. J., Bauer, K. R., Bolick-Aldrich, S., Chen, V. W., Finch, J. L., . . . Yin, X. (2008). The impact of socioeconomic status on survival after cancer in the United States: Findings from the National Program of Cancer Registries Patterns of Care Study. *Cancer, 113,* 582–591.

Corral, I., & Landrine, H. (2008). Acculturation and ethnic-minority health behavior: A test of the operant model. *Health Psychology, 27,* 737–745.

Cyrus-David, M., King, J., Bevers, T., & Robinson, E. (2009). Validity assessment of the Breast Cancer Risk Reduction Health Belief scale. *Cancer, 115,* 4907–4916.

Faggiano, F., Partanen, T., Kogevinas, M., & Boffetta, P. (1997). Socioeconomic differences in cancer incidence and mortality. *IARC Scientific Publications,* 65–176.

Faulkner, D. L., & Merritt, R. K. (1998). Race and cigarette smoking among United States adolescents: The role of lifestyle behaviors and demographic factors. *Pediatrics, 101,* E4.

Ford, A. F., Reddick, K., Browne, M. C., Robins, A., Thomas, S. B., & Crouse, Q. S. (2009). Beyond the cathedral: Building trust to engage the African American community in health promotion and disease prevention. *Health Promotion Practice, 10,* 485–489.

Freedman, L. S., Simon, R., Foulkes, M. A., Friedman, L., Geller, N. L., Gordon, D. J., & Mowery, R. (1995). Inclusion of women and minorities in clinical trials and the NIH Revitalization Act of 1993—The perspective of NIH clinical trialists. *Controlled Clinical Trials, 16,* 277–285.

Freeman, H. P. (1998). The meaning of race i n science—Considerations for cancer research: Concerns of special populations in the National Cancer Program. *Cancer, 82,* 219–225.

Fry, W. A., Menck, H. R., & Winchester, D. P. (1996). The National Cancer Data Base report on lung cancer. *Cancer, 77,* 1947–1955.

Fujimura, J. H., & Rajagopalan, R. (2011). Different differences: The use of 'genetic ancestry' versus race in biomedical human genetic research. *Social Studies of Science, 241*(1), 5–30.

Gaskin, D. J., Price, A., Brandon, D. T., & Laveist, T. A. (2009). Segregation and disparities in health services use. *Med Care Research and Review, 66,* 578–589.

Goldson, A., Henschke, U., Leffall, L. D., & Schneider, R. L. (1981). Is there a genetic basis for the differences in cancer incidence between Afro-Americans and Euro-Americans? *Journal of the National Medical Association, 73,* 701–706.

Gordon, N. H. (1995). Association of education and income with estrogen receptor status in primary breast cancer. *American Journal of Epidemiology, 142,* 796–803.

Gordon, N. H. (2003). Socioeconomic factors and breast cancer in black and white Americans. *Cancer Metastasis Review, 22,* 55–65.

Greenberg, C. C., Weeks, J. C., & Stain, S. C. (2008). Disparities in oncologic surgery. *World Journal of Surgery, 32,* 522–528.

Griggs, J. J., Culakova, E., Sorbero, M. E., van Ryn, M., Poniewierski, M. S., Wolff, D. A., . . . Lyman, G. H. (2007). Effect of patient socioeconomic status and body mass index on the quality of breast cancer adjuvant chemotherapy. *Journal of Clinical Oncology, 25,* 277–284.

Harlan, L., Brawley, O., Pommerenke, F., Wali, P., & Kramer, B. (1995). Geographic, age, and racial variation in the treatment of local/regional carcinoma of the prostate. *Journal of Clinical Oncology, 13,* 93–100.

Harlan, L.C., Coates, R.J., Block, G., Greenberg, R. S., Ershow, A., Forman, M., . . . Heymsfield, S. B. (1993). Estrogen receptor status and dietary intakes in breast cancer patients. *Epidemiology, 4,* 25–31.

Henschke, U. K., Leffall, L. D., Jr., Mason, C. H., Reinhold, A. W., Schneider, R. L., & White, J. E. (1973). Alarming increase of the cancer mortality in the U.S. Black population (1950–1967). *Cancer, 31*, 763–768.

Kaufman, J. S., Cooper, R. S., & McGee, D. L. (1997). Socioeconomic status and health in blacks and whites: The problem of residual confounding and the resiliency of race. *Epidemiology, 8*, 621–628.

Lafleur, J., Said, Q., McAdam-Marx, C., Jackson, K., & Mortazavi, M. (2007). Problems in studying the association between race and pain in outcomes research. *Journal of Pain and Palliative Care Pharmacotherapy, 21*, 57–62.

Law, M. R., & Morris, J. K. (1998). Why is mortality higher in poorer areas and in more northern areas of England and Wales? *Journal of Epidemiol Community Health, 52*, 344–352.

Lund, M. J., Brawley, O. P., Ward, K. C., Young, J. L., Gabram, S. S., & Eley, J. W. (2008). Parity and disparity in first course treatment of invasive breast cancer. *Breast Cancer Research and Treatment, 109*, 545–557.

Lund, M. J., Trivers, K. F., Porter, P. L., Coates, R. J., Leyland-Jones, B., Brawley, O.W., . . . Eley, J. W. (2009). Race and triple negative threats to breast cancer survival: A population-based study in Atlanta, GA. *Breast Cancer Research and Treatment, 113*, 357–370.

Mayer, K. H., Bradford, J. B., Makadon, H. J., Stall, R., Goldhammer, H., & Landers, S. (2008). Sexual and gender minority health: What we know and what needs to be done. *American Journal of Public Health, 98*, 989–995.

Nkwa-Mullan, I., Rhee, K. B., Williams, K., Sanchez, I., Sy, F. S., Stinson, N., Jr., & Ruffin, J. (2010). The science of eliminating health disparities: Summary and analysis of the NIH summit recommendations. *American Joirnal of Public Health, 100*(Suppl 1), S12–S18.

Offit, K., Gilewski, T., McGuire, P., Schluger, A., Hampel, H., Brown, K., . . . Goldgar, D. (1996). Germline *BRCA1 185delAG* mutations in Jewish women with breast cancer. *Lancet, 347*, 1643–1645.

Satia-Abouta, J, Patterson, R. E., Neuhouser, M. L., & Elder, J. (2002). Dietary acculturation: Applications to nutrition research and dietetics. *Journal of the American Dietetic Association, 102*, 1105–1118.

Shavers, V. L., & Brown, M. L. (2002). Racial and ethnic disparities in the receipt of cancer treatment. *Journal of the National Cancer Institute, 94*, 334–357.

Spangler, E., Zeigler-Johnson, C. M., Coomes, M., Malkowicz, S. B., Wein, A., Rebbeck, T. R. (2007). Association of obesity with tumor characteristics and treatment failure of prostate cancer in African-American and European American men. *Journal of Urology, 178*, 1939–1944.

Thomson, C. S., Hole, D. J., Twelves, C. J., Brewster, D. H., & Black, R. J. (2001). Prognostic factors in women with breast cancer: Distribution by socioeconomic status and effect on differences in survival. *Journal of Epidemiology and Community Health, 55*, 308–315.

Ward, E., Jemal, A., Cokkinides, V., et al. (2004). Cancer disparities by race/ethnicity and socioeconomic status. *CA: A Cancer Journal for Clinicians, 54*, 78–93.

Witzig, R. (1996). The medicalization of race: Scientific legitimization of a flawed social construct. *Annals of Internal Medicine, 125*, 675–679.

I

UNDERSTANDING CANCER DISPARITIES

1

The Biology of Cancer and Its Relationship to Disparities in Cancer Occurrence and Outcomes

*Brooke Sylvester, Olufunmilayo I. Olopade,
and Margaret K. Offermann*

DNA DAMAGE AND THE DEVELOPMENT OF CANCER

Cancer is a group of diseases in which cells have developed the ability to invade into surrounding tissues and potentially metastasize to distant sites (Kessenbrock, Plaks, & Werb, 2010; Talmadge & Fidler, 2010). There are many different types of cancer, but they all occur as a consequence of acquired mistakes in the DNA, including epigenetic changes (Hoeijmakers, 2009). The DNA provides the master plan for all organisms in which four nucleotide bases (guanine, cytosine, adenine, and thymine) occur in specific arrangements and spell out the exact instructions required to create a particular organism with its own unique traits. The coding contained in the DNA is responsible for the formation and function of the complete spectrum of different cells and organs, as well as the biologic changes that occur as we age. The changes in the DNA that lead to cancer alter critical cellular processes that govern cell behavior, leading to cells that can invade and move to places where they do not belong (Markowitz & Bertagnolli, 2009; Michor, Iwasa, Vogelstein, Lengauer, & Nowak, 2005; Vogelstein & Kinzler, 2004). The different types of cancer reflect the different types of cells that undergo changes in their programming as a consequence of the alterations in the DNA (Aranda, Nolan, & Muthuswamy, 2008; Asselin-Labat et al., 2008; Lindvall, Bu, Williams, & Li, 2007; Lukacs et al., 2008; Mishra, Glod, & Banerjee, 2009). For example, kidney cancer occurs when the DNA in kidney cells changes to allow cells to invade and metastasize (Valladares Ayerbes et al., 2008), whereas breast cancer occurs when breast cells develop critical changes in their DNA (Lindvall et al., 2007; Turner & Grose, 2010). The types of mistakes that lead to cancer create additional subtypes of cancer. For example, breast cancer with amplification of the *HER-2/neu* gene is different from breast cancer that over expresses the estrogen receptor (Charafe-Jauffret et al., 2005; Livasy et al., 2006). Thus, cancer is hundreds of different diseases, and knowledge of the shared and unique features of the different types of cancer is leading to more effective strategies for prevention, early detection, and treatment.

To understand why some people get cancer and others do not, it is important to understand that people are protected against cancer by many biologic processes designed to ensure that the more than 3 billion nucleotides in the DNA are properly copied each time a cell divides (Bartek & Lukas, 2007; de Bruin & Wittenberg, 2009; Talos & Moll, 2010). Both genetic and environmental factors affect the likelihood that mistakes will occur, and both contribute to disparities in cancer occurrence and outcome in various populations.

There are many different types of errors that can occur when DNA is replicated, and when they are not corrected, the changes are usually detrimental to the cell, but occasionally they give a growth advantage. While nearly all cells have the same DNA, different types of cells use distinct portions of the DNA for defining cellular characteristics and behavior, and making proteins that address each cell's specific needs. Access to distinct portions of the DNA code are regulated through a process called epigenetics, in which the ability to read the DNA code is changed without changing the DNA sequence, and epigenetic changes can also contribute to cancer (Clark, 2007; Omura & Goggins, 2009; Weidman, Dolinoy, Murphy, & Jirtle, 2007). Most cancers also contain alterations in the DNA sequence. Simple substitutions of nucleotides can lead to mutations that alter proteins or change regulatory regions in the DNA (Lee et al., 2010; Salk, Fox, & Loeb, 2010). Sometimes changes involve large portions of DNA, including duplications, deletions, inversions, or movement of DNA to distant regions (called translocations); these changes often affect hundreds of genes simultaneously (Argos et al., 2008; Dreyling et al., 1995; Grushko et al., 2002; Murnane, 2010; Nussenzweig & Nussenzweig, 2010; Turner & Grose, 2010). Changes in DNA that are detrimental to the cells usually are eliminated, whereas changes that give cells a growth and survival advantage can rapidly be propagated and set the stage for the development of cancer.

The development of cancer generally requires multiple changes in the DNA, and cells that undergo many divisions are at increased risk for cancer, especially if they are exposed to carcinogenic agents that induce DNA damage (Rajaraman, Guernsey, Rajaraman, & Rajaraman, 2006). The likelihood of multiple mistakes happening within a single cell increases over time and with multiple cell divisions. Thus, the overall risk of cancer increases with age and is more likely to occur in cells that are programmed to undergo frequent replacement, such as skin cells or cells lining the colon (Hoeijmakers, 2009). There can be more than 1,000 mutations and other genetic mistakes within some cancers (Kwei, Kung, Salari, Holcomb, & Pollack, 2010; Lee et al., 2010), indicating that many biologic processes are likely to be altered and making simple fixes difficult. Cancer cells continue to evolve and acquire additional changes in their DNA (Kwei et al., 2010; Negrini, Gorgoulis, & Halazonetis, 2010; Talos & Moll, 2010). As new variants arise, those that offer survival advantage become more prevalent in the population. The ongoing evolution of tumors can lead to resistance to treatment and clinical relapses, even when the original cancer shows a complete clinical response.

Despite the huge number of changes in DNA that have been identified in some cancers, critical changes converge on a limited number of biologic processes. Pathways that are commonly involved include those that allow replication of damaged DNA, those that promote cellular replication, those that inhibit programmed cell death, those that immortalize cells, and those that stimulate environments favorable for tumor cell growth (Kessenbrock et al., 2010; Tammela & Alitalo, 2010; Turner & Grose, 2010).

DISPARITIES IN CANCER INCIDENCE AND OUTCOME

The incidence and outcome of cancer differ in various segments of the U.S. population, with socioeconomic status, race/ethnicity, residence, gender, and sexual orientation all having an impact (American Cancer Society, 2010). Data from the Surveillance, Epidemiology, and End Results (SEER) program show that African Americans have the highest incidence and mortality rates of cancer compared to other racial and ethnic groups within the United States. The mortality rate for African American males is 34% higher than among Caucasian males; African American females display a 17% higher mortality rate when compared to Caucasian females. The causes of the increased mortality depend on the type of cancer and involve differences in tumor biology, timeliness of diagnosis, approach to cancer management, and presence of coexisting diseases. Hispanics, Asians/Pacific Islanders, and American Indians/Alaska Natives in the United States have lower incidence rates when compared to Caucasians and African Americans for the most common cancer types. In contrast, Asians/Pacific Islanders display the highest incidence and mortality rates for liver and stomach cancers, cancers that are initiated by infectious agents that are more prevalent in Asia than in the United States, suggesting that immigrants from these areas might be contributing to the higher incidence (Kimura, 2000; Tsai & Chung, 2010). To understand and correct the disparities that exist, it is important to incorporate our evolving knowledge of the complex biologic processes that are affected by various forms of cancer into the analysis of the disparities that exist.

INHERITED SUSCEPTIBILITY TO CANCER

While cancer is due to acquired mistakes in the DNA, the likelihood of acquiring these changes can be affected by inherited factors in the DNA. It is currently estimated that more than 90% of cancers are sporadic and are not due to an inherited susceptibility, whereas 5%–10% of cancers are linked to an inherited susceptibility. The prevalence of some of the inherited factors differs in various populations, thereby contributing to some cancer disparities (Markowitz & Bertagnolli, 2009; Petrucelli, Daly, & Feldman, 2010; Rebbeck, Halbert, & Sankar, 2006). For those who have inherited a defective copy of a gene that increases cancer risk, the development of cancer is still dependent on acquiring additional changes in the DNA, with various environmental factors affecting the likelihood that cancer-causing changes will occur.

Some inherited cancer-susceptibility genes confer risk for many forms of cancer, whereas others confer risk for only a specific type of cancer (Markowitz & Bertagnolli, 2009; Petrucelli et al., 2010; Rebbeck et al., 2006). Inherited defects in the *BRCA1* and *BRCA2* genes increase risk for both breast and ovarian cancers (about 80% lifetime risk in some carriers), whereas they confer a much smaller risk of developing other cancers, including pancreatic cancer (Petrucelli et al., 2010). The BRCA1 and BRCA2 proteins play a role in DNA repair, and when the proteins are defective, damaged DNA is more likely to persist and accumulate multiple changes that can culminate in cancer (Kwei et al., 2010; Olopade, Grushko, Nanda, & Huo, 2008; Powell & Kachnic, 2008; Zhang & Powell, 2005). Inherited mutations in the *BRCA* genes are found most often in people of Ashkenazi Jewish decent, but they may also contribute to breast cancer in young African American women, as will be discussed later in the chapter.

Some people inherit defective forms of one of the enzymes in the DNA mismatch repair system, and this predisposes to hereditary nonpolyposis colorectal cancer (Lynch syndrome), with endometrial cancer and ovarian cancer also occurring at increased frequency (Hampel et al., 2005). Many other genes that predispose to cancer have been identified, but most of the inherited cancer syndromes are relatively rare, and thus do not play a large role in overall disparities in the occurrence and outcome of cancer in various populations.

ENVIRONMENTAL FACTORS CONTRIBUTING TO CANCER

Tumorigenesis is a multistage process that usually happens over many years, making it difficult to pinpoint the specific environmental agents responsible for the multiple changes that lead to cancer. Broadly defined, environmental factors include all external forces that act upon an organism, including dietary factors, infectious agents, sunlight, occupational exposures, pollutants, and all other agents encountered throughout a lifetime, some of which might increase risk for cancer (Chameides, 2010; Clavel, 2007; Monforton, 2006; Robinson, 2002; Tominaga, 1999; Weidman et al., 2007; Zhao, Shi, Castranova, & Ding, 2009). Exposure to carcinogens at a young age is generally more problematic than for older individuals, due to the higher rate of cell division in younger people who are growing and due to the many years over which additional mistakes can accumulate (Barton et al., 2005). Some environmental factors increase the risk of cancer by directly inducing DNA damage, whereas others increase the likelihood that a cell with damaged DNA will survive, proliferate, and go on to develop more damage that leads to cancer.

Cancer clusters that are associated with specific occupations, specific geographic sites, and/or use of specific products have played an important role in identifying carcinogenic agents. For example, boys who served as chimney sweeps in the 18th century were observed to develop scrotal cancer, an otherwise rare form of cancer that was triggered by some of the chemicals in the soot that came in contact with their tissues (Cherniack, 1992; Hall, 1998). In the late 19th century, epidemiologic studies identified an excessive occurrence of bladder cancer among workers in the aniline dye industry. Since that time, multiple studies have firmly established that the risk of bladder cancer increases with exposure to a variety of industrial chemicals known to have carcinogenic effects, including naphthylamine, methylene dianiline, and toluidine (Golka, Wiese, Assennato, & Bolt, 2004). Ship workers and others exposed to asbestos fibers are at increased risk of mesothelioma and of lung cancer, with the inflammation triggered by the fibers playing a large role in tumor development many years after the exposure (Gibbs & Berry, 2008; Maeda et al., 2010). The Environmental Protection Agency, the Consumer Product Safety Commission, the Occupational Safety and Health Administration, and other federal and state groups have enacted regulations to limit exposure to many carcinogenic substances. These regulations reduce risk, but exposures to carcinogens continue to occur, with some occupations and geographic areas posing greater risk than others, and with lower socioeconomic groups proportionally having greater exposures (Steenland, Burnett, Lalich, Ward, & Hurrell, 2003).

Tobacco

Some chemicals that are present in tobacco are carcinogenic, and the risk that they pose increases with exposure (Secretan et al., 2009). Some people also inherit an increased risk to becoming addicted to nicotine and hence are at increased risk of heavy smoking, which thereby increases their cancer risk (Stevens et al., 2008). There are multiple genes that affect the likelihood that someone will become addicted, and the role of these in racial differences in tobacco use and dependence is only starting to be explored (Sherva et al., 2010). In addition, some people inherit genes that modulate their risk of cancer through differences in their ability to metabolize and clear carcinogens, through differences in their ability to recognize and repair damaged DNA, and through other mechanisms (Weisberg, Tran, Christensen, Sibani, & Rozen, 1998; Wu et al., 2002). The tissues that are most at risk for damage from the carcinogens in cigarettes are those within the respiratory track, mouth, and upper digestive tract, which are exposed to the chemicals in smoke. Some chemicals in smoke get absorbed and are excreted through the kidneys and bladder, which contributes to an increased risk of kidney and bladder cancer in smokers (Green et al., 2000; Lodovici & Bigagli, 2009). Most smokers start as teenagers; the incidence of lung cancer, however, peaks after age 60, which indicates that it often takes a long time for carcinogenic agents to cause damage to the DNA that is sufficient to cause cancer. Quitting smoking reduces but does not eliminate risk, because some of the damage that has occurred is permanent, and these cells remain at increased risk for acquiring additional changes in the DNA (Ebbert et al., 2003). Some agents enhance the carcinogenic nature of tobacco. For example, the combination of heavy tobacco and alcohol poses a greater risk of developing cancers of the oral cavity and esophagus than either agent alone (Scully & Bedi, 2000; Secretan et al., 2009). The mechanisms responsible for these combined effects are not known and are being investigated. The combination of asbestos and tobacco leads to a much higher risk of lung cancer than either agent alone (O'Reilly, McLaughlin, Beckett, & Sime, 2007). Some of the cancers that are induced by tobacco can also occur in nonsmokers. Sometimes, these tumors are linked to secondhand smoke, but some of them have molecular features that indicate that distinct mechanisms are involved in their initiation. For example, while most head and neck cancer in the United States is due to heavy use of tobacco and alcohol, an increasing number are due to infection with human papillomavirus (HPV) (Settle et al., 2009). Many cases of lung cancer in nonsmokers have molecular features that differ dramatically from lung cancer in smokers, pointing to distinct mechanisms involved in their development.

Dietary Factors

Dietary factors can either increase or decrease the risk of cancer through a variety of different mechanisms (Ahn et al., 2007; Carpenter, Yu, & London, 2009; Huxley et al., 2009). People with diets that are low in fruits and vegetables are at increased risk for cancer, yet people who consume high amounts of fruits and vegetables do not appear to be at less risk for cancer than those who consume moderate amounts. Very low consumption of fruits and vegetables can lead to vitamin deficiencies, including folate, vitamin B6, vitamin B12, and vitamin A, and these can increase mutation rates (Ames, 1999). Several randomized studies indicate that supplementation with micronutrients is often not sufficient to reduce risk, and may increase risk in some situations (Goodman, Alberts, & Meyskens, 2008). For example, deficiencies in beta-carotene (a precursor to vitamin A) have been associated with an increased risk of cancer in people exposed to the carcinogens in tobacco, but randomized trials in high-risk populations have shown that supplementation with beta-carotene increased rather than decreased cancer incidence and cancer mortality among smokers (Bardia et al., 2008). The form in which a micronutrient is delivered can also make a difference. Vitamin C from dietary sources, but not from supplements, is associated with a reduced risk of oral premalignant lesions (Maserejian, Giovannucci, Rosner, & Joshipura, 2007). Consumers are often led to believe that such supplements are safe and effective, but many do not help, and some may be causing harm.

Some studies show that the manner in which the food is prepared plays an important role in the increased risk that is linked to consumption of some foods. For example, grilling of red meats at high temperatures can generate heterocyclic amine carcinogens that would be absent or at lower levels with meat prepared in different manners (Alaejos, Gonzalez, & Afonso, 2008; Cross & Sinha, 2004). This is thought to contribute to some of the increased risk of cancer in people who consume large quantities of red meat. Smoking and salt preservation are thought to contribute to the high rate of stomach cancer in Japan, especially when the bacteria *Helicobacter pylori* (HP) is present (Kimura, 2000). A diet high in fresh fruits and vegetables reduces the risk of stomach cancer in people with HP who consume high quantities of salted and pickled foods, illustrating the complexity of how diet affects cancer risk.

While some methods of food preservation are associated with increased risk of cancer, foods that are free of preservatives are not always better than those that have preservatives, especially if the food is at risk for contamination with microorganisms. Several fungi that grow on grains produce potent carcinogens, with fumonisen and aflatoxin increasing the risk of liver cancer (Larsen, 2010; Moore, 2009; Murphy et al., 1996; Preston & Williams, 2005). Levels of these toxins are carefully monitored and regulated in the United States, but are often found in the food supplies of developing nations, especially those with poor storage facilities. Susceptibility to carcinogens found in food can be modified by many dietary factors. For example, the chlorophyll found in green plants reduces absorption of aflatoxin, thereby offering some protection from this potent carcinogen (Preston & Williams, 2005).

Some advocacy groups have raised concern that milk products, especially those from cows that receive bovine growth factor, increase the risk of breast cancer. Bovine growth hormone is biologically inactive in humans, and data from multiple epidemiologic studies as well as laboratory studies do not show that dairy products increase risk of breast cancer (Parodi, 2005).

Obesity

There is an increased rate of some forms of cancer in individuals who are obese (Ahn et al., 2007; Brown & Simpson, 2010; Calle, Rodriguez, Walker-Thurmond, & Thun, 2003; van Kruijsdijk, van der Wall, & Visseren, 2009). There are multiple biologic changes that can occur during obesity, including insulin resistance, elevated levels of circulating cellular growth factors, elevated levels of estrogen, and increased inflammation (van Kruijsdijk et al., 2009). These may be working with carcinogens, viruses, and other factors to increase the risk of DNA damage, thereby enhancing the risk of tumor development. Fat also serves as a reservoir for certain types of chemicals, some of which are carcinogenic.

The multiple changes in DNA that lead to cancer generally occur over many years, and thus it is likely that the age at which someone becomes obese and the duration of the obesity both have an impact on cancer risk. Some ethnic and racial groups are at increased risk of obesity, with genetic, cultural, and environmental factors all contributing to variations in its prevalence. Dieting reverses obesity in only a small fraction of people who attempt it, and studies that have looked at the consequences of weight loss in large populations did not show a reduction in mortality, most likely because some of the weight loss was triggered by disease processes rather than by individual choice (Bamia et al., 2010; Dixon, 2010; Eckel, 2008; Nanri et al., 2010). Nonsurgical methods for planned weight loss have been disappointing, with a low percentage of subjects achieving and sustaining the desired weight, but subjects often show improvement in cholesterol and markers of inflammation, providing evidence of probable clinical benefit (Dansinger, Gleason, Griffith, Selker, & Schaefer, 2005; Eckel, 2008; Franco et al., 2007; Rapp et al., 2008; Sacks et al., 2009). One 10-year prospective interventional study showed that bariatric surgery on morbidly obese patients in Sweden led to major sustained weight loss, with a modest reduction in cancer rates in women but not men (Sjostrom et al., 2009). Thus, while obesity may increase the risk of cancer, weight loss in adults is disappointing in its ability to reduce risk. Ideally, efforts should be focused on preventing obesity to reduce short- and long-term health effects, including cancer.

Inflammation

The immune system is designed to respond to infection or injury, and in most cases it protects the host, but it can sometimes contribute to tumor formation and propagation (Grivennikov, Greten, & Karin, 2010; Sgambato & Cittadini, 2010; Wang & DuBois, 2008). This occurs in part because cells of the immune system are designed to attach and kill foreign organisms, but they can also damage normal cells when inflammation is prolonged. The duration of inflammation is linked to the risk of cancer, with the site of the inflammation being linked to where cancer occurs. The inflammation can be in response to inflammatory diseases, such as ulcerative colitis, which increases the risk of colon cancer (Markowitz & Bertagnolli, 2009). Prolonged stomach acid reflux can lead to chronic irritation of the esophagus that causes cellular changes recognized as Barrett's esophagus, a premalignant condition in which inflammation plays an important role in the subsequent development of esophageal cancer (Edelstein, Farrow, Bronner, Rosen, & Vaughan, 2007; Sharma, 2009a, 2009b). Particle irritation, as occurs with asbestos, triggers an inflammatory response that plays an important role in the development of mesothelioma and lung cancer (Antonescu-Turcu & Schapira, 2010; Heintz, Janssen-Heininger, & Mossman, 2010; Maeda et al., 2010). Prolonged infection, as occurs with some viral, bacterial, or parasitic infections, also plays an important role in the development of some forms of cancer (Heintz et al., 2010; Maeda et al., 2010).

Infectious Agents

Some reports estimate that 20%–30% of human cancers are initiated by an infectious agent, with specific viruses, bacteria, and parasites serving as carcinogens (Morris, Young, & Dawson, 2008). Some viruses directly contribute to human cancers by bringing genetic materials into cells that permanently alter cellular programming, thereby increasing the likelihood that cells will acquire additional changes that sometimes result in cancer (Morris et al., 2008). Tumorigenic viruses that directly alter cellular programming as an early event in tumor development include HPV, Epstein–Barr virus (EBV), the Kaposi's sarcoma herpesvirus (KSHV), hepatitis B, human T cell leukemia virus, and Merkel cell carcinoma polyoma virus (Carbone, Cesarman, Spina, Gloghini, & Schulz, 2009; Chang et al., 1994; Feng, Shuda, Chang, & Moore, 2008; Kalland, Ke, & Oyan, 2009; Klass & Offermann, 2005; Morris et al., 2008; Ruprecht, Mayer, Sauter, Roemer, & Mueller-Lantzsch, 2008). The inflammatory response that accompanies chronic infection can also lead to some forms of cancer, as occurs with HP and schistosomiasis (Kimura, 2000; Mostafa, Sheweita, & O'Connor, 1999). HP is a bacterium that contributes to the development of most cases of stomach cancer (Perrin, Ruskin, & Niwa,

2010), and the parasite schistosomiasis causes bladder cancer in parts of the world where infection is common (Mostafa et al., 1999). Infections that suppress immune function, including the human immunodeficiency virus (HIV), also contribute to tumorigenesis by reducing the ability of the immune system to suppress or kill tumorigenic viruses and developing tumors (Carbone et al., 2009; Crum-Cianflone et al., 2009). The importance of recognizing the role of infectious agents in tumorigenesis relates to the potential for preventing or clearing the infectious agent, thereby reducing cancer risk.

The likelihood that someone will develop a cancer as a consequence of an infectious agent is affected by place of birth, racial or ethnic background, sexual orientation, socioeconomic status, access to state-of-the-art health care and other factors. For example, hepatitis B is a vaccine-preventable disease that is endemic to certain parts of Asia and Africa (Lee & Lee, 2007; Tsai & Chung, 2010). Women who are carriers can transmit the virus to their newborn offspring, and the virus is also transmitted sexually or through contact with infected blood. People who develop chronic active hepatitis as a consequence of hepatitis B infection are at increased risk for hepatocellular cancer, with most tumors arising after 30 years or more of infection, since tumor development remains dependent on the acquisition of additional changes in the DNA. The risk of hepatitis B infection can be reduced through vaccination, screening of blood products to ensure that the products are free of the virus, using sterile needles for injections and infusions, and educating the public on how to reduce the risk of sexually transmitted diseases. When someone is found to be a chronic carrier and has chronic active hepatitis, treatments are available that clear infection in a high percentage of carriers. These measures are disparately used to prevent and control infection within various populations within the United States, and many of them are not available in poor countries.

In addition to differences in prevalence of infection with tumorigenic agents in different populations, there are differences in exposure to agents that serve as co-carcinogens. For example, nearly 100% of cervical cancers and anal cancers are initiated by HPV, but only a subset of people who are infected with tumorigenic strains of HPV go on to develop cancer (Longworth & Laimins, 2004; Settle et al., 2009; Stanley, Pett, & Coleman, 2007; Woodman, Collins, & Young, 2007). Both smoking and obesity increase the likelihood that someone with HPV infection will go on to develop cervical cancer (Rieck & Fiander, 2006). Screening through the use of Pap smears detects HPV-induced premalignant and malignant changes that can be treated before they become advanced, but the use of these methods and the use of vaccination against HPV is not consistent across various populations.

Infection with HIV increases the risk for cancer, with the greatest risk from cancers linked to tumorigenic viruses such as HPV, EBV, and KSHV

(Carbone et al., 2009; Crum-Cianflone et al., 2009). HIV infection increases the risk for the development of Kaposi's sarcoma 20,000–80,000-fold, with people who acquired HIV through homosexual activity at greater risk than those who acquired HIV through intravenous drug use. Not all people infected with HIV are at equal risk for the development of cancer, in part because lifestyle factors affect the risk of co-infection with HPV and KSHV, and they also affect exposure to co-carcinogens.

Radiation

Ionizing radiation can induce DNA damage, thereby increasing risk for cancer development (Bolus, 2008; Wall et al., 2006; Williams, 2008). Higher risks are associated with younger age at exposure, and females have somewhat higher risks of cancer from radiation exposure than males do. Some occupations and geographic sites are associated with increased levels of exposure, but the role of ionizing radiation in cancer disparities has not been well studied. Several recent studies report greater occupational exposure among African American than Caucasian workers in the Savannah River Site nuclear power plant, with African Americans more likely to have detectable radiation exposure on their monitors (Angelon-Gaetz, Richardson, & Wing, 2010). Ionizing radiation is used in a variety of screening and diagnostic tests at doses designed to minimize patient risk, but the cumulative effects are not negligible, especially in individuals who have frequent and/or numerous tests at a young age (Wall et al., 2006). The radiation exposure that occurs with CAT scans, angiograms, and nuclear medicine studies is much higher than with mammograms or simple X-rays, and their long-term risk is not fully known, in part because cumulative exposure is not generally tracked in the United States, but exposures from imaging tests can be substantial (Goodman et al., 2008). Ionizing radiation is used at high doses to treat some forms of cancer. It increases the risk of secondary cancers, and thus its use is generally restricted to life-threatening diseases in which the benefit of radiation far outweighs the risks (Doi, Mieno, Shimada, & Yoshinaga, 2009; Li et al., 2010; Shuryak, Hahnfeldt, Hlatky, Sachs, & Brenner, 2009). Improvements in the methods used to deliver therapeutic radiation have reduced its carcinogenicity by more effectively focusing its delivery to the cancers being targeted, with less damage to normal cells. Ultraviolet (UV) radiation in sunlight can also cause DNA damage, thereby increasing the risk of several forms of skin cancer (McPhail, 1997). Skin pigment reduces the ability of UV radiation to penetrate skin and cause damage; thus, light-skinned individuals are more at risk for damage through sunburn and excessive tanning, and this can lead to premalignant conditions such as actinic keratosis, as well as skin cancers.

Chemotherapy

Therapies that damage DNA remain a primary modality for treating many types of cancer, with the hope that cancer cells, due to their higher growth rates, will be more affected than normal cells. These therapies increase the risk of secondary cancers, with some combinations being more carcinogenic than others (Gururangan, 2009). People with inherited defects in DNA repair are at increased risk for secondary cancers induced by chemotherapy and/or radiation. The treatment for many forms of cancer includes the use of radiation and/or cytotoxic chemotherapy, recognizing that the greatest chances of cure are dependent on eradication of all cancer cells. The numbers of long-term cancer survivors have increased steadily, but this trend comes at a price. The cumulative incidence of subsequent cancers approaches 15% at 20 years after diagnosis of primary cancer, representing a three- to tenfold increased risk compared with the general population. Some treatment programs have a much higher risk of subsequent cancers, and when possible, less carcinogenic treatment options have replaced some that have especially high rates of secondary malignancies.

BIOLOGY OF BREAST CANCER DISPARITIES

Disparate Incidence and Mortality Rates

Breast cancer is the most commonly reported cancer of women in the United States, with an estimated 230,480 new cases of invasive cancer expected to affect women in 2011 (American Cancer Society, 2011). Overall mortality rates for breast cancer began a steady decline in the 1990s, due to a combination of increased screening and the utilization of therapies that were developed in response to improved understanding of breast tumor biology and the molecular mechanisms driving disease progression (Newman & Martin, 2007). Caucasian women have the highest age-adjusted incidence rates of breast cancer in comparison with all racial/ethnic groups over the age of 45 years. However, African American women have the highest incidence rates among women under the age of 45 years (Amend, Hicks, & Ambrosone, 2006; Newman & Martin, 2007; Polite, Dignam, & Olopade, 2005). Furthermore, African American women have the highest mortality rates from breast cancer and a lower 5-year survival than Caucasian women (American Cancer Society, 2010; Field et al., 2005). By contrast, Hispanic, Asian/Pacific Islander, and American Indian/Alaska Native women have lower incidence and mortality rates of breast cancer than both Caucasian and African American women (American Cancer Society, 2010).

Disparities in Breast Cancer Stage and Tumor Characteristics

Early studies undertaken to examine the impact of race and ethnicity on breast cancer were carried out when characterization of breast cancer primarily involved staging and microscopic appearance of the tumors. These studies demonstrated that African American and Hispanic patients were more likely to present with advanced tumors that had more aggressive histologic features than Caucasian patients, but they were unable to determine whether this was due to delays in seeking medical intervention or whether there were biologic differences in the forms of breast cancer that developed. For example, the National Cancer Institute's Black/White Cancer Survival Study, which was a cohort of 1,130 women (518 Caucasian and 612 African American) aged 20–79 diagnosed with primary breast cancer between January 1, 1985 and December 31, 1986 (Eley et al., 1994), reported that African American women were almost twice as likely as Caucasian women to be diagnosed at advanced stages: 30% of African Americans presented with stage III or IV cancers compared to 18% of Caucasians. The microscopic appearance of breast cancer reports the degree to which breast cancers resemble normal breast structures (differentiation), how rapidly the cells are replicating (mitotic index), and how much the normal architecture of cells is altered (atypia). The Black/White Cancer Survival Study reported that African Americans more commonly had poorly differentiated tumors (20% vs. 14%) and tumors with high-grade nuclear atypia (15% vs. 10%) in comparison to Caucasians, and 18% of African Americans had high-grade mitotic activity in comparison to 10% of Caucasians, following adjustment for age and stage (Chen et al., 1994; Eley et al., 1994).

Recent studies continue to show that African American women are significantly more likely to present with later-stage tumors than Caucasian women, and are also more likely to display tumor characteristics associated with a poor prognosis, irrespective of age and stage of disease (Curtis, Quale, Haggstrom, & Smith-Bindman, 2008; Porter et al., 2004). African American women are also more likely to be diagnosed with breast cancer at a younger age than Caucasian women, with 35% of African Americans diagnosed under the age of 50 years compared to 21% of Caucasians (Fiel et al., 2005). This raises the possibility that hereditary syndromes and/or distinct environmental exposures might be contributing to earlier development of breast cancer and the worse outcome in African Americans compared to Caucasians. In addition, African Americans are 40% more likely to be diagnosed with inflammatory breast cancer when compared to Caucasians. Inflammatory breast cancer is a very aggressive form of breast cancer in which tumor cells grow and spread to remote sites very rapidly. Prolonged inflammation is well known to increase the risk of developing certain forms of cancer, but the inflammation in this condition is not known to precede the development of cancer. Inflammatory breast cancer makes up approximately 2% of total breast cancer cases and thus plays only a minor role in the disparities in outcome that occur (Hance, Anderson, Devesa, Young, & Levine, 2005).

Older African Americans often have a worse outcome when diagnosed with breast cancer compared to their Caucasian counterparts (Curtis et al., 2008). African Americans on Medicare had a 30% increased risk of death from breast cancer when compared to Caucasian patients, after adjustment for hormone receptor status, tumor size, nodal status, and menopausal status.

There is considerable variability in how patients with breast cancer are managed throughout the United States, but this variability is eliminated for patients on clinical trials, who are closely monitored while following strict protocols. When African American patients on clinical trials were compared to Caucasian patients on the same trials, they experienced worse disease-free survival [HR = 1.56; 95% CI (1.15–2.11)] and overall survival [HR = 1.95; 95% CI (1.36–2.78)] after adjusting for hormone receptor status, tumor size, menopausal status, nodal status, and baseline absolute neutrophil count (Hershman et al., 2009). Collectively, these and other studies suggest that there may be differences in breast cancer biology and progression that contribute to the disparities in disease outcome.

While Hispanic women have a lower incidence of and mortality rate for breast cancer than Caucasians, those who develop breast cancer tend to have a more aggressive breast cancer phenotype. When the tumors of 4,885 Caucasian women, 1,016 African American women, and 777 Hispanic women were collected from 31 hospitals nationwide, both African American (49%) and Hispanic (48%) women were more likely than Caucasian women (39%) to have high levels of cell replication and less cellular differentiation seen within their tumors (Elledge, Clark, Chamness, & Osborne, 1994).

The Role of Inherited Genes in Disparities

BRCA1 and BRCA2 are proteins that play an important role in DNA repair (Kwei et al., 2010; Olopade et al., 2008; Powell & Kachnic, 2008; Zhang & Powell, 2005). People who inherit mutant forms of either *BRCA1* or *BRCA2* have a 40%–80% lifetime risk of developing breast cancer. *BRCA1* and *BRCA2* mutation frequencies vary by geographic region and ethnicity (Fackenthal & Olopade, 2007). Within the United States, the Ashkenazi Jewish population has the highest reported frequencies of *BRCA1* and *BRCA2* mutations, mainly due to three founder mutations (*BRCA1* 187delAG and 5385insC, *BRCA2* 6174delT) that have a combined carrier frequency of 1 in 40 for this population. By comparison, the overall prevalence of *BRCA1* and *BRCA2* mutations is estimated to be between 1 in 400 and 1 in 800 (Petrucelli et al., 2010).

Patients taken from the Northern California Breast Cancer Family Registry were used to assess the *BRCA1* mutation carrier frequency within various racial and ethnic groups who developed breast cancer within the United States. These patients were under the age of 65 and were diagnosed with invasive breast cancer between January 1, 1995 and December 31, 2003. Five racial/ ethnic groups, including 549 Caucasians (encompassing both Ashkenazi Jewish Caucasians and non-Ashkenazi Jewish Caucasians), 444 Asians, 393 Hispanics, and 341 African Americans, were tested for *BRCA1* mutations. After the Ashkenazi Jewish patient population (8.3%), Hispanics (3.5%) had the highest frequency of inherited *BRCA1* mutations, followed by non-Ashkenazi Caucasians (2.2%), African Americans (1.3%), and then Asians (0.5%). Interestingly, this study also reported that African American patients (17%) diagnosed under the age of 35 had a significantly higher *BRCA1* mutation frequency when compared to the other non-Ashkenazi Jewish populations (Hispanics [8.9%], Asians [2.4%], Caucasians [7.2%]) in the same age range. Additionally, this study found that the types of *BRCA1* mutations varied among the different racial/ethnic groups. The most frequent *BRCA1* alterations in Hispanics and Caucasians (including both the Ashkenazi Jewish and non-Ashkenazi Jewish populations) were frame-shift mutations, whereas in African Americans, the most prevalent *BRCA1* alterations were missense mutations (John et al., 2007). Other studies have also reported unique and distinct *BRCA1* and *BRCA2* mutations within the African American population (Ademuyiwa & Olopade, 2003; Olopade et al., 2003). Awareness of different types of mutations helps in screening patients for inherited defects that predispose to breast and other cancers. African Americans also appear to have a higher incidence of unclassified variants of *BRCA1* and *BRCA2* in comparison to other racial/ethnic populations. These variants are sequences within the gene that differ from sequences found in most people, yet they are not known to adversely affect the structure of the protein and hence are not currently considered mutations. Due to the undetermined significance of these variants, it is unknown whether they modify breast cancer risk and survival.

With the advent of high-throughput sequencing and whole-genome technologies, studies show that the major genetic component contributing to breast cancer predisposition is likely caused by multiple and common low-penetrance genes that act in conjunction to modify breast cancer risk (Olopade et al., 2008). Genome-wide association studies have led to the identification of single nucleotide polymorphisms (SNPs) within a small number of genes, primarily within Caucasian populations with estrogen receptor positive breast cancers. A primary example of this phenomenon was the identification of four SNPs in the *FGFR2* gene that were highly associated with breast cancer risk in a study of 1,145 postmenopausal women of European ancestry with invasive breast cancer and 1,142 controls (Hunter et al., 2007). Additional SNPs that are significantly associated with breast cancer risk have been identified in four genes (*CASP8, TNRC9, MAP3K1,* and *LSP1*) and three genomic regions (*2q35, 8q24,* and *5p12*). These findings were validated in additional cohorts of Caucasian women; however, in studies of other racial/ethnic populations, the SNPs had a modest effect in an Asian cohort and discordant results in cohorts of African ancestry (Olopade et al., 2008). These studies indicate that associations between genomic variants and cancer risk vary among racial/ethnic populations and, further, they demonstrate the need to assess the relationships between SNPs and disease risk within diverse patient cohorts. The identification of these modifiers of cancer risk may further elucidate why differences exist in genetic susceptibilities to cancer among individuals and populations.

Differences in Proteins That Regulate Cellular Proliferation, Apoptosis, and DNA Repair

The changes in DNA that occur in cells that become cancerous lead to changes in the expression of many proteins, some of which play critical roles in the malignant behavior of the cells. These include cyclins, proteins that serve as co-factors to enzymes that regulate progression through the cell cycle (Malumbres & Barbacid, 2009). Alterations that occur in cancer can lead to high levels of several cyclin proteins independent of the usual signals for their production. In general, women with breast cancer who exhibit low levels of cyclin E expression and high levels of cyclin D1 expression are significantly less likely to die from their breast cancer than women with high levels of cyclin E and low levels of cyclin D1 (Porter et al., 2004). African American women had higher levels of cyclin E (OR [odds ratio] = 4.3) and lower levels of cyclin D1 expression (OR = 0.5) than Caucasian women in their breast cancer cells, potentially contributing to the worse outcome for African American women.

One of the most common events in the development of cancer involves the tumor suppressor protein p53 that is mutated or eliminated in over 50% of human cancers (Green & Kroemer, 2009). Protein p53 is a transcription factor that is induced when abnormal DNA is present or under cellular stress, and it leads to expression of multiple proteins, including proteins that inhibit DNA replication, help repair damaged DNA, and induce programmed cell death—all functions that are designed to protect the integrity of the DNA. When the function of p53 is disrupted, cells with damaged DNA are more likely to be propagated and acquire more mistakes. The mutations in the p53 gene (*TP53*) that most commonly occur in tumors lead to a stabilization of the protein and a loss of its ability to function as a transcription factor, so that high levels of p53 protein reflect loss of p53 function. Patients with stage I and II breast cancers displayed no difference in the frequency of *TP53* gene alterations between African Americans (20%) and Caucasians (19%), but there were differences in the types of *TP53* alterations that were encountered (Blaszyk et al., 1994; Shiao, Chen, Scheer, Wu, & Correa, 1995). When more advanced stages were included in the analysis, tumors of African Americans (OR = 1.7) more frequently displayed high levels of mutant p53 protein expression when compared to the tumors of Caucasians (Porter et al., 2004). In general, tumors that display high levels of mutant p53 have a more aggressive phenotype, are less likely to respond to adjuvant therapy, and thus might contribute to the worse outcome of African American patients.

Differences in Hormonal Factors That Contribute to Breast Cancer Disparities

Estrogen is known to play an important role in the development and progression of many cases of breast cancer, especially those that express high levels of estrogen receptor (ER) and progesterone receptor (PR). Both genetic and environmental factors affect the levels and types of estrogen that are present. Estrogens are synthesized from cholesterol, with estradiol being the predominant form (Taioli et al., 1999, 2010). The ovaries make most of the estradiol until menopause, but estradiol is also made by fat cells and may play a role in the increased rate of ER positive breast cancer in obese postmenopausal women (Brown & Simpson, 2010).

Two mutually exclusive pathways are involved in metabolizing estradiol. One pathway utilizes the enzyme CYP1A1 to generate an inactive metabolite (2-hydroxyestrone), and the other pathway uses CYP3A4 to generate a metabolite that continues to have estrogenic activity (16α-hydroxyestrone) (Masi & Olopade, 2005). There is an inherited variant of CYP3A4 that is more active and leads to higher levels of the 16α-hydroxyestrone metabolite, and it was more common in African American girls (62%), when compared to Hispanic (52%) and Caucasian girls (17%) in a study of 137 healthy 9-year-old girls (Kadlubar et al., 2003). This high-activity variant was associated with earlier onset of puberty. These data suggest that higher physiological levels of active estrogen, along with earlier onset of puberty, may contribute to the higher prevalence of both early onset breast cancer and breast cancer–specific mortality in African American women (Masi & Olopade, 2005).

Differences in Molecular Characteristics of Breast Cancers

The alterations in DNA that lead to breast cancer lead to changes in gene expression, which can be assessed using complementary DNA (cDNA) microarrays, a method that allows evaluation of hundreds of genes simultaneously.

Comparison of breast cancer specimens to normal breast cells has revealed that some breast cancers are derived from cells that line the breast ducts (luminal cells), whereas others arise from cells that are beneath the luminal cells (basal or myoepithelial cells). Six distinct subtypes of breast cancer have been identified that have distinct patterns of gene expression: luminal A, luminal B, HER2-enriched, basal-like, normal breast-like, and claudin-low (Perou et al., 2000; Prat et al., 2010). Luminal A tumors have relatively high expression of genes, such as the *ER* gene, that are normally expressed by cells that line the breast ducts (luminal cells) (Carey et al., 2006; Oh et al., 2006; Prat et al., 2010; Sorlie et al., 2001). Luminal B tumors show low to moderate expression of *ER*, whereas they express high levels of genes that induce cell proliferation and block programmed cell death (apoptosis), reflecting a more aggressive form of breast cancer compared to luminal A cancers. The HER2-enriched subtype demonstrates overexpression of *ERBB2/HER-2/neu* and low levels of *ER* and *ER*-associated genes. The basal-like subtype generally does not express *ER*, *PR*, or *ERBB2/HER-2/neu*, whereas it has high levels of expression of other proteins, such as keratin 5, keratin 17, and laminin. The normal breast-like subtype is distinguished by high expression of genes characteristic of basal epithelial and adipose cells, along with low expression of genes characteristic of luminal epithelial cells.

Of all the subtypes, luminal A tumors have the best prognosis, demonstrating the highest overall survival and relapse-free survival (Prat et al., 2010; Sorlie et al., 2001). The tumors are slower to metastasize than some of the other forms, and treatments that attack the ability of hormones to drive these tumors have been available for many years. Basal-like, claudin-low, and HER2 classified tumors are more aggressive tumors that metastasize more readily, leading to a worse outcome both in terms of overall survival and relapse-free survival (Di Cosimo & Baselga, 2010). The use of herceptin has dramatically improved the prognosis of patients with HER2-classified tumors, indicating that knowledge of factors that drive tumor growth and survival can be exploited for developing new treatments (Mukai, 2010). Basal-type tumors metastasize early and have been especially difficult to treat, but new insights into their biology are leading to more effective treatments, such as the poly ADP-ribose polymerase (PARP) inhibitors in conjunction with new combinations of cytotoxic chemotherapy (Anders et al., 2010; Di Cosimo & Baselga, 2010).

Molecular characterization using cDNA microarrays reveals that African American women are more likely to have basal-like tumors and less likely to have luminal A or B tumors than Caucasians, providing strong evidence that some of the disparities are not just due to differences in access to care and in tumor management. In the Carolina Breast Cancer Study of 496 cases (196 African American and 300 non–African American) of invasive breast cancer, the prevalence of basal-like tumors was significantly higher in African Americans (26%) than in non–African Americans (16%) (Carey et al., 2006). Additionally, this high prevalence of basal-like tumors in African Americans was mainly seen in premenopausal women, irrespective of stage at diagnosis. This study also found that basal-like tumors were more likely to have high nuclear and histological grade, as well as a high mitotic index, than other tumor subtypes, after adjustment for age, race, and stage. Furthermore, the basal (44%) and HER2 (43%) subtypes had a higher percentage of p53 mutations in comparison to luminal subtypes (luminal A, 15%; luminal B, 23%), thereby offering some insights into why early studies showed that African Americans were more likely to have tumors that displayed unfavorable microscopic features. It is currently not known why African Americans are more prone to develop basal-like tumors than Caucasians. It is also not known why luminal A breast cancers predominate in Asian and Caucasian populations, and are more common in postmenopausal than in premenopausal women. However, further study of the mechanisms driving the individual breast cancer subtypes and the environmental exposures that likely modify these processes will lead to improved understanding of this phenomenon.

BIOLOGY OF COLORECTAL CANCER DISPARITIES

Incidence and Mortality Rates

Colorectal cancer is the third leading cause of new cancer cases and cancer deaths in both men and women within the United States, with an estimated 141,210 cases expected to occur in 2011. Overall incidence and mortality have decreased in the past two decades as a result of improved screening and improvements in treatment. Screening can lead to the removal of premalignant polyps, thereby decreasing the likelihood that cancer will develop. However, incidence rates are increasing about 2% per year in adults under the age of 50, a population that is not recommended for screening unless in high-risk circumstances (American Cancer Society, 2010). African Americans have the highest age-adjusted incidence and mortality rates of any other racial/ethnic group, whereas Asians/Pacific Islanders and American Indians/Alaska Natives have the lowest rates. Both incidence and mortality rates within African Americans are declining, but the decline has been slower than in Caucasians, leading to an increasing divergence, especially in mortality rates (American Cancer Society, 2009, 2010). For those who get colorectal cancer, African Americans (OR = 1.2), American Indians (OR = 1.2), Hispanics (especially Mexicans, OR = 1.2), and Hawaiians (OR = 1.3) are more likely to die than Caucasians, with the greatest disparity in risk of death in early-stage cancers (stages I and II), even while adjusting for age, stage, and treatment (African Americans, OR = 1.4; Hispanics, OR=1.4; Hawaiians, OR = 1.4) (Alexander et al., 2004; Chien, Morimoto, Tom, & Li, 2005). In a study of 574 patients (224 African American and 350 Caucasian) from the University of Alabama at Birmingham Hospital and the Birmingham Veterans Affairs Hospital tumor registries, African Americans with high-grade tumors were three times more likely to die of colon cancer within 5 years of surgical resection when compared to Caucasians with high-grade tumors [HR = 3.05, 95% CI (1.32–7.05)], following adjustment for race, gender, age, hospital, stage, and anatomic site. The African Americans and Caucasians within this study had similar proportions of high-grade tumors at diagnosis, a similar prevalence of comorbid conditions, and a similar frequency of deaths due to causes other than colorectal cancer, suggesting that differences in the aggressiveness of the cancers play an important role in the disparate survival outcomes among these populations (Alexander et al., 2005). Furthermore, in a large population study (33,464 Caucasians, 6,024 African Americans, 1,618 Asian/Pacific Islanders, and 911 American Indian/Alaska Natives or other unidentified racial/ethnic groups), patients diagnosed under the age of 50 were more likely to present with distant disease and poorly differentiated tumors and were more likely to be African American (Fairley et al., 2006). SEER data has also shown that the differential in incidence and survival outcome between African American and Caucasian patients is the largest in younger cohorts (under 50 years of age) (Polite, Dignam, & Olopade, 2006). Collectively, these studies suggest that African Americans are developing cancers with more aggressive phenotypes, thereby leading to their escalated rates of colorectal cancer mortality.

The Role of Genetics in Colorectal Cancer Disparities

Approximately 15% of all colorectal cancers occur in people who have an inherited risk for colorectal cancer. The majority of these are due to inherited mutations in one of the DNA mismatch repair genes (*MLH1, MSH2, PMS2,* and *MSH6*) that lead to the development of Lynch syndrome (Kinzler & Vogelstein, 1996). The changes in DNA mismatch repair that occur in this syndrome can affect particular areas of the DNA called "microsatellites," leading to a specific type of genomic instability called microsatellite instability (MSI). MSI can also occur in response to acquired changes in DNA repair, but the presence of MSI within colon cancer cells suggests the presence of either inherited defects in DNA mismatch repair enzymes or acquired mistakes in the function of this pathway. A few studies have examined MSI in colorectal cancers from African Americans and Caucasians to determine if mismatch repair pathway dysfunction is playing a role in the higher rates of young-onset cases and proximally located colon tumors in young African Americans compared to Caucasians. These small studies reported that MSI incidence was more than twofold greater in African Americans when compared to Caucasians (Ashktorab et al., 2005; Ionov, Peinado, Malkhosyan, Shibata, & Perucho, 1993), but larger studies found that the rate in African Americans was approximately 20%, a frequency similar to what has been reported in the U.S. population (Cunningham et al., 2001; Hampel et al., 2005). It remains to be determined whether there are racial differences in the frequency of people harboring defective DNA mismatch repair genes, since not all cases of MSI are due to an inherited defect.

Another genetic syndrome that leads to colorectal cancer is familial adenomatosis polyposis (FAP). The syndrome results from an inherited defect in the *APC* gene, and people who inherit defective *APC* develop hundreds of polyps, each with the potential to progress to cancer. Nearly 100% of people who inherit mutant *APC* develop cancer by the time they are in their forties. The large number of polyps that occur in this syndrome make carriers easy to identify, but FAP is sufficiently rare that it does not play a large role in the racial disparities that exist.

Methylenetetrahydrofolate reductase (MTHFR) is an enzyme involved in folate metabolism, which has been inversely linked to colorectal cancer risk (Le Marchand, Wilkens, Kolonel, & Henderson, 2005). Folate is important in making the building blocks for DNA, and folic acid deficiency leads to double-strand chromosome breaks by extensive incorporation of uracil into DNA. This occurs because there is a deficiency of thymidine when folate is low, so its precursor, uracil, is substituted. Folate also plays a functional role in DNA methylation, so patterns of methylation of the genome change during folate deficiency, and this can alter gene expression (Ames, 1999; Goelz, Vogelstein, Hamilton, & Feinberg, 1985). A common polymorphism, C677T, in the MTHFR gene was previously identified and shown to result in a temperature-sensitive enzyme that functions with decreased activity (Weisberg et al., 1998). In a study of 2,843 cases and controls from the Multiethnic Cohort Study, the MTHFR 677TT genotype was associated with a 23% decreased risk of colorectal cancer (Le Marchand et al., 2005). There was an even stronger association at high levels of folate intake. The study also reported differences in the allele frequency among racial/ethnic groups, with the T allele being the lowest in African Americans and Hawaiians when compared to Hispanics, Japanese, and Caucasians. The differences in the frequency of this allele might contribute to the higher incidences of colorectal cancer in Hawaiian and African American populations.

Environmental Factors Contributing to Colorectal Cancer Disparities

The development of colorectal cancer is dependent on the accumulation of multiple changes in the DNA. Irrespective of whether the colorectal cancer is sporadic or in people with genetic risk, the majority of cancers arise in polyps, so that removal of polyps is likely responsible for the decreasing incidence of colorectal cancer that has occurred in recent years. Insights into the steps involved in the development of cancer come from comparing the DNA in colorectal cancer to DNA in polyps and in unaffected colon or rectum. Such studies show that over 90% of polyps contain an acquired change in the *APC* gene (either genetic or epigenetic), and additional changes in the DNA are found when polyps grow very large. Not all polyps progress to cancer, but those that do contain many more genetic changes that are responsible for the ability of cells to invade and metastasize.

Epidemiologic studies have shown that alcohol consumption, smoking, diabetes, obesity, and high meat intake are associated with increased risks of colorectal cancer (Akhter et al., 2007; Gapstur, Potter, & Folsom, 1994; Huxley et al., 2009). These exposures can lead to inappropriate DNA methylation and alkylation that promote carcinogenesis (Cross & Sinha, 2004; Slattery, Schaffer, & Edwards, 1997). Therefore, the dietary and lifestyle patterns that are common to specific racial/ethnic populations may induce altered frequencies and/or spectra in genetic alterations among different populations, leading to variations in cancer risk and clinicopathologic features.

Whole-genome analysis of tumors offers insights into some of the changes that occur in colorectal cancer in different patient populations. When 15 colorectal cancer samples taken from African American patients at Howard University Hospital were compared to a previously published analysis of 22 Caucasian colorectal cancer cases from Germany, many of the genetic changes were similar, but there were a few differences (Ashktorab et al., 2010; Lassmann et al., 2007). The *ATM* gene, whose encoded protein functions in the DNA damage response, was frequently amplified in Caucasian tumors but not in any of the African American tumors. In addition, the *DCC* gene, whose encoded protein functions as a receptor that can induce programmed cell death (Rodrigues, De Wever, Bruyneel, Rooney, & Gespach, 2007), was primarily amplified in Caucasians but deleted in African Americans (Takayama, Miyanishi, Hayashi, Sato, & Niitsu, 2006). They also reported that the *STS* gene, involved in promoting the growth of human breast cancer cells, was deleted in Caucasians and amplified in African Americans (Ashktorab et al., 2010). The functional consequences of these differences are not known, but they indicate that differences exist in the types of changes that occur in tumors from various patients, underscoring the need for characterizing both the causes and the consequences of these differences.

CONCLUSIONS

Researchers have made tremendous progress in understanding many of the biologic changes that occur in cancer and some of the factors that initiate and perpetuate various forms of cancer. Vaccines, antibiotics, and other interventions are helping reduce some of the cancers that are initiated by infectious agents, and government regulations are reducing exposures to known carcinogens that once were more commonly encountered by the public. Multiple genes that are inherited and lead to increased risk for cancer have been identified, offering the opportunity to screen for people who are at increased risk. Screening for some forms of cancer has improved outcome through identifying cancers before they have spread, and clinical trials have helped define combinations of treatment that improve outcome. Knowledge of how specific genes and biologic processes contribute to tumorigenesis offers the opportunity for developing interventions that reduce risk and/or allow early detection of premalignant and malignant changes. Various forms of cancer are being characterized by some of the specific mutations and changes in gene expression that occur, offering more detailed understanding of biologic similarities and differences in cancers that were previously only characterized by their microscopic appearance. For those who get cancer, specific pathways that are critical to tumor cell survival and growth are now being targeted in many forms of cancer, leading to more effective treatments, with fewer long-term side effects. These and other advances in detection and treatment are responsible for the more than 10 million cancer survivors in the United States today.

Population studies have alerted the nation to the disparities in cancer incidence and mortality rates among the diverse racial/ethnic populations within the United States. Health care access plays a vital role in cancer health disparities, as unequal access plagues many, especially minority and impoverished populations. Biologic factors also contribute to the differences in incidence and outcome of cancer in different racial and ethnic groups. Racial and ethnic classifications do not necessarily align with population ancestry and hence are limited in their ability to identify people who might have some shared genetic background. African Americans are a heterogeneous group with admixture from African, European, and American Indian populations. Asian/Pacific Islander and Hispanic designations include a variety of ancestries within each racial/ethnic construct. To begin to refine our understanding of how genes contribute to tumor risk, researchers have begun to incorporate ancestry informative markers (AIMs) into their analysis of diverse populations, as a method to reduce bias associated with population stratification (Nassir et al., 2009).

Elimination of the disparities that exist in cancer incidence and outcome is an important goal, but it is not sufficient. There are approximately

1.5 million people who get cancer in the United States each year, and more than 550,000 people die of it. Elimination of cancer disparities would have a valuable impact on reducing these numbers. Through knowledge, it should be possible to develop more effective interventions that decrease incidence and mortality from cancer, to benefit people from all racial and ethnic groups.

REFERENCES

Ademuyiwa, F. O., & Olopade, O. I. (2003). Racial differences in genetic factors associated with breast cancer. *Cancer and Metastasis Reviews, 22*(1), 47–53.

Ahn, J., Schatzkin, A., Lacey, J. V., Jr., Albanes, D., Ballard-Barbash, R., Adams, K. F., . . . Leitzmann, M. F. (2007). Adiposity, adult weight change, and postmenopausal breast cancer risk. *Archives of Internal Medicine, 167*(19), 2091–2102.

Akhter, M., Kuriyama, S., Nakaya, N., Shimazu, T., Ohmori, K., Nishino, Y., . . . Tsuji, I. (2007). Alcohol consumption is associated with an increased risk of distal colon and rectal cancer in Japanese men: The Miyagi Cohort Study. *European Journal of Cancer, 43*(2), 383–390.

Alaejos, M. S., Gonzalez, V., & Afonso, A. M. (2008). Exposure to heterocyclic aromatic amines from the consumption of cooked red meat and its effect on human cancer risk: A review. *Food Additives and Contaminant Part A Chemistry, Analysis, Control, Exposure and Risk Assessment, 25*(1), 2–24.

Alexander, D., Chatla, C., Funkhouser, E., Meleth, S., Grizzle, W. E., & Manne, U. (2004). Postsurgical disparity in survival between African Americans and Caucasians with colonic adenocarcinoma. *Cancer, 101*(1), 66–76.

Alexander, D., Jhala, N., Chatla, C., Steinhauer, J., Funkhouser, E., Coffey, C. S., . . . Manne, U. (2005). High-grade tumor differentiation is an indicator of poor prognosis in African Americans with colonic adenocarcinomas. *Cancer, 103*(10), 2163–2170.

Amend, K., Hicks, D., & Ambrosone, C. B. (2006). Breast cancer in African-American women: Differences in tumor biology from European-American women. *Cancer Research, 66*(17), 8327–8330.

American Cancer Society. (2009). *Cancer facts & figures for African Americans 2009–2010* (pp. 1–28). Atlanta, GA: Author.

American Cancer Society (2011). *Cancer facts and figures*. Atlanta, GA: Author.

Ames, B. N. (1999). Micronutrient deficiencies. A major cause of DNA damage. *Annals of the New York Academy of Sciences, 889*, 87–106.

Anders, C. K., Winer, E. P., Ford, J. M., Dent, R., Silver, D. P., Sledge, G. W., & Carey, L. A. (2010). Poly(ADP-Ribose) polymerase inhibition: "Targeted" therapy for triple-negative breast cancer. *Clinical Cancer Research, 16*(19), 4702–4710.

Angelon-Gaetz, K. A., Richardson, D. B., & Wing, S. (2010). Inequalities in the nuclear age: Impact of race and gender on radiation exposure at the Savannah River Site (1951–1999). *New Solutions, 20*(2), 195–210.

Antonescu-Turcu, A. L., & Schapira, R. M. (2010). Parenchymal and airway diseases caused by asbestos. *Current Opinion in Pulmonary Medicine, 16*(2), 155–161.

Aranda, V., Nolan, M. E., & Muthuswamy, S. K. (2008). Par complex in cancer: A regulator of normal cell polarity joins the dark side. *Oncogene, 27*(55), 6878–6887.

Argos, M., Kibriya, M. G., Jasmine, F., Olopade, O. I., Su, T., Hibshoosh, H., & Ahsan, H. (2008). Genomewide scan for loss of heterozygosity and chromosomal amplification in breast carcinoma using single-nucleotide polymorphism arrays. *Cancer Genetics and Cytogenetics, 182*(2), 69–74.

Ashktorab, H., Schaffer, A. A., Daremipouran, M., Smoot, D. T., Lee, E., & Brim, H. (2010). Distinct genetic alterations in colorectal cancer. *PLoS One, 5*(1), e8879.

Ashktorab, H., Smoot, D. T., Farzanmehr, H., Fidelia-Lambert, M., Momen, B., Hylind, L., . . . Giardiello, F. M. (2005). Clinicopathological features and microsatellite instability (MSI) in colorectal cancers from African Americans. *International Journal of Cancer, 116*(6), 914–919.

Asselin-Labat, M. L., Vaillant, F., Shackleton, M., Bouras, T., Lindeman, G. J., & Visvader, J. E. (2008). Delineating the epithelial hierarchy in the mouse mammary gland. *Cold Spring Harbor Symposia on Quantitative Biology, 73,* 469–478.

Bamia, C., Halkjaer, J., Lagiou, P., Trichopoulos, D., Tjonneland, A., Berentzen, T. L., . . . Trichopoulou, A. (2010). Weight change in later life and risk of death amongst the elderly: The European Prospective Investigation into Cancer and Nutrition-Elderly Network on Ageing and Health study. *Journal of Internal Medicine, 268*(2), 133–144.

Bardia, A., Tleyjeh, I. M., Cerhan, J. R., Sood, A. K., Limburg, P. J., Erwin, P. J., & Montori, V. M. (2008). Efficacy of antioxidant supplementation in reducing primary cancer incidence and mortality: systematic review and meta-analysis. *Mayo Clinic Proceedings, 83*(1), 23–34.

Bartek, J., & Lukas, J. (2007). DNA damage checkpoints: From initiation to recovery or adaptation. *Current Opinion in Cell Biology, 19*(2), 238–245.

Barton, H. A., Cogliano, V. J., Flowers, L., Valcovic, L., Setzer, R. W., & Woodruff, T. J. (2005). Assessing susceptibility from early-life exposure to carcinogens. *Environmental Health Perspectives, 113*(9), 1125–1133.

Blaszyk, H., Vaughn, C. B., Hartmann, A., McGovern, R. M., Schroeder, J. J., Cunningham, J., . . . Kovach, J. S. (1994). Novel pattern of p53 gene mutations in an American black cohort with high mortality from breast cancer. *Lancet, 343*(8907), 1195–1197.

Bolus, N. E. (2008). Review of common occupational hazards and safety concerns for nuclear medicine technologists. *Journal of Nuclear Medicine Technology, 36*(1), 11–17.

Brown, K. A., & Simpson, E. R. (2010). Obesity and breast cancer: Progress to understanding the relationship. *Cancer Research, 70*(1), 4–7.

Calle, E. E., Rodriguez, C., Walker-Thurmond, K., & Thun, M. J. (2003). Overweight, obesity, and mortality from cancer in a prospectively studied cohort of U.S. adults. *New England Journal of Medicine, 348*(17), 1625–1638.

Carbone, A., Cesarman, E., Spina, M., Gloghini, A., & Schulz, T. F. (2009). HIV-associated lymphomas and gamma-herpes viruses. *Blood, 113*(6), 1213–1224.

Carey, L. A., Perou, C. M., Livasy, C. A., Dressler, L. G., Cowan, D., Conway, K., . . . Millikan, R. C. (2006). Race, breast cancer subtypes, and survival in the Carolina Breast Cancer Study. *Journal of the American Medical Association, 295*(21), 2492–2502.

Carpenter, C. L., Yu, M. C., & London, S. J. (2009). Dietary isothiocyanates, glutathione S-transferase M1 (GSTM1), and lung cancer risk in African Americans and Caucasians from Los Angeles County, California. *Nutrition and Cancer, 61*(4), 492–499.

Chameides, W. L. (2010). Environmental factors in cancer: Focus on air pollution. *Reviews on Environmental Health, 25*(1), 17–22.

Chang, Y., Cesarman, E., Pessin, M. S., Lee, F., Culpepper, J., Knowles, D. M., & Moore, P. S. (1994). Identification of herpes virus-like DNA sequences in AIDS-associated Kaposi's sarcoma. *Science, 266*(5192), 1865–1869.

Charafe-Jauffret, E., Ginestier, C., Monville, F., Fekairi, S., Jacquemier, J., Birnbaum, D., & Bertucci, F. (2005). How to best classify breast cancer: Conventional and novel classifications (review). *International Journal of Oncology, 27*(5), 1307–1313.

Chen, V. W., Correa, P., Kurman, R. J., Wu, X. C., Eley, J. W., Austin, D., . . . Edward, B. K. (1994). Histological characteristics of breast carcinoma in blacks and whites. *Cancer Epidemiology, Biomarkers & Prevention, 3*(2), 127–135.

Cherniack, M. G. (1992). Diseases of unusual occupations: An historical perspective. *Occupational Medicine, 7*(3), 369–384.

Chien, C., Morimoto, L. M., Tom, J., & Li, C. I. (2005). Differences in colorectal carcinoma stage and survival by race and ethnicity. *Cancer, 104*(3), 629–639.

Clark, S. J. (2007). Action at a distance: Epigenetic silencing of large chromosomal regions in carcinogenesis. *Human Molecular Genetics, 16*(Special No. 1), R88–R95.

Clavel, J. (2007). Progress in the epidemiological understanding of gene–environment interactions in major diseases: Cancer. *Comptes Rendu Biologies, 330*(4), 306–317.

Cross, A. J., & Sinha, R. (2004). Meat-related mutagens/carcinogens in the etiology of colorectal cancer. *Environmental and Molecular Mutagenesis, 44*(1), 44–55.

Crum-Cianflone, N., Hullsiek, K. H., Marconi, V., Weintrob, A., Ganesan, A., Barthel, R. V., . . . Wegner, S. (2009). Trends in the incidence of cancers among HIV-infected persons and the impact of antiretroviral therapy: A 20-year cohort study. *AIDS, 23*(1), 41–50.

Cunningham, J. M., Kim, C. Y., Christensen, E. R., Tester, D. J., Parc, Y., Burgart, L. J., . . . Thibodeau, S. N. (2001). The frequency of hereditary defective mismatch repair in a prospective series of unselected colorectal carcinomas. *American Journal of Human Genetics, 69*(4), 780–790.

Curtis, E., Quale, C., Haggstrom, D., & Smith-Bindman, R. (2008). Racial and ethnic differences in breast cancer survival: How much is explained by screening, tumor severity, biology, treatment, comorbidities, and demographics? *Cancer, 112*(1), 171–180.

Dansinger, M. L., Gleason, J. A., Griffith, J. L., Selker, H. P., & Schaefer, E. J. (2005). Comparison of the Atkins, Ornish, Weight Watchers, and Zone diets for weight loss and heart disease risk reduction: A randomized trial. *Journal of the American Medical Association, 293*(1), 43–53.

de Bruin, R. A., & Wittenberg, C. (2009). All eukaryotes: Before turning off G1-S transcription, please check your DNA. *Cell Cycle, 8*(2), 214–217.

Di Cosimo, S., & Baselga, J. (2010). Management of breast cancer with targeted agents: importance of heterogeneity [corrected]. *Nature Reviews Clinical Oncology, 7*(3), 139–147.

Dixon, J. B. (2010). The effect of obesity on health outcomes. *Molecular and Cellular Endocrinology, 316*(2), 104–108.

Doi, K., Mieno, M. N., Shimada, Y., & Yoshinaga, S. (2009). Risk of second malignant neoplasms among childhood cancer survivors treated with radiotherapy: Meta-analysis of nine epidemiological studies. *Paediatric and Perinatal Epidemiology, 23*(4), 370–379.

Dreyling, M. H., Kobayashi, H., Olopade, O. I., Le Beau, M. M., Rowley, J. D., & Bohlander, S. K. (1995). Detection of 9p deletions in leukemia cell lines by interphase fluorescence in situ hybridization with YAC-derived probes. *Cancer Genetics and Cytogenetics, 83*(1), 46–55.

Ebbert, J. O., Yang, P., Vachon, C. M., Vierkant, R. A., Cerhan, J. R., Folsom, A. R., & Sellers, T. A. (2003). Lung cancer risk reduction after smoking cessation:

Observations from a prospective cohort of women. *Journal of Clinical Oncology, 21*(5), 921–926.

Eckel, R. H. (2008). Clinical practice. Nonsurgical management of obesity in adults. *New England Journal of Medicine, 358*(18), 1941–1950.

Edelstein, Z. R., Farrow, D. C., Bronner, M. P., Rosen, S. N., & Vaughan, T. L. (2007). Central adiposity and risk of Barrett's esophagus. *Gastroenterology, 133*(2), 403–411.

Eley, J. W., Hill, H. A., Chen, V. W., Austin, D. F., Wesley, M. N., Greenberg, R. S., . . . Kurman, R. (1994). Racial differences in survival from breast cancer. Results of the National Cancer Institute Black/White Cancer Survival Study. *Journal of the American Medical Association, 272*(12), 947–954.

Elledge, R. M., Clark, G. M., Chamness, G. C., & Osborne, C. K. (1994). Tumor biologic factors and breast cancer prognosis among white, Hispanic, and black women in the United States. *Journal of the National Cancer Institute, 86*(9), 705–712.

Fackenthal, J. D., & Olopade, O. I. (2007). Breast cancer risk associated with BRCA1 and BRCA2 in diverse populations. *Nature Reviews Cancer, 7*(12), 937–948.

Fairley, T. L., Cardinez, C. J., Martin, J., Alley, L., Friedman, C., Edwards, B., & Jamison, P. (2006). Colorectal cancer in U.S. adults younger than 50 years of age, 1998–2001. *Cancer, 107*(5 Suppl), 1153–1161.

Feng, H., Shuda, M., Chang, Y., & Moore, P. S. (2008). Clonal integration of a polyomavirus in human Merkel cell carcinoma. [Research Support, N.I.H., Extramural Research Support, Non-U.S. Gov't]. *Science, 319*(5866), 1096–1100.

Field, T. S., Buist, D. S., Doubeni, C., Enger, S., Fouayzi, H., Hart, G., . . . Yao, J. (2005). Disparities and survival among breast cancer patients. *Journal of the National Cancer Institute Monographs* (35), 88–95.

Franco, M., Ordunez, P., Caballero, B., Tapia Granados, J. A., Lazo, M., Bernal, J. L., . . . Cooper, R. S. (2007). Impact of energy intake, physical activity, and population-wide weight loss on cardiovascular disease and diabetes mortality in Cuba, 1980–2005. *American Journal of Epidemiology, 166*(12), 1374–1380.

Gapstur, S. M., Potter, J. D., & Folsom, A. R. (1994). Alcohol consumption and colon and rectal cancer in postmenopausal women. *International Journal of Epidemiology, 23*(1), 50–57.

Gibbs, G. W., & Berry, G. (2008). Mesothelioma and asbestos. *Regulatory Toxicology and Pharmacology, 52*(1 Suppl), S223–S231.

Goelz, S. E., Vogelstein, B., Hamilton, S. R., & Feinberg, A. P. (1985). Hypomethylation of DNA from benign and malignant human colon neoplasms. *Science, 228*, 187–190.

Golka, K., Wiese, A., Assennato, G., & Bolt, H. M. (2004). Occupational exposure and urological cancer. *World Journal of Urology, 21*(6), 382–391.

Goodman, G. E., Alberts, D. S., & Meyskens, F. L. (2008). Retinol, vitamins, and cancer prevention: 25 years of learning and relearning. *Journal of Clinical Oncology, 26*(34), 5495–5496.

Green, D. R., & Kroemer, G. (2009). Cytoplasmic functions of the tumour suppressor p53. *Nature, 458*(7242), 1127–1130.

Green, J., Banks, E., Berrington, A., Darby, S., Deo, H., & Newton, R. (2000). N-acetyltransferase 2 and bladder cancer: An overview and consideration of the evidence for gene–environment interaction. *British Journal of Cancer, 83*(3), 412–417.

Grivennikov, S. I., Greten, F. R., & Karin, M. (2010). Immunity, inflammation, and cancer. *Cell, 140*(6), 883–899.

Grushko, T. A., Blackwood, M. A., Schumm, P. L., Hagos, F. G., Adeyanju, M. O., Feldman, M. D., . . . Olopade, O. I. (2002). Molecular–cytogenetic analysis of HER-2/neu gene in BRCA1-associated breast cancers. *Cancer Research, 62*(5), 1481–1488.

Gururangan, S. (2009). Late effects of chemotherapy. *Cancer Treatment and Research, 150,* 43–65.

Hall, E. J. (1998). From chimney sweeps to astronauts: Cancer risks in the work place: The 1998 Lauriston Taylor lecture. *Health Physics, 75*(4), 357–366.

Hampel, H., Frankel, W. L., Martin, E., Arnold, M., Khanduja, K., Kuebler, P., . . . de la Chapelle, A. (2005). Screening for the Lynch syndrome (hereditary nonpolyposis colorectal cancer). *New England Journal of Medicine, 352*(18), 1851–1860.

Hance, K. W., Anderson, W. F., Devesa, S. S., Young, H. A., & Levine, P. H. (2005). Trends in inflammatory breast carcinoma incidence and survival: The surveillance, epidemiology, and end results program at the National Cancer Institute. *Journal of the National Cancer Institute, 97*(13), 966–975.

Heintz, N. H., Janssen-Heininger, Y. M., & Mossman, B. T. (2010). Asbestos, lung cancers, and mesotheliomas: From molecular approaches to targeting tumor survival pathways. *American Journal of Respiratory Cell and Molecular Biology, 42*(2), 133–139.

Hershman, D. L., Unger, J. M., Barlow, W. E., Hutchins, L. F., Martino, S., Osborne, C. K., . . . Albain, K. S. (2009). Treatment quality and outcomes of African American versus white breast cancer patients: Retrospective analysis of Southwest Oncology studies S8814/S8897. *Journal of Clinical Oncology, 27*(13), 2157–2162.

Hoeijmakers, J. H. (2009). DNA damage, aging, and cancer. *New England Journal of Medicine, 361*(15), 1475–1485.

Hunter, D. J., Kraft, P., Jacobs, K. B., Cox, D. G., Yeager, M., Hankinson, S. E., . . . Chanock, S. J. (2007). A genome-wide association study identifies alleles in *FGFR2* associated with risk of sporadic postmenopausal breast cancer. *Nature Genetics, 39*(7), 870–874.

Huxley, R. R., Ansary-Moghaddam, A., Clifton, P., Czernichow, S., Parr, C. L., & Woodward, M. (2009). The impact of dietary and lifestyle risk factors on risk of colorectal cancer: A quantitative overview of the epidemiological evidence. *International Journal of Cancer, 125*(1), 171–180.

Ionov, Y., Peinado, M. A., Malkhosyan, S., Shibata, D., & Perucho, M. (1993). Ubiquitous somatic mutations in simple repeated sequences reveal a new mechanism for colonic carcinogenesis. *Nature, 363*(6429), 558–561.

John, E. M., Miron, A., Gong, G., Phipps, A. I., Felberg, A., Li, F. P., . . . Whittemore, A. S. (2007). Prevalence of pathogenic BRCA1 mutation carriers in 5 US racial/ethnic groups. *Journal of the American Medical Association, 298*(24), 2869–2876.

Kadlubar, F. F., Berkowitz, G. S., Delongchamp, R. R., Wang, C., Green, B. L., Tang, G., . . . Wolff, M. S. (2003). The *CYP3A4*1B* variant is related to the onset of puberty, a known risk factor for the development of breast cancer. *Cancer Epidemiology, Biomarkers & Prevention, 12*(4), 327–331.

Kalland, K. H., Ke, X. S., & Oyan, A. M. (2009). Tumour virology—History, status and future challenges. *Acta Pathologica, Microbiologica et Immunologica Scandinavica, 117*(5–6), 382–399.

Kessenbrock, K., Plaks, V., & Werb, Z. (2010). Matrix metalloproteinases: Regulators of the tumor microenvironment. *Cell, 141*(1), 52–67.

Kimura, K. (2000). Gastritis and gastric cancer. Asia. *Gastroenterology Clinics of North America, 29*(3), 609–621.

Kinzler, K. W., & Vogelstein, B. (1996). Lessons from hereditary colorectal cancer. *Cell, 87*(2), 159–170.

Klass, C. M., & Offermann, M. K. (2005). Targeting human herpesvirus-8 for treatment of Kaposi's sarcoma and primary effusion lymphoma. *Current Opinion in Oncology, 17*(5), 447–455.

Kwei, K. A., Kung, Y., Salari, K., Holcomb, I. N., & Pollack, J. R. (2010). Genomic instability in breast cancer: Pathogenesis and clinical implications. *Molecular Oncology, 4*(3), 255–266.

Larsen, L. (2010). *Environmental health sourcebook: Basic consumer health information about the environment and its effects on human health* (3rd ed.). Detroit, MI: Omnigraphics.

Lassmann, S., Weis, R., Makowiec, F., Roth, J., Danciu, M., Hopt, U., & Werner, M. (2007). Array CGH identifies distinct DNA copy number profiles of oncogenes and tumor suppressor genes in chromosomal- and microsatellite-unstable sporadic colorectal carcinomas. *Journal of Molecular Medicine, 85*(3), 293–304.

Le Marchand, L., Wilkens, L. R., Kolonel, L. N., & Henderson, B. E. (2005). The MTHFR C677T polymorphism and colorectal cancer: The multiethnic cohort study. *Cancer Epidemiology, Biomarkers & Prevention, 14*(5), 1198–1203.

Lee, A. T., & Lee, C. G. (2007). Oncogenesis and transforming viruses: The hepatitis B virus and hepatocellularcarcinoma—the etiopathogenic link. *Frontiers in Bioscience, 12*, 234–245.

Lee, W., Jiang, Z., Liu, J., Haverty, P. M., Guan, Y., Stinson, J., . . . Zhang, Z. (2010). The mutation spectrum revealed by paired genome sequences from a lung cancer patient. *Nature, 465*(7297), 473–477.

Li, C. I., Nishi, N., McDougall, J. A., Semmens, E. O., Sugiyama, H., Soda, M., . . . Kopecky, K. J. (2010). Relationship between radiation exposure and risk of second primary cancers among atomic bomb survivors. *Cancer Research, 70*(18), 7187–7198.

Lindvall, C., Bu, W., Williams, B. O., & Li, Y. (2007). Wnt signaling, stem cells, and the cellular origin of breast cancer. *Stem Cell Review, 3*(2), 157–168.

Livasy, C. A., Karaca, G., Nanda, R., Tretiakova, M. S., Olopade, O. I., Moore, D. T., & Perou, C. M. (2006). Phenotypic evaluation of the basal-like subtype of invasive breast carcinoma. *Modern Pathology, 19*(2), 264–271.

Lodovici, M., & Bigagli, E. (2009). Biomarkers of induced active and passive smoking damage. *International Journal of Environmental Research and Public Health, 6*(3), 874–888.

Longworth, M. S., & Laimins, L. A. (2004). Pathogenesis of human papillomaviruses in differentiating epithelia. *Microbiology and Molecular Biology Reviews, 68*(2), 362–372.

Lukacs, R. U., Lawson, D. A., Xin, L., Zong, Y., Garraway, I., Goldstein, A. S., . . . Witte, O. N. (2008). Epithelial stem cells of the prostate and their role in cancer progression. *Cold Spring Harbor Symposia on Quantitative Biology, 73*, 491–502.

Maeda, M., Nishimura, Y., Kumagai, N., Hayashi, H., Hatayama, T., Katoh, M., . . . Otsuki, T. (2010). Dysregulation of the immune system caused by silica and asbestos. *Journal of Immunotoxicology, 7*(4), 268–278.

Malumbres, M., & Barbacid, M. (2009). Cell cycle, CDKs and cancer: A changing paradigm. *Nature Reviews Cancer, 9*(3), 153–166.

Markowitz, S. D., & Bertagnolli, M. M. (2009). Molecular origins of cancer: Molecular basis of colorectal cancer. *New England Journal of Medicine, 361*(25), 2449–2460.

Maserejian, N. N., Giovannucci, E., Rosner, B., & Joshipura, K. (2007). Prospective study of vitamins C, E, and A and carotenoids and risk of oral premalignant lesions in men. *International Journal of Cancer, 120*(5), 970–977.

Masi, C. M., & Olopade, O. I. (2005). Racial and ethnic disparities in breast cancer: A multilevel perspective. *Medical Clinics of North America, 89*(4), 753–770.

McPhail, G. (1997). There's no such thing as a healthy glow: Cutaneous malignant melanoma—the case against suntanning. *European Journal of Cancer Care (England), 6*(2), 147–153.

Michor, F., Iwasa, Y., Vogelstein, B., Lengauer, C., & Nowak, M. A. (2005). Can chromosomal instability initiate tumorigenesis? *Seminars in Cancer Biology, 15*(1), 43–49.

Mishra, P. J., Glod, J. W., & Banerjee, D. (2009). Mesenchymal stem cells: Flip side of the coin. *Cancer Research, 69*(4), 1255–1258.

Monforton, C. (2006). Weight of the evidence or wait for the evidence? Protecting underground miners from diesel particulate matter. *American Journal of Public Health, 96*(2), 271–276.

Moore, M. A. (2009). Diverse influences of dietary factors on cancer in Asia. *Asian Pacific Journal of Cancer Prevention, 10*(6), 981–986.

Morris, M. A., Young, L. S., & Dawson, C. W. (2008). DNA tumour viruses promote tumour cell invasion and metastasis by deregulating the normal processes of cell adhesion and motility. *European Journal of Cell Biology, 87*(8–9), 677–697.

Mostafa, M., Sheweita, S., & O'Connor, P. (1999). Relationship between schistosomiasis and bladder cancer. *Clinical Microbiology Reviews, 12*, 97–111.

Mukai, H. (2010). Treatment strategy for HER2-positive breast cancer. *International Journal of Clinical Oncology, 15*(4), 335–340.

Murnane, J. P. (2010). Telomere loss as a mechanism for chromosome instability in human cancer. *Cancer Research, 70*(11), 4255–4259.

Murphy, P. A., Hendrich, S., Hopmans, E. C., Hauck, C. C., Lu, Z., Buseman, G., & Munkvold, G. (1996). Effect of processing on fumonisin content of corn. *Advances in Experimental Medicine and Biology, 392*, 323–334.

Nanri, A., Mizoue, T., Takahashi, Y., Noda, M., Inoue, M., & Tsugane, S. (2010). Weight change and all-cause, cancer and cardiovascular disease mortality in Japanese men and women: The Japan Public Health Center-Based Prospective Study. *International Journal of Obesity (London), 34*(2), 348–356.

Nassir, R., Kosoy, R., Tian, C., White, P. A., Butler, L. M., Silva, G., . . . Seldin, M. F. (2009). An ancestry informative marker set for determining continental origin: Validation and extension using human genome diversity panels. *BMC Genetics, 10*, 39.

Negrini, S., Gorgoulis, V. G., & Halazonetis, T. D. (2010). Genomic instability—An evolving hallmark of cancer. *Nature Reviews Molecular Cell Biology, 11*(3), 220–228.

Newman, L. A., & Martin, I. K. (2007). Disparities in breast cancer. *Current Problems in Cancer, 31*(3), 134–156.

Nussenzweig, A., & Nussenzweig, M. C. (2010). Origin of chromosomal translocations in lymphoid cancer. *Cell, 141*(1), 27–38.

O'Reilly, K. M., McLaughlin, A. M., Beckett, W. S., & Sime, P. J. (2007). Asbestos-related lung disease. *American Family Physician, 75*(5), 683–688.

Oh, D. S., Troester, M. A., Usary, J., Hu, Z., He, X., Fan, C., . . . Perou, C. M. (2006). Estrogen-regulated genes predict survival in hormone receptor-positive breast cancers. *Journal of Clinical Oncology, 24*(11), 1656–1664.

Olopade, O. I., Fackenthal, J. D., Dunston, G., Tainsky, M. A., Collins, F., & Whitfield-Broome, C. (2003). Breast cancer genetics in African Americans. *Cancer, 97* (1 Suppl), 236–245.

Olopade, O. I., Grushko, T. A., Nanda, R., & Huo, D. (2008). Advances in breast cancer: pathways to personalized medicine. *Clinical Cancer Research, 14*(24), 7988–7999.

Omura, N., & Goggins, M. (2009). Epigenetics and epigenetic alterations in pancreatic cancer. *International Journal of Clinical and Experimental Pathology, 2*(4), 310–326.

Parodi, P. W. (2005). Dairy product consumption and the risk of breast cancer. *Journal of the American College of Nutrition, 24*(6 Suppl), 556S–568S.

Perou, C. M., Sorlie, T., Eisen, M. B., van de Rijn, M., Jeffrey, S. S., Rees, C. A., . . . Botstein, D. (2000). Molecular portraits of human breast tumours. *Nature, 406*(6797), 747–752.

Perrin, D., Ruskin, H. J., & Niwa, T. (2010). Cell type-dependent, infection-induced, aberrant DNA methylation in gastric cancer. *Journal of Theoretical Biology, 264*(2), 570–577.

Petrucelli, N., Daly, M. B., & Feldman, G. L. (2010). Hereditary breast and ovarian cancer due to mutations in *BRCA1* and *BRCA2*. *Genetics in Medicine, 12*(5), 245–259.

Polite, B. N., Dignam, J. J., & Olopade, O. I. (2005). Colorectal cancer and race: Understanding the differences in outcomes between African Americans and whites. *Medical Clinics of North America, 89*(4), 771–793.

Polite, B. N., Dignam, J. J., & Olopade, O. I. (2006). Colorectal cancer model of health disparities: Understanding mortality differences in minority populations. *Journal of Clinical Oncology, 24*(14), 2179–2187.

Porter, P. L., Lund, M. J., Lin, M. G., Yuan, X., Liff, J. M., Flagg, E. W., . . . Eley, J. W. (2004). Racial differences in the expression of cell cycle-regulatory proteins in breast carcinoma. *Cancer, 100*(12), 2533–2542.

Powell, S. N., & Kachnic, L. A. (2008). Therapeutic exploitation of tumor cell defects in homologous recombination. *Anti-Cancer Agents in Medical Chemistry, 8*(4), 448–460.

Prat, A., Parker, J. S., Karginova, O., Fan, C., Livasy, C., Herschkowitz, J. I., . . . Perou, C. M. (2010). Phenotypic and molecular characterization of the claudin-low intrinsic subtype of breast cancer. *Breast Cancer Research, 12*(5), R68.

Preston, R. J., & Williams, G. M. (2005). DNA-reactive carcinogens: Mode of action and human cancer hazard. *Critical Reviews in Toxicology, 35*(8–9), 673–683.

Rajaraman, R., Guernsey, D. L., Rajaraman, M. M., & Rajaraman, S. R. (2006). Stem cells, senescence, neosis and self-renewal in cancer. *Cancer Cell International, 6*, 25.

Rapp, K., Klenk, J., Ulmer, H., Concin, H., Diem, G., Oberaigner, W., & Schroeder, J. (2008). Weight change and cancer risk in a cohort of more than 65,000 adults in Austria. *Annals of Oncology, 19*(4), 641–648.

Rebbeck, T. R., Halbert, C. H., & Sankar, P. (2006). Genetics, epidemiology, and cancer disparities: Is it black and white? *Journal of Clinical Oncology, 24*(14), 2164–2169.

Rieck, G., & Fiander, A. (2006). The effect of lifestyle factors on gynaecological cancer. *Best Practice & Research in Clinical Obstetrics & Gynaecology, 20*(2), 227–251.

Robinson, D. (2002). Cancer clusters: Findings vs feelings. *MedGenMed, 4*(4), 16.

Rodrigues, S., De Wever, O., Bruyneel, E., Rooney, R. J., & Gespach, C. (2007). Opposing roles of netrin-1 and the dependence receptor DCC in cancer cell invasion, tumor growth and metastasis. *Oncogene, 26*(38), 5615–5625.

Ruprecht, K., Mayer, J., Sauter, M., Roemer, K., & Mueller-Lantzsch, N. (2008). Endogenous retroviruses and cancer. *Cellular and Molecular Life Sciences, 65*(21), 3366–3382.

Sacks, F. M., Bray, G. A., Carey, V. J., Smith, S. R., Ryan, D. H., Anton, S. D., . . . Williamson, D. A. (2009). Comparison of weight-loss diets with different compositions of fat, protein, and carbohydrates. *New England Journal of Medicine, 360*(9), 859–873.

Salk, J. J., Fox, E. J., & Loeb, L. A. (2010). Mutational heterogeneity in human cancers: Origin and consequences. *Annual Review of Pathology, 5*, 51–75.

Scully, C., & Bedi, R. (2000). Ethnicity and oral cancer. *Lancet Oncology, 1*(1), 37–42.

Secretan, B., Straif, K., Baan, R., Grosse, Y., El Ghissassi, F., Bouvard, V., . . . Cogliano, V. (2009). A review of human carcinogens—Part E: Tobacco, areca nut, alcohol, coal smoke, and salted fish. *Lancet Oncology, 10*(11), 1033–1034.

Settle, K., Posner, M. R., Schumaker, L. M., Tan, M., Suntharalingam, M., Goloubeva, O., . . . Cullen, K. J. (2009). Racial survival disparity in head and neck cancer results from low prevalence of human papillomavirus infection in black oropharyngeal cancer patients. *Cancer Prevention Research (Philadelphia, PA), 2*(9), 776–781.

Sgambato, A., & Cittadini, A. (2010). Inflammation and cancer: A multifaceted link. *European Review for Medical and Pharmacological Sciences, 14*(4), 263–268.

Sharma, P. (2009a). Barrett's esophagus and cancer. Preface. *Surgical Oncology Clinics of North America, 18*(3), xv–xvi.

Sharma, P. (2009b). Clinical practice. Barrett's esophagus. *New England Journal of Medicine, 361*(26), 2548–2556.

Sherva, R., Kranzler, H. R., Yu, Y., Logue, M. W., Poling, J., Arias, A. J., . . . Gelernter, J. (2010). Variation in nicotinic acetylcholine receptor genes is associated with multiple substance dependence phenotypes. *Neuropsychopharmacology, 35*(9), 1921–1931.

Shiao, Y. H., Chen, V. W., Scheer, W. D., Wu, X. C., & Correa, P. (1995). Racial disparity in the association of p53 gene alterations with breast cancer survival. *Cancer Research, 55*(7), 1485–1490.

Shuryak, I., Hahnfeldt, P., Hlatky, L., Sachs, R. K., & Brenner, D. J. (2009). A new view of radiation-induced cancer: Integrating short- and long-term processes. Part II: Second cancer risk estimation. *Radiation and Environmental Biophysics, 48*(3), 275–286.

Sjostrom, L., Gummesson, A., Sjostrom, C. D., Narbro, K., Peltonen, M., Wedel, H., . . . Carlsson, L. M. (2009). Effects of bariatric surgery on cancer incidence in obese patients in Sweden (Swedish Obese Subjects Study): A prospective, controlled intervention trial. *Lancet Oncology, 10*(7), 653–662.

Slattery, M. L., Schaffer, D., & Edwards, S. L. (1997). Are dietary factors involved in DNA methylation associated with colon cancer? *Nutrition and Cancer, 28*, 52–62.

Sorlie, T., Perou, C. M., Tibshirani, R., Aas, T., Geisler, S., Johnsen, H., . . . Borresen-Dale, A. L. (2001). Gene expression patterns of breast carcinomas distinguish tumor subclasses with clinical implications. *Proceedings of the National Academy of Sciences of the United States of America, 98*(19), 10869–10874.

Stanley, M. A., Pett, M. R., & Coleman, N. (2007). HPV: From infection to cancer. *Biochemical Society Transactions, 35*(6), 1456–1460.

Steenland, K., Burnett, C., Lalich, N., Ward, E., & Hurrell, J. (2003). Dying for work: The magnitude of US mortality from selected causes of death associated with occupation. *American Journal of Industrial Medicine, 43*(5), 461–482.

Stevens, V. L., Bierut, L. J., Talbot, J. T., Wang, J. C., Sun, J., Hinrichs, A. L., . . . Calle, E. E. (2008). Nicotinic receptor gene variants influence susceptibility to heavy smoking. *Cancer Epidemiology, Biomarkers & Prevention, 17*(12), 3517–3525.

Taioli, E., Bradlow, H. L., Garbers, S. V., Sepkovic, D. W., Osborne, M. P., Trachman, J., . . . Garte, S. J. (1999). Role of estradiol metabolism and *CYP1A1* polymorphisms in breast cancer risk. *Cancer Detection and Prevention, 23*(3), 232–237.

Taioli, E., Im, A., Xu, X., Veenstra, T. D., Ahrendt, G., & Garte, S. (2010). Comparison of estrogens and estrogen metabolites in human breast tissue and urine. *Reproductive Biology and Endocrinology, 8*, 93.

Takayama, T., Miyanishi, K., Hayashi, T., Sato, Y., & Niitsu, Y. (2006). Colorectal cancer: Genetics of development and metastasis. *Journal of Gastroenterology, 41*(3), 185–192.

Talmadge, J. E., & Fidler, I. J. (2010). AACR centennial series: The biology of cancer metastasis: Historical perspective. *Cancer Research, 70*(14), 5649–5669.

Talos, F., & Moll, U. M. (2010). Role of the p53 family in stabilizing the genome and preventing polyploidization. *Advances in Experimental Medicine and Biology, 676*, 73–91.

Tammela, T., & Alitalo, K. (2010). Lymphangiogenesis: Molecular mechanisms and future promise. *Cell, 140*(4), 460–476.

Tominaga, S. (1999). Major avoidable risk factors of cancer. *Cancer Letters, 143*(Suppl 1), S19–S23.

Tsai, W. L., & Chung, R. T. (2010). Viral hepatocarcinogenesis. *Oncogene, 29*(16), 2309–2324.

Turner, N., & Grose, R. (2010). Fibroblast growth factor signalling: From development to cancer. *Nature Reviews Cancer, 10*(2), 116–129.

Valladares Ayerbes, M., Aparicio Gallego, G., Diaz Prado, S., Jimenez Fonseca, P., Garcia Campelo, R., & Anton Aparicio, L. M. (2008). Origin of renal cell carcinomas. *Clinical and Translational Oncology, 10*(11), 697–712.

van Kruijsdijk, R. C., van der Wall, E., & Visseren, F. L. (2009). Obesity and cancer: The role of dysfunctional adipose tissue. *Cancer Epidemiology, Biomarkers & Prevention, 18*(10), 2569–2578.

Vogelstein, B., & Kinzler, K. W. (2004). Cancer genes and the pathways they control. *Nature Medicine, 10*(8), 789–799.

Wall, B. F., Kendall, G. M., Edwards, A. A., Bouffler, S., Muirhead, C. R., & Meara, J. R. (2006). What are the risks from medical X-rays and other low dose radiation? *British Journal of Radiology, 79*(940), 285–294.

Wang, D., & DuBois, R. N. (2008). Pro-inflammatory prostaglandins and progression of colorectal cancer. *Cancer Letters, 267*(2), 197–203.

Weidman, J. R., Dolinoy, D. C., Murphy, S. K., & Jirtle, R. L. (2007). Cancer susceptibility: Epigenetic manifestation of environmental exposures. *Cancer Journal, 13*(1), 9–16.

Weisberg, I., Tran, P., Christensen, B., Sibani, S., & Rozen, R. (1998). A second genetic polymorphism in methylenetetrahydrofolate reductase (MTHFR) associated with decreased enzyme activity. *Molecular Genetics and Metabolism, 64*(3), 169–172.

Williams, D. (2008). Radiation carcinogenesis: Lessons from Chernobyl. *Oncogene, 27*(Suppl 2), S9–S18.

Woodman, C. B., Collins, S. I., & Young, L. S. (2007). The natural history of cervical HPV infection: Unresolved issues. *Nature Reviews Cancer, 7*(1), 11–22.

Wu, X., Zhao, H., Amos, C. I., Shete, S., Makan, N., Hong, W. K., . . . Spitz, M. R. (2002). p53 Genotypes and haplotypes associated with lung cancer susceptibility and ethnicity. *Journal of the National Cancer Institute, 94*(9), 681–690.

Zhang, J., & Powell, S. N. (2005). The role of the *BRCA1* tumor suppressor in DNA double-strand break repair. *Molecular Cancer Research, 3*(10), 531–539.

Zhao, J., Shi, X., Castranova, V., & Ding, M. (2009). Occupational toxicology of nickel and nickel compounds. *Journal of Environmental Pathology, Toxicology and Oncology, 28*(3), 177–208.

2

Racial/Ethnic and Socioeconomic Disparities in Cancer Incidence, Stage, Survival, and Mortality in the United States

Jiemin Ma, Rebecca Siegel, and Ahmedin Jemal

Cancer is the second most common cause of death in the United States, following heart disease. The American Cancer Society projected that about 1,596,670 new cancer cases will be diagnosed and about 571,950 Americans will die of cancer in 2011 (American Cancer Society, 2011). The cancer burden varies considerably by race/ethnicity and socioeconomic status. Eliminating these disparities has been stated as an overarching objective of the Federal Healthy People 2010 initiative (U.S. Department of Health and Human Services, 2000) and the Society's 2015 challenge goal (American Cancer Society Board of Directors, 1996). This chapter reviews trends in cancer incidence, stage at diagnosis, survival, and mortality in the United States by race/ethnicity and socioeconomic status.

MEASUREMENTS AND DEFINITIONS

Incidence and mortality (or death) rates are two commonly used measurements of cancer burden. They are usually defined as the number of new cancer cases or deaths, respectively, per 100,000 persons over a specified time period. In cancer statistics, age-standardized rates are usually reported in order to minimize the effect of age when comparing rates between populations with different age structures.

Survival, a measure of disease prognosis, is the proportion of cancer patients surviving for a specified time interval after diagnosis, usually 5 years. In cancer statistics, a commonly reported survival estimate is relative survival rate, which is defined as the ratio of the observed proportion of survivors (all causes of death) among a cohort of cancer patients to the proportion of expected survivors among a comparable cohort of the general population, such that relative survival removes the effect of other causes of death. In the United States, the relative survival estimate is not available for some subpopulations, such as small racial/ethnic groups, because suitable life tables are unavailable for them. In this case, cause-specific survival, which represents a net survival of a specified disease in the absence of other causes of death, may serve as an alternative to relative survival, although cause-specific survival requires accurate classification of cause of death (Howlader et al., 2010).

The stage of cancer at the time of diagnosis is an important determinant of the choice of therapy and disease prognosis. In general, earlier stage at diagnosis is associated with better survival. In cancer registry, a summary staging scheme is applied to group invasive tumors into one of four categories: localized, regional, distant, and unstaged.

DATA COLLECTION AND REPORTING

Incidence, Stage at Diagnosis, and Survival

Since 1973, the Surveillance, Epidemiology, and End Results (SEER) Program of the National Cancer Institute (NCI) has been collecting information on the demographic characteristics of new cancer patients, extent of disease at time of diagnosis, first course of treatment, and follow-up for vital status (National Cancer Institute, 2010). Over the years, SEER has expanded from nine population-based cancer registries covering 10% of the U.S. population to 17 registries covering 28% of the population. The National Program of Cancer Registries (NPCR) (Centers for Disease Control and Prevention, 2010b) of the Centers for Disease Control and Prevention (CDC) was established by Congress through the Cancer Registries Amendment Act in 1992, and also routinely collects data on cancer occurrence, extent of disease, and initial treatment. The NPCR currently funds statewide population-based registries in 45 states, the District of Columbia, Puerto Rico, and the U.S. Pacific Island jurisdictions. The NPCR, together with SEER, currently cover the entire U.S. population.

Neither SEER nor NPCR collect individual-level socioeconomic indicators; therefore, use of SEER and NPCR data to examine disparities in cancer incidence in the United States is largely limited to analysis based on area-level indicators of socioeconomic status (SES), such as poverty rate by county, zip code, or census tract. The limitation of these ecological studies, which use aggregate data to make inferences about individuals, is that the populations within a given area may not be homogenous with respect to the particular SES variable of interest (MacRae, 1994).

Mortality

Cancer mortality data covering the entire U.S. population have been collected by the National Vital Statistics System, which is administered by the National Center for Health Statistics (NCHS) of the CDC, since 1930 (Centers for Disease Control and Prevention, 2010a). Based on information from death certificates, underlying causes of death are selected and coded according to the selection and coding rules of the revision of the International Classification of Diseases (ICD) at the time of death; the ICD is revised about every 10 years. The classification of death due to cancer is generally accurate for major cancer sites (e.g., the lung, prostate, female breast, and colorectal) (German et al., 2010; Kircher, Nelson, & Burdo, 1985). However, for some cancer sites, such as cancers in the oral cavity and pharynx, it is less consistent between the underlying cause of death and cancer registry diagnosis (German et al., 2010). NCHS has also been collecting educational attainment on death certificates, beginning in 1989 in some states and from 1993 in all states. This information has been used to describe differences in cancer mortality rates and trends by educational level (Albano et al., 2007; Kinsey, Jemal, Liff, Ward, & Thun, 2008).

RACIAL/ETHNIC DISPARITIES

In cancer statistics, cancer cases and deaths are commonly grouped into four major racial groups—White; Black, or African American (AA); Asian and Pacific Islander (API); and American Indian/Alaska Native (AI/AN)—and into two ethnic origins: non-Hispanic/Latino and Hispanic/Latino. Notably, race classification of the AI/AN group may be problematic in some cancer registries. Linkage of cancer registry data with the Indian Health Service (IHS) patient database is an effective method to reduce misclassification of the AI/AN population. However, cancer rates among AI/AN groups should still be interpreted with caution, because the IHS-linked cancer registry data are thought to lack complete representation of the AI/AN population. This linkage covers about 55% of the U.S. AI/AN population.

Incidence

Cancer incidence rates vary markedly between racial and ethnic groups (Table 2.1) (Edwards et al., 2010). For all cancers combined, Black men have a 14% higher incidence rate than White men, whereas Black women have a 7% lower incidence rate than White women (Jemal, Siegel, Xu, & Ward, 2010). For the specific cancer sites listed in Table 2.1, Blacks consistently have higher incidence rates than Whites, except for cancers of the lung and breast among

TABLE 2.1 Cancer Incidence Rate[a] by Site, Race, and Ethnicity in the United States, 2002–2006

	White	AA	API	AI/AN[b]	Hispanic/Latino[c]
All sites					
Male	550.1	626.0	334.5	441.2	430.3
Female	420.0	389.5	276.3	369.3	326.8
Lung and bronchus					
Male	85.9	104.8	50.6	78.0	49.2
Female	57.1	50.7	27.6	56.1	26.5
Prostate	146.3	231.9	82.3	108.8	131.1
Breast (female)	123.5	113.0	81.6	91.7	90.2
Colon and rectum					
Male	58.2	68.4	44.1	55.0	50.0
Female	42.6	51.7	33.1	44.7	35.1
Kidney and renal pelvis					
Male	19.7	20.6	9.0	24.5	18.2
Female	10.3	10.6	4.5	15.6	10.3
Liver and bile duct					
Male	8.0	12.5	21.4	12.9	15.9
Female	2.8	3.8	8.1	6.8	6.2
Stomach					
Male	8.9	16.7	17.5	14.7	14.3
Female	4.2	8.5	9.8	7.3	8.6
Uterine cervix	7.9	11.1	7.6	9.4	12.7

Incidence rates were calculated based on the registry data in 43 states.

AA, African American; API, Asian American and Pacific Islander; AI/AN, American Indian and Alaska Native.

[a]Per 100,000, age adjusted to the 2000 U.S. standard population.

[b]Data based on Contract Health Service Delivery Areas, comprising about 55% of the U.S. American Indian/Alaska Native population.

[c]Persons of Hispanic/Latino origin may be of any race.

Source: From "Annual report to the nation on the status of cancer, 1975–2006, featuring colorectal cancer trends and impact of interventions (risk factors, screening, and treatment) to reduce future rates" by B. K. Edwards, E. Ward, B. A. Kohler, C. Eheman, A. G. Zauber, R. N. Anderson, et al., 2010, *Cancer*, 116, pp. 544–573. Used with permission.

women. The higher breast cancer incidence rates among White women may be attributable to the combined effect of cancer screening (e.g., more frequent mammography in White women) and exposure to risk factors (e.g., later age at first birth and greater use of menopausal hormone therapy among White compared to Black women) (Ghafoor et al., 2003).

Compared to Whites and Blacks, other racial/ethnic groups have a lower incidence rate for all cancers combined (Table 2.1). With respect to site-specific cancer incidence, these minority groups have a lower rate than Whites for most of the common cancer sites, but typically have a higher rate for cancer sites related to infectious agents, such as the uterine cervix, liver, and stomach. For example, the incidence rate for cancer of the uterine cervix is 60% higher among Hispanics/Latinos than among Whites. Asian American/Pacific Islanders have the highest incidence rates for both liver and stomach cancers in both men and women. Higher stomach and liver cancer incidence rates in the API population may reflect an increased prevalence of chronic infection with *Helicobacter pylori* and hepatitis B and C viruses, respectively, in this population (Ward et al., 2004). American Indians and Alaska Natives have a higher incidence rate for kidney cancer than other racial/ethnic group. The higher prevalence of obesity and smoking among American Indians and Alaska Natives may contribute to this disparity (Espey et al., 2007).

Although cancer incidence varies largely across racial/ethnic groups, prostate, lung, and colorectal cancer in men, and breast, lung, and colorectal cancer in women, without specific rank order, are the three most commonly diagnosed cancers in each racial/ethnic group (Edwards et al., 2010).

Stage at Diagnosis and Survival

African Americans and other minority groups are more likely than Whites to be diagnosed at a later stage of disease for all the four major cancers: lung, colorectal, female breast, and prostate cancers (Figure 2.1) (Altekruse et al., 2010). For lung cancer, the proportion of distant stage diagnoses is 2%–8% points higher in minority groups than in Whites; for breast cancer, the percentage of localized stage diagnoses is 10% points higher in White women than in Black women.

Since 1975, survival rates for the four common cancer sites, with the exception of the lung, have substantially improved among both African Americans and Whites (Table 2.2) (Altekruse et al., 2010). However, African American men and women continue to have poorer survival than their White counterparts for nearly every cancer site. During the period from 1999 to 2006, the relative 5-year survival rate in African Americans was at least 10% points lower than in Whites for all cancers combined (59.2% in Blacks vs. 69.1% in Whites) and cancers of the colorectum (56.7% in Blacks vs. 67.9% in Whites) and female breast (78.4% in Blacks vs. 91.2% in Whites). Because accurate life expectancies are not available for racial and ethnic groups other than Whites and Blacks, relative survival rates cannot be calculated for those minority populations. However, an analysis of cause-specific survival rates among cancer patients diagnosed between 1999 and 2006 in 17 SEER areas reported that all minority male populations (Blacks, Asians/Pacific Islanders, American Indians/Alaska Natives, and Hispanics) had a greater probability of dying from cancer within 5 years of diagnosis

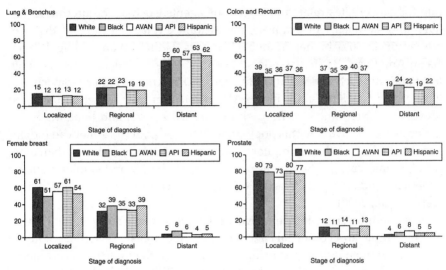

FIGURE 2.1 The Distribution of Selected Cancers by Race/Ethnicity and Stage at Diagnosis, United States, 1999–2006

For each cancer type, stage categories do not total 100% because insufficient information is available to assign a stage to all cancer cases.
Source: From *SEER cancer statistics review, 1975–2007* by S. F. Altekruse, C. L., Kosary, M. Krapcho, N. Neyman, R. Aminou, W. Waldron, et al., 2010, Bethesda, MD: National Cancer Institute. Used with permission.

than White men. Among women, Asians/Pacific Islanders have the highest (68.2%) and African Americans have the lowest 5-year cancer-specific survival rate (56.0%) (Table 2.3) (Altekruse et al., 2010).

Mortality

For all cancers combined, Black men have a 34% higher death rate than White men; and Black women have a 17% higher death rate than White women (Jemal et al., 2010). For the specific cancer sites listed in Table 2.4, African Americans consistently have higher death rates than Whites, except for lung cancer among women and kidney cancer among both men and women.

Racial/ethnic groups other than Blacks have a lower death rate than Whites for all cancers combined and for most of the common cancer sites. However, they have higher death rates for cancers of the liver, kidney, and uterine cervix. For example, death rates for both liver and stomach cancer among Asian Americans and Pacific Islanders are almost twice as high as those in Whites. The death rate from kidney cancer in American Indians and Alaska Natives is about 1.5 times as high as that in Whites.

Similar to the incidence data, lung, prostate, and colorectal cancer in men and lung, breast, and colorectal cancer in women, are the three

TABLE 2.2 Five-Year Relative Survival Rates (%) by Race and Year of Diagnosis, United States, 1975–2006

	All Cancers Combined		Lung Cancer		Colorectal Cancer		Breast Cancer (Female)		Prostate Cancer	
	White	Black	White	Black	White	Black	White	Black	White	Black
1975–1977	51.2	39.9	12.8	11.6	51.2	46.3	76.1	62.4	70.2	61.4
1978–1980	51.3	39.6	13.4	12.0	52.7	46.2	75.5	63.9	72.9	62.8
1981–1983	52.6	39.6	13.9	11.7	55.6	47.5	77.6	64.1	74.6	63.7
1984–1986	54.8	40.8	13.6	11.4	59.4	49.2	80.5	65.3	77.6	66.3
1987–1989	57.8	43.6	13.8	11.2	61.1	53.3	85.4	71.3	85.3	72.1
1990–1992	62.3	48.1	14.4	10.7	63.0	53.6	86.7	71.7	94.8	85.2
1993–1995	63.6	53.1	15.1	13.2	61.7	52.9	88.0	72.8	96.6	92.2
1996–1998	65.8	55.7	15.5	12.7	64.3	55.1	89.7	76.4	98.6	95.2
1999–2006	69.1	59.2	16.8	13.2	67.9	56.7	91.2	78.4	99.9	97.3
Absolute change	17.9	19.3	4.0	1.6	16.7	10.4	15.1	16.0	29.7	35.9
Relative change[a]	35.0	48.4	31.3	13.8	32.6	22.5	19.8	25.6	42.3	58.5

[a]Relative change = absolute difference in 5-year relative survival rates between 1975–1977 and 1999–2006, as a percentage of the rate of 1975–1977.

Source: From *SEER cancer statistics review, 1975–2007* by S. F. Altekruse, C. L., Kosary, M. Krapcho, N. Neyman, R. Aminou, W. Waldron, et al., 2010, Bethesda, MD: National Cancer Institute. Used with permission.

TABLE 2.3   Five-Year Cause-Specific Survival[a] (%) for All Cancers Combined and Selected Cancers, 1999–2006

	White	AA	API	AI/AN[b]	Hispanic/Latino[c]
All cancers combined					
Male	65.6	60.9*	59.8*	53.5*	63.3*
Female	65.6	56.0*	68.2*	60.6*	65.5
Lung cancer					
Male	15.0	12.5*	16.0	12.0	13.6*
Female	19.7	16.1*	22.1*	12.5*	17.2*
Colorectal cancer					
Male	64.9	55.7*	67.5*	59.0*	61.6*
Female	63.7	56.7*	68.6*	65.5	62.4
Breast cancer (female)	88.3	77.5*	90.3*	84.6*	85.3*
Prostate cancer	93.5	91.2*	93.8	89.7*	92.3*

AA, African American; API, Asian American and Pacific Islander; AI/AN, American Indian and Alaska Native.
[a]Five-Year Cause-Specific Survival was calculated by actuarial method using diagnosis years 1999–2006, with follow-up through 2007.
[b]Data based on Contract Health Service Delivery Areas.
[c]Persons of Hispanic/Latino origin may be of any race.
*Statistically significantly different from the rate of Whites ($p < .05$).
Source: From *SEER cancer statistics review, 1975–2007* by S. F. Altekruse, C. L., Kosary, M. Krapcho, N. Neyman, R. Aminou, W. Waldron, et al., 2010, Bethesda, MD: National Cancer Institute. Used with permission.

leading causes of cancer death in all racial/ethnic groups, except in API men, in which liver cancer, but not prostate cancer, is among the three leading causes of cancer death (Edwards et al., 2010).

It is important to note that the cancer disparities described earlier are based on broad racial/ethnic groups that are not homogenous; thus, differences in the cancer burden also exist within each racial/ethnic group. For example, among Asian Americans and Pacific Islanders, native Hawaiians and Samoans have the highest overall cancer incidence and death rates, which are two to three times those for Asian Indians; Chinese and Vietnamese have the highest incidence of and death rates from nasopharyngeal cancer; Vietnamese women are three times as likely to be diagnosed with cervical cancer as Chinese and Japanese women; and Laotians and Samoans have lower percentages of early-stage cancers of the colorectum, breast (female), and cervix uteri, compared with other API groups (American Cancer Society, 2010; Miller, Chu, Hankey, & Ries, 2008).

Racial/ethnic cancer disparities are thought to result from a complex interplay of numerous factors affecting cancer occurrence and outcomes. Minority groups often face obstacles to receiving health care services related to cancer prevention, early detection, and high-quality treatment because of low income, inadequate health insurance, cultural and language barriers, and racial bias. According to data from the National Health Interview Survey

TABLE 2.4 Cancer Death Rate[a] by Site, Race, and Ethnicity
in the United States, 2002–2006

	White	AA	API	AI/AN[b]	Hispanic/Latino[c]
All sites					
Male	226.7	304.2	135.4	183.3	154.8
Female	157.3	183.7	95.1	140.1	103.9
Lung and bronchus					
Male	69.9	90.1	36.9	48.0	33.9
Female	41.9	40.0	18.2	33.5	14.4
Prostate	23.6	56.3	10.6	20.0	19.6
Breast (female)	23.9	33.0	12.5	17.6	15.5
Colon and rectum					
Male	21.4	31.4	13.8	20.0	16.1
Female	14.9	21.6	10.0	13.7	10.7
Kidney and renal pelvis					
Male	6.1	6.0	2.4	9.0	5.2
Female	2.8	2.7	1.2	4.2	2.4
Liver and bile duct					
Male	6.8	10.8	15.0	10.3	11.3
Female	2.9	3.9	6.6	6.5	5.1
Stomach					
Male	4.8	11.0	9.6	9.8	8.3
Female	2.4	5.3	5.8	4.6	4.8
Uterine cervix	2.2	4.6	2.2	3.4	3.1

AA, African American; API, Asian American and Pacific Islander; AI/AN, American Indian and Alaska Native.
[a]Per 100,000, age adjusted to the 2000 U.S. standard population.
[b]Data based on Contract Health Service Delivery Areas, comprising about 55% of the U.S. American Indian/Alaska Native population.
[c]Persons of Hispanic/Latino origin may be of any race.
Source: From "Annual report to the nation on the status of cancer, 1975–2006, featuring colorectal cancer trends and impact of interventions (risk factors, screening, and treatment) to reduce future rates" by B. K. Edwards, E. Ward, B. A. Kohler, C. Eheman, A. G. Zauber, R. N. Anderson, et al., 2010, *Cancer*, 116, pp. 544–573. Used with permission.

(NHIS) in 2009, poverty rates and the likelihood of being medically uninsured are approximately two to three times higher for African Americans and Hispanics/Latinos than for non-Hispanic Whites (Cohen, Martinez, & Ward, 2010). In addition, minority groups often have lower education levels, which are associated with a higher prevalence of risk factors for cancer (Centers for Disease Control and Prevention, 2009, 2010c) and less access to timely or high-quality treatment (Berry et al., 2009; Rolnick et al., 2005). Overall, these socioeconomic disadvantages lead to increased risk of cancer occurrence, more advanced stage at cancer diagnosis, and poorer survival among minority groups, especially African Americans. In addition to social factors, genetic variations are also thought to contribute to the disproportionate cancer burden between racial/ethnic groups; however, genetic differences are thought to make only a minor contribution to cancer disparities (Hemminki, Forsti, & Lorenzo Bermejo, 2008). Detailed descriptions of disparities in cancer risk factors, screening, treatment, and genetic variations can be found in other chapters.

SOCIOECONOMIC DISPARITIES

Socioeconomic status (SES), which is a multidimensional construct of a complex set of factors, including education, income, employment, and other social indicators, is a strong predictor of behavioral risk factors for cancer, as well as a major determinant of insurance status and access to health care. No single indicator of SES fully captures all of the important characteristics that may influence the association between SES and cancer risk, but a consistent pattern emerges across studies of cancer disparity, in which lower SES is related to higher cancer incidence and mortality, regardless of which indicator is used (Aarts, Lemmens, Louwman, Kunst, & Coebergh, 2010; Cheng et al., 2009; Clegg et al., 2009; Marcella & Miller, 2001). These socioeconomic differences in cancer explain a substantial part of the cancer disparities between racial/ethnic groups. In addition, recent studies have shown that the association between SES and cancer is independent of race/ethnicity (Albano et al., 2007; Yin et al., 2010).

Incidence

People with lower SES are more likely to use tobacco, be physically inactive, follow an unhealthy diet, and consume alcohol excessively, partly due to less awareness of the risks of these unhealthy lifestyles, industries' marketing strategies that target socioeconomically disadvantaged populations, and environmental or community factors that provide fewer places for physical activity and less access to fresh fruits and vegetables (American Cancer Society, 2010). For example, data from the NHIS showed that in 2008, the smoking prevalence among persons with less than a high school diploma (27.5%) was 2.6 times higher than that in college graduates (10.6%); and persons living in a family below the poverty line had a 60% higher smoking prevalence (31.5%) than those living at or above the poverty line (19.6%) (Centers for Disease Control and Prevention, 2009). In addition, lower SES appears to be associated with increased exposure to environmental toxins (Evans & Kantrowitz, 2002), as well as reduced adherence to cancer screening recommendations that would help identify precancerous lesions (Blackwell, Martinez, & Gentleman, 2008). As a result, persons with lower SES are more likely to develop cancer than those with higher SES. In an analysis of SEER National Longitudinal Mortality Study (SEER–NLMS) data (Clegg et al., 2009), apparent gradients in incidence rates by educational attainment, family income, and poverty status were observed for all cancers combined in males and for lung cancer in both genders. Lung cancer incidence rates for men and women with less than a high school education were three and two times that of their college-educated counterparts, respectively; and those with family annual incomes less than $12,500 were 1.7 times more likely to be diagnosed with lung cancer than those with annual incomes of $50,000 or higher (Table 2.5). Incidence rates for all cancers combined were 11% and 7% higher in high-poverty areas (census tracts) than in low-poverty areas, for non-Hispanic White and Black men, respectively, and substantial area socio-economic gradients in incidence were also observed for some specific cancer sites (Singh, Miller, Hankey, & Edwards, 2003).

TABLE 2.5   Age-Adjusted Incidence Rates by Selected Socioeconomic Characteristics, 1973–2001 (SEER–NLMS data)

	All Cancers Combined		Lung Cancer	
	Male	**Female**	**Male**	**Female**
Educational attainment (years of education)				
Less than high school graduates (≤11)	730.3	478.5	166.6	71.6
High school graduates (12)	694.7	475.3	123.9	59.1
Some post high school education (13–15)	658.0	481.4	93.6	56.4
College education or beyond (16+)	602.3	443.3	57.6	35.9
Family income (1990 dollars)				
<$12,500	729.5	499.8	150.9	81.4
$12,500–$24,999	712.8	475.3	142.8	62.2
$25,000–$34,999	711.0	461.4	143.5	51.0
$35,000–$49,999	634.7	485.4	93.5	58.8
$50,000+	637.2	448.6	91.0	45.9
Poverty status (ratio of family income to poverty threshold)				
At or below 100%	723.9	492.5	151.4	69.8
100–200%	677.5	449.8	144.6	62.9
200–400%	688.8	447.9	119.6	57.7
400–600%	642.9	481.0	105.7	54.4
Above 600%	653.0	459.6	90.3	47.7

SEER–NLMS, Surveillance, Epidemiology, and End Results—National Longitudinal Mortality Study.
Source: From "Impact of socioeconomic status on cancer incidence and stage at diagnosis: Selected findings from the surveillance, epidemiology, and end results: National Longitudinal Mortality Study" by L. X. Clegg, M. E. Reichman, B. A. Miller, B. F. Hankey, G. K. Singh, Y. D. Lin, et al., 2009, *Cancer Causes and Control*, 20, pp. 417–435. Used with permission.

Stage at Diagnosis and Survival

Both individual- and area-level data showed that the proportions of late-stage diagnoses were higher in patients with lower SES than in those with higher SES, for most common cancer sites, such as the lung, colon and rectum, female breast, cervix, and prostate (Clegg et al., 2009; Schwartz, Crossley-May, Vigneau, Brown, & Banerjee, 2003; Singh et al., 2003). For example, among colorectal cancer patients, the proportions of distant-stage diagnosis for men and women who live in more affluent census tracts are 19.0% and 18.5%, respectively. In contrast, for men and women who live in poorer census tracts, the respective percentages are 23.7% and 22.1%. For female breast cancer, 67% of patients in more affluent census tracts were diagnosed at localized stage; the percentage was 59.0% for patients in poorer census tracts. As a result, more deprived cancer patients have worse outcomes than their more affluent counterparts (Byers et al., 2008; Gordon, 2003). Among male cancer patients, the 5-year survival rate for all cancers combined was 49% in high-poverty areas, contrasting with 61% in low-poverty areas. Among women diagnosed with cancer, the 5-year survival rates for all cancers combined were 53% and 63% in high- and low-poverty areas, respectively.

Disparities in stage at diagnosis and survival were also extensively reported by health insurance status, which is a major determinant of receipt of cancer screening and access to health care services, and is highly correlated with socioeconomic status. Analyses of the National Cancer Data Base (NCDB) revealed that individuals without insurance or with Medicaid insurance were more likely to be diagnosed with cancer in a later stage, or with a larger tumor size, than those with private insurance (Chen, Schrag, Halpern, Stewart, & Ward, 2007; Halpern, Bian, Ward, Schrag, & Chen, 2007; Halpern et al., 2008). Importantly, many cancer patients who are Medicaid-insured are uninsured at the time of diagnosis. For all cancers combined, patients without insurance or with Medicaid insurance were 1.6 times as likely to die in 5 years as those with private insurance (Ward et al., 2008). For both White and African American patients diagnosed with colorectal cancer in 1999–2000, privately insured patients with stage II disease had higher survival rates than patients with stage I disease who were Medicaid-insured or uninsured. Similarly, patients with stage III disease who were privately insured had survival rates similar to those for patients with stage II disease who were Medicaid-insured or uninsured (Figure 2.2) (Ward et al., 2008).

Mortality

Higher cancer mortality rates are consistently observed in populations of lower SES than in those with higher SES, because socioeconomically disadvantaged people are more likely to develop cancer, be diagnosed at

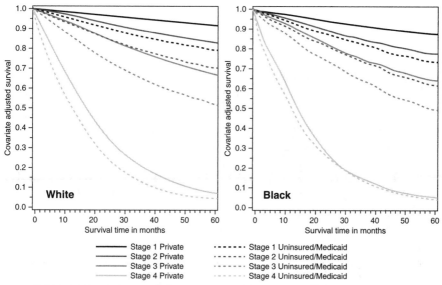

FIGURE 2.2 Colorectal Cancer Survival by Stage and Insurance Status

Source: From "Association of insurance with cancer care utilization and outcomes" by E. Ward, M. Halpern, N. Schrag, V. Cokkinides, C. DeSantis, P. Bandi, et al., 2008, *CA: A Cancer Journal for Clinicians,* 58, pp. 9–31. Used with permission.

a later stage, receive less optimal treatment, and have poorer survival. This observation is consistent across studies regardless of whether individual- or area-level socioeconomic indicators are used. In an analysis of the U.S. mortality data for 2001, Albano et al. (2007) reported that educational attainment was strongly inversely associated with mortality from all cancers combined in both men and women aged 24–65 years, regardless of race. Among Black and White men, those with 12 or fewer years of education were more than twice as likely to die of cancer as those with more than 12 years of education. Cancer death rates among women with 12 or fewer years of education group were 1.8 (White) and 1.4 (Black) times those of their more educated counterparts. Elevated risks of death were also observed for the four most common cancer sites (lung, colorectal, breast, and prostate), among those with less education (Figure 2.3). Notably, disparities by educational attainment are generally larger than those by race. For example, Albano et al. also reported that for all cancers combined and for lung and colorectal cancers, the relative risks of death comparing less-educated (12 or fewer years of education) with highly educated (more than 12 years of education) individuals within each race group were larger than the relative risks of death comparing Blacks with Whites within each educational level, for both men and women (Albano et al., 2007). In addition to educational disparities, disproportionate cancer mortality rates are observed across area-based poverty

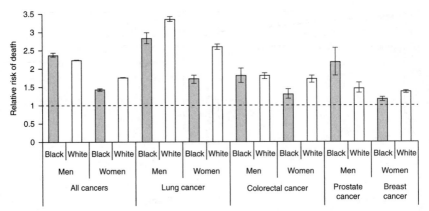

FIGURE 2.3   Relative Risk of Death and 95% Confidence Interval
From Cancer According to Education (≤12 years vs. >12 years),
United States, 2001

Source: From "Cancer mortality in the United States by education level and race" by J. D. Albano,
E. Ward, A. Jemal, R. Anderson, V. E. Cokkinides, T. Murray, et al., 2007, *Journal of the National Cancer
Institute*, 99, pp. 1384–1394. Used with permission.

levels. For example, the overall cancer mortality rate for men in high-
poverty counties was 13% greater than that for men in low-poverty counties
in 1999 (Singh et al., 2003).

TRENDS IN CANCER DISPARITIES

Tracking and monitoring temporal trends in cancer disparities are crucial
for evaluating efforts to reduce these disparities. However, the interpretation
of how disparities have changed over time depends on whether absolute or
relative differences are measured. For example, if mortality rates among two
groups decrease annually by the same absolute value, the absolute disparity
(the arithmetic difference in the rates) remains constant over time, but the relative disparity (the rate ratio) increases continuously. To fully monitor health
disparities, the general consensus is that both relative and absolute measures
are required. However, from the public health point of view, absolute change
in disparities should be emphasized because it reflects the magnitude of disparities in the population and is more relevant to decision making about resource allocation for cancer disparity reduction (Harper & Lynch, 2005).

Trends in Racial/Ethnic Disparities

Figure 2.4 depicts the age-standardized sex- and race-specific incidence and
death rates for all cancers combined between 1975 and 2007 (Altekruse et al.,
2010). Among men, the Black–White disparity in incidence and death rates

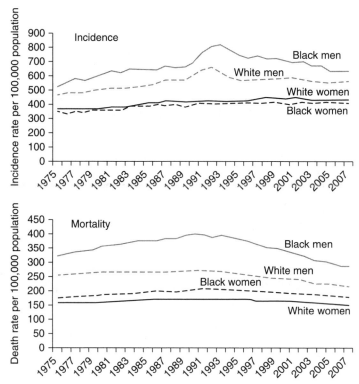

FIGURE 2.4   Cancer Incidence and Mortality Rates for African Americans and Whites for All Cancers Combined in the United States, 1975–2007

Age adjusted to the 2000 US standard population.
Source: From *SEER cancer statistics review, 1975–2007* by S. F. Altekruse, C. L., Kosary, M. Krapcho, N. Neyman, R. Aminou, W. Waldron, et al., 2010, Bethesda, MD: National Cancer Institute. Used with permission.

for all cancers combined widened from 1975 until the early 1990s, and then continuously narrowed up to 2007. Among women, overall cancer incidence rates have remained similar, and the gap in mortality rates between the two races has remained relatively stable over time; Black women continue to experience higher cancer mortality rates than White women, despite lower incidence rates. However, the temporal pattern of disparities in overall cancer incidence and mortality rates masks changes in racial disparities for specific cancer sites.

The Black–White disparities in lung cancer incidence and mortality have been narrowing since the early 1990s, due to more favorable downward trends in tobacco use by African American men in the last decades of the twentieth century (Figures 2.5 and 2.6) (Altekruse et al., 2010). Notably, the disparities in lung cancer death rates between Whites and Blacks under the age of 40 have been eliminated in both men and women (Figure 2.7)

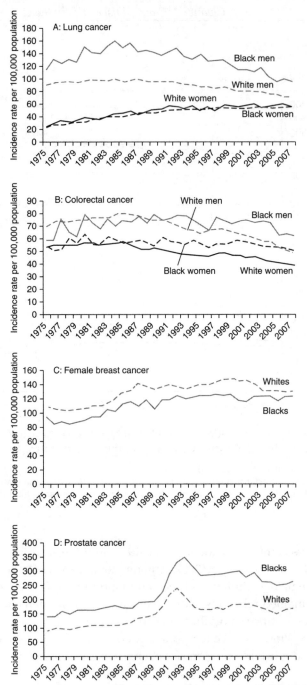

FIGURE 2.5 Cancer Incidence Rates for African Americans and Whites for Lung, Colorectal, Female Breast, and Prostate Cancers in the United States, 1975–2007

Age adjusted to the 2000 U.S. standard population.
Source: From *SEER cancer statistics review, 1975–2007* by S. F. Altekruse, C. L., Kosary, M. Krapcho, N. Neyman, R. Aminou, W. Waldron, et al., 2010, Bethesda, MD: National Cancer Institute. Used with permission.

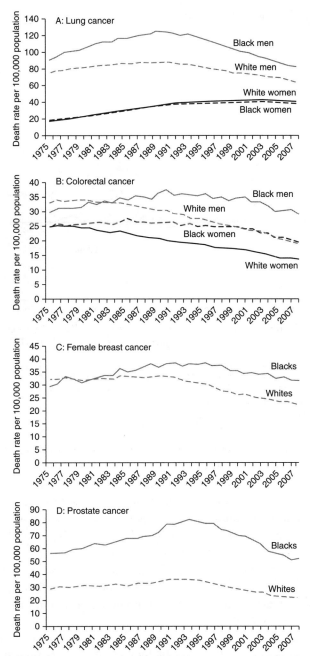

FIGURE 2.6 Cancer Mortality Rates for African American and Whites for Lung, Colorectal, Female Breast, and Prostate Cancers in the United States, 1975–2007

Age adjusted to the 2000 U.S. standard population.
Source: From *SEER cancer statistics review, 1975–2007* by S. F. Altekruse, C. L., Kosary, M. Krapcho, N. Neyman, R. Aminou, W. Waldron, et al., 2010, Bethesda, MD: National Cancer Institute. Used with permission.

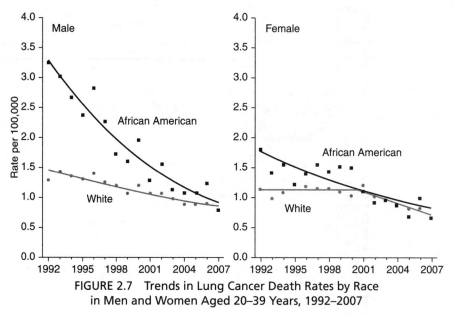

FIGURE 2.7   Trends in Lung Cancer Death Rates by Race in Men and Women Aged 20–39 Years, 1992–2007

Dots represent observed data; lines represent fitted data.
Source: From "The convergence of lung cancer rates between Blacks and Whites under the age of 40, United States" by A. Jemal, M. M. Center, and E. Ward, 2009, *Cancer Epidemiology, Biomarkers & Prevention*, 18, pp. 3349–3352. Used with permission.

(Jemal, Center, & Ward, 2009). The convergence of cancer rates in Blacks and Whites for smoking-related cancers (DeLancey, Thun, Jemal, & Ward, 2008) largely explains the recently narrowed racial gaps in overall cancer incidence and mortality. In contrast, for cancers that are affected by improved screening and/or treatment (female breast, colorectal, and prostate cancers), the Black–White disparities in mortality have been widening over the past three decades (Figures 2.5 and 2.6). This suggests that improvements in early detection and treatment have not equally reached all segments of the population; targeted programs directed at disadvantaged populations to improve access to early detection and treatment are essential to eliminate racial disparities in cancer mortality.

For stomach and liver cancer, minority populations (API, Hispanic, and AI/AN) continue to have disproportionately higher death rates than Whites, although these disparities have been narrowing in recent years for some minority groups (Edwards et al., 2010). For example, between 1997 and 2006, the liver cancer death rate annually increased by an average of 2.2% in White men, whereas the rate increased 1.3% in Hispanic men and decreased 1.3% in API men. For stomach cancer, although the death rates were falling in all racial/ethnic groups between 1997 and 2006, a quicker drop occurred in the API population than in Whites.

Trends in Socioeconomic Disparities

Data on trends in socioeconomic disparities in cancer incidence and mortality are limited in the United States. Using area-level poverty as an indicator of SES, Singh et al. (2003) did not observe consistent socioeconomic gradients in cancer incidence over time. Kinsey et al. (2008) examined the trend in mortality for the major cancer sites between 1993 and 2001 among working-aged (25–64 years) populations and found that the recent declines in death rates from major cancers in the United States mainly reflect declines in more-educated individuals, regardless of race. Except for lung cancer in Black women, death rates for the four major cancers decreased significantly from 1993 to 2001 in persons with at least 16 years of education among Blacks and Whites of both sexes. In contrast, among persons with less than 12 years of education, death rates decreased only for breast cancer in White women; death rates increased for lung cancer in White women and for colon cancer in Black men (Kinsey et al., 2008). These results indicate that socioeconomic disparities in cancer morality, at least through 2001, were widening, rather than narrowing, in working-age populations in the United States.

Using area-level poverty as an SES indicator, Singh et al. (2003) also reported widening area socioeconomic gradients in all-cancer mortality among U.S. men from 1975 to 1999, and reversed socioeconomic gradients in all-cancer mortality over time among U.S. women; among men, the death rate for all cancers combined was 2% higher in poorer areas than in more affluent counties in 1975, but increased to 13% by 1999. Contrastingly, in women, all-cancer mortality was 3% lower in poorer areas compared with more affluent counties in 1975, but in 1999, the rate was 3% higher in poorer areas. Mortality trends for the specific cancer sites showed similar patterns over time, with widening area socioeconomic disparities observed for male lung and prostate cancers and a reversal in the disparities for female colorectal and breast cancer mortality rates.

CONCLUSION

African Americans continue to bear a disproportionally greater cancer burden than Whites in the United States, largely due to differences in access to health services for cancer prevention, early detection, and treatment. While the Black–White disparities in mortality rates have narrowed for smoking-related cancers, in the most recent time period, they continued to increase for cancers affected by screening and/or treatment, including colorectal, female breast, and prostate cancers. It is also noteworthy that the disparities by socioeconomic status are larger than those by race. Therefore, more emphasis should be placed on improving access to screening and treatment among all disadvantaged segments of the population, in order to narrow or eliminate cancer disparities. In addition, primary prevention focusing on modifiable risk factors should be emphasized, as incidence continues to be higher in Blacks for most cancer sites and in other ethnic groups for infection-related cancers, such as liver, stomach, and cervical cancer. Importantly, effective implementation and evaluation of efforts to reduce disparities depend on timely collection and analysis of reliable surveillance data. This requires an improvement of the current data collection system, in which detailed and systematic data on race/ethnicity, socioeconomic status, insurance status, and quality of care are still lacking. The goal of eliminating disparities can only be achieved by coordinated and sustained efforts on the part of governmental, academic, and private organizations, as well as individuals devoted to cancer prevention.

REFERENCES

Aarts, M. J., Lemmens, V. E., Louwman, M. W., Kunst, A. E., & Coebergh, J. W. (2010). Socioeconomic status and changing inequalities in colorectal cancer? A review of the associations with risk, treatment and outcome. *European Journal of Cancer, 46*(15), 2681–2695.

Albano, J. D., Ward, E., Jemal, A., Anderson, R., Cokkinides, V. E., Murray, T., . . . Thun, M. J. (2007). Cancer mortality in the United States by education level and race. *Journal of the National Cancer Institute, 99*(18), 1384–1394.

Altekruse, S. F., Kosary, C. L., Krapcho, M., Neyman, N., Aminou, R., Waldron, W., . . . Edwards, B. K. (2010). *SEER cancer statistics review, 1975–2007.* Bethesda, MD: National Cancer Institute.

American Cancer Society. (2010). *Cancer facts & figures 2010.* Atlanta, GA: Author.

American Cancer Society. (2011). *Cancer facts & figures 2011.* Atlanta, GA: Author.

American Cancer Society Board of Directors. (1996). *ACS challenge goals for U.S. cancer mortality for the year 2015. Proceedings of the Board of Directors.* Atlanta, GA: American Cancer Society.

Berry, J., Bumpers, K., Ogunlade, V., Glover, R., Davis, S., Counts-Spriggs, M., . . . Flowers, C. (2009). Examining racial disparities in colorectal cancer care. *Journal of Psychosocial Oncology, 27*(1), 59–83.

Blackwell, D. L., Martinez, M. E., & Gentleman, J. F. (2008). Women's compliance with public health guidelines for mammograms and Pap tests in Canada and the United States: An analysis of data from the Joint Canada/United States Survey Of Health. *Women's Health Issues, 18*(2), 85–99.

Byers, T. E., Wolf, H. J., Bauer, K. R., Bolick-Aldrich, S., Chen, V. W., Finch, J. L., . . . Yin, X. (2008). The impact of socioeconomic status on survival after cancer in the United States: Findings from the National Program of Cancer Registries Patterns of Care Study. *Cancer, 113*(3), 582–591.

Centers for Disease Control and Prevention. (2009). Cigarette smoking among adults and trends in smoking cessation—United States, 2008. *Morbidity and Mortality Weekly Report, 58*(44), 1227–1232.

Centers for Disease Control and Prevention. (2010a). About the National Vital Statistics System. Retrieved October 6, 2010, from http://www.cdc.gov/nchs/nvss/about_nvss.htm

Centers for Disease Control and Prevention. (2010b). National Program of Cancer Registries (NPCR). Retrieved October 6, 2010, from http://www.cdc.gov/cancer/npcr/about.htm

Centers for Disease Control and Prevention. (2010c). Vital signs: State-specific obesity prevalence among adults—United States, 2009. *Morbidity and Mortality Weekly Report, 59*(30), 951–955.

Chen, A. Y., Schrag, N. M., Halpern, M., Stewart, A., & Ward, E. M. (2007). Health insurance and stage at diagnosis of laryngeal cancer: Does insurance type predict stage at diagnosis? *Archives of Otolaryngology—Head & Neck Surgery, 133*(8), 784–790.

Cheng, I., Witte, J. S., McClure, L. A., Shema, S. J., Cockburn, M. G., John, E. M., & Clarke, C. A. (2009). Socioeconomic status and prostate cancer incidence and mortality rates among the diverse population of California. *Cancer Causes and Control, 20*(8), 1431–1440.

Clegg, L. X., Reichman, M. E., Miller, B. A., Hankey, B. F., Singh, G. K., Lin, Y. D., . . . Edwards, B. K. (2009). Impact of socioeconomic status on cancer incidence and stage at diagnosis: Selected findings from the surveillance, epidemiology, and end results: National Longitudinal Mortality Study. *Cancer Causes and Control, 20*(4), 417–435.

Cohen, R. A., Martinez, M. E., & Ward, B. W. (2010, June). Health insurance coverage: Early release of estimates from the National Health Interview Survey, 2009. National Center for Health Statistics. Retrieved from http://www.cdc.gov/nchs/nhis.htm

DeLancey, J. O., Thun, M. J., Jemal, A., & Ward, E. M. (2008). Recent trends in Black–White disparities in cancer mortality. *Cancer Epidemiology, Biomarkers & Prevention, 17*(11), 2908–2912.

Edwards, B. K., Ward, E., Kohler, B. A., Eheman, C., Zauber, A. G., Anderson, R. N., . . . Ries, L. A. G. (2010). Annual report to the nation on the status of cancer, 1975–2006, featuring colorectal cancer trends and impact of interventions (risk factors, screening, and treatment) to reduce future rates. *Cancer, 116*(3), 544–573.

Espey, D. K., Wu, X. C., Swan, J., Wiggins, C., Jim, M. A., Ward, E., . . . Edwards, B. K. (2007). Annual report to the nation on the status of cancer, 1975–2004, featuring cancer in American Indians and Alaska Natives. *Cancer, 110*(10), 2119–2152.

Evans, G. W., & Kantrowitz, E. (2002). Socioeconomic status and health: The potential role of environmental risk exposure. *Annual Review of Public Health, 23*, 303–331.

German, R. R., Fink, A. K., Heron, M., Stewart, S. L., Johnson, C. J., Finch, J. L., & Yin, D. (2010). The accuracy of cancer mortality statistics based on death certificates in the United States. *Cancer Epidemiology, 35*(2), 126–131.

Ghafoor, A., Jemal, A., Ward, E., Cokkinides, V., Smith, R., & Thun, M. (2003). Trends in breast cancer by race and ethnicity. *CA: A Cancer Journal for Clinicians, 53*(6), 342–355.

Gordon, N. H. (2003). Socioeconomic factors and breast cancer in Black and White Americans. *Cancer and Metastasis Reviews, 22*(1), 55–65.

Halpern, M. T., Bian, J., Ward, E. M., Schrag, N. M., & Chen, A. Y. (2007). Insurance status and stage of cancer at diagnosis among women with breast cancer. *Cancer, 110*(2), 403–411.

Halpern, M. T., Ward, E. M., Pavluck, A. L., Schrag, N. M., Bian, J., & Chen, A. Y. (2008). Association of insurance status and ethnicity with cancer stage at diagnosis for 12 cancer sites: a retrospective analysis. *Lancet Oncology, 9*(3), 222–231.

Harper, S., & Lynch, J. (2005). *Methods for measuring cancer disparities: Using data relevant to Healthy People 2010 cancer-related objectives* (NCI Cancer Surveillance Monograph Series, No. 6). Bethesda, MD: National Cancer Institute.

Hemminki, K., Forsti, A., & Lorenzo Bermejo, J. (2008). Etiologic impact of known cancer susceptibility genes. *Mutation Research, 658*(1–2), 42–54.

Howlader, N., Ries, L. A., Mariotto, A. B., Reichman, M. E., Ruhl, J., & Cronin, K. A. (2010). Improved estimates of cancer-specific survival rates from population-based data. *Journal of the National Cancer Institute, 102*(20), 1584–1598.

Jemal, A., Center, M. M., & Ward, E. (2009). The convergence of lung cancer rates between Blacks and Whites under the age of 40, United States. *Cancer Epidemiology, Biomarkers & Prevention, 18*(12), 3349–3352.

Jemal, A., Siegel, R., Xu, J., & Ward, E. (2010). Cancer statistics, 2010. *CA: A Cancer Journal for Clinicians, 60*(5), 277–300.

Kinsey, T., Jemal, A., Liff, J., Ward, E., & Thun, M. (2008). Secular trends in mortality from common cancers in the United States by educational attainment, 1993–2001. *Journal of the National Cancer Institute, 100*(14), 1003–1012.

Kircher, T., Nelson, J., & Burdo, H. (1985). The autopsy as a measure of accuracy of the death certificate. *New England Journal of Medicine, 313*(20), 1263–1269.

MacRae, K. (1994). Socioeconomic deprivation and health and the ecological fallacy. *British Medical Journal, 309*(6967), 1478–1479.

Marcella, S., & Miller, J. E. (2001). Racial differences in colorectal cancer mortality. The importance of stage and socioeconomic status. *Journal of Clinical Epidemiology, 54*(4), 359–366.

Miller, B. A., Chu, K. C., Hankey, B. F., & Ries, L. A. (2008). Cancer incidence and mortality patterns among specific Asian and Pacific Islander populations in the U.S. *Cancer Causes and Control, 19*(3), 227–256.

National Cancer Institute. (2010). Overview of the SEER program. Retrieved October 6, 2010, from http://seer.cancer.gov/about

Rolnick, S., Hensley A. S., Kucera, G. P., Fortman, K., Ulcickas Y. M., Jankowski, M., & Johnson, C. C. (2005). Racial and age differences in colon examination surveillance following a diagnosis of colorectal cancer. *Journal of the National Cancer Institute Monographs,* (35), 96–101.

Schwartz, K. L., Crossley-May, H., Vigneau, F. D., Brown, K., & Banerjee, M. (2003). Race, socioeconomic status and stage at diagnosis for five common malignancies. *Cancer Causes and Control, 14*(8), 761–766.

Singh, G. K., Miller, B. A., Hankey, B. F., & Edwards, B. K. (2003). *Area socioeconomic variations in U.S. cancer incidence, mortality, stage, treatment, and survival, 1975–1999* (NCI Cancer Surveillance Monograph Series, No. 4). Bethesda, MD: National Cancer Institute.

U.S. Department of Health and Human Services. (2000, November). *Healthy People 2010: Understanding and improving health* (2nd ed.). Washington, DC: U.S. Government Printing Office.

Ward, E., Halpern, M., Schrag, N., Cokkinides, V., DeSantis, C., Bandi, P., . . . Jemal, A. (2008). Association of insurance with cancer care utilization and outcomes. *CA: A Cancer Journal for Clinicians, 58*(1), 9–31.

Ward, E., Jemal, A., Cokkinides, V., Singh, G. K., Cardinez, C., Ghafoor, A., & Thun, M. (2004). Cancer disparities by race/ethnicity and socioeconomic status. *CA: A Cancer Journal for Clinicians, 54*(2), 78–93.

Yin, D., Morris, C., Allen, M., Cress, R., Bates, J., & Liu, L. (2010). Does socioeconomic disparity in cancer incidence vary across racial/ethnic groups? *Cancer Causes and Control, 21*(10), 1721–1730.

3

Disparities in Cancer Risk Factors and Cancer Screening in the United States

Vilma Cokkinides, J. Lee Westmaas, Priti Bandi, and Elizabeth Ward

Much progress has been made over the past three decades in understanding, preventing, detecting, diagnosing, and treating cancer (Curry, Byers, & Hewitt, 2003; Jemal, Ward, & Thun, 2010). Cancer prevention, as a public health strategy based on research evidence, is the first line of defense in reducing the number of deaths resulting from cancer. It includes medical approaches (i.e., use of recommended cancer screenings) as well as environmental and behavioral interventions to modify risk factors. While many factors contribute to cancer risk, the chief behavioral (modifiable) risk factors are tobacco use, obesity, physical inactivity, and diet (Curry et al., 2003; World Cancer Research Fund/American Institute for Cancer Research, 2007). These behavioral risk factors also have a large impact on the incidence of other major chronic illnesses, such as cardiovascular disease and diabetes (Curry et al., 2003; World Cancer Research Fund/American Institute for Cancer Research, 2007). Moreover, comprehensive reviews have documented disparities in these risk factors among racial, ethnic, and socioeconomically vulnerable populations (Ward et al., 2004), and by geographic region ("Vital Signs," 2010). Though not fully understood, the causes of disparities in behavioral risk factors for cancer appear to be multifaceted and complex; experts suggest that cancer disparities are partly due to lack of access to medical care, including preventive care and state-of-the-art cancer services, environmental factors that deter adoption of healthful behaviors, or that facilitate unhealthful ones (e.g., the higher prevalence of fast-food outlets in segregated Black neighborhoods), and the interplay of low socioeconomic class, culture, and social injustice. On the other hand, inherent biological characteristics are not considered key factors in influencing cancer disparities (Ward et al., 2004). In this chapter, we discuss the major (modifiable) risk factors for the most common cancers in the United States as well as disparities in their prevalence among sociodemographic groups (i.e., race/ethnicity, gender, and socioeconomic status). We also summarize research on interventions with the potential to reduce disparities among special populations (as defined by race/ethnicity, sexual orientation, etc.) in tobacco smoking, the single preventable risk factor responsible for the majority of cancer cases.

Various national survey data are routinely used to monitor health status, medical conditions, and health services utilization in the United States. These provide prevalence estimates (proportion of the population) of behavioral risk factors for groups belonging to the major sociodemographic categories (age, race/ethnicity, gender, income, and education). Three national government-sponsored surveys are the National Health Interview Survey, the National Health and Nutrition Examination Survey, and the Behavioral Risk Factor Surveillance System. It is important to recognize some limitations of estimates from national surveys, however, that may result in less accurate information for some racial/ethnic or other categories. These include the exclusion of: (i) cell phone–only households (which tend to be of lower socioeconomic status); (ii) respondents for whom Spanish and English is not their primary spoken language (and which could result in inflated or depressed estimates for some racial/ethnic groups); and (iii) military and institutionalized populations. Smaller sample sizes for some racial/ethnic groups, such as American Indian or Alaska Natives, also hinder the precision of their estimates of smoking prevalence. Moreover, ethnic categories used in national surveys (e.g., Asian) may not capture the heterogeneity present among various groups within that category. This is illustrated by data from California, which collects more detailed information on behavioral risk factors among its large Asian populations; for example, whereas the prevalence of smoking among Japanese American females (15.6%) is similar to that for non-Hispanic Whites (15.9%), the rate for Chinese American females is substantially lower (2.2%) ("Vital Signs," 2010). Underreporting of unhealthful behaviors such as smoking may also occur for some ethnic groups, depending on the sampling methodology used. Specifically, there is evidence that the prevalence of tobacco smoking is substantially higher among African Americans when random household sampling using same-race interviewers and neighborhood factors are considered; rates of smoking as high as 59% among Black men in high-poverty/high-segregated neighborhoods have been observed using these methods (Landrine, 2010).

TOBACCO SMOKING

Tobacco Smoking and Cancer Risk

Tobacco use is a major cause of disease and premature death in the United States and many other countries (Centers for Disease Control and Prevention, 2008). Each year, more than 150,000 smokers in the United States die from smoking-attributable cancer, with about 80% of these deaths from lung cancer. Smoking also accounts for $193 billion in health care expenditures and productivity losses (Centers for Disease Control and Prevention, 2008).

Tobacco smoking is causally related to at least 16 types of cancers (International Agency for Research on Cancer, 2004), including cancers of the lung, colon and rectum, oral cavity, nasal cavities and nasal sinuses, pharynx, larynx, esophagus (squamous cell carcinoma and adenocarcinoma), stomach, pancreas, liver, urinary bladder, kidney (adenocarcinoma and transitional cell carcinoma), and the uterine cervix, and myeloid leukemia. Among these, the strongest association is with lung cancer (U.S. Department of Health and Human Services, 2004). Environmental tobacco smoke is responsible for an additional 3,000 lung cancer deaths among nonsmokers (Centers for Disease Control and Prevention, 2002). The health risks of tobacco use are not limited to cigarette smoking. Cigar, pipe, and smokeless tobacco use also increase the risk of cancer (U.S. Department of Health and Human Services, 2004). In addition to cancer, smoking is linked with the risk of other chronic conditions such as cardiovascular disease (Eyre et al., 2004).

Disparities in Prevalence of Tobacco Smoking

Over the past four decades, public health efforts have led to enormous reductions in tobacco use in the United States (Centers for Disease Control and Prevention, 2008). Still, 1 in 5 adults in the United States continues to smoke, with some subgroups smoking at even greater levels. An estimated 20.9% of U.S. adults currently smoke, but rates are higher among men (23.2%) than among women (18.1%). Although the prevalence of adult cigarette smoking varies by gender, as well as race or ethnic group, it is important to note age-group differences within these categories (see Table 3.1). For example, in considering race/ethnicity alone, smoking prevalence is similar for White and African American males (25% and 23.5%, respectively). Among White males, however, 31- to 44-year-olds smoke at higher rates (31.6%) compared to males 45 years or older (20.0%). In contrast, for African American males, the rates are more similar for the two age groups (21.7% and 25.5%) (see Table 3.1).

The prevalence of smoking also varies by level of educational attainment, with the highest prevalence of cigarette smoking among individuals who have only attended or completed high school. Also, men and women whose income is less than twice the poverty level are much more likely to be current smokers compared to those with higher incomes (see Table 3.1). Regional differences in tobacco use have also been noted, with smoking prevalence generally higher in the Southern states, including traditionally tobacco-growing states, and the Midwest (Jemal et al., 2008). These geographic differences have been correlated with less stringent tobacco control laws and policies (Jemal, Cokkinides, Shafey, & Thun, 2003).

TABLE 3.1 The Proportion of Persons Who Were Current Smokers by Race/Ethnicity, Age, Education Level, and Income Level, Adults 18 and Older, United States

Characteristic	% Current Smokers[a]	
	Males	Females
Race/ethnicity by age		
White	25.0	20.8
18–34	31.6	23.8
35–44	27.8	25.1
45 years or older	20.0	16.7
African American	23.5	18.7
18–34	21.7	17.5
35–44	25.8	20.2
45 years or older	25.5	19.7
Hispanic	17.7	9.5
18–34	20.6	8.9
35–44	20.5	12.6
45 years or older	15.9	9.1
Asian American	16.5	7.3
18–34	21.0	7.6
35–44	15.8	3.4
45 years or older	15.0	9.4
American Indian and Alaska Native[b]	31.0	17.7
18–34	35.5	20.0
35–44	21.5	7.9
45 years or older	33.6	19.7
Income[c]		
Below poverty level	34.2	29.4
At 100% to 200% above poverty level	29.2	22.9
>200% of poverty level	20.5	15.1
Education (years)[d]		
8 or fewer	24.2	12.0
9–11	37.0	31.9
12 or GED	31.4	26.1
13–15	23.0	20.0
16	12.0	9.3
More than 16	4.8	6.6

Percentages are age adjusted to the 2000 U.S. standard population.
[a]Smoking is defined as persons who reported having smoked at least 100 cigarettes or more and who reported now smoking every day or some days.
[b]American Indian/Alaska Native only, the estimated smoking prevalence should be interpreted with caution because of the small sample sizes.
[c]Family income estimates are based on reported family income and poverty thresholds published by the U.S. Census Bureau.
[d]Prevalence by education level is for those ≥25 years.
Source: Smoking and physical inactivity data are from the National Health Interview Survey, 2009, National Center for Chronic Disease Prevention and Health Promotion, Centers for Disease Control and Prevention.

Reducing Initiation and Prevalence of Tobacco Smoking

Tobacco control policies and laws, along with educational and clinical strategies—all with a solid evidence base—can prevent the initiation of smoking or help smokers quit. As is the case for cardiovascular disease, many of the risks associated with tobacco use decrease after cessation. Interventions that encourage quit attempts or assist smokers in quitting thus represent the surest short-term strategies to reduce lung cancer mortality at the population level (Curry et al., 2003; Doll, Peto, Boreham, & Sutherland, 2004; U.S. Department of Health and Human Services, 2000). To sustainably reduce the level of tobacco consumption and diseases in the long term, however, population-level strategies to prevent the initiation of smoking among youth are needed. This is most effectively achieved by strong advocacy that leads to legislative changes. Policies with demonstrated effects in reducing the initiation into smoking include limiting youth access and marketing of tobacco products, legislating smoke-free environments, increasing tobacco taxes, and conducting antismoking campaigns (Bala, Strzeszynski, & Cahill, 2008). In addition, because of the tobacco industry's predatory practices in encouraging youth initiation, monitoring of their new products and promotions, and the heft of the law to curtail them, are needed. The new Family Smoking Prevention and Tobacco Control Act enacted in 2009 is a step in this direction.

Advocacy for and the implementation of legislation at the population level is also crucial to help reduce tobacco consumption by helping smokers quit. Health care reform that includes reimbursement for cessation treatments, or increasing taxes on cigarettes, strongly motivates many smokers to quit. For example, in anticipation of cigarette tax increases, thousands of smokers in the state of Michigan inundated the state-sponsored telephone counseling quit line, which led to its closure for several weeks in 2009 ("Quit-Smoking Hotline," March, 2009). This example also illustrates that once smokers are motivated to quit, individual-level interventions, which are characterized by higher levels of personal interaction between the targets of the interventions and their providers, are needed to provide smokers with the tools to help them do so successfully. Individual-level interventions are based on psychosocial or biomedical explanations for behavior, and include cognitive–behavioral strategies implemented in a variety of settings, as well as pharmacologic treatment. These methods can effectively double or triple smokers' ability to quit, and thus play an important role in reducing the prevalence of smoking.

Reducing Disparities in Initiation and Prevalence of Tobacco Smoking

Although we know what interventions effectively prevent or reduce smoking prevalence, more research is needed to investigate the extent to which they reduce or eliminate *disparities* in tobacco consumption and cessation.

Reducing the burden of tobacco for all individuals, regardless of minority status, is an overarching goal (Zhu, Hebert, Wong, Cummins, & Gamst, 2010) and so investigators have typically not geared population-level interventions to reduce disparities in tobacco use or cessation. Nevertheless, researchers have begun reporting the results of more in-depth analyses that determine whether the effects of broad-based, population-level interventions have similar or pronounced effects among certain sociodemographic or economically vulnerable groups. Evidence that population-level strategies not targeted to specific populations can nevertheless disproportionately impact them is illustrated by the finding that the substantial gap in lung cancer death rates between Black and White young adults (20–39 years) in the early 1990s was virtually eliminated by the mid-2000s, a result attributed to cigarette price increases and other intervention strategies that strongly impacted Black young adults (Jemal, Center, & Ward, 2009).

The lethal effect of disparities in tobacco use (e.g., higher lung cancer rates in older African American smokers) has also encouraged investigators to examine whether *individual-level* interventions that acknowledge or incorporate the differing experiences, attitudes, and knowledge of a particular group will be more powerful—and thus more successful—in achieving behavior change compared to interventions that do not. An example of such cultural adaptation would be a counseling program to help African American smokers quit that includes strategies to help them better cope with stressors resulting from racial discrimination, a possible trigger of urges to smoke and relapse.

In the sections that follow, we first review *population-level* interventions that, while not necessarily targeted toward vulnerable populations, nonetheless have been evaluated for their ability to reduce disparities in tobacco use. We then review the evidence for the effectiveness of *individual-level* smoking cessation interventions among populations experiencing disparities in tobacco use and cessation. We briefly describe how these treatments have been modified or expanded in attempts to increase the likelihood of cessation among these populations, and we discuss their impact, if any, in changing disparities in tobacco use or cessation.

Effects of Population-Level Interventions in Reducing Disparities

Some interventions with the largest impact have been at the population level, which recognizes that behavior change is a result of social and environmental influences. As noted earlier, the reduction in tobacco prevalence from its high of 64% to its current 20% of the population can be attributed to a number of population-level strategies that effectively reduce the likelihood of smoking initiation. For example, higher tobacco taxes make the cost of cigarettes prohibitive for youth and have been shown to be associated with lower uptake of smoking in this population (Levy, Cummings, & Hyland, 2000a, 2000b). Tobacco taxes thus represent an effective primary prevention tool to reduce smoking consumption in the long term. Young Black adults may be particularly sensitive to these increases, which could explain the recent convergence in lung cancer rates between Black and White young adults (Jemal et al., 2009). In general, however, data is lacking on whether higher tobacco taxes prevent initiation to a greater or lesser degree among youth belonging to other groups that have traditionally experienced disparities.

Higher cigarette prices also lead to reductions in prevalence by encouraging existing smokers to quit (Farrelly, 2001; Farrelly, Pechacek, Thomas, & Nelson, 2008). Studies have now also documented that cigarette price increases have larger impacts on socioeconomically vulnerable populations, such as those from lower-income brackets and minority populations (Farrelly, 2001; Siahpush, Wakefield, Spittal, Durkin, & Scollo, 2009). These effects are reliable and have been reported in samples from Canada, the United Kingdom (U.K.), the United States, and other countries. A particularly well-designed study in Australia using monthly (rather than yearly) data on smoking prevalence and cigarette prices (because such data allow for greater sensitivity in detecting causal associations) found that lower-income groups were most responsive to increases in price, as evidenced by their greatest reduction in prevalence. The effect of tobacco taxes in reducing disparities can be striking. For example, Farrelly et al. found that compared to Whites, responsivity to price increases was two times greater for African Americans, and six times greater for Hispanics (Farrelly, 2001).

Antitobacco-advertising campaigns also play a role in preventing initiation into smoking (Emery et al., 2005; Farrelly, Davis, Haviland, Healton, & Messeri, 2005; Siegel & Biener, 2000), although the extent to which they limit initiation among members of special populations has not been investigated. There is evidence, however, that antitobacco campaigns have the potential to reduce disparities in the likelihood of cessation, but that the content of antitobacco-advertising messages appears to be a crucial factor. In a longitudinal study that examined the effects of 134 different antitobacco television advertisements broadcast in Massachusetts over a 2-year period, advertisements that were "highly emotional," where the narrator described the negative health effects of smoking on oneself or family members, or that included personal testimonials, had the strongest effects on quitting among low- and middle-SES (socioeconomic status) groups. In contrast, for high-income individuals (at least some college and >$50,000 per year), there were no differences between the type of advertisements and the likelihood of quitting (Durkin, Biener, & Wakefield, 2009). Differential effects of the advertisements as a function of ethnicity or race were not reported, however.

Considering that African American communities are disproportionately targeted by tobacco industry advertising (Primack, Bost, Land, & Fine, 2007), it will be imperative that counter-advertising has similar or stronger effects on African American smokers if disparities in tobacco use and its effects are to be eliminated for this group.

Effects of Community-Level Interventions in Reducing Disparities

Community-level interventions aimed at preventing smoking initiation among children and adolescents are typically school based. Multicomponent programs that include education combined with learning to resist social influences to smoke, deconstructing media influences promoting tobacco use, skills training, and helping to construct and deliver the intervention have shown positive short-term effects (i.e., between 1 and 3 years) (Dobbins, DeCorby, Manske, & Goldblatt, 2008). Effects are even greater when 15 or more sessions up to the ninth grade are delivered (Flay, 2009), and when combined with media and policy interventions such as smoking bans and increased taxation (Dobbins et al., 2008). Data is lacking, however, on whether the efficacy of school-based prevention programs differ as a function of gender, racial/ethnic group, or other sociodemographic variables (Dobbins et al., 2008).

For individuals who already smoke, one of the most popular community-level interventions is the Quit and Win contests held in many communities in North America, and now internationally in about 80 countries. The contests originated from the Minnesota Heart Health Program, are publicized through mass media outlets, and attempt to engage smokers from entire communities by offering incentives and prizes to those who successfully quit (Cahill & Perera, 2008). In one randomized controlled trial of a Quit and Win contest, women and lower-income smokers, who typically have lower quit rates compared with men and higher-income smokers, were equally likely to successfully stop smoking (Hahn et al., 2005). The homogeneity of participants in many Quit and Win contests, however (i.e., predominantly White, younger, greater educational attainment) (Cahill & Perera, 2008), makes it difficult to determine whether special populations are, in general, equally likely to benefit from them. Other methodological concerns have plagued evaluations of the effects of community interventions other than Quit and Win in reducing smoking prevalence. For example, in a review of community interventions in general, Secker-Walker and colleagues pointed out that many studies were underpowered, did not use randomization to interventions, or used the individual as the unit of analysis when the community was the unit of assignment (Secker-Walker, Gnich, Platt, & Lancaster, 2002). In the most methodologically rigorous study of the set of studies that they examined (the COMMIT study), however, men appeared to benefit somewhat more than women, and lighter smokers more than heavier smokers (Fisher, 1995).

Individual-Level Interventions in Reducing Disparities in Tobacco Smoking

Current Smoking Cessation Treatments

As noted earlier, whereas population-level interventions are instrumental in *preventing* the uptake of smoking or in *motivating* smokers to consider quitting, individual-level interventions for cessation provide smokers with the tools to successfully quit. By definition, individual-level interventions are characterized by increased contact between the provider and recipient, and currently there are several treatments that a smoker can use to help him or her quit. The extent to which these are also effective for members of groups that have experienced disparities is now receiving greater research attention. Moreover, standard behavioral treatments are now more commonly subjected to cultural tailoring, with the aim of enhancing cessation rates and ultimately reducing prevalence in, and disparities resulting from, tobacco use. Groups that have been the target of cultural tailoring of smoking cessation treatments include African Americans, members of the gay/lesbian/bisexual community, and psychiatric populations.

Interventions to reduce disparities in prevalence by facilitating cessation are based on principles outlined in the updated (2008) *Clinical Practice Guideline: Treating Tobacco Use and Dependence* by the U.S. Department of Health and Human Services (Fiore et al., 2008). The guideline states that "Tobacco dependence is a chronic disease that often requires repeated intervention and multiple attempts to quit" and that "Effective treatments exist that can significantly increase rates of long-term abstinence." In addition to recommending first-line medications such as NRT (nicotine replacement therapy), bupropion (Zyban), and varenicline (Chantix), the guideline panel concluded that, based on results of their meta-analyses, "Individual, group, and telephone counseling are effective, and their effectiveness increases with treatment intensity." As described in the guideline, counseling consists of helping smokers "recognize danger situations" (that increase the risk of relapse), "develop coping skills" (to learn how to handle danger situations), and to "provide basic information about smoking and successful quitting." The guideline panel also recommended that smokers receive intra-treatment support from their provider that entails encouraging a quit attempt, communicating caring and concern, and facilitating dialogue with the smoker about the quitting process. These basic principles of tobacco treatment represent the protocol used in behavioral treatments found to be most effective in helping smokers quit. In addition to forming the basis of individual counseling by health professionals, they are incorporated into group programs for cessation and in telephone counseling protocols.

Recently, the format of delivery of tobacco cessation treatment has been expanded to include the Internet as well as mobile phones. Using automated algorithms, Internet programs for smoking cessation attempt to replicate the activities, information, and social support that smokers typically receive from in-person behavioral treatments. They also overcome some of the practical issues that smokers might have with using telephone counseling or attending group meetings (e.g., cost, or distance from treatment location). Reviews and meta-analyses of Internet-based treatments for tobacco use or other health behaviors have concluded that these programs are effective compared to minimal or no treatments (Portnoy, Scott-Sheldon, Johnson, & Carey, 2008; Webb, Joseph, Yardley, & Michie, 2010). There is, however, room for improvement; for example, by capitalizing on the interactive capabilities of the Internet and providing adequate follow-up contact or treatment (Bock et al., 2004).

In addition to the above treatments, the *Clinical Practice Guideline* also found that less intense interventions, such as being asked about one's smoking status, or being advised to quit by a doctor, are associated with higher odds of quitting compared to controls. Individuals from ethnic-minority groups are less likely to be the recipients of these interventions (Cokkinides, Halpern, Barbeau, Ward, & Thun, 2008); however, a difference that studies have shown is related to socioeconomic factors such as lack of access to health insurance or to health systems (Koh et al., 2010). The remainder of this section will focus on the effectiveness of multisession behavioral treatments, which offer smokers the greatest chance of quitting, in reducing disparities in smoking prevalence.

Adapting Current Tobacco Treatments to Reduce Disparities in Special Populations

One reason for the relative paucity of research on the effectiveness of standard cessation treatments for special populations has been their underrepresentation in these studies, a case that is particularly true for African American smokers (Webb, 2008). Reduced participation unfortunately precludes analyses of a treatment's effect as a function of minority or racial/ ethnic categories. Research is also needed on whether cultural tailoring of standard treatments to special populations increases the reach of treatments in these populations, or produces higher quit rates. Fortunately, research on cultural tailoring of cessation treatments is increasing, as evidenced by the number of presentations at the first pre-conference workshop on reducing disparities in smoking cessation at the 2010 annual meeting of the Society for Nicotine and Tobacco Research (Fagan, 2010).

Cultural adaptation, according to Borrelli, "involves any modification of an EBT's [evidence-based treatment's] design, treatment components, approach to delivery, or nature of the therapeutic relationship, in order to accommodate the cultural beliefs, values, attitudes, and behaviors of the target population" (Borrelli, 2010). In the process of adapting an intervention to a particular group, researchers attend to its members' common historical, environmental, and social influences. Borrelli proposed four phases of cultural adaptation. Phase 1 consists of information gathering from the community, focus groups, and archival historical data to best determine how the intervention can be made culturally specific. Phase 2 consists of modifying the intervention both at the surface level (i.e., so that intervention materials and messages are pertinent to "the observable social and behavioral characteristics of the group e.g., people, places, language, music, foods, brand names, locations, and clothing") (Resnicow, Braithwaite, Ahluwalia, & Butler, 2000), and at a deeper level (by incorporating the shared cultural values of the group) (Resnicow et al., 2000). Phases 3 and 4 consist of pilot-testing the culturally adapted intervention and measuring outcomes, respectively. An example of applying these principles in a group program for urban African American smokers would be to use images of African Americans in written materials, quotes from smokers who have quit using a vernacular that may be more common to members of this group, and addressing the types of stressors faced by the African American community as a factor in smoking (e.g., racial discrimination).

African American and Other Racial/Minority Smokers

To examine whether standard current cessation treatments are effective among African American smokers, and whether cultural tailoring can increase cessation rates, Webb conducted a meta-analysis of interventions in which approximately 50% of the participants were African Americans. Treatments that were ethno-culturally tailored were also included. Results of her analyses indicated that standard treatments were indeed effective for this population in increasing long-term quitting. Culturally tailored interventions, however, were superior only in facilitating short-term quitting. In addition, Church-based treatments were significantly better than others in producing short-term quitting, a finding that confirmed the importance of the Church as a socially supportive and socially cohesive institution that can facilitate positive health behavior change among African Americans (Pederson, Ahluwalia, Harris, & McGrady, 2000). The meta-analysis also found that group counseling programs were of particular benefit. Taken together, these findings indicate that social support during the quitting process may need to be an important component of tobacco treatment for African American smokers, and that cultural tailoring may demonstrate its greatest benefit in the early stages of the quitting process. Specifically, at least for African American smokers, cultural tailoring may increase the appeal of the program and its ability to recruit and retain smokers.

Several studies have documented higher rates of tobacco use among American Indian/Alaska Native populations, but lacking are interventions that are targeted or culturally tailored to members of this ethnic group. Although initial attempts to treat tobacco dependence in this population showed moderate success (Johnson, Lando, Schmid, & Solberg, 1997), subsequent tobacco control efforts recognized the ultimate importance of understanding cultural factors that could impact the success of treatments. These include ascribing an important role for elders (Varcoe, Bottorff, Carey, Sullivan, & Williams, 2010) and gaining a thorough understanding of other traditions, taboos, and religious beliefs and practices that could impact the success of tobacco treatment (Oberly & Macedo, 2004).

Low-SES Smokers

At the current time, we could find no published studies that examined whether standard cognitive–behavioral counseling used in in-person, group, or quit-line counseling programs are equally effective for low-income individuals, or those with lower levels of educational attainment, as compared with higher-income groups. Moreover, descriptions of cessation treatments adapted for this group are lacking. Nevertheless, attention to barriers that low-SES individuals face would likely result in greater use of treatments, improved motivation to quit, and possibly an equivalent or greater rate of quitting as compared with higher-SES individuals. Increasing health insurance coverage, particularly for cessation treatments, would remove several important barriers. Overall, offering free cessation counseling, in addition to NRT or other cessation medications, dispelling myths about the effects of NRT (Shiffman, Ferguson, Rohay, & Gitchell, 2008), making treatments more convenient, such as providing them at the workplace, and addressing coping with peer smoking, are likely to result in great uptake of treatments and cessation among low-SES smokers. Other forms of tobacco use (e.g., chewing tobacco) are also more prevalent among some groups of low-SES individuals and would thus need to be addressed in treatments.

Gay and Lesbian Smokers

Although, to date, national surveys have not asked respondents about their sexual orientation, extant studies have found a greater prevalence of smoking among gay men, and lesbian and bisexual women, compared with the general population. For example, in the California Health Interview Survey, a population-based sample of men and women, the prevalence of smoking among gay men was 33.2%, a rate that was 55.9% higher than that for heterosexual men (Tang et al., 2004). These results were consistent with those of another large-scale probability study of lesbian, gay, and bisexual (LGB) individuals (Gruskin, Greenwood, Matevia, Pollack, & Bye, 2007) in which the prevalence of daily smoking among gay men was 27.3%, as compared to 19.7% for heterosexual men. Similar findings have been obtained in samples from other large urban centers (Greenwood et al., 2005). These surveys also found elevated rates of smoking among lesbians and bisexual women, but the discussion below focuses on gay men due to the lack of reports of cessation interventions for, or attended by, lesbian and bisexual women.

The literature is sparse on reports investigating the success of standard smoking cessation interventions for gay men, or whether interventions tailored to this population can achieve comparable or higher quit rates. Only recently have steps been taken to understand disparities in smoking between gay and heterosexual men, and to incorporate these into culturally tailored interventions. Cultural tailoring of cessation interventions for gay men involves acknowledging the unique stressors that gay men face related to their sexual orientation that may explain their higher smoking rates, and their possibly greater difficulty quitting. These include internalized homophobia, expectations of stigma, and experiences with prejudice and rejection over their sexual orientation (Meyer, 2003). For example, in one study of LGB (lesbian, gay, and bisexual) youth, the experience of rejection after disclosing sexual orientation predicted subsequent smoking levels (Rosario, Schrimshaw, & Hunter, 2009). Recent data also suggests that young gay men may smoke when attempting to conceal their sexual orientation (Pachankis, Westmaas, & Dougherty, 2010). Other factors implicated in gay men's higher smoking rates include the strong presence of tobacco promotional campaigns in gay venues (Dilley, Spigner, Boysun, Dent, & Pizacani, 2008; Smith, Offen, & Malone, 2005) and the centrality of places in the LGB community where smoking is more tolerated, such as bars (Trocki, Drabble, & Midanik, 2009).

Although there are many ways in which a standard intervention can be adapted to the experiences, values, and beliefs of a particular population, research on efforts to culturally tailor cessation interventions to gay men is sparse. Interventions that have done so have found promising results, however. In one study conducted in the U.K., a group cessation program that was facilitated by gay men for gay men, and that included "group discussion and processes" and "culturally specific contexts" for gay men, found quit rates comparable to those of the national population (Harding, Bensley, & Corrigan, 2004). Also tested have been Internet-based interventions tailored for gay men (e.g., www.iquit.medschool.ucsf.edu).

Although gay men appear to prefer interventions specifically tailored for them (Schwappach, 2008, 2009), comparisons between standard and tailored treatments will be needed to determine whether tailored treatments are indeed the best strategy for reducing disparities in this population. Treatments tailored or targeted to lesbian and bisexual women should also be a priority in efforts to reduce disparities in the prevalence of smoking among LGB individuals.

Psychiatric Populations

Population-based studies of smoking prevalence have typically not included assessments of mental illness diagnoses. The rate of smoking among individuals with a history of mental illness (lifetime or past-month), however, is almost double that compared with those who report no history of mental illness (Lasser et al., 2000). Moreover, individuals with mental illness are estimated to consume about 44.3% of cigarettes sold in the United States (Lasser et al., 2000). Reasons for psychiatric populations' greater prevalence are varied, and include the perception that smoking alleviates psychiatric symptoms or side effects of medications, genetic susceptibility, the reluctance of addictions counselors to treat tobacco dependence for fear of diminishing the success of treatment for co-occurring disorders, use of cigarettes in token economies in psychiatric settings, and special promotional efforts by the tobacco industry (Hall & Prochaska, 2009; Winterer, 2010). There has also been an implicit assumption by health care providers that depression-prone smokers will not be successful in quitting. According to a recent meta-analysis, however, a lifetime history of major depressive disorder does *not* decrease the likelihood of cessation using standard behavioral treatments for cessation (Hitsman, Borrelli, McChargue, Spring, & Niaura, 2003). Still, this may not be the case for individuals with recurring depression, or those who report depressive symptoms at the beginning of treatment (Brown et al., 2001; Glassman et al., 1993; Seidman et al., 2010). In any event, smoking cessation interventions have been adapted to address these smokers' depressed mood, or diminished positive affect. These activities include identifying life goals and values, monitoring and incorporating enjoyable activities consistent with these goals and values into daily activities, strategies to increase positive thoughts and decrease negative ones, and social skills and assertiveness training. Interventions with such tailoring improve cessation rates compared to those that do not (Brown et al., 2001; MacPherson et al., 2010).

Schizophrenic patients also smoke at substantially higher rates compared with controls (Leonard & Adams, 2006). While bupropion seems to be clearly superior to placebo in helping schizophrenic patients achieve abstinence (Tsoi, Porwal, & Webster, 2010a), very few studies have reported on the effectiveness of standard *behavioral* treatments in this population, as is also the case for treatments specifically tailored to this group (Tsoi, Porwal, & Webster, 2010b). Of the studies that have done so, adaptations have included the use of contingency reinforcement with money, deeper emphasis on motivating smokers, or more intense social skills training. These have not shown to be superior to standard treatments in producing short- and long-term quitting rates, however (Tsoi et al., 2010b). Still, the small number of studies in this area, and their inherent methodological problems, preclude conclusions about whether adapting current cessation treatments for schizophrenic patients can reduce disparities in tobacco prevalence (Tsoi et al., 2010b). Data is also lacking on cessation interventions for smokers who have co-occurring substance use disorders, such as alcohol or other drug dependence (Hall & Prochaska, 2009).

The Future of Disparities in Tobacco Use

Recent attention to the problem of disparities in tobacco consumption, and in its effects, has led to a greater focus on whether interventions reduce to-bacco prevalence to the same degree among members of special populations, particularly ethnic-minority groups, as compared to the general population. Results for population- and community-level interventions thus far have been encouraging. Moreover, cultural tailoring of individual-level interventions, though in its nascent stages, shows promise in attracting smokers to treatments, and in helping them quit, at least in the short term. Research on the development and testing of culturally tailored interventions, and on understanding the causes of disparities, remains a priority for the American Cancer Society (ACS) and for other funding agencies, as this knowledge will lead to better strategies to reduce disparities. For example, research funded by the ACS has examined how the tobacco industry has targeted young African American adults of low socioeconomic status. This research is important in helping develop effective counter-strategies to discourage tobacco use in this and other vulnerable populations, such as LGB smokers and psychiatric patients. Prevention programs to reduce initiation of tobacco use in special populations, and in the general public, should also be a strong component of public health initiatives. Public health policies that also include improving access to care for tobacco-related diseases, as well as psychosocial and medical treatments for tobacco dependence, will effect the greatest reduction in tobacco prevalence and hopefully the elimination of disparities.

OBESITY, PHYSICAL ACTIVITY, AND NUTRITION

Obesity, physical inactivity, and poor nutrition are major risk factors for cancer, second only to tobacco use (World Cancer Research Fund/American Institute for Cancer Research, 2007). In the United States and in many developed nations, the prevalence of overweight (defined as a body mass index [BMI] greater or equal to 25 kg/m² and less than 30 kg/m²) and obesity (BMI greater or equal to 30 kg/m²) has increased dramatically in recent decades, and much of the increase has been attributed to changes in diet and physical activity in Westernized societies (Hedley et al., 2004; Kumanyika et al., 2008; Ogden, Carroll, McDowell, & Flegal, 2007). In the United States, overweight and obesity contribute to 14–20% of all cancer-related mortality (Calle, Rodriguez, Walker-Thurmond, & Thun, 2003). Overweight and obesity are clearly associated with increased risk for developing cancers of the breast (in postmenopausal women), colon, endometrium, kidney, gallbladder, liver, and adenocarcinoma of the esophagous (World Cancer Research Fund/American Institute for Cancer Research, 2007); (Calle et al., 2003). In addition, excess body weight is an independent risk factor for cardiovascular disease and type 2 diabetes (Eyre et al., 2004).

Excessive weight gain is a direct function of an imbalance between the amount of calories consumed and the amount of calories expended by an individual; therefore, physical inactivity and poor nutrition play important roles in maintaining a healthy weight (Kushi et al., 2006; World Cancer Research Fund/American Institute for Cancer Research, 2007). The increasing trends in unhealthy eating and physical inactivity and resultant increases in overweight and obesity have largely been influenced by the environments in which people live, learn, work, and play (Kumanyika et al., 2008). For example, unhealthy eating trends have been driven by the greater availability and marketing of pre-packaged processed foods, low-cost/big-portion restaurant meals, and soft drinks, all of which may be high in sugar, calories, and/or fat; this is compounded by fewer opportunities to be regularly active as a result of our modes of transportation, sedentary jobs, and forms of entertainment during leisure time. Hence, to more effectively control overweight and obesity, experts recommend a public health approach that promotes environmental changes for healthy eating and increased physical activity, in addition to targeted behavioral and medical interventions (Eyre et al., 2004; Kumanyika et al., 2008; Kushi et al., 2006).

Physical activity has numerous mental and physical health benefits, including reductions in the risk of premature mortality, cardiovascular disease, hypertension, diabetes, and osteoporosis (Haskell et al., 2007; International Agency for Research on Cancer, 2002). Physical inactivity is an important risk factor for many chronic diseases and plays an important role in certain cancers (breast and colorectal cancer) (International Agency for Research on Cancer, 2002). Epidemiologic evidence shows that the risk of breast and colon cancers is reduced by physical activity (International Agency for Research on Cancer, 2002), and an active rather than sedentary lifestyle might also reduce the risk of other types of cancer, such as prostate, lung, and endometrial cancers, as well as the risk of dying from cancer (Calle et al., 2003). Physical activity contributes to the reduction in cancer risk through a range of pathways; supporting evidence continues to accumulate that physical activity reduces chronic disease risk both directly through its impact on hormones and indirectly through its impact on weight control (International Agency for Research on Cancer, 2002; Kushi et al., 2006). Although much remains to be learned about the role of specific nutrients—or the combination of nutrients—in decreasing the risk of chronic disease, however, dietary patterns are emerging as an important consideration. A balanced eating pattern emphasizing whole-grain foods, legumes, vegetables, and fruits, and limiting the intake of saturated fats, trans fats, cholesterol, and added sugars and salt, is associated with decreased risk of a variety of chronic diseases (Kushi et al., 2006). Population studies have shown that people who have a high intake of vegetables and fruits and a lower intake of animal fat, meat, or calories have a reduced risk of some of the most common types of cancer (International Agency for Research on Cancer, 2002; Kushi et al., 2006). Diets high in fruits and vegetables may have a protective effect against many cancers (International Agency for Research on Cancer, 2002). Conversely, excess consumption of red and processed meat may be associated with an increased risk of colorectal cancer (International Agency for Research on Cancer, 2002).

Based upon a comprehensive review of the evidence, the ACS has published guidelines on nutrition and physical activity for cancer prevention (Kushi et al., 2006). To all individuals seeking to reduce their cancer risk, it recommends the following individual choices: maintaining a healthy weight throughout life, adopting a physically active lifestyle, following a healthy diet, and limiting consumption of alcoholic beverages.

Racial/Ethnic and Socioeconomic Disparities in Obesity and Related Risk Factors

During the past decade, based on the National Health and Nutrition Examination Survey, which has collected objectively measured height and weight information from participants, the obesity (BMI ≥ 30 kg/m^2) trends in women have increased nonsignificantly, from 33.4% in 1999–2000 to 36.1% in 2007–2008; among men, the prevalence rose from 27.5% to 32.6% in this period. Compared to White men and women, African American and Hispanic men and women have higher rates of obesity (over 34%) (see Table 3.2). The prevalence of obesity varies slightly with the level of education in men, and strongly with the level of education in women. Prevalence ranges from 23.4% in women with more than 16 years of education to 44.0% in women with 8 or fewer years of education. Variations in obesity prevalence by income are also greater among women than for men (see Table 3.2).

TABLE 3.2   Prevalence of Obesity and Related Risk Factors by Race/Ethnicity, Education Level, and Income Level, Adults 18 and Older, United States

Characteristic	% No Leisure-Time Physical Activity[a]		% Obese[b]		% Five or More Fruit or Vegetable Servings a Day	
	Males	Females	Males	Females	Males	Females
Race/ethnicity						
Hispanic	40.5	47.6	34.8	43.3	17.2	24.1
White	27.4	29.5	32.6	33.6	18.2	26.7
African American	34.7	44.8	37.6	49.9	18.3	23.6
Asian American	32.1	39.9	—	—	23.9	30.6
American Indian and Alaska Native[c]	36.3	36.4	—	—	16.4	27.8
Income						
Below poverty level	46.2	52.8	28.9	42.1	16.0	22.6
100–200% above poverty level	42.4	45.5	35.1	40.0	17.5	25.1
> 200% of poverty level	24.9	27.6	33.0	32.8	20.7	30.3
Education (years)[d]						
8 or fewer	57.0	61.6	31.7	44.0	15.0	22.3
9–11	47.7	53.7	32.2	46.3	14.0	19.3
12 or GED	39.4	45.2	33.4	40.3	14.3	21.0
13–15	27.9	31.1	37.8	38.1	17.4	26.3
16*[1]	20.2	21.5	26.7	23.4	22.7	34.5
More than 16	15.1	17.1	—	—	—	—
Total	**30.4**	**34.6**	**32.6**	**36.1**	**18.4**	**26.2**

Percentages are age adjusted to the 2000 U.S. standard population.
[a]No leisure time physical activity is defined as not engaging in any regular leisure time physical activities.
[b]Obese is defined as Body Mass Index (BMI) $\geq$30 kg.m².
[c]The estimate should be interpreted with caution because of the small sample sizes.
[d]Prevalence by education level is for those $\geq$25 years.
*[1]Percent obese in the "16 years" educational category includes also those with more than 16 years of education.
— Data not available due to insufficient sample size.
Source: Physical inactivity data are from the National Health Interview Survey, 2009, National Center for Chronic Disease Prevention and Health Promotion, Centers for Disease Control and Prevention. Obesity data are from National Health and Nutrition Examination Survey, 2007–08, National Center for Health Statistics, Centers for Disease Control and Prevention. Data on consumption of daily servings of fruit and vegetables are from the Behavioral Risk Factor Surveillance System, 2009, Centers for Disease Control and Prevention.

Compared to White men and women, all racial and ethnic groups show higher levels of inactivity during leisure time. Moreover, there are strong gradients in levels of inactivity during leisure time by income and education status; for example, over half (57%) of those with less education (eighth grade education) report no physical activity while 15% of those with higher education do so (see Table 3.2). However, it should be noted that this survey only collects information on physical activity at leisure and may considerably underestimate total physical activity. Hence, for segments of the population that are employed in industries with physically demanding jobs, a more comprehensive assessment of total physical activity should consider physical activity at both work and leisure.

Currently, the proportion of the adult population that reports consuming five or more fruit or vegetable servings daily is low: 26.2% in women and 18.4% in men. Except in Asian men and women, all race and ethnic groups also show low prevalence levels of fruit and vegetable consumption. Further, there are variations in reported levels of consumption, which are lowest among those at less than twice the poverty rate, and in those who are less educated (see Table 3.2).

Contextual factors that have been described to affect poorer and minority communities include: fewer neighborhood resources, such as inadequate housing; fewer opportunities for safer recreational environments; lower access to fresh foods and healthy nutrition; greater exposure to environmental carcinogens; and selective marketing strategies of tobacco companies and fast-food chains (Kumanyika et al., 2008; Larson, Story, & Nelson, 2008; Ward et al., 2004). Additionally, cultural factors and health literacy, such as attitudes and beliefs about preventive behaviors (Ward et al., 2004), may play a role in health behaviors.

Policies and programs that support healthy behaviors throughout the life cycle are needed to counteract socioenvironmental factors that reduce individuals' opportunities to eat well and be physically active (Kumanyika et al., 2008; Kushi et al., 2006). Schools and child care facilities, workplaces, and health care facilities are important settings for the implementation of policies and programmatic initiatives. For instance, in the clinical setting, primary care providers play an important role in the clinical management of obesity and in assisting patients on weight management strategies. The appeal of setting-based approaches includes the ability to implement effective strategies to target populations (i.e., students, employees, or patients) and to also influence social norms within the setting, with possible transfer to outside settings through linkage with community-based prevention programs. In order to foster and support public policy and wellness initiatives in schools, workplaces, and communities, the nutrition and physical activity guidelines of the ACS call attention to community action strategies that can lead to improved access to nutritious food or provide safer environments for physical activity. For example, at the state and local level, community leaders can promote policy changes that may include regulation of the school food environments and zoning changes that bring grocery stores into poor neighborhoods (Kumanyika et al., 2008; Kushi et al., 2006).

RACIAL/ETHNIC AND SOCIOECONOMIC DISPARITIES
IN CANCER SCREENING

Reducing cancer risk through modifiable lifestyle factors (tobacco use, obesity, nutrition, and physical activity) does not eliminate the risk of disease entirely. Thus, early detection of some chronic conditions could alter the natural history of the disease through implementation of therapeutic interventions that treat either precursor lesions or early-stage disease. Early detection of cancer through established screening methods has been shown to reduce mortality from cancer of the colon and rectum (with the use of the fecal occult blood test and/or endoscopic visual examinations of the large intestine), and uterine cervix (with the Pap test) and breast cancer (with the mammogram) (Smith, Cokkinides, & Brawley, 2009). Screening refers to testing in individuals who are asymptomatic for a particular disease (i.e., they have no symptoms that may indicate the presence of disease) and age is their only (known) factor that puts them at average risk. In addition to detecting cancer early, screening for colorectal or cervical cancers can identify and result in the removal of precancerous abnormalities, preventing cancer altogether (Smith et al., 2009).

The ACS publishes updates to cancer screening guidelines for adults at high and at average risk, respectively, on an ongoing basis (Smith et al., 2009; Smith, Cokkinides, Brooks, Saslow, & Brawley, 2010). The ACS screening guidelines for average-risk individuals recommend that all adults age 50 years and older be screened periodically for colorectal cancer, and that women of designated ages be screened regularly for breast and cervical cancer. On the other hand, due to the complexities regarding early detection for prostate cancer screening, the ACS states that men who have at least a 10-year life expectancy should have an opportunity to make an informed decision with their health care provider about whether to be screened for prostate cancer, after receiving information about the benefits, risks, and uncertainties associated with prostate cancer screening. Prostate cancer screening should not occur without an informed decision-making process (Smith et al., 2009).

High rates of screening utilization throughout the population are important to accomplish the goal of reducing the rate of late-stage or advanced cancers, which affects cancer prognosis and survival. Published studies have described the many factors that account for the underutilization of cancer screening in the United States (Smith et al., 2009; Ward et al., 2004, 2008). Of these factors, the prominent ones associated with the receipt of (routine) cancer screening rates are having health insurance status and socioeconomic factors. Another key factor that also influences the use of cancer screening is receiving a recommendation to get screened from a medical health care professional (Smith et al., 2009).

Although 68% of non-Hispanic White women over 40 years of age reported having a mammogram in the past 2 years, only 52.2% reported a mammogram within the past year (see Table 3.3). Since the ACS breast cancer screening guidelines recommend yearly mammograms among average-risk 40-year-old women, there still remains a large portion of the age-eligible population that does not receive screening regularly, or at all. In addition, mammography usage appears lowest in American Indian/Alaska Native women; only 55.3% had a mammogram within 2 years and only 42.2% in the past year (see Table 3.3). Mammography within the past year was even lower among women who had immigrated to the United States in the past 10 years (39.6%) or who lacked health insurance coverage (26.0%). Rates were only slightly higher for mammography within the past 2 years (49.7% for recent immigrants and 35.6% for women with no health insurance) (see Table 3.3).

The percentage of women aged 18 years and older who reported having a Pap test in the past 3 years was 79.6% in non-Hispanic Whites and 81.5% in African Americans, but lower in Hispanics (75.0%), American Indians/Alaska Natives (65.2%), and Asians (63.8%), as well as recent immigrants (60.1%) and those with no health insurance (60.6%) (see Table 3.3).

Research supports the use of several screening tests for colorectal cancer, including the less invasive fecal occult blood test (FOBT), on a yearly basis and/or invasive endoscopy procedures (flexible sigmoidoscopy every 5 years or colonoscopy every 10 years) of the lower intestine (Smith et al., 2009). National survey data tracks colorectal cancer screening utilization by total test use (combined FOBT and/or endoscopy) and separately for the two specific tests. However, it should be noted that these surveys may underestimate utilization of colorectal cancer screening, as they do not assess other available testing modalities for colorectal cancer screening, such as double contrast barium enema and the virtual colonoscopy. Relative to other established breast and cervical screening, the utilization of any colorectal cancer screening among adults aged 50 and older is lower—50.2% of women and 54.9% of men reported being up to date with colorectal cancer screening testing in 2008 (see Table 3.3). The use of colorectal cancer screening (by FOBT in the past year) and/or endoscopy in the past 10 years) does not differ by gender, but varies widely by race/ethnicity: the lowest rates are seen among American Indians/Alaska Natives and among Hispanic/Latinos compared with non-Hispanic Whites. In addition, individuals with fewer years of education and no health insurance coverage, and recent (10 years or less) immigrants were the least likely to report having FOBT in the past year or endoscopy within 10 years (see Table 3.3).

It is clear from this data that significant disparities persist in screening among various population subgroups, including non-White, less educated, and lower-income individuals, and those with no access to health care and immigrant status. Though health insurance status is strongly related to use

TABLE 3.3 Prevalent Use of Cancer Screening by Selected Characteristics, Adults, National Health Interview Survey, 2008

Characteristic	Breast Cancer Screening: Mammography Prevalence (%) in Women ≥40 years		Cervical Cancer: Pap Test Prevalence (%) in Women ≥18 years	Colorectal Cancer Screening Prevalence (%) in Adults ≥50 years		
	Within past 2 years	Within past years	Within past 3 years	Fecal occult blood test[a]	Endoscopy[b]	Combined FOBT/ endoscopy[c]
Gender						
Male	—	—	—	10.3	52.2	54.9
Female	—	—	—	9.7	48.6	52.0
Race/ethnicity						
Hispanic/Latino	61.5	46.8	75.0	7.8	34.6	37.2
White	68.0	54.2	79.6	10.3	52.7	56.0
African American	67.7	52.2	81.5	8.9	47.3	48.9
Asian American	65.1	52.2	63.8	12.1	42.6	47.8
American Indian and Alaska Native[†]	55.3	42.2	65.2	4.5	31.7	33.1
Education (years)						
11 or fewer	53.9	40.1	69.1	8.1	34.0	37.3
12	64.3	49.2	73.9	8.1	48.1	50.8
13–15	69.1	55.2	82.4	12.9	52.2	56.3
16 or more	77.9	64.5	86.8	10.8	61.9	64.5
Health insurance coverage						
No	35.6	26.0	60.6	8.8	12.7	19.5
Yes	70.5	56.2	81.0	10.3	52.6	55.7
Immigration status						
Born in United States	67.6	53.5	79.7	10.1	51.9	55.0
In United States ≤10 years	49.7	39.6	60.1	8.0	22.5	28.0
In United States 10+ years	65.8	51.8	74.3	9.7	38.7	41.9
Total	**67.1**	**53.0**	**78.3**	**10.0**	**50.2**	**53.2**

Percentages are adjusted to the 2000 U.S. standard population.

[a]Fecal occult blood test: a home fecal occult blood test within the past year.

[b]Endoscopy: a sigmoidoscopy test within the past 5 years or a colonoscopy within the past 10 years.

[c]Combined FOBT/endoscopy: a fecal occult blood test within the past year, a sigmoidoscopy test within the past 5 years, or a colonoscopy within the past 10 years.

[†]Estimates should be interpreted with caution because of small sample size.

—Data not applicable.

Source: Data are from the National Health Interview Survey, 2008, National Center for Health Statistics, Centers for Disease Control and Prevention.

of preventive services, other contextual factors may also influence the use of medical services (i.e., the distribution and accessibility of health services and the medical workforce) (Ward et al., 2008). In addition, based on more in-depth investigations of psychosocial factors, there are other potential factors to consider, such as differences in knowledge about cancer prevention, culture, or other barriers to care (Ward et al., 2004). Such cultural and contextual factors should be considered when adapting evidence-based interventions in cancer screening in order to better promote adherence to recommended cancer screening guidelines, particularly among medically underserved populations and vulnerable populations. A number of national initiatives and community-based programs are making contributions in addressing the cancer disparities noted among racial and ethnically diverse populations; for example, the National Breast and Cervical Cancer Early Detection Program (NBCCEDP) is perhaps one of the most visible programs devoted to the early detection of breast cancer among low-income, underinsured, and underserved women (see Chapter 11, "Racial Disparities in Breast and Cervical Cancer: Can Legislative Action Work?").

Clinicians and the health care systems play a major role in enabling patient participation in cancer screening. For example, studies have shown that people who receive a clinician's recommendation for cancer screening are more likely to be screened than those who do not receive a recommendation ("Recommendations," 2008). The Task Force on Community Preventive Services recommends that to maximize the potential impact of interventions for improving cancer screening, a diverse set of strategies should be implemented. These include centralized or office-based systems, including computer-based reminder systems, to assist clinicians in counseling age-/risk-eligible patients about screening, as well as organizational support systems to help manage referrals and follow-up of cancer screening tests ("Recommendations," 2008). In addition, as people who lack health insurance have less access to preventive care and are less likely to get timely cancer screening, access to affordable, quality health care continues to be a fundamental policy priority. The newly enacted health care reform legislation includes several provisions (i.e., increasing the emphasis on prevention services) that will likely improve access to and the quality of health care to many Americans.

Disparities in health outcomes will persist as long as large segments of the U.S. population have limited or no access to prevention and early detection intervention programs. There is a need to build programs for prevention and early detection based on the existing research evidence. With more systematic and targeted efforts to reduce tobacco use, improve diet and physical activity, reduce obesity, and expand the use of established screening tests, there is a great potential to further prevent cancer and save lives.

REFERENCES

Bala, M., Strzeszynski, L., & Cahill, K. (2008). Mass media interventions for smoking cessation in adults. *Cochrane Database Systematic Review*, (1), CD004704.

Bock, B., Graham, A., Sciamanna, C., Krishnamoorthy, J., Whiteley, J., Carmona-Barros, R., . . . Abrams, D. B. (2004). Smoking cessation treatment on the Internet: Content, quality, and usability. *Nicotine & Tobacco Research*, 6(2), 207–219.

Borrelli, B. (2010). Smoking cessation: Next steps for special populations research and innovative treatments. *Journal of Consulting and Clinical Psychology*, 78(1), 1–12.

Brown, R. A., Kahler, C. W., Niaura, R., Abrams, D. B., Sales, S. D., Ramsey, S. E., . . . Miller, I. (2001). Cognitive–behavioral treatment for depression in smoking cessation. *Journal of Consulting and Clinical Psychology*, 69(3), 471–480.

Cahill, K., & Perera, R. (2008). Quit and Win contests for smoking cessation. *Cochrane Database Systematic Review* (4), CD004986.

Calle, E. E., Rodriguez, C., Walker-Thurmond, K, & Thun, M. J. (2003). Overweight, obesity, and mortality from cancer in a prospectively studied cohort of U.S. adults. *New England Journal of Medicine*, 348, 1625–1638.

Centers for Disease Control and Prevention. (2002). Smoking-attributable mortality, morbidity, and economic costs (SAMMEC): Adult SAMMEC and maternal and child health (MCH) SAMMEC software. Retrieved from http://www.cdc.gov/tobacco/sammec

Centers for Disease Control and Prevention. (2008). Smoking-attributable mortality, years of potential life lost, and productivity losses—United States, 2000–2004. *Morbidity and Mortality Weekly Report*, 57(45), 1226–1228.

Cokkinides, V. E., Halpern, M. T., Barbeau, E. M., Ward, E., & Thun, M. J. (2008). Racial and ethnic disparities in smoking-cessation interventions: Analysis of the 2005 National Health Interview Survey. *American Journal of Preventive Medicine*, 34(5), 404–412.

Curry, S. J., Byers, T., & Hewitt, M. (Eds). (2003). *Fulfilling the potential of cancer prevention and early detection.* Washington, DC: National Academies Press.

Dilley, J. A., Spigner, C., Boysun, M. J., Dent, C. W., & Pizacani, B. A. (2008). Does tobacco industry marketing excessively impact lesbian, gay and bisexual communities? *Tobacco Control*, 17(6), 385–390.

Dobbins, M., DeCorby, K., Manske, S., & Goldblatt, E. (2008). Effective practices for school-based tobacco use prevention. *Preventive Medicine*, 46(4), 289–297.

Doll, R., Peto, R., Boreham, J., & Sutherland, I. (2004). Mortality in relation to smoking: 50 years' observation on male British doctors. *British Medicine Journal*, 328, 1519–1527.

Durkin, S. J., Biener, L., & Wakefield, M. A. (2009). Effects of different types of antismoking ads on reducing disparities in smoking cessation among socioeconomic subgroups. *American Journal of Public Health*, 99(12), 2217–2223.

Emery, S., Wakefield, M. A., Terry-McElrath, Y., Saffer, H., Szczypka, G., O'Malley, P. M., . . . Flay, B. (2005). Televised state-sponsored antitobacco advertising and youth smoking beliefs and behavior in the United States, 1999–2000. *Archive of Pediatric & Adolescent Medicine*, 159(7), 639–645.

Eyre, H., Kahn, R., Robertson, R. M., Clark, N. G., Doyle, C., Hong, Y., . . . Thun, M. J. (2004). Preventing cancer, cardiovascular disease, and diabetes: A common agenda for the American Cancer Society, the American Diabetes Association, and the American Heart Association. *CA: A Cancer Journal for Clinicians*, 54(4), 190–207.

Fagan, P. (2010). *Cultural tailoring and eliminating disparities in smoking cessation in the next decade.* Paper presented at the Society for Research on Nicotine and Tobacco, Baltimore, MD.

Farrelly, M. C. (2001). Response by adults to increases in cigarette prices by sociode-mographic characteristics [Article]. *Southern Economic Journal, 68*(1), 156.

Farrelly, M. C., Davis, K. C., Haviland, M. L., Healton, C. G., & Messeri, P. (2005). Evidence of a dose–response relationship between "truth" antismoking ads and youth smoking prevalence [Article]. *American Journal of Public Health, 95*(3), 425–431.

Farrelly, M. C., Pechacek, T. F., Thomas, K. Y., & Nelson, D. (2008). The impact of tobacco control programs on adult smoking. *American Journal of Public Health, 98*(2), 304–309.

Fiore, M. C., Jaen, C. R., Baker, T. B., Bailey, W. C., Benowitz, N. L., Curry, S. J., . . . Wewers, M. E. (2008). *Clinical practice guideline: Treating tobacco use and dependence: 2008 update.* Rockville, MD: U.S. Department of Health and Human Services. Public Health Service.

Fisher, E. B., Jr. (1995). The results of the COMMIT trial. Community Intervention Trial for Smoking Cessation. *American Journal of Public Health, 85*(2), 159–160.

Flay, B. R. (2009). The promise of long-term effectiveness of school-based smoking pre-vention programs: A critical review of reviews. *Tobacco Induced Diseases, 5*(1), 7.

Glassman, A. H., Covey, L. S., Dalack, G. W., Stetner, F., Rivelli, S. K., Fleiss, J., & Cooper, T. B. (1993). Smoking cessation, clonidine, and vulnerability to nicotine among dependent smokers. *Clinical Pharmacology & Therapeutics, 54*(6), 670–679.

Greenwood, G. L., Paul, J. P., Pollack, L. M., Binson, D., Catania, J. A., Chang, J., . . . Stall, R. (2005). Tobacco use and cessation among a household-based sample of U.S. urban men who have sex with men. *American Journal of Public Health, 95*(1), 145–151.

Gruskin, E. P., Greenwood, G. L., Matevia, M., Pollack, L. M., & Bye, L. L. (2007). Disparities in smoking between the lesbian, gay, and bisexual population and the general population in California. *American Journal of Public Health, 97*(8), 1496–1502.

Hahn, E. J., Rayens, M. K., Warnick, T. A., Chirila, C., Rasnake, R. T., Paul, T. P., . . . Christie, D. (2005). A controlled trial of a Quit and Win contest. *American Journal of Health Promotion, 20*(2), 117–126.

Hall, S. M., & Prochaska, J. J. (2009). Treatment of smokers with co-occurring disor-ders: Emphasis on integration in mental health and addiction treatment settings. *Annual Review of Clinical Psychology, 5*, 409–431.

Harding, R., Bensley, J., & Corrigan, N. (2004). Targeting smoking cessation to high prev-alence communities: Outcomes from a pilot intervention for gay men. *BMC Public Health, 4*, 43.

Haskell, W. L., Lee, I. M., Pate, R. R., Powell, K. E., Blair, S. N., Franklin, B. A., . . . Bauman, A. (2007). Physical activity and public health: updated recommendation for adults from the American College of Sports Medicine and the American Heart Association. *Medicine & Science in Sports & Exercise, 39*(8), 1423–1434.

Hedley, A. A., Ogden, C. L., Johnson, C. L., Carroll, M. D., Curtin, L. R., & Flegal, K. M. (2004). Prevalence of overweight and obesity among U.S. children, adoles-cents, and adults, 1999–2002. *Journal of the American Medical Association, 291*(23), 2847–2850.

Hitsman, B., Borrelli, B., McChargue, D. E., Spring, B., & Niaura, R. (2003). History of depression and smoking cessation outcome: A meta-analysis. *Journal of Consulting and Clinical Psychology, 71*(4), 657–663.

International Agency for Research on Cancer. (2002). *IARC Handbooks of cancer prevention. Volume 6: Weight control and physical activity.* Lyon, France: IARC Press.

International Agency for Research on Cancer. (2004). *IARC monographs on the evaluation of carcinogenic risks to humans. Volume 83: Tobacco smoke and involuntary smoking.* Lyon, France: IARC Press.

Jemal, A., Center, M. M., & Ward, E. (2009). The convergence of lung cancer rates between Blacks and Whites under the age of 40, United States. *Cancer Epidemiology, Biomarkers & Prevention, 18*(12), 3349–3352.

Jemal, A., Cokkinides, V. E., Shafey, O., & Thun, M. J. (2003). Lung cancer trends in young adults: An early indicator of progress in tobacco control (United States). *Cancer Causes and Control, 14*(6), 579–585.

Jemal, A., Thun, M. J., Ries, L. A., Howe, H. L., Weir, H. K., Center, M. M., . . . Edwards, B. K. (2008). Annual report to the nation on the status of cancer, 1975–2005, featuring trends in lung cancer, tobacco use, and tobacco control. *Journal of the National Cancer Institute, 100*(23), 1672–1694.

Jemal, A., Ward, E., & Thun, M. (2010). Declining death rates reflect progress against cancer. *PLoS One, 5*(3), e9584.

Johnson, K. M., Lando, H. A., Schmid, L. S., & Solberg, L. I. (1997). The GAINS project: Outcome of smoking cessation strategies in four urban Native American clinics. *Addictive Behaviors, 22*(2), 207–218.

Koh, H. K., Oppenheimer, S. C., Massin-Short, S. B., Emmons, K. M., Geller, A. C., & Viswanath, K. (2010). Translating research evidence into practice to reduce health disparities: A social determinants approach. *American Journal of Public Health, 100*(Suppl. 1), S72–S80.

Kumanyika, S. K., Obarzanek, E., Stettler, N., Bell, R., Field, A. E., Fortmann, S. P., . . . Hong, Y. (2008). Population-based prevention of obesity: The need for comprehensive promotion of healthful eating, physical activity, and energy balance: A scientific statement from American Heart Association Council on Epidemiology and Prevention, Interdisciplinary Committee for Prevention (formerly the expert panel on population and prevention science). *Circulation, 118*(4), 428–464.

Kushi, L. H., Byers, T., Doyle, C., Bandera, E. V., McCullough, M., McTiernan, A., . . . Thun, M. J. (2006). American Cancer Society Guidelines on Nutrition and Physical Activity for cancer prevention: Reducing the risk of cancer with healthy food choices and physical activity. *CA: A Cancer Journal for Clinicians, 56*(5), 254–281; quiz 313–254.

Landrine, H. (2010). *Understanding & reducing cancer disparities: The Georgia Community Health Survey Project.* Atlanta, GA: American Cancer Society.

Larson, N. I., Story, M. T., & Nelson, M. C. (2008). Neighborhood environments: Disparities in access to healthy foods in the U.S. *American Journal of Preventive Medicine, 36*, 74–81.

Lasser, K., Boyd, J. W., Woolhandler, S., Himmelstein, D. U., McCormick, D., & Bor, D. H. (2000). Smoking and mental illness: A population-based prevalence study. *Journal of the American Medical Association, 284*(20), 2606–2610.

Leonard, S., & Adams, C. E. (2006). Smoking cessation and schizophrenia. *American Journal of Psychiatry, 163*(11), 1877.

Levy, D. T., Cummings, K. M., & Hyland, A. (2000a). Increasing taxes as a strategy to reduce cigarette use and deaths: Results of a simulation model. *Preventive Medicine, 31*(3), 279–286.

Levy, D. T., Cummings, K. M., & Hyland, A. (2000b). A simulation of the effects of youth initiation policies on overall cigarette use. *American Journal of Public Health, 90*(8), 1311–1314.

MacPherson, L., Tull, M. T., Matusiewicz, A. K., Rodman, S., Strong, D. R., Kahler, C. W., . . . Lejuez, C. W. (2010). Randomized controlled trial of behavioral activation smoking cessation treatment for smokers with elevated depressive symptoms. *Journal of Consulting and Clinical Psychology, 78*(1), 55–61.

Meyer, I. H. (2003). Prejudice, social stress, and mental health in lesbian, gay, and bisexual populations: Conceptual issues and research evidence. *Psychological Bulletin, 129*(5), 674–697.

Oberly, J., & Macedo, J. (2004). The R word in Indian country: Culturally appropriate commercial tobacco-use research strategies. *Health Promotion Practice, 5*(4), 355–361.

Ogden, C. L., Carroll, M. D., McDowell, M. A., & Flegal, K. M. (2007). *Obesity among adults in the United States–no statistically significant change since 2003–2004* (NCHS Data Brief No. 1). National Center for Health Statistics, Hyattsville, MD.

Pachankis, J. E., Westmaas, J. L., & Dougherty, L. (2011). The influence of sexual orientation and masculinity on young men's tobacco smoking. *Journal of Consulting Clinical Psychology, 79*(2), 142–152.

Pederson, L. L., Ahluwalia, J. S., Harris, K. J., & McGrady, G. A. (2000). Smoking cessation among African Americans: What we know and do not know about interventions and self-quitting. *Preventive Medicine, 31*(1), 23–38.

Portnoy, D. B., Scott-Sheldon, L. A. J., Johnson, B. T., & Carey, M. P. (2008). Computer-delivered interventions for health promotion and behavioral risk reduction: A meta-analysis of 75 randomized controlled trials, 1988–2007. *Preventive Medicine, 47*(1), 3–16.

Primack, B. A., Bost, J. E., Land, S. R., & Fine, M. J. (2007). Volume of tobacco advertising in African American markets: Systematic review and meta-analysis. *Public Health Reports, 122*(5), 607–615.

Quit-smoking hotline shuts as free products run out. (March, 2009). National Tobacco Cessation Collaborative Online Newsletter.

Recommendations for client- and provider-directed interventions to increase breast, cervical, and colorectal cancer screening. (2008). *American Journal of Preventive Medicine, 35*(1, Suppl. 1), S21–S25. doi: 10.1016/j.amepre.2008.04.004

Resnicow, K., Braithwaite, R. L., Ahluwalia, J. S., & Butler, J. (2000). Cultural sensitivity in substance abuse prevention. *Journal of Community Psychology, 28*, 271–290.

Rosario, M., Schrimshaw, E. W., & Hunter, J. (2009). Disclosure of sexual orientation and subsequent substance use and abuse among lesbian, gay, and bisexual youths: Critical role of disclosure reactions. *Psychology of Addictive Behaviors, 23*(1), 175–184.

Schwappach, D. L. (2008). Smoking behavior, intention to quit, and preferences toward cessation programs among gay men in Zurich, Switzerland. *Nicotine & Tobacco Research, 10*(12), 1783–1787.

Schwappach, D. L. (2009). Queer quit: Gay smokers' perspectives on a culturally specific smoking cessation service. *Health Expectations, 12*(4), 383–395.

Secker-Walker, R. H., Gnich, W., Platt, S., & Lancaster, T. (2002). Community interventions for reducing smoking among adults. *Cochrane Database Systematic Review* (3), CD001745.

Seidman, D. F., Westmaas, J. L., Goldband, S., Rabius, V., Katkin, E. S., Pike, K. J., . . . Sloan, R. P. (2010). Randomized controlled trial of an interactive Internet smoking cessation program with long-term follow-up. *Annals of Behavioral Medicine, 39*(1), 48–60.

Shiffman, S., Ferguson, S. G., Rohay, J., & Gitchell, J. G. (2008). Perceived safety and efficacy of nicotine replacement therapies among U.S. smokers and ex-smokers: Relationship with use and compliance. *Addiction, 103*(8), 1371–1378.

Siahpush, M., Wakefield, M. A., Spittal, M. J., Durkin, S. J., & Scollo, M. M. (2009). Taxation reduces social disparities in adult smoking prevalence. *American Journal of Preventive Medicine, 36*(4), 285–291. doi: 10.1016/j.amepre.2008.11.013

Siegel, M., & Biener, L. (2000). The impact of an antismoking media campaign on progression to established smoking: Results of a longitudinal youth study. *American Journal of Public Health, 90*(3), 380–386.

Smith, E. A., Offen, N., & Malone, R. E. (2005). What makes an ad a cigarette ad? Commercial tobacco imagery in the lesbian, gay, and bisexual press. *Journal of Epidemiology and Community Health, 59*(12), 1086–1091.

Smith, R. A., Cokkinides, V., & Brawley, O. W. (2009). Cancer screening in the U.S., 2009: A review of current American Cancer Society guidelines and issues in cancer screening. *CA: A Cancer Journal for Clinicians, 59*(1), 27–41.

Smith, R. A., Cokkinides, V., Brooks, D., Saslow, D., & Brawley, O. W. (2010). Cancer screening in the United States, 2010: A review of current American Cancer Society guidelines and issues in cancer screening. *CA: A Cancer Journal for Clinicians, 60*(2), 99–119.

Tang, H., Greenwood, G. L., Cowling, D. W., Lloyd, J. C., Roeseler, A. G., & Bal, D. G. (2004). Cigarette smoking among lesbians, gays, and bisexuals: How serious a problem? (United States). *Cancer Causes and Control, 15*(8), 797–803.

Trocki, K. F., Drabble, L. A., & Midanik, L. T. (2009). Tobacco, marijuana, and sensation seeking: Comparisons across gay, lesbian, bisexual, and heterosexual groups. *Psychology of Addictive Behaviors, 23*(4), 620–631.

Tsoi, D. T., Porwal, M., & Webster, A. C. (2010a). Efficacy and safety of bupropion for smoking cessation and reduction in schizophrenia: Systematic review and meta-analysis. *British Journal of Psychiatry, 196*(5), 346–353.

Tsoi, D. T., Porwal, M., & Webster, A. C. (2010b). Interventions for smoking cessation and reduction in individuals with schizophrenia. *Cochrane Database Systematic Review, (6),* CD007253.

U.S. Department of Health and Human Services. (2000). *Reducing tobacco use: A report of the Surgeon General.* Atlanta, GA: U.S. Department of Health and Human Services, Centers for Disease Control and Prevention, National Center for Chronic Disease Prevention and Health Promotion, Office on Smoking and Health.

U.S. Department of Health and Human Services. (2004). *The health consequences of smoking: A report from the Surgeon General.* Washington, DC: U.S. Department of Health and Human Services, Centers for Disease Control and Prevention, National Center for Chronic Disease Prevention and Health Promotion, Office of Smoking and Health.

Varcoe, C., Bottorff, J. L., Carey, J., Sullivan, D., & Williams, W. (2010). Wisdom and influence of elders: Possibilities for health promotion and decreasing tobacco exposure in First Nations communities. *Canadian Journal of Public Health, 101*(2), 154–158.

Vital signs: Current cigarette smoking among adults aged ≥ 18 years—United States, 2009. (2010). *Morbidity and Mortality Weekly Report (MMWR), 59*(35), 1135–1140.

Ward, E., Halpern, M., Schrag, N., Cokkinides, V., DeSantis, C., Bandi, P., . . . Jemal, A. (2008). Association of insurance with cancer care utilization and outcomes. *CA: A Cancer Journal for Clinicians, 58*(1), 9–31.

Ward, E., Jemal, A., Cokkinides, V., Singh, G. K., Cardinez, C., Ghafoor, A., & Thun, M. (2004). Cancer disparities by race/ethnicity and socioeconomic status. *CA: A Cancer Journal for Clinicians, 54*(2), 78–93.

Webb, M. S. (2008). Treating tobacco dependence among African Americans: A meta-analytic review. *Health Psychology, 27*(3 Suppl.), S271–S282.

Webb, T. L., Joseph, J., Yardley, L., & Michie, S. (2010). Using the Internet to promote health behavior change: A systematic review and meta-analysis of the impact of theoretical basis, use of behavior change techniques, and mode of delivery on efficacy. *Journal of Medical Internet Research, 12*(1), e4.

Winterer, G. (2010). Why do patients with schizophrenia smoke? *Current Opinion in Psychiatry, 23*(2), 112–119.

World Cancer Research Fund/American Institute for Cancer Research. (2007). *Expert Report, Food, Nutrition, Physical Activity and the Prevention of Cancer: A Global Perspective.* Washington DC: AICR.

Zhu, S. H., Hebert, K., Wong, S., Cummins, S., & Gamst, A. (2010). Disparity in smoking prevalence by education: Can we reduce it? *Global Health Promotion, 17* (1 Suppl.), 29–39.

4

Disparities in Cancer Treatment: Factors That Impact Health Equity in Breast, Colon, and Lung Cancer

Ronit Elk, Arden Morris, Tracy L. Onega, Pamela Ganschow, Dawn Hershmann, Otis W. Brawley, and Samuel Cykert

The lower survival of Black patients compared to White patients with cancer has been reported for many cancer sites and stages (Bach, Cramer, Warren, & Begg, 1999; Bach et al., 2002). Awareness of cancer mortality disparities has generated nearly 20 years of research to identify the underlying causes (Dayal, Polissar, Yang, & Dahlberg, 1987; Freeman, 2004; Institute of Medicine, 2003; Mayberry et al., 1995). Evidence continues to mount indicating disparities in cancer care, especially in the treatment of breast, colon, and lung cancers. The challenge to isolate the root causes of racial/ethnic treatment inequalities in cancer remains, but is likely multifactorial. Any factor evaluated must account for stage at diagnosis, socioeconomic status (SES), health insurance coverage, biologic differences, effective screening, and diagnosis and surveillance, and scores of other potentially contributing and confounding factors. In this chapter, we focus on disparities in the treatment of the three common cancers—breast, colon, and lung—that constitute three of the four leading causes of mortality. We describe the evidence indicating disparities, examine potential contributory factors, discuss successful interventions in reducing disparities, and end with research and policy implications.

DISPARITIES IN TREAMENT DETERMINED BY ANALYIS OF DATABASES

Differences in treatment have been the focus of an extensive literature based on retrospective observational studies over the past 20 years. Taken together, these studies provide strong evidence that cancer treatment disparities contribute to excess mortality in racial minorities, even when adjusting for sociodemographic and clinical factors.

Breast Cancer

Despite a lower incidence of breast cancer than in White women, Black women in the United States experience a higher mortality. From 2003 to 2007, the mortality for Black patients with breast cancer was 32.4/100,000 compared to 23.4/100,000 in White patients, which is all the more notable since incidence in Whites was 7% higher than for Blacks (Altekruse et al., 2010). Black women also present with more advanced disease and more aggressive tumors than their White counterparts. For example, only 48% of Black women have advanced breast cancer, compared to 38% of Whites at the time of diagnosis (Altekruse et al., 2010). Similarly, tumor types with a better prognosis (receptor positive) are found less often in Black women (65% of breast cancers) compared to White women (80% of breast cancers) (Chu, Anderson, Fritz, Ries, & Brawley, 2001). These differences in stage and tumor biology explain some of the difference in mortality, but certainly not all. Several studies using population-based data delineate important variation in treatment patterns according to race. Among the 22,701 women with breast cancer reported in the merged Surveillance, Epidemiology, and End Results database (SEER)–Medicare dataset between 1992 and 1999, Black and Hispanic women were significantly less likely than White to receive adequate care across the cancer control continuum, including breast-conserving surgery, radiation, estrogen receptor testing, and surveillance mammography (Haggstrom, Quale, & Smith-Bindman, 2005). In a SEER study of women diagnosed under age 35, African American and Hispanic women received surgery and radiation less frequently after undergoing breast-conserving surgery (Shavers, Harlan, & Stevens, 2003). Even in an integrated health care system, Black women are less likely to receive adjuvant radiotherapy (31% Black, 23% White, $P = .03$) following breast-conserving surgery, a known indicator of quality care and survival (Hershman et al., 2005).

Colon Cancer

Disparities in mortality are also evident for colon cancer, with a 10% higher death rate for Black men than White and a 7% higher rate in Black women compared to their White counterparts (Altekruse et al., 2010). Studies have found similar survival rates of colorectal cancer when African American and White patients received the same treatment, and controlling for other factors (Bach et al., 1999; Dignam et al., 1999, 2003), suggesting a strong role for treatment differences in the excess mortality experienced by Black patients with colorectal cancer. In fact, treatment patterns reported from observational studies confirm inferior colon cancer treatments in African American patients with the disease (Ayanian et al., 2003). Despite definitive standards of care for colorectal cancer that have been widely disseminated, population-based studies have consistently shown lower use of appropriate therapies in minority patients. A SEER study (1987–1995) showed that adjuvant therapy for colorectal cancer was 75% more likely to be received by White patients compared to Black (Potosky, Harlan, Kaplan, Johnson, & Lynch, 2002). A study from the California Cancer Registry (1996–1997) also found that recommended adjuvant radiation therapy occurred less frequently.

Racial/ethnic differences in surveillance post treatment for recurrence have been reported. African Americans were less likely than Hispanics, and both groups were less likely than Caucasians, to receive surveillance for recurrence after curative bowel resection for colon cancer, even after accounting for SES and other factors (Ellison, Warren, Knopf, & Brown, 2003).

Lung Cancer

Lung cancer is the leading cause of cancer mortality in the United States, with mortality rates in men of 87.5/100,000 for Black patients compared to 68.3/100,000 in White patients (Bach et al., 1999). These mortality rate disparities typify the past several decades (Jemal et al., 2004), and when considered in absolute terms—in terms of lives lost—correspond to tremendous and tragic population impacts.

Some non-small-cell lung cancers are potentially curable if resected at an early stage; thus surgical treatment can be critical to survival. Black patients with lung cancer were 13% less likely than Whites to receive surgical treatment (64.0% vs. 76.7%, respectively), which explained most of the excess mortality in early-stage disease experienced by Blacks (Altekruse et al., 2010). A study published 9 years later showed a similar under use of surgery by Blacks (44.7% Blacks compared with 63.4% Whites) (Cykert, Dilworth-Anderson, et al., 2010; Esnaola et al., 2008). In a large SEER–Medicare study examining treatment trends by race over 12 years (1991–2002), significant disparities were seen by race for almost all major lung cancer treatment modalities and were undiminished over time. For early-stage, non-small-cell lung cancer, Blacks were 37% less likely to receive surgery, 42% less likely to receive chemotherapy, and, for later stages, 57% less likely to receive chemotherapy compared with Whites (Hardy et al., 2009). Such pervasive differences across the treatment spectrum are very likely to contribute to higher mortality for Black patients with lung cancer, and suggest wide-ranging, systemic causes.

Mechanisms Underlying Disparities in Cancer Outcomes

In an effort to understand poorer outcomes for minorities with cancer, observational studies have addressed factors other than treatment. Differences in stage at diagnosis, SES, and quality of care have been examined for breast, colorectal, lung, and other cancers. From these studies, several important themes have emerged. Stage at diagnosis, a factor critical to prognosis, is nearly always more advanced for Blacks compared to Whites (McCann, 2005; Morris, Rhoads, Stain, & Birkmeyer, 2010). Stage at diagnosis is related to tumor biology and use of screening, for breast and colorectal cancers, and to care seeking or access for lung cancer. Many studies show similar breast screening rates for Black and White women (Escarce, 2007; Sabatino et al., 2008), but colorectal cancer screening is markedly underused by minorities (Morris et al., 2010). Lower screening rates are likely to be due to a number of factors, including access to care, financial barriers, and cultural beliefs.

SES is known to contribute to lower screening, inadequate treatment, and higher mortality among individuals with cancer, but is difficult to completely separate from race/ethnicity. In fact, some research suggests that low SES is a proxy for race in the disparities literature. Certainly, most studies show an attenuation of racial disparities in cancer outcomes when accounting for SES (Morris et al., 2010) but do not often show complete resolution. However, a host of studies have also shown a race effect on cancer survival *independent* of SES (Morris et al., 2010; Smedley, Stith, & Nelson, 2003), including analyses that specifically stratify race by SES (LaVeist, 2005).

Quality of care may contribute to disparities in cancer treatment and outcomes, as minority patients disproportionately attend poorer-quality facilities. For example, ample evidence shows that Black and low-income patients are much more likely to receive care at hospitals with fewer resources, higher surgical mortality, and lower volume (Birkmeyer et al., 2002; Neighbors et al., 2007; Onega, Duell, Shi, Demidenko, & Goodman, 2010). The effect of race on mortality seems to be much more attenuated when adjusting for hospital effects than for patient characteristics, suggesting that discrimination may occur not based on who you are but where you go, which indeed is a large-scale systemic issue.

Taken together over the past 20 years, observational research has contributed much to our understanding of cancer disparities based on race/ethnicity and demonstrates inequalities that impact the lives of many individuals. However, given the retrospective nature of these studies, and the limitations of claims and other population-based data at controlling unmeasured co-founders, these data are limited. Retrospective research does not contain the detail required to affect real-time decisions at the point of care. Prospective studies are therefore necessary to answer these questions.

DISPARITIES IN TREAMENT AS ASSESSED BY PROSPECTIVE STUDIES

Over the past few years, prospective studies have been conducted that have shed light on factors contributing to health disparities, often broader than just relating to cancer. Based on the results of these studies, we have identified eight general principles that likely contribute to treatment disparities. These include: (a) biologic response; (b) implicit bias and stereotypes; (c) experiencing racism; (d) psychosocial factors; (e) the patient–provider relationship, trust, and shared communication; (f) respecting patient preferences versus pushing for treatment; (g) physician risk aversion based in perceptions of communication, social support, and adherence to treatment; and (h) access to care. We discuss the potential role of each of these in affecting health disparities outcome.

Biologic Response

Advances in genomics are giving rise to new investigations into genetic components of racial differences in cancer outcomes. Exploring biologic differences is compelling for breast cancer, given the higher incidence of more aggressive tumors among women of African descent. Genomic analyses of breast cancer phenotypes have determined molecular subtypes (Morris & Mitchell, 2008), and studies are identifying genes associated with breast and prostate cancers that are expressed at much higher levels in Black cancer patients than White (Brower, 2008). While this area of research is relatively young, the idea that genetics or biology will explain most of the observed racial disparities is extremely unlikely. Other biologically based differences may be due to differences in metabolism of drugs used in treatment, or biologic resistance to effective treatment. African American women more often have aggressive tumors that are less responsive to treatment compared with White women (Millikan et al., 2003), and have higher rates of estrogen, progesterone, and HER-2 receptor negative tumors that are not amenable to the newer anti-estrogen or anti-HER-2-directed therapies (Millikan et al., 2003). Yet, even when controlling for stage and grade, disparities in survival rates persist, clearly indicating that other factors play a role. Ultimately, most researchers agree that cancer survival disparities are predominantly due to race as a social construct rather than a biologic one (Bach et al., 2002; Brower, 2008). There are some researchers who hope to bridge the social and biologic by examining the complex, multilevel interplay of factors that influence cancer risk, cancer, and mortality (Brower, 2008; Gibbons et al., 2007).

Implicit Bias and Stereotypes

Although future physicians often enter medical school with idealism and positive attitudes about caring for the underserved, implicit bias and stereotyping likely play a role in formulating important medical decisions that add to persisting disparities in cancer care (Crandall, Volk, & Loemker, 1993; Woloschuk, Harasym, & Temple, 2004). Van Ryn and Burke (2000) found that physicians regarded Black patients more negatively than White patients, and their perceptions of patients, including those about "noncompliance," were influenced by the patients' sociodemographic characteristics (van Ryn & Burke, 2000). Schulman and his team reported an increase in cardiologists' decisions against cardiac catheterization when the same hypothetical scenario was linked to a picture of an African American rather than a White patient (Schulman et al., 1999). In another study, researchers measured 287 physicians' "prowhite and problack" bias using Greenwald's Implicit Association Test (IAT) in a group of physicians that held no overt racial bias. They found that physicians' decisions against aggressive cardiac care were more common for African American scenarios when the respondents had a measured, "prowhite" implicit bias (Green et al., 2007). These studies all suggest that an overwhelmingly non–African American provider group may unconsciously use subjective clinical data, such as interpretation of comorbidity information or perceptions of noncompliance, to formulate different recommendations for minority patients compared to Whites.

A recent prospective study (Cykert, Dilworth-Anderson, et al., 2010) showed that decisions about surgical resection for early-stage non-small-cell lung cancer may help us operationalize the concept of implicit bias in cancer care. In this study, African Americans were substantially less likely than Whites to receive potentially lifesaving surgery. With surgery, at least half the patients survive more than 4 years, whereas without it, most will die within a year. Patients who reported that the doctor's communication was ineffective or who misunderstood the improved prognosis of surgery were less likely to proceed with treatment. These findings could be related to implicit bias and physician framing, or could be a reflection of poor communication about the illness, prognosis, and treatment options. However, the finding that African American patients with two or more comorbid illnesses rarely went to surgery, while the surgical rates for White patients with similar conditions were not affected, suggests that physician calculation and decision making played a significant role. The approach to surgical intervention offered to White patients with comorbid illnesses appears to be more evidence based, as Strand, Rostad, Damhuis, and Norstein (2007) demonstrated that age and the extent of the procedure was much more predictive of postoperative mortality than high comorbidity scores.

Unexpectedly, in the Cykert, Dilworth-Anderson, et al. (2010) study, African Americans with higher trust scores also chose surgery less often. Although implicit bias was not formally measured, these findings suggest that physicians advise against surgical intervention when speaking to African Americans with higher risk. Prior studies have shown blind trust to be correlated with patient passivity (Kraetschmer, Sharpe, Urowitz, & Deber, 2004). African American patients have been found to be more passive

(Gordon et al., 2006) and when facing decisions in treating cancer, passive patients want the doctor to make the decision (Salkeld, Solomon, Short, & Butow, 2004).

Experiencing Racism

Patients in minority groups may experience racism or perceive discrimination. Perceived discrimination refers not so much to "everyday unfair treatment" but to major events, such as being denied housing. Either real or perceived racism may result in psychological and physical effects. Even in integrated, economically homogeneous communities, real or perceived discrimination is negatively associated with patient participation in *processes* of medical care—most commonly as a delay in seeking care and nonadherence to medical recommendations (Blanchard et al., 2005; ; Casagrande et al., 2007; Van Houtven et al., 2005). The likelihood of delaying or not adhering to care increases in direct proportion to the volume of major discrimination events reported (Casagrande et al., 2007). Passivity (DiMatteo, Lepper, & Croghan, 2000) and helplessness/hopelessness are also strongly associated with nonadherence (DiMatteo et al., 2000), whereas traits such as resilience and self-efficacy provide a protective effect (Keyes, 2009; Williams, Yu, Jackson, & Anderson, 1997). In contrast to major events of perceived discrimination, perception of everyday unfair treatment, such as being treated discourteously or as a dishonest person (Kessler, Mickelson, & Williams, 1999), has been associated with *outcomes* of care—specifically with poor physical health, reduced well-being, and increased psychological distress (Kressin, Raymond, & Manze, 2008; Krieger, Rowley, Herman, Avery, & Phillips, 1993; Williams, Lavizzo-Mourey, & Warren, 1994). It is likely that chronic stress mediates and moderates this relationship. The association between everyday unfair treatment and poorer health outcomes is strongest among those who internalize or are resigned to the experience (Krieger, 1990; Krieger and Sidney, 1996), and is absent among those who discuss or resist discrimination (Krieger, 1990). Several studies have found that individual psychological traits such as optimism and self-esteem protect against chronic stress (Lutgendorf, Sood, & Antoni, 2010; Segerstrom and Miller, 2004). A small but growing body of work has linked endogenous stress hormones to immune dysregulation and angiogenesis, which are linked in turn to cancer progression (Lutgendorf et al., 2010).

Psychosocial Factors

Lack of attention to patients' psychological and social needs can derail the most sophisticated treatment plans. Unaddressed psychosocial issues may also interfere with the quality or utilization of health care, as well as affecting the progression of cancer through similar stress mechanisms (Institute of Medicine, 2008). Based on theory and empirical work, Magai, Consedine,

Adjei, Hershman, and Neugut (2008) provide a useful conceptual model for psychosocial issues in health. They propose that three domains—cognitive, affective, and social network—account for most of the ethnic variance in both cancer screening and treatment decision making. More importantly, these domains offer potential targets for intervention. The cognitive dimension encompasses the patient's knowledge, attitudes, and beliefs, factors that drive decision making (McDonald, Thorne, Pearson, & Adams-Campbell, 1999). Although cognitive factors are no longer accepted as a sole explanation for health behaviors, they continue to be among the easiest to influence. For example, health literacy is an important cognitive factor that is considered inadequate for more than 20% of adult Americans (about 50% of Americans are estimated to have low literacy, 20% of them with inadequate literacy). Poor health literacy disproportionately affects those of low SES and has a major impact on cancer care communication, physician recommendations, and patient adherence to care (Chew, Bradley, & Boyko, 2004; Davis et al., 2002; Michielutte, Alciati, & el-Arculli, 1999). Interventions to improve health literacy among cancer patients have been eagerly embraced, but fall short if they are focused on information and do not address beliefs (Magai et al., 2008).

The affective dimension, which includes emotion, coping, and emotion regulation, also has a major impact on uptake of cancer care (Ahmed, Lemkau, Nealeigh, & Mann, 2001; Davis et al., 2002; Lynch, Steginga, Hawkes, Pakenham, & Dunn, 2008; Ortiz, Lamdan, Johnson, & Korbage, 2009; Schulz and Beach, 1999; Sherbourne, Hays, Ordway, DiMatteo, & Kravitz, 1992). Overwhelming fear or anxiety has been found to inhibit adherence to cancer treatment, but when these fears are harnessed, they may facilitate adherence (Ahmad, Musil, Zauszniewski, & Resnick, 2005; Magai et al., 2008). Social networks are generally considered helpful in coping, but they may influence disparities in the use of chemotherapy in both positive and negative ways. Although those who receive social support tend to follow the care recommended to them and even have a significant survival advantage (Kroenke, Kubzansky, Schernhammer, Holmes, & Kawachi, 2006), those providing the support tend to delay or neglect their own care (Ortiz et al., 2009; Schulz and Beach, 1999). Black patients are more likely than Whites to be providing social support, heading single-parent households, or caring for grandchildren (Musil et al., 2010). On the other hand, Black patients are also more likely to receive support from a social network, resulting in uptake of care particularly among breast cancer patients (Eng, 1993).

The Patient–Provider Relationship, Trust, and Shared Communication

There are early data to indicate that some patients decline treatment due to aspects of the patient–provider relationship (Morris et al., 2009). This relationship includes two key components, communication and trust.

Communication (which includes information, support, and building of relationships) is usually initiated by the physician and directed toward the patient (Arora, 2003; Galassi, Schanberg, & Ware, 1992; Street, Gordon, & Haidet, 2007). Individual- and group-level differences in communication methods have been well established, and communication that is not aligned with patient preferences is unlikely to be successful (Miller & Beech, 2009; Miller, Marolen, & Beech, 2010). For example, in a study of ways to promote prostate cancer screening in Black men, supportive communication that addressed negative preconceptions such as fear of cancer and distrust of statistics was much more effective than informational counseling (Farrell, Murphy, & Schneider, 2002).

Patient trust in physicians is closely related to patient satisfaction. Trust is a good indicator of the patient–physician relationship, and is even more useful for understanding patients' uptake of medical care. Although there are limited data regarding the specific influence of trust in cancer care (Morris et al., 2009), trust is a powerful mediator of disparities in the treatment of chronic conditions. In a study of patient trust, medication cost, and adherence to care, medication cost was only associated with nonadherence among patients with low trust in physicians (Keating, Gandhi, Orav, Bates, & Ayanian, 2004; Piette, Heisler, Krein, & Kerr, 2005). Trust levels tend to be stable, but they can be affected by the quality of physician's communication behavior as well as the content of the communication (Keating et al., 2004). In a recent study, Black patients required more relationship-building communication before consenting to an invasive procedure (i.e., the clinicians had to build better levels of trust among their Black patients before consent was given), whereas White patients required more informational communication before they consented (Collins, Clark, Petersen, & Kressin, 2002).

Given our historical legacy of racial discrimination and unethical medical practices (Institute of Medicine, 2003), it is hardly surprising that Black patients want more supportive and open communication from their doctors. Ironically, instead of engaging in this kind of communication, physicians may respond to their own discomfort around racial discordance by relying predominantly on informational communication. In a study of race and informed decision making, investigators audio-taped patient–surgeon conversations (Levinson et al., 2008). They found that the informational content of patient–provider conversations did not differ by race. However, relationship-building words and behaviors, such as responsiveness, respect, and listening, from physicians were markedly lower toward Black patients than toward White patients. Another recent study of newly diagnosed breast cancer patients found that, in the first consultation, oncologists were significantly more likely to build relationships with White and affluent patients, and that minority patients were less likely to ask questions and volunteer information (Siminoff, Graham, & Gordon, 2006).

Respecting Patient Preferences Versus Urging Treatment

Although patients' preferences should always be taken into consideration, there are circumstances in which this is especially and even critically important; for example, when considering aggressive cancer care in circumstances of marginal benefit, or when considering palliative care as opposed to salvage chemotherapy and adjuvant chemotherapy (Mandelblatt et al., 2010; Parr et al., 2010). However, many decisions against cancer treatment, especially when examined in the context of race, often reflect patient attitudes, misperceptions, mistrust, or physician miscommunication rather than a clear patient preference. For example, the belief that air exposure spreads lung cancer has been cited as a possible barrier to potentially life saving surgery (DeLisser, Keirns, Clinton, & Margolis, 2009). If an African American patient holds this belief and refuses surgery, should the matter be dropped as a matter of patient preference, given the impact on survival that this decision entails? The literature on quality of communication and shared decision making demonstrates limited questioning, less dialogue, and fewer explanations for African American patients during clinical encounters (Clever et al., 2006). This breakdown in information sharing likely contributes to refusal based on mistrust or misperception rather than an ingrained or rational preference. Instead of accepting reluctance toward care by invoking patient preference, performing an evaluation of barriers to care including health literacy and patient comprehension may reduce care disparities. For instance, Gabrijel and colleagues (Gabrijel et al., 2008) showed that lung cancer patients experience large knowledge gaps about treatment options as early as 3 days after a visit.

The teach-back method, establishing patient comprehension, has been used to improve care in low health literacy populations (Paasche-Orlow et al., 2005; Wilson, Baker, Nordstrom, & Legwand, 2008; Yin et al., 2008). In the teach-back method, the provider asks the patient to repeat what he or she understood about the factual information and recommendations provided by the provider. If misperceptions or other areas of concern arise, these can be immediately clarified and concerns allayed. Yet this simple effective method, illustrated so well in Chapter 16, is used infrequently by physicians in general (Schillinger et al., 2003). In lung cancer care, half of all patients do not understand their treatment options very soon after seeing their doctor (Gabrijel et al., 2008). This is a serious knowledge gap, given the gravity of impending decisions, and could potentially be avoided using the teach-back method. Elements of low health literacy contribute to racial differences in HIV care (Waldrop-Valverde et al., 2010), receipt of preventive care (Bennett, Chen, Soroui, & White, 2009), and poor glycemic control (Osborn, Cavanaugh, Wallston, White, & Rothman, 2009; Schillinger et al., 2003), further supporting the rationale that communication interventions can differentially improve the care of Black patients. In addition to assuring comprehension, interventions that simply enhance fundamental communication have been associated with improved care. In two studies, increasing patient involvement in decisions and increasing perceptions of being treated with dignity led to improvements in depression and preventive care (Beach et al., 2005; Clever et al., 2006). By extrapolating these strategies to cancer care, similar improvements could be expected to occur.

Physician Risk Aversion

Physicians are aware of the risks that surgery entails, and weigh the risks and benefits in making treatment recommendations to patients. However, there are data to indicate that physicians may under-recommend surgery to African American patients compared to their White patients, because of poor communication with their Black patients and their perception that these patients will be noncompliant (Cykert, McGuire, et al., 2010). In this study, Cykert and his team (Cykert, McGuire, et al.) found that a quarter of physicians who took care of patients with lung cancer believed that African American patients received lung surgery less often than White patients because they felt that their communication with the Black patients was more often difficult or inadequate. In fact, half said that they would recommend against surgery because of difficult communication. Apparently connected to this difficult communication dyad, patients' disbelief in their diagnosis was also cited as a reason for Black patients to undergo lung cancer surgery less often than White patients (Cykert, Dilworth-Anderson, et al., 2010).

There are no specific reports that directly connect physician attitudes to less cancer surgery. However, there is evidence linking these physician perceptions, especially negative attitudes about patient compliance, to reductions in other important treatments. For example, researchers examining patients referred for kidney transplantation found that physicians did not refer Black patients for this surgery because they believed that the Black patients would be noncompliant (Ayanian et al., 2004). Similar perceptions have been shown to be associated with delayed prescription of HIV medications for African Americans and Latinos (Stone, 2005; Wong et al., 2004). These reports connecting physicians' perception of noncompliance to limitations in other health states strongly raise the question as to whether reduced rates of cancer surgery indeed mirror physicians' risk aversion to recommending high-risk treatments for patients who suffer from serious illnesses.

Access to Care

Access to care has many dimensions, including individual, health care systems, and geographic (Aday & Andersen, 1974; Andersen, McCutcheon, Aday, Chiu, & Bell, 1983), but in its most simplistic form can be described by availability, proximity, and affordability of care. Studies of geographic access to cancer care in the United States that have examined the interaction of race/ethnicity and place of residence have shown that urban Blacks have similar or better access to specialized cancer care than urban Whites, but rural Blacks have relatively poor access and lower utilization of specialized cancer care compared with all other groups (Onega, Duell, Shi, Demidenko, & Goodman, 2008; Onega, Duell, Shi, Demidenko, & Goodman, 2009). For example, rural Black patients have to travel over 5 hours longer than rural White patients to the nearest National Cancer Institute center (Onega, Duell, Shi, Demidenko, et al., 2008). Disparities in geographic access are most marked for Native Americans, with a median travel time to any oncologist over twice that of any other group (Onega, Duell, Shi, Wang, et al., 2008). Per capita oncologist supply has not been shown to differ for Blacks compared to Whites (Onega, Duell, Shi, Wang, et al., 2008), suggesting that disparities in access to resources may be related to specialized care, advanced technology, and density of providers and services.

FINDINGS ACROSS DISEASES

Table 4.1 summarizes the various factors, grouped into four—(a) patient; (b) provider; (c) health system, and (d) contextual—factors found to have contributed to disparities in cancer treatment. Three cancers—breast, lung, and colorectal—are used here as illustrative examples that can serve as models for disparities in other cancers or other chronic illnesses.

Breast Cancer

Despite a lower incidence of breast cancer among African American women, stage for stage, they are more likely than White women to die from breast cancer (McBride et al., 2007), leaving racial differences in treatment, which have been documented in breast cancer treatment for years, as a likely cause for these persistent disparate outcomes.

Survival outcomes depend on the timeliness, quality, and completeness of treatment. Recent advances in treatment that have the greatest potential to affect breast cancer mortality rates are those involving systemic adjuvant therapy for nonmetastatic patients and may also include benefits from neo-adjuvant chemotherapy. Even in the setting of cooperative group trials, where all women are prescribed identical treatment, disparities exist, despite controlling for tumor characteristics and accesses to care. Disparities in outcome are seen in both pre- and postmenopausal women, and women with and without hormone-sensitive cancer (Albain, Unger, Crowley, Coltman, & Hershman, 2009; Hershman et al., 2010). However, African American women are more likely to miss appointments and discontinue therapy earlier than White women (Hershman et al., 2010).

TABLE 4.1 Factors Potentially Influencing Disparities in Cancer Treatment

Cancer Type	Patient Factors			Provider[1] Factors	Health System Factors	Contextual Factors
	Clinical	Socio-demographic	Psychosocial			
Breast cancer	Genetic factors Screening history Cultural beliefs Fear Resources for accessing health services (e.g., childcare, transport) Access time/time to initiation of care Stage at diagnosis Adherence to evaluation and treatment recommendations Comorbidities Competing needs			See Factors that affect breast, colorectal, and lung cancer (last row of table)	Screening program Accessibility of screening, diagnostic and treatment services Appointment rescheduling Quality of screening and treatment	Geographic location of accessible treatment facilities
Lung cancer	Tobacco use			• Variable interpretation of comorbidities based on implicit biases (in other words, a greater willingness to perform or refer for riskier surgery regarding patients with	• Lack of real-time registries • Lack of systematic scrutiny of no-treatment decisions base on relative (not absolute contraindications) • No systems to confirm patient understanding	As above plus: • Providers who care for African Americans have a lower rate of Board Certification • Less technology

(continued)

TABLE 4.1 *(continued)*

Cancer Type	Patient Factors			Provider[1] Factors	Health System Factors	Contextual Factors
	Clinical	Socio-demographic	Psychosocial			
Lung cancer	Tobacco use			whom physicians are more comfortable) • Lack of health literacy and teach-back training for providers • Reduced patient participation in conversations with African American patients	• Lack of systems to recapture patients who make knee-jerk (or soft) no-surgery decisions and offer second opportunities • Inconsistent navigation systems in depth and completeness • Lack of CQI based on race • Lack of a regular source of care (primary care) to have uncertain patients reengage in care	diffusion in institutions who care for African American patients • Regular source of care less, especially in African American men
Colorectal cancer	Age at diagnosis Gender Comorbidity BMI Cancer stage CRC screening history	Race/ethnicity Income Education Employment context (paid sick leave, flexible work schedule) Marital status Health insurance	Fear/cancer threat appraisal Health literacy Social support Caregiving Perceived discrimination Trust	Race/ethnicity Age Gender General Surgery-board certification Colorectal Surgery board certification Clinical volume Practice patterns Communication style	CRC screening program Specialty care Radiation facilities Patient navigator program Cancer center Nurse:bed ratio	Geographic region Aggregate SES Travel time (rural/urban) Provider supply

Cancer Type	Patient Factors			Provider[1] Factors	Health System Factors	Contextual Factors
	Clinical	Socio-demographic	Psychosocial			
Prostate cancer	Genetic factors				Screening program	
Factors that affect breast, colorectal, and lung cancer	• Age at diagnosis • Gender • Comorbidity • BMI • Cancer stage	• Race/ethnicity • Income • Education • Employment context (paid sick leave, flexible work schedule)[1] • Marital status • Health insurance • Primary language	• Fear/cancer threat appraisal[2] • Health literacy[3] • Social support • Caregiving • Perceived discrimination[4] • Trust • Religiosity/spirituality/resignation • Mental adjustment to cancer scale • Preferences	• Race/ethnicity • Age • Gender • Board certification • Clinical volume • Practice patterns • Communication style • Practice type • Foreign medical graduate	• Specialty care • Radiation facilities • Patient navigator program • Cancer center • Nurse: bed ratio • Number of beds • Teaching/nonteaching	• Geographic region • Aggregate SES • Travel time (rural/urban) • Provider supply

1. "Provider" includes "hospital."

2. *Cancer threat appraisal* is an attitude reflecting distress about a cancer diagnosis and has demonstrated a major impact on uptake of cancer care.

3. *Health literacy* maybe inadequate for more than 20% of adult Americans and has a major impact on cancer care communication, recommendations, and adherence.

4. *Perceived discrimination* is a belief reflecting general perception of unfair treatment associated with discrimination due to membership in a socially vulnerable group.

A number of studies have demonstrated that under use of adjuvant treatment plays an important role among various subpopulations of minority women (Bickell et al., 2006; Prehn et al., 2002), including data showing that African American women are more likely to discontinue treatment (Griggs, Sorbero, Stark, Heininger, & Dick, 2003; Hershman et al., 2009; Li, Malone, & Daling, 2003; Mandelblatt et al., 2000).

The presence of comorbid conditions (such as obesity, diabetes, or hypertension) may also influence the range of treatments offered to women with breast cancer and contribute to both higher breast cancer mortality rates and higher rates of death from competing causes among Black women (Schairer, Mink, Caroll, & Devesa, 2004; Tammemagi, Nerenz, Neslund-Dudas, Feldkamp, & Nathanson, 2005). As survival rates from breast cancer improve due to advances in screening and treatment, the influence of comorbid conditions is emerging as a competing cause of death among breast cancer survivors and highlights yet another racial inequity.

While differences in patterns of care in breast cancer treatment have been established, why they occur and how to overcome them has not. In the past few years, much attention has been paid to the dramatic geographic differences in the magnitude of the African American/White breast cancer mortality, with cities such as Chicago and Houston experiencing some of the greatest disparities and New York City exhibiting some of the lowest differences in the United States (McBride et al., 2007). These data suggest that health system and contextual factors, such as the location, accessibility, and quality of screening, diagnostic, and treatment facilities, are potentially some of the largest contributors to racial disparities in breast cancer mortality (Ansell et al., 2009).

Colorectal Cancer

Although colorectal cancer screening and treatment regimens have become increasingly effective, African American patients continue to experience about 20% higher cancer-specific mortality than their White counterparts (American Cancer Society, 2009; Chien, Morimoto, Tom, & Li, 2005; Morris, Wei, Birkmeyer, & Birkmeyer, 2006). This disparity persists even after adjusting for stage of disease and comorbidities, implying that under treatment and poorer quality of care may play a major explanatory role. In fact, most previous research into mechanisms underlying disparate colorectal cancer outcomes has simply measured race-related differences in use of care—and found them abundant. Previous studies have found that Black patients were considerably less likely than Whites to undergo colectomy for colon cancer (Ball & Elixhauser, 1996; Lee, Gehlbach, Hosmer, Reti, & Baker, 1997). National data indicate that Black patients with advanced colorectal cancer are 20%–50% less likely than Whites to undergo adjuvant treatment after surgery (Ayanian et al., 2003; Baldwin et al., 2005; Baxter, Rothenberger, Morris, & Bullard, 2005; Govindarajan, Shah, Erkman, & Hutchins, 2003; Morris, Billingsley, Baxter, & Baldwin, 2004; Morris et al., 2006; Potosky et al., 2002;). Although some have suggested that Black patients are inherently less likely than Whites to benefit from standard colon cancer chemotherapy regimens (Jessup, Stewart, Greene, & Minsky, 2005), the results of rigorously conducted multicenter randomized controlled trials negate such claims (Bach et al., 2002; Dignam et al., 1999, 2003; McCollum et al., 2002). Additionally, among a national cohort of veterans with colorectal cancer, no racial difference in colorectal cancer mortality was identified after controlling for other patient characteristics, stage of disease, and surgical and adjuvant therapy (Dominitz, Samsa, Landsman, & Provenzale, 1998). Taken together, these and similar population-based studies (Bach et al., 2002; Schwartz, Crossley-May, Vigneau, Brown, & Banerjee, 2003) imply that identical treatment of Black and White colorectal cancer patients leads to identical cancer outcomes. Conversely, the unexplained variation or absence of evidence-based treatment among Black colorectal cancer patients results in higher cancer mortality or poorer outcomes.

Reasons for under use of adjuvant therapy among Black patients are largely unknown. To determine whether access to care was part of the problem, Morris et al. (2008) reviewed SEER–Medicare data linked to American Medical Association and American Hospital Association data for incident rectal cancer cases over a 6-year interval, and found that Black and White patients were equally likely to see a medical oncologist postoperatively (73.1% vs. 74.9%). However, among patients who saw a medical oncologist, African American patients were substantially less likely than Whites to use chemotherapy (54.1% vs. 70.2%). Examination of baseline patient characteristics that might account for these discrepancies in treatment revealed that individual demographic and clinical variables had minimal influence. For example, as age at diagnosis and comorbidities increased, use of chemotherapy by White patients declined as expected. By contrast, among Black patients in the cohort, those with the lowest comorbidity scores were the least likely to receive treatment. A similar study recently evaluated the use of chemotherapy among stage III colon cancer patients (Baldwin et al., 2005). Again, although Black and White patients were equally likely to be referred to an oncologist, the youngest Black patients in the cohort were the least likely to undergo chemotherapy. Taken together, these data imply that Black patients who are younger and healthier—that is, those who have the most to gain from chemotherapy—are the least likely to receive it.

In exploring reasons for why these disparities were present, studies have found poorer adherence to medical recommendations among healthier patients in general, due to decreased experience with medical encounters (Carlos, Fendrick, Patterson, & Bernstein, 2005; Carlos, Underwood, Fendrick, & Bernstein, 2005) or increased family caregiver responsibilities (Ahmed et al., 2001; Kim, Kabeto, Wallace, & Langa, 2004; Ortiz et al., 2009; Schulz & Beach, 1999). In addition, in spite of access to an initial consultation, Black patients in the study may have been less likely to undergo adjuvant treatment because of difficulty or unfamiliarity with navigating the medical system (Freeman, 2006), lack of transportation (Guidry, Aday, Zhang, & Winn, 1997; Lutgendorf et al., 2010), or lack of available specialist providers (Bach, Pham, Schrag, Tate, & Hargreaves, 2004). Finally, Black patients may be more likely than White patients to refuse adjuvant therapy for social or cultural reasons, such as reduced risk tolerance, lack of trust in medical treatment, or resignation to a disease state. Previous studies of colorectal and prostate cancer have indicated that a greater proportion of Black than White patients may delay or refuse surgical care until the disease has become relatively acute or advanced (Demissie et al., 2004; Shavers et al., 2004). It follows that Black patients are more likely to undergo urgent or emergent surgery, a well-defined risk factor for early recurrence and mortality (Ball & Elixhauser, 1996). In another study, the perceptions of African Americans who considered their physicians uninterested and less engaging led to a lack of understanding of their treatment options and less adherence to physician recommendations (Gordon, Street, Sharf, Kelly, & Souchek, 2006). Thus, poorer colorectal cancer outcomes are primarily influenced by how well (and if at all) each aspect of care is delivered, which in turn is influenced by patient characteristics and by the characteristics of providers and hospitals.

Lung Cancer

Decisions against lung cancer surgery in early stage, non-small-cell disease serves as nearly a guarantee of death within 4 years, with half these deaths occurring within a year of diagnosis (Bach et al., 1999). Patients' perceptions of progressive lung cancer are that the prognosis for this disease is exceedingly poor and the disease is thus very much feared (Cykert & Phifer, 2003). Only very few patients with early-stage disease have absolute contraindications for surgery, so why are decisions against surgery so common and strongly associated with African Americans? Several reasons are possible. African Americans often hold beliefs that could potentially delay diagnosis or impede treatment of lung cancer (Margolis et al., 2003). Lack of trust, superstitions, religiosity, and fatalism have all been proposed (Cykert, Dilworth-Anderson, et al., 2010; Gordon et al., 2006) as cultural barriers to recommended care. However, although surgical refusal by African Americans has been reported as equal (Cykert, Dilworth-Anderson, et al., 2010) or marginally higher than for Whites (Lathan, Neville, & Earle, 2006), frank refusal only explains a tiny fraction of the treatment gap.

A recent prospective study (Cykert, Dilworth-Anderson, et al., 2010) found that when patients perceived their communication with their physician, and perceived their prognosis to be poor, they were more likely to decide against surgery, regardless of race. Another complicating factor in physician–patient communication about lung cancer surgery is that nearly one-fifth of physicians who provide lung cancer care underestimate survival relative to treatment (Schroen, Detterbeck, Crawford, Rivera, & Socinksi, 2000).

System factors have also been associated with sub-optimal care for African Americans. For instance, low hospital volume for lung cancer procedures predicts poor lung cancer outcomes (Strand et al., 2007). African Americans received proportionately more care at such facilities (Epstein, Gray, & Schlesinger, 2010; Lucas, Stukel, Morris, Siewers, & Birkmeyer, 2006). Yet another contributing factor is lack of regular care. Even when insured, African American patients have less access to primary care (Corbie-Smith, Flagg, Doyle, & O'Brien, 2002) and, in early-stage lung cancer, having this access to continuing care seems to provide the possibility of reevaluation and the opportunity to reengage in cancer treatment.

INTERVENTIONS DESIGNED TO REDUCE DISPARITIES IN CANCER OUTCOME

Although there has been an accumulation of studies indicating disparities in treatment, there is a dearth of studies focusing on strategies to reduce such disparities. One of the most well-known and very effective studies has been conducted by Bickell and her team (Bickell et al., 2008). They instituted a tracking and feedback registry across six unaffiliated hospitals in New York City, designed to target a cause of treatment under use that was more common among minority women. Their system tracked patients referred to oncologists by the surgeon and closed the loop by informing the surgeons' office if the patient had kept the appointment. Surgeons were repeatedly reminded to call those patients who had not, thus spurring the surgical office to encourage the patients to follow up with their next stage of treatment. Overall, rates of oncology consultations, chemotherapy, and hormonal therapy were higher in the post-intervention groups. Among Black and Hispanic women, there was a significant increase in oncology consultations (86% before vs. 96% after the intervention), decreases in under-use of radiotherapy (23% before vs. 10% after), chemotherapy (26% before vs. 6% after), and hormonal therapy (27% before vs. 11% after). Overall rates of missing appointments dropped for all groups (from 34% to 14% in African American women, from

23% to 13% in Hispanic women, and from 17% to 14% in White women). This exciting study illustrates how a simple system, implemented to help all patients, but designed specifically to target causes of under treatment most common in minority women, was successful in reducing treatment under use and in eliminating racial disparity in adjuvant under use.

There are currently several studies examining the effectiveness of patient navigator programs in reducing health disparities during screening and treatment, but no data has been published yet on effectiveness on reducing disparities during treatment. Two published studies have examined the effectiveness of patient navigators in the diagnostic phase following mammography screening in minority populations. Both studies demonstrated the effectiveness of the patient navigator program in enhancing timely follow-up of breast abnormalities (Battaglia, Roloff, Posner, & Freund, 2007) and timeliness to diagnostic resolution (Ferrante, Chen, & Kim, 2008).

In Chapter 16 of this book, Vanessa Sheppard and her team describe a study focusing on empowering African American women, newly diagnosed with breast cancer, to become involved in their treatment decision making, with the goal of improving outcomes in African American breast cancer patients. The Sisters Informing Sisters[SM] intervention is a culturally appropriate empowerment model in which peers, African American women who had completed breast cancer treatment, were trained in T.A.L.K. Back![©], a shared decision-making approach. A very high degree of satisfaction was reported by patients; most (86%) reported that they found this model helped them communicate better with the provider, and that the program guidebook increased their understanding of treatment options.

DIRECTIONS FOR THE FUTURE

Disparities in treatment across ethnic groups in the United States have clearly been demonstrated. It is also clear that the factors that contribute to the less than optimal care received by some populations in the United States are multiple, complex, and potentially overlapping. What is not clear is why the path to finding solutions to rectify this morally reprehensible situation has not been more widely studied, and why effective strategies to eradicate inequities have not been widely implemented.

Key lessons for the future are apparent. The successful elimination of disparities in cancer care and outcomes will require change at multiple levels (Morris et al., 2010), with a concomitant need for (a) additional research dedicated to effective interventions, (b) specific application in clinical practice, and (c) implementation of transparent effective systems and policy change.

Future Research

Despite the numerous studies that have documented disparities, there is a need for several additional research directions. Although there are many reports comparing the treatment of African Americans with White groups, similar research focusing on the care of other ethnic groups, including Hispanics and Native Americans, is lacking and must be conducted. Research is needed to better clarify mechanisms of care that can be targeted for intervention with prospectively identified metrics. Studies that examine the effectiveness of interventions to reduce treatment disparities are imperative and urgent, yet rare. Systemic change in provider patterns, health care systems, and other contextual factors are more likely to be implemented once there is clear evidence that such interventions result in health equity. The funding of such studies by organizations such as the American Cancer Society and the National Cancer Institute should be a major priority.

Shift in Clinical Practice

Enhanced communication models, enhanced patient involvement, quality improvement techniques, real-time, point-of-care informatics, and other effective practices must be specifically applied in clinical practice to reduce cancer care disparities. Institutional and payer policies that align financial incentives around evidence-based care should include measures for equity in care. (a) Enhanced communication models: Poor doctor–patient communication has been demonstrated to negatively affect patient treatment choices, resulting in poorer outcome. The need to enhance provider–patient communication has been clearly demonstrated across multiple studies. The reality is that physicians are often encumbered by time constraints, so an alternative of a cancer educator has been recommended (Cykert, Dilworth-Anderson, et al., 2010). The teach-back method, proven to result in improved care in patients with low health (Paasche-Orlow et al., 2005; Wilson et al., 2008; Yin et al., 2008), is yet another effective strategy that is relatively simple to implement. Other such strategies exist; they simply need to be implemented. (b) Enhanced patient involvement: Prior studies have demonstrated that by increasing patient involvement in decisions and by increasing perceptions of being treated with dignity, improvements in care resulted (Beach et al., 2005; Clever et al., 2006). Extrapolating these to cancer treatment decisions should improve similarly. (c) Quality improvement and informatics: Audit and data feedback have been associated with improved patient outcomes in practice (Abreu, 1999). When coupled with quality improvement interventions, improved outcomes have been documented in the management of chronic diseases (Strand et al., 2007) and hospital care, including a reduction in mortality (Jamtvedt, Young, Kristoffersen, O'Brien, & Oxman, 2006;

Sequist, Adams, Zhang, Ross-Degnan, & Ayanian, 2006). In the lung cancer setting where unidirectional, implicit bias has been insinuated, addressing this in a systematic manner beyond diversity training is needed, including standardization and transparency in the process of care.

Implementation of Systems Change

Current data suggest that health system and contextual factors, such as the location, accessibility, and quality of screening, diagnostic, and treatment facilities, are potentially some of the largest contributors to racial disparities in breast cancer mortality (Ansell et al., 2009). Other systemic changes needed include the following: (a) Access to high-quality facilities is therefore a crucial factor. (b) Accrual of race-specific data by institutions and provision of race-specific feedback has been demonstrated (Bickell et al., 2008) to overcome implicit bias—the collection of such data by all institutions that care for cancer patients is a necessary first step. (c) A tracking and feedback registry to increase patients' connection with oncologists has demonstrated a significant decrease in under-use of appropriate treatment for breast cancer (Bickell et al., 2008). This system was implemented in multiple hospitals, including municipal hospitals, indicating that such implementation is possible across a variety of settings. (d) Patient navigator programs have been demonstrated to enhance timely resolution of abnormal mammographies (Battaglia et al., 2007; Ferrante et al., 2008) in minority, urban populations, and could be applied to reduce disparities in cancer control and cancer care. The American Cancer Society sponsors such programs in many areas around the country. We recognize that establishing such programs requires considerable planning and resources, and therefore encourage providers, health systems, patients, and communities to coordinate and optimize efforts. The informatics support provided by the HITECH portion of the American Recovery and Reinvestment Act and the expanded health insurance coverage and reimbursement changes provided by the Accountable Care Act should be leveraged as building blocks for these new systems of care. The guiding compass in implementing all future research, clinical care, and policy efforts should be our urgent quest to ensure that all members of our society receive equal and excellent medical care.

REFERENCES

Abreu, J. M. (1999). Conscious and nonconscious African American stereotypes: Impact on first impression and diagnostic ratings by therapists. *Journal of Consulting and Clinical Psychology, 67*(3), 387–393.

Aday, L. A., & Andersen, R. (1974). A framework for the study of access to medical care. *Health Services Research, 9*(3), 208–220.

Ahmad, M. M., Musil, C. M., Zauszniewski, J., & Resnick, M. (2005). Prostate cancer: Appraisal, coping, and health status. *Journal of Gerontological Nursing, 31*(10), 34–43.

Ahmed, S. M., Lemkau, J. P., Nealeigh, N., & Mann, B. (2001). Barriers to healthcare access in a non-elderly urban poor American population. *Health and Social Care in the Community, 9*(6), 445–453.

Albain, K. S., Unger, J. M., Crowley, J., Coltman, C., Jr., & Hershman, D. (2009). Racial disparities in cancer survival among randomized clinical trials patients of the Southwest Oncology Group. *Journal of the National Cancer Institute, 101*(14), 984–992.

Altekruse, S. F., Kosay, C. L., Krapcho, M., Neyman, N., Aminou, R., Waldron, W., . . . Edwards, B. K. (Eds.). (2010). *SEER cancer statistics review, 1975–2007.* Bethesda, MD: National Cancer Institute. Retrieved from http://seer.cancer.gov/csr/1975_2007/, based on November 2009 SEER data submission, posted to the SEER web site.

American Cancer Society (2009). *Colorectal cancer facts and figures.* Atlanta, GA: Author.

Andersen, R. M., McCutcheon, A., Aday, L., Chiu, G. Y., & Bell, R. (1983). Exploring dimensions of access to medical care. *Health Services Research, 18*(1), 49–74.

Ansell, D., Grabler, P., Whitman, S., Ferrans, C., Burgess-Bishop, J., Murray, L. R., . . . Marcus, E. (2009). A community effort to reduce the Black/White breast cancer mortality disparity in Chicago. *Cancer Causes and Control, 20*(9), 1681–1688.

Arora, N. K. (2003). Interacting with cancer patients: The significance of physicians' communication behavior. *Social Science and Medicine, 57*(5), 791–806.

Ayanian, J. Z., Cleary, P. D., Keogh, J. H., Noonan, S. J., David-Kasdan, J. A., & Epstein, A. M. (2004). Physicians' beliefs about racial differences in referral for renal transplantation. *American Journal of Kidney Diseases, 43*(2), 350–357.

Ayanian, J. Z., Zaslavsky, A. M., Fuchs, C. S., Guadagnoli, E., Creech, C. M., Cress, R. D., . . . Wright, W. E. (2003). Use of adjuvant chemotherapy and radiation therapy for colorectal cancer in a population-based cohort. *Journal of Clinical Oncology, 21*(7), 1293–1300.

Bach, P. B., Cramer, L. D., Warren, J. L., & Begg, C. B. (1999). Racial differences in the treatment of early-stage lung cancer. *New England Journal of Medicine, 341*(16), 1198–1205.

Bach, P. B., Pham, H. H., Schrag, D., Tate, R. C., & Hargraves, J. L. (2004). Primary care physicians who treat Blacks and Whites. *New England Journal of Medicine, 351*(6), 575–584.

Bach, P. B., Schrag, D., Brawley, O. W., Galaznik, A., Yakren, S., & Begg, C. B. (2002). Survival of Blacks and Whites after a cancer diagnosis. *Journal of the American Medical Association, 287*(16), 2106–2113.

Baldwin, L. M., Dobie, S. A., Billingsley, K., Cai, Y., Wright, G. E., Dominitz, J. A., . . . Taplin, S. H. (2005). Explaining Black–White differences in receipt of recommended colon cancer treatment. *Journal of the National Cancer Institute, 97*(16), 1211–1220.

Ball, J. K., & Elixhauser, A. (1996). Treatment differences between Blacks and Whites with colorectal cancer. *Medical Care, 34*(9), 970–984.

Battaglia, T. A., Roloff, K., Posner, M. A., & Freund, K. M. (2007). Improving follow-up to abnormal breast cancer screening in an urban population. A patient navigation intervention. *Cancer, 109*(2 Suppl.), 359–367.

Baxter, N. N., Rothenberger, D. A., Morris, A. M., & Bullard, K. M. (2005). Adjuvant radiation for rectal cancer: Do we measure up to the standard of care? An epidemiologic analysis of trends over 25 years in the United States. *Diseases of the Colon and Rectum, 48*(1), 9–15.

Beach, M. C., Sugarman, J., Johnson, R. L., Arbelaez, J. J., Duggan, P. S., & Cooper, L. A. (2005). Do patients treated with dignity report higher satisfaction, adherence, and receipt of preventive care?" *Annals of Family Medicine, 3*(4), 331–338.

Bennett, I. M., Chen, J., Soroui, J. S., & White, S. (2009). The contribution of health literacy to disparities in self-rated health status and preventive health behaviors in older adults. *Annals of Family Medicine, 7*(3), 204–211.

Bickell, N. A., Shastri, K., Fei, K., Oluwole, S., Godfrey, H., Hiotis, K., . . . Guth, A. (2008). A tracking and feedback registry to reduce racial disparities in breast cancer care. *Journal of the National Cancer Institute, 100*(23), 1717–1723.

Bickell, N. A., Wang, J. J., Oluwole, S., Schrag, D., Godfrey, H., Hiotis, K., . . . Guth, A. A. (2006). Missed opportunities: Racial disparities in adjuvant breast cancer treatment. *Journal of Clinical Oncology, 24*(9), 1357–1362.

Birkmeyer, J. D., Siewers, A. E., Finlayson, E. V. A., Stukel, T. A., Lucas, F. L., Batista, I., . . . Wennberg, D. E. (2002). Hospital volume and surgical mortality in the United States. *New England Journal of Medicine, 346*(15), 1128–1137.

Blanchard, J. C., Haywood, Y., Stein, B. D., Tanielian, T. L., Stoto, M., & Lurie, N. (2005). In their own words: Lessons learned from those exposed to anthrax. *American Journal of Public Health, 95*(3), 489–495.

Brower, V. (2008). Cancer disparities: Disentangling the effects of race and genetics. *Journal of the National Cancer Institute, 100*(16), 1126–1129.

Carlos, R. C., Fendrick, A. M., Patterson, S. K., & Bernstein, S. J. (2005). Associations in breast and colon cancer screening behavior in women. *Academic Radiology, 12*(4), 451–458.

Carlos, R. C., Underwood, W., III, Fendrick, A. M., & Bernstein, S. J. (2005). Behavioral associations between prostate and colon cancer screening. *Journal of the American College of Surgeons, 200*(2), 216–223.

Casagrande, S. S., Gary, T. L., LaVeist, T. A., Gaskin, D. J., & Cooper, L. A. (2007). Perceived discrimination and adherence to medical care in a racially integrated community. *Journal of General Internal Medicine, 22*(3), 389–395.

Chew, L. D., Bradley, K. A., & Boyko, E. J. (2004). Brief questions to identify patients with inadequate health literacy. *Family Medicine, 36*(8), 588–594.

Chien, C., Morimoto, L. M., Tom, J., & Li, C. I. (2005). Differences in colorectal carcinoma stage and survival by race and ethnicity. *Cancer, 104*(3), 629–639.

Chu, K. C., Anderson, W. F., Fritz, A., Ries, L. A., & Brawley, O. W. (2001). Frequency distributions of breast cancer characteristics classified by estrogen receptor and progesterone receptor status for eight racial/ethnic groups. *Cancer, 92*(1), 37–45.

Clever, S. L., Ford, D. E., Rubenstein, L. V., Rost, K. M., Meredith, L. S., Sherbourne, C. D., . . . Cooper, L. A. (2006). Primary care patients' involvement in decision-making is associated with improvement in depression. *Medical Care, 44*(5), 398–405.

Collins, T. C., Clark, J. A., Petersen, L. A., & Kressin, N. R. (2002). Racial differences in how patients perceive physician communication regarding cardiac testing. *Medical Care, 40*(1 Suppl.), I27–34.

Corbie-Smith, G., Flagg, E. W., Doyle, J. P., & O'Brien, M. A. (2002). Influence of usual source of care on differences by race/ethnicity in receipt of preventive services. *Journal of General Internal Medicine, 17*(6), 458–464.

Crandall, S. J., Volk, R. J., & Loemker, V. (1993). Medical students' attitudes toward providing care for the underserved. Are we training socially responsible physicians?" *Journal of the American Medical Association, 269*(19), 2519–2523.

Cykert, S., Dilworth-Anderson, P., Monroe, M. H., Walker, P., McGuire, F. R., Corbie-Smith, G., . . . Bunton, A. J. (2010). Factors associated with decisions to undergo surgery among patients with newly diagnosed early-stage lung cancer. *Journal of the American Medical Association, 303*(23), 2368–2376.

Cykert, S., McGuire, F., Walker, P., Monroe, M., Corbie-Smith, G., Dilworth-Anderson, P., & Edwards, L. (2010). Physicians' attitudes about recommending surgery for early stage lung cancer and possible reasons for treatment disparities [Abstract]. *Journal of General Internal Medicine, 26*(1 Suppl.), 87.

Cykert, S., & Phifer, N. (2003). Surgical decisions for early stage, non-small cell lung cancer: Which racially sensitive perceptions of cancer are likely to explain racial variation in surgery?" *Medical Decision Making, 23*(2), 167–176.

Davis, T. C., Williams, M. V., Marin, E., Parker, R. M., & Glass, J. (2002). Health literacy and cancer communication. *CA: A Cancer Journal for Clinicians, 52*(3), 134–149.

Dayal, H., Polissar, L., Yang, C. Y., & Dahlberg, S. (1987). Race, socioeconomic status, and other prognostic factors for survival from colorectal cancer. *Journal of Chronic Diseases, 40*(9), 857–864.

DeLisser, H. M., Keirns, C. C., Clinton, E. A., & Margolis, M. L. (2009). "The air got to it": Exploring a belief about surgery for lung cancer. *Journal of the National Medical Association, 101*(8), 765–771.

Demissie, K., Oluwole, O. O., Balasubramanian, B. A., Osinubi, O. O., August, D., & Rhoads, G. G. (2004). Racial differences in the treatment of colorectal cancer: A comparison of surgical and radiation therapy between Whites and Blacks. *Annals of Epidemiology, 14*(3), 215–221.

Dignam, J. J., Colangelo, L., Tian, W., Jones, J., Smith, R., Wickerham, D. L., & Wolmark, N. (1999). Outcomes among African-Americans and Caucasians in colon cancer adjuvant therapy trials: Findings from the National Surgical Adjuvant Breast and Bowel Project. *Journal of the National Cancer Institute, 91*(22), 1933–1940.

Dignam, J. J., Ye, Y., Colangelo, L., Smith, R., Mamounas, E. P., Wieand, H. S., & Wolmark, N. (2003). Prognosis after rectal cancer in Blacks and Whites participating in adjuvant therapy randomized trials. *Journal of Clinical Oncology, 21*(3), 413–420.

DiMatteo, M. R., Lepper, H. S., & Croghan, T. W. (2000). Depression is a risk factor for noncompliance with medical treatment: A meta-analysis of the effects of anxiety and depression on patient adherence. *Archives of Internal Medicine, 160*(14), 2101–2107.

Dominitz, J. A., Samsa, G. P., Landsman, P., & Provenzale, D. (1998). Race, treatment, and survival among colorectal carcinoma patients in an equal-access medical system. *Cancer, 82*(12), 2312–2320.

Ellison, G. L., Warren, J. L., Knopf, K. B., & Brown, M. L. (2003). Racial differences in the receipt of bowel surveillance following potentially curative colorectal cancer surgery. *Health Services Research, 38*(6 Pt. 2), 1885–1903.

Eng, E. (1993). The Save our Sisters project. A social network strategy for reaching rural Black women. *Cancer, 72*(3 Suppl.), 1071–1077.

Epstein, A. J., Gray, B. H., & Schlesinger, M. (2010). Racial and ethnic differences in the use of high-volume hospitals and surgeons. *Archives of Surgery, 145*(2), 179–186.

Escarce, J. J. (2007, September). *Racial and ethnic disparities in access to and quality of health care* (Research Synthesis Report No. 12). Princeton, NJ: Robert Wood Johnson Foundation.

Esnaola, N. F., Gebregziabher, M., Knott, K., Finney, C., Silvestri, G. A., Reed, C. E., & Ford, M. E. (2008). Under use of surgical resection for localized, non-small cell lung cancer among Whites and African Americans in South Carolina. *Annals of Thoracic Surgery, 86*(1), 220–226; discussion 227.

Farrell, M. H., Murphy, M. A., & Schneider, C. E. (2002). How underlying patient beliefs can affect physician–patient communication about prostate-specific antigen testing. *Effective Clinical Practice, 5*(3), 120–129.

Ferrante, J. M., Chen, P. H., & Kim, S. (2008). The effect of patient navigation on time to diagnosis, anxiety, and satisfaction in urban minority women with abnormal mammograms: A randomized controlled trial. *Journal of Urban Health, 85*(1), 114–124.

Freeman, H. P. (2004). Poverty, culture, and social injustice: Determinants of cancer disparities. *CA: A Cancer Journal for Clinicians, 54*(2), 72–77.

Freeman, H. P. (2006). Patient navigation: A community centered approach to reducing cancer mortality. *Journal of Cancer Education, 21*(1 Suppl.), S11–S14.

Gabrijel, S., Grize, L., Helfenstein, E., Brutsche, M., Grossman, P., Tamm, M., & Kiss, A. (2008). Receiving the diagnosis of lung cancer: Patient recall of information and satisfaction with physician communication. *Journal of Clinical Oncology, 26*(2), 297–302.

Galassi, J. P., Schanberg, R., & Ware, W. B. (1992). The Patient Reactions Assessment: A brief measure of the quality of the patient–provider medical relationship. *Psychological Assessment, 4*(3), 346–351.

Gibbons, M. C., Brock, M., Alberg, A. J., Glass, T., LaVeist, T. A., Baylin, S., . . . Fox, C. E. (2007). The sociobiologic integrative model (SBIM), enhancing the integration of sociobehavioral, environmental, and biomolecular knowledge in urban health and disparities research. *Journal of Urban Health, 84*(2), 198–211.

Gordon, H. S., Street, R. L., Jr., Sharf, B. F., Kelly, P. A., & Souchek, J. (2006). Racial differences in trust and lung cancer patients' perceptions of physician communication. *Journal of Clinical Oncology, 24*(6), 904–909.

Govindarajan, R., Shah, R. V., Erkman, L. G., & Hutchins, L. F. (2003). Racial differences in the outcome of patients with colorectal carcinoma. *Cancer, 97*(2), 493–498.

Green, A. R., Carney, D. R., Pallin, D. J., Ngo, L. H., Raymond, K. L., Iezzoni, L. I., & Banaji, M. R. (2007). Implicit bias among physicians and its prediction of thrombolysis decisions for Black and White patients. *Journal of General Internal Medicine, 22*(9), 1231–1238.

Griggs, J. J., Sorbero, M. E., Stark, A. T., Heininger, S. E., & Dick, A. W. (2003). Racial disparity in the dose and dose intensity of breast cancer adjuvant chemotherapy. *Breast Cancer Research and Treatment, 81*(1), 21–31.

Guidry, J. J., Aday, L. A., Zhang, D., & Winn, R. J. (1997). Transportation as a barrier to cancer treatment. *Cancer Practice, 5*(6), 361–366.

Haggstrom, D. A., Quale, C., & Smith-Bindman, R. (2005). Differences in the quality of breast cancer care among vulnerable populations. *Cancer, 104*(11), 2347–2358.

Hardy, D., Liu, C. C., Xia, R., Cormier, J. N., Chan, W., White, A., . . . Du, X. L. (2009). Racial disparities and treatment trends in a large cohort of elderly Black and White patients with nonsmall cell lung cancer. *Cancer, 115*(10), 2199–2211.

Hershman, D., McBride, R., Jacobson, J. S., Lamerato, L., Roberts, K., Grann, V. R., & Neugut, A. I. (2005). Racial disparities in treatment and survival among women with early-stage breast cancer. *Journal of Clinical Oncology, 23*(27), 6639–6646.

Hershman, D. L., Kushi, L. H., Shao, T., Buono, D., Kershenbaum, A., Tsai, W. Y., . . . Neugut, A. I. (2010). Early discontinuation and nonadherence to adjuvant hormonal therapy in a cohort of 8, 769 early-stage breast cancer patients. *Journal of Clinical Oncology, 28*(27), 4120–4128.

Hershman, D. L., Unger, J. M., Barlow, W. E., Hutchins, L. F., Martino, S., Osborne, C. K., . . . Albain, K. S. (2009). Treatment quality and outcomes of African American versus White breast cancer patients: Retrospective analysis of Southwest Oncology studies S8814/S8897. *Journal of Clinical Oncology, 27*(13), 2157–2162.

Institute of Medicine (2003). *Unequal treatment: Confronting racial and ethnic disparities in health care.* Washington, DC: National Academies Press.

Institute of Medicine. (2008). In N. E. Adler & A. E. Page (Eds.), *Cancer care for the whole patient: Meeting psychosocial health needs.* Washington, DC: National Academies Press.

Jamtvedt, G., Young, J. M., Kristoffersen, D., O'Brien, M. A., & Oxman, A. D. (2006). Audit and feedback: Effects on professional practice and health care outcomes. *Cochrane Database Systematic Reviews* (2), CD000259.

Jemal, A., Clegg, L. X., Ward, E., Ries, L. A., Wu, X., Jamison, P. M., . . . Edwards B. K. (2004). Annual report to the nation on the status of cancer, 1975–2001, with a special feature regarding survival. *Cancer, 101*(1), 3–27.

Jessup, J. M., Stewart, A., Greene, F. L., & Minsky, B. D. (2005). Adjuvant chemotherapy for stage III colon cancer: Implications of race/ethnicity, age, and differentiation. *Journal of the American Medical Association, 294*(21), 2703–2711.

Keating, N. L., Gandhi, T. K., Orav, E. J., Bates, D. W., & Ayanian, J. Z. (2004). Patient characteristics and experiences associated with trust in specialist physicians. *Archives of Internal Medicine, 164*(9), 1015–1020.

Kessler, R. C., Mickelson, K. D., & Williams, D. R. (1999). The prevalence, distribution, and mental health correlates of perceived discrimination in the United States. *Journal of Health and Social Behavior, 40*(3), 208–230.

Keyes, C. L. (2009). The Black–White paradox in health: Flourishing in the face of social inequality and discrimination. *Journal of Personality, 77*(6), 1677–1706.

Kim, C., Kabeto, M. U., Wallace, R. B., & Langa, K. M. (2004). Quality of preventive clinical services among caregivers in the health and retirement study. *Journal of General Internal Medicine, 19*(8), 875–878.

King, M. L. Speaking before the Second National Convention for Medical Committee for Human Rights. Chicago, Illinois. March 25, 1966.

Kraetschmer, N., Sharpe, N., Urowitz, S., & Deber, R. B. (2004). How does trust affect patient preferences for participation in decision-making?*Health Expectations, 7*(4), 317–326.

Kressin, N. R., Raymond, K. L., & Manze, M. (2008). Perceptions of race/ethnicity-based discrimination: A review of measures and evaluation of their usefulness for the health care setting. *Journal of Health Care for the Poor and Underserved, 19*(3), 697–730.

Krieger, N. (1990). Racial and gender discrimination: Risk factors for high blood pressure?*Social Science & Medicine, 30*(12), 1273–1281.

Krieger, N., Rowley, D. L., Herman, A. A., Avery, B., & Phillips M. T. (1993). Racism, sexism, and social class: Implications for studies of health, disease, and well-being. *American Journal of Preventive Medicine, 9*(6 Suppl.), 82–122.

Krieger, N., & Sidney, S. (1996). Racial discrimination and blood pressure: The CARDIA Study of young Black and White adults. *American Journal of Public Health, 86*(10), 1370–1378.

Kroenke, C. H., Kubzansky, L. D., Schernhammer, E. S., Holmes, M. D., & Kawachi, I. (2006). Social networks, social support, and survival after breast cancer diagnosis. *Journal of Clinical Oncology, 24*(7), 1105–1111.

Lathan, C. S., Neville, B. A., & Earle, C. C. (2006). The effect of race on invasive staging and surgery in non-small-cell lung cancer. *Journal of Clinical Oncology, 24*(3), 413–418.

LaVeist, T. A. (2005). Disentangling race and socioeconomic status: A key to understanding health inequalities. *Journal of Urban Health, 82*(2 Suppl. 3), 26–34.

Lee, A. J., Gehlbach, S., Hosmer, D., Reti, M., & Baker, C. S. (1997). Medicare treatment differences for Blacks and Whites. *Medical Care, 35*(12), 1173–1189.

Levinson, W., Hudak, P. L., Feldman, J. J., Frankel, R. M., Kuby, A., Bereknyei, S., & Braddock, C., III (2008). "It's not what you say . . .": Racial disparities in communication between orthopedic surgeons and patients. *Medical Care, 46*(4), 410–416.

Li, C. I., Malone, K. E., & Daling, J. R. (2003). Differences in breast cancer stage, treatment, and survival by race and ethnicity. *Archives of Internal Medicine, 163*(1), 49–56.

Lucas, F. L., Stukel, T. A., Morris, A. M., Siewers, A. E., & Birkmeyer J. D. (2006). Race and surgical mortality in the United States. *Annals of Surgery, 243*(2), 281–286.

Lutgendorf, S. K., Sood, A. K., & Antoni, M. H. (2010). Host factors and cancer progression: Biobehavioral signaling pathways and interventions. *Journal of Clinical Oncology, 28*(26), 4094–4099.

Lynch, B. M., Steginga, S. K., Hawkes, A. L., Pakenham, K. I., & Dunn, J. (2008). Describing and predicting psychological distress after colorectal cancer. *Cancer, 112*(6), 1363–1370.

Magai, C., Consedine, N. S., Adjei, B. A., Hershman, D., & Neugut, A. (2008). Psychosocial influences on suboptimal adjuvant breast cancer treatment adherence among African American women: Implications for education and intervention. *Health Education & Behavior, 35*(6), 835–854.

Mandelblatt, J. S., Hadley, J., Kerner, J. F., Schulman, K. A., Gold, K., Dunmore-Griffith, J., . . . Winn, R. (2000). Patterns of breast carcinoma treatment in older women: Patient preference and clinical and physical influences. *Cancer, 89*(3), 561–573.

Mandelblatt, J. S., Sheppard, V. B., Hurria, A., Kimmick, G., Isaacs, C., Taylor, K., . . . Muss, H. (2010). Breast cancer adjuvant chemotherapy decisions in older women: The role of patient preference and interactions with physicians. *Journal of Clinical Oncology, 28*(19), 3146–3153.

Margolis, M. L., Christie, J. D., Silvestri, G. A., Kaiser, L., Santiago, S., & Hansen-Flaschen, J. (2003). Racial differences pertaining to a belief about lung cancer surgery: Results of a multicenter survey. *Annals of Internal Medicine, 139*(7), 558–563.

Mayberry, R. M., Coates, R. J., Hill, H. A., Click, L. A., Chen, V. W., Austin, D. F., . . . Edwards, B. K. (1995). Determinants of Black/White differences in colon cancer survival. *Journal of the National Cancer Institute, 87*(22), 1686–1693..

McBride, R., Hershman, D., Tsai, W. Y., Jacobson, J. S., Grann, V., & Neugut, A. I. (2007). Within-stage racial differences in tumor size and number of positive lymph nodes in women with breast cancer. *Cancer, 110*(6), 1201–1208.

McCann, J., Artinian, V., Duhaime, L., Lewis, J. W., Jr., Kvale, P. A., & DiGiovine, B. (2005). Evaluation of the causes for racial disparity in surgical treatment of early stage lung cancer. *Chest, 128*, 3440–3446.

McCollum, A. D., Catalano, P. J., Haller, D. G., Mayer, R. J., Macdonald, J. S., Benson, A. B., III, & Fuchs, C. S. (2002). Outcomes and toxicity in African-American and Caucasian patients in a randomized adjuvant chemotherapy trial for colon cancer. *Journal of the National Cancer Institute, 94*(15), 1160–1167.

McDonald, P. A., Thorne, D. D., Pearson, J. C., & Adams-Campbell, L. L. (1999). Perceptions and knowledge of breast cancer among African-American women residing in public housing. *Ethnicity & Disease, 9*(1), 81–93.

Michielutte, R., Alciati, M. H., & el-Arculli, R. (1999). Cancer control research and literacy. *Journal of Health Care for the Poor and Underserved, 10*(3), 281–297.

Miller, S. T., & Beech, B. M. (2009). Rural healthcare providers question the practicality of motivational interviewing and report varied physical activity counseling experience. *Patient Education and Counseling, 76*(2), 279–282.

Miller, S. T., Marolen, K. N., & Beech, B. M. (2010). Perceptions of physical activity and motivational interviewing among rural African-American women with type 2 diabetes. *Women's Health Issues, 20*(1), 43–49.

Millikan, R., Eaton, A., Worley, K., Biscocho, L., Hodgson, E., Huang, W. Y., . . . Dressler, L. (2003). HER2 codon 655 polymorphism and risk of breast cancer in African Americans and whites. *Breast Cancer Research and Treatment, 79*(3), 355–364.

Morris, A. M., Alexander, G., Murphy, M., Thompson, P., Elston-Lafata, J., & Birkemer, J. (2009, June). *Race and patient perspectives on chemotherapy for colorectal cancer*. Paper presented at Academy Health, 26th Annual Research Meeting, Chicago, IL.

Morris, A. M., Billingsley, K. G., Baxter, N. N., & Baldwin, L. M. (2004). Racial disparities in rectal cancer treatment: A population-based analysis. *Archives of Surgery, 139*(2), 151–155; discussion 156.

Morris, A. M., Billingsley, K. G., Hayanga, A. J., Matthews, B., Baldwin, L. M., & Birkmeyer, J. D. (2008). Residual treatment disparities after oncology referral for rectal cancer. *Journal of the National Cancer Institute, 100*(10), 738–744.

Morris, A. M., Rhoads, K. F., Stain, S. C., & Birkmeyer, J. D. (2010). Understanding racial disparities in cancer treatment and outcomes. *Journal of the American College of Surgeons, 211*(1), 105–113.

Morris, A. M., Wei, Y., Birkmeyer, N. J., & Birkmeyer, J. D. (2006). Racial disparities in late survival after rectal cancer surgery. *Journal of the American College of Surgeons, 203*(6), 787–794.

Morris, G. J., & Mitchell, E. P. (2008). Higher incidence of aggressive breast cancers in African-American women: A review. *Journal of the National Medical Association, 100*(6), 698–702.

Musil, C. M., Gordon, N. L., Warner, C. B., Zauszniewski, J. A., Standing, T., & Wykle, M. (2010). Grandmothers and caregiving to grandchildren: Continuity, change, and outcomes over 24 months. *Gerontologist, 51*(1), 86–100.

Neighbors, C. J., Rogers, M. L., Shenassa, E. D., Sciamanna, C. N., Clark, M. A., & Novak, S. P. (2007). Ethnic/racial disparities in hospital procedure volume for lung resection for lung cancer. *Medical Care, 45*(7), 655–663.

Onega, T., Duell, E. J., Shi, X., Demidenko, E., & Goodman, D. (2008). Influence of place of residence in access to specialized cancer care for African Americans. *Journal of Rural Health, 26*, 12–19.

Onega, T., Duell, E. J., Shi, X., Demidenko, E., & Goodman, D. (2009). Determinants of NCI Cancer Center attendance in Medicare patients with lung, breast, colorectal, or prostate cancer. *Journal of General Internal Medicine, 24*(2), 205–210.

Onega, T., Duell, E. J., Shi, X., Demidenko, E., & Goodman, D. C. (2010). Race versus place of service in mortality among Medicare beneficiaries with cancer. *Cancer, 116*(11), 2698–2706; PMID 20309847

Onega, T., Duell, E. J., Shi, X., Wang, D., Demidenko, E., & Goodman, D. (2008). Geographic access to cancer care in the U.S. *Cancer, 112*(4), 909–918.

Onega, T. L., Weiss, J., & Jenkyn, A. (2010, September 30–October 3). *The influence of race/ethnicity on facility use and post-surgical utilization among Medicare beneficiaries with breast cancer.* Paper presented at the American Association for Cancer Research (AACR), The Science of Cancer Health Disparities.

Ortiz, N., Lamdan, R., Johnson, S., & Korbage, A. (2009). Caregiver status: A potential risk factor for extreme self-neglect. *Psychosomatics, 50*(2), 166–168.

Osborn, C. Y., Cavanaugh, K., Wallston, K. A., White, R. O., & Rothman, R. L. (2009). Diabetes numeracy: An overlooked factor in understanding racial disparities in glycemic control. *Diabetes Care, 32*(9), 1614–1619.

Paasche-Orlow, M. K., Riekert, K. A., Bilderback, A., Chanmugam, A., Hill, P., Rand, C. S., . . . Krishnan, J. A. (2005). Tailored education may reduce health literacy disparities in asthma self-management. *American Journal of Respiratory and Critical Care Medicine, 172*(8), 980–986.

Parr, J. D., Zhang, B., Nilsson, M. E., Wright, A., Balboni, T., Duthie, E., . . . Prigerson, H. G. (2010). The influence of age on the likelihood of receiving end-of-life care consistent with patient treatment preferences. *Journal of Palliative Medicine, 13*(6), 719–726.

Piette, J. D., Heisler, M., Krein, S., & Kerr, E. A. (2005). The role of patient–physician trust in moderating medication nonadherence due to cost pressures. *Archives of Internal Medicine, 165*(15), 1749–1755.

Potosky, A. L., Harlan, L. C., Kaplan, R. S., Johnson, K. A., & Lynch, C. F. (2002). Age, sex, and racial differences in the use of standard adjuvant therapy for colorectal cancer. *Journal of Clinical Oncology, 20*(5), 1192–1202.

Prehn, A. W., Topol, B., Stewart, S., Glaser, S. L., O'Connor, L., & West, D. W. (2002). Differences in treatment patterns for localized breast carcinoma among Asian/Pacific islander women. *Cancer, 95*(11), 2268–2275.

Sabatino, S. A., Coates, R. J., Uhler, R. J., Breen, N., Tangka, F., & Shaw, K. M. (2008). Disparities in mammography use among US women aged 40–64 years, by race, ethnicity, income, and health insurance status, 1993 and 2005. *Medical Care, 46*(7), 692–700.

Salkeld, G., Solomon, M., Short, L., & Butow, P. N. (2004). A matter of trust—patient's views on decision-making in colorectal cancer. *Health Expectations, 7*(2), 104–114.

Schairer, C., Mink, P. J., Caroll, L., & Devesa, S. S. (2004). Probabilities of death from breast cancer and other causes among female breast cancer patients. *Journal of the National Cancer Institute, 96*(17), 1311–1321.

Schillinger, D., Piette, J., Grumbach, K., Wang, F., Wilson, C., Daher, C., . . . Bindman, A. (2003). Closing the loop: Physician communication with diabetic patients who have low health literacy. *Archives of Internal Medicine, 163*(1), 83–90.

Schroen, A. T., Detterbeck, F. C., Crawford, R., Rivera, P., & Socinski, M. A. (2000). Beliefs among pulmonologists and thoracic surgeons in the therapeutic approach to non-small cell lung cancer. *Chest, 118*(1), 129–137.

Schulman, K. A., Berlin, J. A., Harless, W., Kerner, J. F., Sistrunk, S., & Gersh, B. J. (1999). The effect of race and sex on physicians' recommendations for cardiac catheterization. *New England Journal of Medicine, 340*(8), 618–626.

Schulz, R., & Beach, S. R. (1999). Caregiving as a risk factor for mortality: The Caregiver Health Effects Study. *Journal of the American Medical Association, 282*(23), 2215–2219.

Schwartz, K. L., Crossley-May, H., Vigneau, F. D., Brown, K., & Banerjee, M. (2003). Race, socioeconomic status and stage at diagnosis for five common malignancies. *Cancer Causes and Control, 14*(8), 761–766.

Segerstrom, S. C., & Miller, G. E. (2004). Psychological stress and the human immune system: A meta-analytic study of 30 years of inquiry. *Psychological Bulletin, 130*(4), 601–630.

Sequist, T. D., Adams, A., Zhang, F., Ross-Degnan, D., & Ayanian, J. Z. (2006). Effect of quality improvement on racial disparities in diabetes care. *Archives of Internal Medicine, 166*(6), 675–681.

Shavers, V. L., Brown, M. L., Potosky, A. L., Klabunde, C. N., Davis, W., Moul, J. W., & Fahey, A. (2004). Race/ethnicity and the receipt of watchful waiting for the initial management of prostate cancer. *Journal of General Internal Medicine, 19*(2), 146–155.

Shavers, V. L., Harlan, L. C., & Stevens, J. L. (2003). Racial/ethnic variation in clinical presentation, treatment, and survival among breast cancer patients under age 35. *Cancer, 97*(1), 134–147.

Sherbourne, C. D., Hays, R. D., Ordway, L., DiMatteo, M. R., & Kravitz, R. L. (1992). Antecedents of adherence to medical recommendations: Results from the Medical Outcomes Study. *Journal of Behavioral Medicine, 15*(5), 447–468.

Siminoff, L. A., Graham, G. C., & Gordon, N. H. (2006). Cancer communication patterns and the influence of patient characteristics: Disparities in information-giving and affective behaviors. *Patient Education and Counseling, 62*(3), 355–360.

Smedley, B., Stith, A. Y., & Nelson, A. (Eds.) (2003). *Unequal treatment: Confronting racial and ethnic disparities in health care.* Washington, DC: National Academies Press.

Stone, V. E. (2005). Physician contributions to disparities in HIV/AIDS care: The role of provider perceptions regarding adherence. *Current HIV/AIDS Reports, 2*(4), 189–193.

Strand, T. E., Rostad, H., Damhuis, R. A., & Norstein, J. (2007). Risk factors for 30-day mortality after resection of lung cancer and prediction of their magnitude. *Thorax, 62*(11), 991–997.

Street, R. L., Jr., Gordon, H., & Haidet, P. (2007). Physicians' communication and perceptions of patients: Is it how they look, how they talk, or is it just the doctor? *Social Science & Medicine, 65*(3), 586–598.

Tammemagi, C. M., Nerenz, D., Neslund-Dudas, C., Feldkamp, C., & Nathanson, D. (2005). Comorbidity and survival disparities among Black and White patients with breast cancer. *Journal of the American Medical Association, 294*(14), 1765–1772.

Van Houtven, C. H., Voils, C. I., Oddone, E. Z., Weinfurt, K. P., Friedman, J. Y., Schulman, K. A., and Bosworth, H. B. (2005). Perceived discrimination and reported delay of pharmacy prescriptions and medical tests. *Journal of General Internal Medicine, 20*(7), 578–583.

van Ryn, M., & Burke, J. (2000). The effect of patient race and socio-economic status on physicians' perceptions of patients. *Social Science & Medicine, 50*(6), 813–828.

Waldrop-Valverde, D., Osborn, C. Y., Rodriguez, A., Rothman, R. L., Kumar, M., & Jones, D. L. (2010). Numeracy skills explain racial differences in HIV medication management. *AIDS and Behavior, 14*(4), 799–806.

Williams, D. R., Lavizzo-Mourey, R., & Warren, R. C. (1994). The concept of race and health status in America. *Public Health Reports, 109*(1), 26–41.

Williams, D. R., Yu, Y., Jackson, J. S., & Anderson, N. B. (1997). Racial differences in physical and mental health: Socio-economic status, stress and discrimination. *Journal of Health Psychology, 2*(3), 335–351.

Wilson, F. L., Baker, L. M., Nordstrom, C. K., & Legwand, C. (2008). Using the teach-back and Orem's Self-Care Deficit Nursing theory to increase childhood immunization communication among low-income mothers. *Issues in Comprehensive Pediatric Nursing, 31*(1), 7–22.

Woloschuk, W., Harasym, P. H., & Temple, W. (2004). Attitude change during medical school: A cohort study. *Medical Education, 38*(5), 522–534.

Wong, M. D., Cunningham, W. E., Shapiro, M. F., Andersen, R. M., Cleary, P. D., Duan, N., . . . Wenger, N. S., for the HCSUS Consortium. (2004). Disparities in HIV treatment and physician attitudes about delaying protease inhibitors for nonadherent patients. *Journal of General Internal Medicine, 19*(4), 366–374.

Yin, H. S., Dreyer, B. P., van Schaick, L., Foltin, G. L., Dinglas, C., & Mendelsohn, A. L. (2008). Randomized controlled trial of a pictogram-based intervention to reduce liquid medication dosing errors and improve adherence among caregivers of young children. *Archives of Pediatrics & Adolescent Medicine, 162*(9), 814–822.

5

Racial, Ethnic, and Socioeconomic Health Disparities Among Cancer Survivors and Informal Caregivers

Tenbroeck Smith, Kevin Stein, Youngmee Kim, Dexter Cooper,
Katherine Virgo, Irma Corral, and Hope Landrine

Cancer survivors are a group with unique health needs, and cancer survivorship is an area in need of better scientific understanding. First, cancer survivors experience the distress of a cancer diagnosis, the physical consequences of the disease, the complexity of treatment decisions, and the side effects of treatment. After completing initial treatment, cancer survivors face physical and psychological sequalae as well as the social and financial impact of the cancer, all of which can persist for years after the completion of treatment. Reports such as the Institute of Medicine's *From Cancer Patient to Cancer Survivor: Lost in Transition* (2006) and the Centers for Disease Control and Prevention's *The National Action Plan for Cancer Survivorship* (2004) highlight the growing clinical, public health, research, and policy efforts to better understand and meet the needs of survivors. The cancer survivor movement has identified family members and informal cancer caregivers as another population with unique needs resulting from the impact of cancer on their lives. Though still relatively young in academic terms, the field of cancer survivorship research has identified health-related quality of life, continuing care, employment and financial issues, and health behaviors as areas in which cancer survivors can experience negative health outcomes.

Racial/ethnic and socioeconomic cancer health disparities are relatively well described in preventive health behaviors, early detection, incidence, and mortality, but little research to date describes disparities among cancer survivors (Aziz & Rowland, 2002). Non-White race/ethnicity and lower socioeconomic status (SES)—which includes income, education, and employment—are predictive of poorer survival rates, less access to quality health care, and socio-ecological burdens (Ashing-Giwa, 2005). The conceptual models of adjustment to cancer implicit in much of survivorship research to date focus on individual demographic, medical, and attitudinal factors. Of these factors, socioeconomic status (SES)—which includes income, education, and employment status—is an important aspect of health disparities, thought by some to be more predictive of health outcomes than race or ethnicity.

Ashing-Giwa (2005) outlined a model for understanding health disparities among cancer survivors that included environmental, cultural, and health system factors. Environmental factors include variables such as neighborhood characteristics, which may impair accessibility to needed specialists, services, or medications. The model includes social support and spirituality, which can act as buffers to decrease the impact of negative life events. Cultural differences in ethnicity, ethnic identity, or acculturation can lead to different prioritization of outcomes, different medical decision-making processes, differences in the use of spirituality and social support, communication difficulties, or avoidance of health care providers. A prominent health system issue related to access to care is insurance coverage, lack of which can lead to late-stage cancer at diagnosis, sub-optimal treatment, and higher mortality rates. Health provider biases, such as lower likelihood of prescribing needed pain medications, must also be considered. The intersection of survivor and caregivers' unique and increased medical needs with the factors that cause health disparities suggests that unique disparities may exist among survivors and caregivers.

This chapter provides an overview of the issues faced by cancer survivors and literature describing racial/ethnic and SES disparities among survivors and caregivers. Those interested in intervention should read Chapters 7–21 in this book, which are devoted to interventions designed to reduce cancer disparities; Chapters 19–21 specifically target reductions in survivorship disparities. While health disparities exist for various gender, age, and sexual orientation groups, they are not described in this chapter. Each section of this chapter starts by providing an overview of the given issue faced by survivors and then describes the extent of research on racial/ethnic and SES disparities relevant to that issue.

DEFINITIONS AND DEMOGRAPHICS

In this chapter, the term "cancer survivor" will apply to people from the time of cancer diagnosis through the balance of their lives (Mullan, 1985), a definition that became widespread with the growth of the field of survivorship in the late 20th and early 21st centuries. The number of cancer survivors in the United States has grown steadily, from 3 million in 1971 to 11.7 million in 2007 (SEER, 2010), as a result of improving survival rates garnered from advances in cancer treatment and screening.

Other contributing factors include increased life expectancy, overall population growth, and increasing numbers of older people. Given the ongoing nature of these trends, the number of cancer survivors is expected to continue to rise (Institute of Medicine, 2006).

In 2007, an estimated 88% of survivors were White (10.3 million), 8% were African American (942,000), and 4% were from other ethnic groups (SEER, 2010). Survivors are less diverse than the general U.S. population which, in 2007, was 66% White, 15% Hispanic, 13% African American, and 4% Asian (U.S. Census Bureau, 2008). The lower levels of diversity among survivors likely reflect increased mortality rates among certain racial/ethnic groups as well as less diversity among older Americans—cancer is more likely to occur in older people and the majority of survivors (60%) are 65 or older. The most common initial diagnoses among survivors are breast (23%), prostate (20%), or colorectal cancer (10%), which varies by racial/ethnic group (Schultz, Stava, Beck, & Vassilopoulou-Sellin, 2004). Most survivors have completed initial curative treatment and are disease-free. Those under treatment for a new diagnosis, recurrence, or metastatic disease make up smaller fractions. In recognition of this, the rest of this chapter will focus primarily on disease-free, post-treatment survivors.

HEALTH-RELATED QUALITY OF LIFE AND LATE EFFECTS

Health-related quality of life (HRQOL) is a multidimensional construct that includes physical, emotional, social, and functional well-being and is, perhaps, the best studied aspect of survivorship. While deficits in HRQOL may be considerable during curative treatment and immediately thereafter, the majority of disease-free long-term cancer survivors (e.g., those more than 5 years from diagnosis) report overall HRQOL that is comparable to similarly aged peers with no history of cancer (Ganz et al., 2002; Tomich, Helgeson, & Nowak Vache, 2005). However, a significant proportion of long-term survivors continue to experience diminished functioning, such that survivors in the National Health Interview Survey (NHIS) report deficits in self-rated health (Schootman, Deshpande, Pruitt, Aft, & Jeffe, 2010). In the NHIS, African American survivors' self-rated health is somewhat poorer, but their level of psychological distress is modestly better than for Whites (Schootman et al., 2010; Short & Mallonee, 2006). Some studies report lower levels of physical well-being among African American cancer survivors and better psychological functioning (Ashing-Giwa & Lim, 2009; Bowen et al., 2007), while others report no racial differences in HRQOL. HRQOL in non-White survivors has been related to concerns about money, housing, and neighborhood characteristics (Ashing-Giwa, Ganz, & Petersen, 1999; Ashing-Giwa, Tejero,

Kim, Padilla, & Hellemann, 2007), and African American/White HRQOL disparities may be explained by disease characteristics, comorbidities, and neighborhood characteristics (e.g., segregated neighborhoods) (Hao et al., 2010). Cancer survivors with less education and low incomes are at risk of poor HRQOL (Clauser et al., 2008). Even within racial/ethnic groups, SES can impact HRQOL. African American survivors with lower SES have poorer health than African American survivors with higher SES (Ashing-Giwa, 2005), suggesting that the effects of race/ethnicity and SES play an important role in survivor HRQOL that may be additive.

Symptoms and side effects of cancer and cancer treatment are important determinants of survivors' HRQOL. Some symptoms (e.g., pain and urinary incontinence) may arise during treatment and persist over time. Other side effects (i.e., late effects) have a later onset, typically surfacing months or even years after the cessation of therapy (Stein, Smith, Sharpe, Zhao, & Kirch, 2008). Late effects manifest as both physical and emotional deficits, including toxicity to the cardiac, pulmonary, and renal systems, neurocognitive impairment, hormonal deficiency, and diminished endocrine and reproductive functioning (Institute of Medicine, 2006). While little research describes disparities in survivor late effects, Schultz et al. (2004) found that Hispanic survivors were more likely to report abdominal pain, diabetes mellitus, frequent infections, and migraine headaches, whereas African American survivors were more likely to cite circulatory problems, dizziness, heart disease, memory loss, and lung problems. For an in-depth review of long-term late effects, see *From Cancer Patient to Cancer Survivor: Lost in Transition* (Institute of Medicine, 2006). This chapter provides an overview of several of the most common, well-researched effects.

Cancer survivors are at risk for recurrence of the original cancer or the development of a new, biologically distinct, second primary cancer. Recurrence is not uncommon among survivors, with rates varying depending upon type of cancer, stage of disease, and treatments received (Duncan et al., 1993; Martini et al., 1995). Higher rates of recurrence among African Americans are generally attributed to more advanced stage at diagnosis and/or receipt of less complete treatment (Moran et al., 2008; Vicini et al., 2010). After adjusting for SES, African American and White colorectal cancer patients with the same stage of disease and treatment have similar survival and recurrence-free survival rates (Dimou, Syrigos, & Saif, 2009), suggesting that these factors play an important role in explaining racial/ethnic recurrence disparities.

An estimated 8% of cancer survivors have second primary cancers (Mariotto, Rowland, Ries, Scoppa, & Feuer, 2007). The high rate of second primary cancers has been attributed to late effects of treatment and the same risk factors that led to the first cancer. African Americans have higher incidence rates for second cancers (SEER, 2006), but lower prevalence rates than Whites (Mariotto et al., 2007). This counterintuitive finding is similar to African Americans' higher incidence and lower prevalence rates for first primary cancers, which has been attributed to African Americans' higher cancer mortality rates and lower life expectancy. Because of the threat of cancer returning, survivors never really "get over" cancer (Mullan, 1985) and recurrence is one of the most common concerns of cancer survivors (Baker, Denniston, Smith, & West, 2005).

The best-studied side effect of cancer may be pain, which is highly feared, has barriers to its management, and impacts HRQOL (Caraceni & Portenoy, 1999). Though pain is most common during treatment (59%), it is also prevalent among survivors who have completed treatment (33%) (van den Beuken-van Everdingen et al., 2007). Research on pain disparities suggests that African Americans and other non-Whites typically report higher levels of cancer-related pain, and have fewer resources and more barriers to adequate pain management (Cleeland, Gonin, Baez, Loehrer, & Pandya, 1997; Yoon et al., 2008). Compared to Whites, African Americans are more likely to have their physicians underestimate their pain (Anderson et al., 2000). Likewise, African Americans and Hispanic cancer survivors reported experiencing more barriers to the management of their cancer pain (Stein et al., 2010). Higher levels of current pain among African American than White survivors have been explained by a combination of demographics, education, disease, and neighborhood characteristics (Smith, Crammer, & Stefanek, 2010).

Other common long-term effects include fatigue, which is among the most common and distressing symptoms of cancer patients during active treatment (Richardson & Ream, 1996; Stone, Richards, A'Hern, & Hardy, 2000) and can be quite persistent following the completion of initial treatment (Bower et al., 2006). Cancer survivors may have difficulty adjusting to life after treatment (Mullan, 1985) and experience depression, cognitive impairment, or other psychological sequalae (Bender et al., 2006; Bower, 2008). Cancer can also affect sexual functioning and interest in sex for both genders (Schover, 2005). Further, lower-SES survivors have been shown to have worse physical functioning (Bowen et al., 2007) and an increased number of symptoms such as pain, fatigue, and depression (Eversley et al., 2005; Mao et al., 2007).

While the impact of the disease is mostly negative, some studies have demonstrated benefits from the cancer experience among some survivors. Survivors may gain a greater appreciation for life, improve relationships with family and friends, and have a sense of increased meaning, purpose, or spirituality (Foley et al., 2006; Tomich et al., 2005). One study found Hispanic survivors more likely to report that their family relationships improved

(Schultz et al., 2004). There is a growing body of research describing long-term late effects among survivors, with a few studies directly examining disparities. Given that racial/ethnic disparities in cancer recurrence and pain appear to be accounted for by SES, access to care, and neighborhood characteristics, future efforts to investigate HRQOL and late-effect disparities should include these factors whenever possible.

SURVEILLANCE AND CONTINUING CARE

After cancer survivors complete initial treatment and begin to return to their former roles, they continue to need cancer care due to persistent symptoms as well as their risk of recurrence and second cancers (Oeffinger & McCabe, 2006). Follow-up care, at minimum, involves the survivors seeing a physician every 3 to 4 months for 2 or 3 years to check for recurrence, metastasis, and side effects (National Cancer Institute, 2010). Survivors may also talk to their physicians about developing survivorship care plans that cover physical, emotional, social, and spiritual needs. Survivors continue to experience significant informational needs about cancer tests and treatment (70.8%), ways to increase health or reduce cancer risk (67.8%), side effects of cancer (63.3%), cancer-related psychological issues (54.4%), insurance (42.1%), and sex and fertility (30.9%) (Beckjord et al., 2008).

There are guidelines for surveillance—searching for the recurrence of the original cancer—and screening—the search for new cancers. These forms of early detection can improve treatment efficacy, quality of life, and overall prognosis. Surveillance is particularly important for survivors. Mammography utilization has been shown to decrease from 79.8% among 1-year breast cancer survivors to 62.6% at 5 years, suggesting that rates may be lower than expected among long-term survivors (Doubeni et al., 2006). Studies have shown lower breast and colorectal cancer surveillance rates among non-Whites than Whites and, for breast only, among those with lower SES (Ellison, Warren, Knopf, & Brown, 2003; Keating, Landrum, Guadagnoli, Winder, & Ayanian, 2006), which may partly result from lack of access to oncologists and diagnostic equipment. Non-White survivors rely on primary care physicians (PCP) rather than oncologists more than Whites (Mao et al., 2009; Snyder et al., 2008). Those from lower-SES groups are less likely to see physicians, more likely to utilize urgent care (e.g., emergency rooms), and have greater need of assistance with appointments, transportation, and out-of-pocket costs (Dwight-Johnson, Ell, & Lee, 2005; Ng et al., 2008). Other factors such as fear of recurrence may influence disparities in surveillance rates (Ashing-Giwa et al., 2010). There is a need to improve surveillance for survivors generally, and among non-White and low-SES groups in particular.

One model of survivorship care calls for oncologists to follow survivors for 5 years, but does not clearly delineate when and how responsibility for care should be transferred to PCP (Oeffinger & McCabe, 2006). Unfortunately, many patients are "lost in transition" and do not receive the care they should when they move from their oncologist to their PCP (IOM, 2006). This model may be impractical given that the supply of oncologists is insufficient to meet the medical needs of the growing population of cancer survivors (Institute of Medicine, 2006). Results suggest that the majority of survivors—even those only a few years from diagnosis—do not see an oncologist annually (Keating et al., 2007; Snyder et al., 2008). Thus, much of the responsibility for survivor care belongs to PCP. Most PCP are willing to take this responsibility, but many express uncertainties about guidelines for survivor care (Nissen et al., 2007), which may reflect the lack of guidelines for many relatively well-studied areas of survivorship care such as cardiac and pulmonary late effects (Earle, 2007). Further, survivors seen by PCP are less likely to be up to date with surveillance tests than those seen by oncologists (Field et al., 2008; Keating et al., 2006). On the other hand, survivors seen by PCP are more likely to receive noncancer preventive services, such as influenza vaccines, than those seen by oncologists (Snyder et al., 2009). Together, these results suggest that a coordinated effort where oncologists provide for cancer-related needs and PCP for other health concerns may provide the best survivor care (Kantsiper et al., 2009). The coordination of care that such a model would require is complicated by confusion among survivors and health providers as to who should provide which aspect of follow-up care (Edwards et al., 2002; Hewitt, Bamundo, Day, & Harvey, 2007). Furthermore, many PCP report that oncologists do a poor job transferring survivors to their care (Hewitt et al., 2007; Nissen et al., 2007). One potential solution to these problems is the use of cancer treatment summaries and survivorship care plans (Ganz & Hahn, 2008). One study found that survivors seen by PCP provided with surveillance guidelines had rates of recurrence and levels of HRQOL equivalent to those seen by oncologists (Grunfeld et al., 2006).

Another area of concern is patient–provider communication. Non-White women report that physicians do not discuss survivorship care plans or permit patient input (Burg, Lopez, Dailey, Keller, & Prendergast, 2009; Royak-Schaler et al., 2008). Cancer survivors from lower-SES groups experience less frequent communication with providers, as well as delays in diagnostic and therapeutic care, resulting in lower-quality care (Ashing-Giwa et al., 2010; Ok, Marks, & Allegrante, 2008). Improving patient–provider communication among underserved groups, perhaps through increasing provider cultural competency, is an important strategy to improving survivor care. The continuing care of survivors is an emerging field that has yet to define and implement optimal care models and is in need of further research; even so, early evidence suggests that there are health disparities in cancer survivor follow-up care.

HEALTH BEHAVIOR

Health behaviors—exercise, diet, smoking—may be especially important for survivors due to their increased risk for cancer and other conditions (e.g., fatigue, cardiovascular disease, and depression). These behaviors are related to cancer outcomes among survivors: post-treatment physical activity may improve recurrence-free and overall survival (Meyerhardt et al., 2006); decreasing consumption of Western foods may lower risk of recurrence and overall mortality (Meyerhardt et al., 2007); and continued smoking after treatment may increase risk of smoking-related second cancers (Do et al., 2004). Health behaviors may also improve survivor functioning and quality of life (Blanchard et al., 2004). Clinical trials demonstrate that exercise can improve cardiopulmonary function, and quality of life (Courneya et al., 2003), and cancer-related fatigue among survivors, though accrual, reten-tion, and affect maintenance are issues (Mustian et al., 2007). The growing evidence that primary preventive health behaviors are beneficial to survivors has led the American Cancer Society to develop a guide for physical activ-ity and nutrition during and after cancer treatment (Doyle et al., 2006). The importance of health behaviors among survivors is complemented by sug-gestion that the time after the completion of treatment may be a "teachable moment" when survivors are especially receptive to interventions intended to improve health behavior (Ganz, 2005).

The cancer experience may influence health behavior through in-creasing perceptions of vulnerability and enhancing the priority placed on health among survivors and family members. Consistent with survivors' higher risk of cancer, they perceive higher levels of absolute and relative risk than those that are cancer free (Mayer et al., 2007). On the other hand, survivors may be more fatalistic than those with no cancer history (Lykins et al., 2008). Most survivors and family members report that can-cer led them to make positive changes (Bellizzi, Miller, Arora, & Rowland, 2007; Humpel, Magee, & Jones, 2007), though some report no or negative changes. Negative changes in behavior may be due to losses in functional ability experienced by some survivors (Hawkins et al., 2010). Research suggests that cancer survivors have higher cancer screening rates and are more likely to meet physical activity recommendations than controls, but may have similar or higher rates of smoking (Bellizzi, Rowland, Jeffery, & McNeel, 2005). Although results are not consistent across health behav-iors or studies, the evidence suggests that the cancer experience improves health behavior more often than not.

Although a robust literature describes health behavior disparities among cancer-free low-SES and non-White groups, studies of health beha-vior disparities among survivors are scant. NHIS results showed that African American survivors and no-cancer controls were less likely to be physically active than White survivors and controls, and that African American survivors were more likely to be overweight or obese than African American controls or Whites (Schootman et al., 2010). Survivors in lower-SES groups may be less physically active and more likely to smoke (Ng et al., 2008). Changes in diet and physical activity after a diagnosis appear to vary for different racial/ethnic and SES groups (Satia, Walsh, & Pruthi, 2009; Stolley, Sharp, Wells, Simon, & Schiffer, 2006). Possible elements of interventions are suggested by African American survivor barriers to improving health behavior (e.g., pain, lack of an exercise partner or pleasing walking areas) (Stolley et al., 2006) and associations between positive health behavior change and spiritual well-being (Hawkins et al., 2010).

EMPLOYMENT, INSURANCE, AND FINANCE

The impact of cancer on survivors' financial well-being, health coverage, and careers can persist for years after their treatment ends. Cancer treatment can lead to large medical debts and loss of income (Gordon, Scuffham, Hayes, & Newman, 2007). Cancer may cause survivors to exhaust savings, be unable to pay for basic necessities, borrow from relatives or banks, seek charity or public aid, or declare bankruptcy, burdens which disproportionately affect those with lower SES (Himmelstein, Thorne, Warren, & Woolhandler, 2009; *USA Today*, Henry J. Kaiser Family Foundation, & Harvard School of Public Health, 2006). Underserved African American women report that inability to pay medical bills, lack of insurance, long-term financial burdens, and nonmedical expenses are extremely stressful (Darby, Davis, Likes, & Bell, 2009). According to NHIS, non-White and low-income survivors are more likely to be uninsured or have public insurance compared to Whites and those with higher incomes (Sabatino, Coats, Uhler, Alley, & Pollack, 2006). While many survivors of local cancer return to normal employment within a year of diagnosis, those with more advanced disease or disability are more likely to have difficulty returning to work, and African Americans and lower-income survivors may be more likely to lose employment than Whites (Smith, Kaw, & Love-Ghaffari, 2010).

FAMILY MEMBERS AND INFORMAL CAREGIVERS

Cancer affects not only the individual with the disease, but also their family members and close friends, often for years after the diagnosis (Kim & Given, 2008). The impact is greatest among family members providing informal care to the person with cancer (i.e., caregivers). Cancer caregivers often provide a greater intensity of care over a shorter period than those caring for elderly family members, including those with dementia (Kim & Schulz, 2008). Cancer caregivers monitor treatment; manage symptoms; provide emotional, financial, and spiritual support; and assist with personal and instrumental care (Given, Given, & Kozachik, 2001). The strain of this role is associated with caregiver problems with social roles, restrictions of activities, family relationship strain, psychological distress, and diminished physical health (Given et al., 2001; Kim, Baker, Spillers, & Wellisch, 2006; Kim & Schulz, 2008; Nijboer et al., 1998; Weitzner, McMillan, & Jacobsen, 1999; Williamson, Shaffer, & Schulz, 1998). The negative impact of cancer caregiving is offset to some degree by benefit finding (McCausland & Pakenham, 2003) and post-traumatic growth (Kim, Schulz, & Carver, 2007). A thorough review of cancer caregiving is provided by Kim and Given (2008). The review concluded that the psychological, social, and physical impact on caregivers' quality of life (QOL) is significant throughout the trajectory of the illness, though greatest around the time of initial treatment. One major gap identified was a lack of research on non-White cancer caregivers. Research on caregivers of non-cancer diseases finds that African American, and Hispanics are more likely to be single, younger, have less education, have less income, and provide high-intensity care when compared to Whites (National Alliance in Caregiving & AARP, 2009).

Most existing cancer caregiving research investigates spousal caregivers. As a result, little is known about other types of family caregivers. This limitation is especially relevant for non-Whites, who often received care from offspring, parents, siblings, and friends. As the age and diversity of the U.S. population grows, the proportion of older individuals cared for by spouses is expected to decrease and the proportion cared for by adult children to increase (Emanuel et al., 1999; Given, Given, & Stommel, 1994). This trend is likely to have the greatest impact on adult daughters, because caregiving falls disproportionately to women (National Alliance in Caregiving & AARP, 2009). The few existing studies suggest that adult offspring caregivers report higher levels of caregiving stress than spouses or other caregivers (Chumbler, Grimm, Cody, & Beck, 2003). These results are attributed, in part, to the multiple, competing roles that offspring caregivers must balance— employee, spouse, and parent— with caregiving duties.

Cancer also places a financial and economic burden on the family. A few studies have documented family caregivers' loss of employment benefits and health insurance due to their involvement with cancer care (Blank, Clark, Longman, & Atwood, 1989; Jansen, Halliburton, Dibble, & Dodd, 1993; Longo, Fitch, Deber, & Williams, 2006). One study demonstrates that the economic effect of cancer on the family extends beyond the time of diagnosis and treatment (Yabroff & Kim, 2009). Families often assist in managing survivors' late effects, which may carry a financial burden. Further, the survivor's disability may have decreased family income. Together, these factors may have a significant financial impact on the family, particularly among those in lower-SES groups.

Health behaviors may be particularly important to those with a family history of cancer since, for a number of cancers, first-degree relatives are at increased risk. Family members' direct experience with cancer in a loved one should make health behaviors especially salient to them. Although some studies have shown improved health behaviors among those with a family member with cancer (Son et al., 2010), caregivers may neglect their own health, including good nutrition, exercise, and adherence to cancer screening guidelines (Beach, Schulz, Yee, & Jackson, 2000). Health behaviors may be particularly important for non-White caregivers who belong to groups with higher cancer mortality rates.

CONCLUSION

The description of racial/ethnic and SES disparities among cancer survivors is new, with early evidence suggesting that health disparities exist in survivor HRQOL, follow-up care, health behavior, and the financial/career outcomes (for a summary of key findings, see Table 5.1). The reader should note that the existence of racial/ethnic and SES disparities remains practically unexplored in many areas of survivorship research (e.g., fatigue, sexual functioning, and impact on informal caregivers). These results suggest the need for more research to expand understanding of disparities among racial/ethnic and low-income survivors and to develop interventions to address the disparities thus uncovered.

Both descriptive and intervention research are best when informed by theoretical models that describe relevant person, system, and environmental factors and how they impact health outcomes. Conceptual models for explaining HRQOL and late effects disparities must account for potential "ethnic variability in the associations among the individual- and systemic-level" variables that influence HRQOL (Ashing-Giwa & Lim, 2010). These models can build on the relatively well-developed disparities research in self-reported health, cancer recurrence, and pain. Neighborhood factors have been shown to play a role in survivor self-reported health disparities. Access to care, stage of disease at diagnosis, and treatment received appear to explain racial/ethnic recurrence disparities. Pain disparities research describes how specific barriers to pain control vary by group, including a number of system and environmental factors.

These theories should account for other key factors. Too often, studies have a singular focus on racial/ethnic disparities, while ignoring SES disparities or the role of SES as a potential causal factor. The cancer experience appears to have both positive and negative influences on health beliefs (e.g., cancer worry, fatalism) and behaviors. Age is another important factor, because survivors tend to be older and deficits associated with normal

TABLE 5.1 Key Points

Areas of Concern in Survivorship	Related Disparities Issues
Population Survivors are a large (11.7 million) and growing segment of the U.S. population, with unique health and public health needs.	Approximately 8% of U.S. survivors are African American and 4% are a combination of other racial/ethnic groups.
Health-related quality of life and late effects Cancer survivors experience a variety of long-term and late effects that impact their functioning and HRQOL. Examples include cancer recurrence, pain, emotional distress, and cardiovascular problems.	Limited work suggests that African American survivors report worse physical health and pain, but better mental health, than White survivors. Low-SES survivors are more likely to report symptoms or problems with functioning. The research describing disparities in HRQOL and late effects is scant.
Continuing care Survivors need follow-up care by health providers knowledgeable about their risk for the return of cancer, other late effects, and surveillance guidelines. The continuing care of survivors is an emerging field that has yet to define and implement optimal care models.	Limited research suggests that African American and low-SES survivors are less likely to see oncologists for follow-up care and less likely to be up to date with surveillance tests.
Financial concerns Cancer and its treatment can impact the survivors' ability to work, earn an income, obtain health or life insurance, and/or can leave the survivor with significant medical debts.	These problems fall disproportionately on non-White and low-SES groups.
Health behaviors Due to their increased risk of cancer and other health concerns, health behavior is especially important among both survivors and family members. The cancer experience impacts both health beliefs and health behaviors.	Racial/ethnic and SES disparities in health behavior are well-documented well-studied in the general public, but less well studied among survivors.
Informal caregivers The diagnosis of cancer affects the entire family. The stress associated with providing care for a loved one with cancer can negatively affect caregiver QOL and the costs of cancer can impact family finances.	There is practically no work regarding health disparities among family members and informal caregivers.

aging can be misattributed to cancer. Few studies to date have addressed the degree to which racial/ethnic disparities among survivors are a result of cancer diagnosis and treatment, as opposed to simply reflecting similar disparities in those who are cancer free. The question remains: To what degree are disparities among survivors attributable to the cancer experience?

Research on survivor disparities will need to employ techniques to overcome inherent challenges. Oversampling of non-White and low-SES survivors is needed to overcome their relative scarcity and the lower likelihood that they will respond to surveys (Smith et al., 2007). Use of appropriate, culturally sensitive research methods and materials will increase response rates and the validity of results (Hahn et al., 2010). This includes accounting for differences in literacy level and native language as well as validation of measurement scales for specific ethnic groups. Furthermore, consideration must be given to differences in cultural norms, attitudes, and beliefs about cancer.

In conclusion, cancer survivors are a large and growing group with unique health issues. Early evidence suggests that racial/ethnic and SES disparities exist among survivors, though many areas remain under-studied. Culturally appropriate interventions based on theoretical models that take into account the important cultural, environmental, and health system factors that contribute to these disparities are needed.

REFERENCES

Anderson, K. O., Mendoza, T. R., Valero, V., Richman, S. P., Russell, C., Hurley, J., . . . Cleeland, C. S. (2000). Minority cancer patients and their providers: Pain management attitudes and practice. *Cancer, 88,* 1929–1938.

Ashing-Giwa, K. T. (2005). The contextual model of HRQoL: A paradigm for expanding the HRQoL framework. *Quality of Life Research, 14,* 297–307.

Ashing-Giwa, K. T., Ganz, P. A., & Petersen, L. (1999). Quality of life of African-American and White long term breast carcinoma survivors. *Cancer, 85,* 418–426.

Ashing-Giwa, K. T., Gonzalez, P., Lim, J. W., Chung, C., Paz, B., Somlo, G., & Wakabayashi, M. T. (2010). Diagnostic and therapeutic delays among a multiethnic sample of breast and cervical cancer survivors. *Cancer, 116,* 3195–3204.

Ashing-Giwa, K. T., & Lim, J. W. (2009). Examining the impact of socioeconomic status and socioecologic stress on physical and mental health quality of life among breast cancer survivors. *Oncology Nursing Forum, 36,* 79–88.

Ashing-Giwa, K. T., & Lim, J. W. (2010). Predicting physical quality of life among a multiethnic sample of breast cancer survivors. *Quality of Life Research, 19,* 789–802.

Ashing-Giwa, K. T., Tejero, J. S., Kim, J., Padilla, G. V., & Hellemann, G. (2007). Examining predictive models of HRQOL in a population-based, multiethnic sample of women with breast carcinoma. *Quality of Life Research, 16,* 413–428.

Aziz, N. M., & Rowland, J. H. (2002). Cancer survivorship research among ethnic minority and medically underserved groups. *Oncology Nursing Forum, 29,* 789–801.

Baker, F., Denniston, M., Smith, T., & West, M. M. (2005). Adult cancer survivors: How are they faring? *Cancer, 104,* 2565–2576.

Beach, S. R., Schulz, R., Yee, J. L., & Jackson, S. (2000). Negative and positive health effects of caring for a disabled spouse: Longitudinal findings from the caregiver health effects study. *Psychology and Aging, 15,* 259–271.

Beckjord, E. B., Arora, N. K., McLaughlin, W., Oakley-Girvan, I., Hamilton, A. S., & Hesse, B. W. (2008). Health-related information needs in a large and diverse sample of adult cancer survivors: Implications for cancer care. *Journal of Cancer Survivorship, 2,* 179–189.

Bellizzi, K. M., Miller, M. F., Arora, N. K., & Rowland, J. H. (2007). Positive and negative life changes experienced by survivors of non-Hodgkin's lymphoma. *Annals of Behavioral Medicine, 34,* 188–199.

Bellizzi, K. M., Rowland, J. H., Jeffery, D. D., & McNeel, T. (2005). Health behaviors of cancer survivors: Examining opportunities for cancer control intervention. *Journal of Clinical Oncology, 23,* 8884–8893.

Bender, C. M., Sereika, S. M., Berga, S. L., Vogel, V. G., Brufsky, A. M., Paraska, K. K., & Ryan, C. M. (2006). Cognitive impairment associated with adjuvant therapy in breast cancer. *Psychooncology, 15,* 422–430.

Blanchard, C. M., Stein, K. D., Baker, F., Dent, M., Denniston, M., Courneya, K. S., & Nehl, E. (2004). Association between current lifestyle behaviors and health-related quality of life in breast, colorectal, and prostate cancer survivors. *Psychology & Health, 19,* 1–13.

Blank, J. J., Clark, L., Longman, A. J., & Atwood, J. R. (1989). Perceived home care needs of cancer patients and their caregivers. *Cancer Nursing, 12,* 78–84.

Bowen, D. J., Alfano, C. M., McGregor, B. A., Kuniyuki, A., Bernstein, L., Meeske, K., . . . Barbash, R. B. (2007). Possible socioeconomic and ethnic disparities in quality of life in a cohort of breast cancer survivors. *Breast Cancer Research and Treatment, 106,* 85–95.

Bower, J. E. (2008). Behavioral symptoms in patients with breast cancer and survivors. *Journal of Clinical Oncology, 26,* 768–777.

Bower, J. E., Ganz, P. A., Desmond, K. A., Bernaards, C., Rowland, J. H., Meyerowitz, B. E., & Belin, T. R. (2006). Fatigue in long-term breast carcinoma survivors: A longitudinal investigation. *Cancer, 106,* 751–758.

Burg, M. A., Lopez, E. D., Dailey, A., Keller, M. E., & Prendergast, B. (2009). The potential of survivorship care plans in primary care follow-up of minority breast cancer patients. *Journal of General Internal Medicine, 24*(Suppl. 2), S467–S471.

Caraceni, A., & Portenoy, R. K. (1999). An international survey of cancer pain characteristics and syndromes. IASP Task Force on Cancer Pain. International Association for the Study of Pain. *Pain, 82,* 263–274.

Centers for Disease Control and Prevention. (2004). *The national action plan for cancer survivorship: Advancing public health strategies.* Retrieved from http://www.cdc.gov/cancer/survivorship/pdf/plan.pdf

Chumbler, N. R., Grimm, J. W., Cody, M., & Beck, C. (2003). Gender, kinship and caregiver burden: The case of community-dwelling memory impaired seniors. *International Journal of Geriatric Psychiatry, 18,* 722–732.

Clauser, S. B., Arora, N. K., Bellizzi, K. M., Haffer, S. C., Topor, M., & Hays, R. D. (2008). Disparities in HRQOL of cancer survivors and non-cancer managed care enrollees. *Health Care Financing Review, 29,* 23–40.

Cleeland, C. S., Gonin, R., Baez, L., Loehrer, P., & Pandya, K. J. (1997). Pain and treatment of pain in minority patients with cancer. The Eastern Cooperative

Oncology Group Minority Outpatient Pain Study. *Annals of Internal Medicine, 127,* 813–816.

Courneya, K. S., Mackey, J. R., Bell, G. J., Jones, L. W., Field, C. J., & Fairey, A. S. (2003). Randomized controlled trial of exercise training in postmenopausal breast cancer survivors: Cardiopulmonary and quality of life outcomes. *Journal of Clinical Oncology, 21,* 1660–1668.

Darby, K., Davis, C., Likes, W., & Bell, J. (2009). Exploring the financial impact of breast cancer for African American medically underserved women: A qualitative study. *Journal of Health Care for the Poor and Underserved, 20,* 721–728.

Dimou, A., Syrigos, K. N., & Saif, M. W. (2009). Disparities in colorectal cancer in African-Americans vs Whites: Before and after diagnosis. *World Journal of Gastroenterology, 15,* 3734–3743.

Do, K. A., Johnson, M. M., Lee, J. J., Wu, X. F., Dong, Q., Hong, W. K., . . . Spitz, M. R. (2004). Longitudinal study of smoking patterns in relation to the development of smoking-related secondary primary tumors in patients with upper aerodigestive tract malignancies. *Cancer, 101,* 2837–2842.

Doubeni, C. A., Field, T. S., Ulcickas, Y. M., Rolnick, S. J., Quessenberry, C. P., Fouayzi, H., . . . Wei, F. (2006). Patterns and predictors of mammography utilization among breast cancer survivors. *Cancer, 106,* 2482–2488.

Doyle, C., Kushi, L. H., Byers, T., Courneya, K. S., Demark-Wahnefried, W., Grant, B., . . . Andrews. K. S. (2006). Nutrition and physical activity during and after cancer treatment: An American Cancer Society guide for informed choices. *CA: A Cancer Journal for Clinicians, 56,* 323–353.

Duncan, W., Warde, P., Catton, C. N., Munro, A. J., Lakier, R., Gadalla, T., & Gospodarowicz, M. K. (1993). Carcinoma of the prostate: Results of radical radiotherapy (1970–1985). *International Journal of Radiation Oncology, Biology, Physics, 26,* 203–210.

Dwight-Johnson, M., Ell, K., & Lee, P. J. (2005). Can collaborative care address the needs of low-income Latinas with comorbid depression and cancer? Results from a randomized pilot study. *Psychosomatics, 46,* 224–232.

Earle, C. C. (2007). Cancer survivorship research and guidelines: Maybe the cart should be beside the horse. *Journal of Clinical Oncology, 25,* 3800–3801.

Edwards, B. K., Howe, H. L., Ries, L. A., Thun, M. J., Rosenberg, H. M., Yancik, R., . . . Feigal, E. G. (2002). Annual report to the nation on the status of cancer, 1973–1999, featuring implications of age and aging on U.S. cancer burden. *Cancer, 94,* 2766–2792.

Ellison, G. L., Warren, J. L., Knopf, K. B., & Brown, M. L. (2003). Racial differences in the receipt of bowel surveillance following potentially curative colorectal cancer surgery. *Health Services Research, 38,* 1885–1903.

Emanuel, E. J., Fairclough, D. L., Slutsman, J., Alpert, H., Baldwin, D., & Emanuel, L. L. (1999). Assistance from family members, friends, paid care givers, and volunteers in the care of terminally ill patients. *New England Journal of Medicine, 341,* 956–963.

Eversley, R., Estrin, D., Dibble, S., Wardlaw, L., Pedrosa, M., & Favila-Penney, W. (2005). Post-treatment symptoms among ethnic minority breast cancer survivors. *Oncology Nursing Forum, 32,* 250–256.

Field, T. S., Doubeni, C., Fox, M. P., Buist, D. S., Wei, F., Geiger, A. M., . . . Silliman, R. A. (2008). Under utilization of surveillance mammography among older breast cancer survivors. *Journal of General Internal Medicine, 23,* 158–163.

Foley, K. L., Farmer, D. F., Petronis, V. M., Smith, R. G., McGraw, S., Smith, K., . . . Avis, N. (2006). A qualitative exploration of the cancer experience among long-term survivors: Comparisons by cancer type, ethnicity, gender, and age. *Psychooncology, 15,* 248–258.

Ganz, P. A. (2005). A teachable moment for oncologists: Cancer survivors, 10 million strong and growing! *Journal of Clinical Oncology, 23,* 5458–5460.

Ganz, P. A., Desmond, K. A., Leedham, B., Rowland, J. H., Meyerowitz, B. E., & Belin, T. R. (2002). Quality of life in long-term, disease-free survivors of breast cancer: A follow-up study. *Journal of the National Cancer Institute, 94,* 39–49.

Ganz, P. A., & Hahn, E. E. (2008). Implementing a survivorship care plan for patients with breast cancer. *Journal of Clinical Oncology, 26,* 759–767.

Given, B. A., Given, C. W., & Kozachik, S. (2001). Family support in advanced cancer. *CA: A Cancer Journal for Clinicians, 51,* 213–231.

Given, C. W., Given, B. A., & Stommel, M. (1994). The impact of age, treatment, and symptoms on the physical and mental health of cancer patients. A longitudinal perspective. *Cancer, 74,* 2128–2138.

Gordon, L., Scuffham, P., Hayes, S., & Newman, B. (2007). Exploring the economic impact of breast cancers during the 18 months following diagnosis. *Psychooncology, 16,* 1130–1139.

Grunfeld, E., Levine, M. N., Julian, J. A., Coyle, D., Szechtman, B., Mirsky, D., . . . Whelan, T. (2006). Randomized trial of long-term follow-up for early-stage breast cancer: A comparison of family physician versus specialist care. *Journal of Clinical Oncology, 24,* 848–855.

Hahn, E. A., Du, H., Garcia, S. F., Choi, S. W., Lai, J. S., Victorson, D., & Cella, D. (2010). Literacy-fair measurement of health-related quality of life will facilitate comparative effectiveness research in Spanish-speaking cancer outpatients. *Medical Care, 48,* S75–S82.

Hao, Y., Landrine, H., Smith, T., Kaw, C., Corral, I., & Stein, K. (2010). Residential segregation and disparities in health-related quality of life among Black and White cancer survivors. *Health Psychology, 30*(2), 137–144.

Hawkins, N. A., Smith, T., Zhao, L., Rodriguez, J., Berkowitz, Z., & Stein, K. D. (2010). Health-related behavior change after cancer: Results of the American Cancer Society's studies of cancer survivors (SCS). *Journal of Cancer Survivorship, 4,* 20–32.

Hewitt, M. E., Bamundo, A., Day, R., & Harvey, C. (2007). Perspectives on post-treatment cancer care: Qualitative research with survivors, nurses, and physicians. *Journal of Clinical Oncology, 25,* 2270–2273.

Himmelstein, D. U., Thorne, D., Warren, E., & Woolhandler, S. (2009). Medical bankruptcy in the United States, 2007: Results of a national study. *American Journal of Medicine, 122,* 741–746.

Humpel, N., Magee, C., & Jones, S. C. (2007). The impact of a cancer diagnosis on the health behaviors of cancer survivors and their family and friends. *Supportive Care in Cancer, 15,* 621–630.

Institute of Medicine. (2006). *From cancer patient to cancer survivor: Lost in transition.* Washington, DC: The National Academies Press.

Jansen, C., Halliburton, P., Dibble, S., & Dodd, M. J. (1993). Family problems during cancer chemotherapy. *Oncology Nursing Forum, 20,* 689–694.

Kantsiper, M., McDonald, E. L., Geller, G., Shockney, L., Snyder, C., & Wolff, A. C. (2009). Transitioning to breast cancer survivorship: Perspectives of patients, cancer specialists, and primary care providers. *Journal of General Internal Medicine, 24*(Suppl. 2), S459–S466.

Keating, N. L., Landrum, M. B., Guadagnoli, E., Winer, E. P., & Ayanian, J. Z. (2006). Factors related to underuse of surveillance mammography among breast cancer survivors. *Journal of Clinical Oncology, 24*, 85–94.

Keating, N. L., Landrum, M. B., Guadagnoli, E., Winer, E. P., & Ayanian, J. Z. (2007). Surveillance testing among survivors of early-stage breast cancer. *Journal of Clinical Oncology, 25*, 1074–1081.

Kim, Y., Baker, F., Spillers, R. L., & Wellisch, D. K. (2006). Psychological adjustment of cancer caregivers with multiple roles. *Psychooncology, 15*, 795–804.

Kim, Y., & Given, B. A. (2008). Quality of life of family caregivers of cancer survivors: Across the trajectory of the illness. *Cancer, 112*, 2556–2568.

Kim, Y., & Schulz, R. (2008). Family caregivers' strains: Comparative analysis of cancer caregiving with dementia, diabetes, and frail elderly caregiving. *Journal of Aging and Health, 20*, 483–503.

Kim, Y., Schulz, R., & Carver, C. S. (2007). Benefit-finding in the cancer caregiving experience. *Psychosomatic Medicine, 69*, 283–291.

Longo, C. J., Fitch, M., Deber, R. B., & Williams, A. P. (2006). Financial and family burden associated with cancer treatment in Ontario, Canada. *Supportive Care in Cancer, 14*, 1077–1085.

Lykins, E. L., Graue, L. O., Brechting, E. H., Roach, A. R., Gochett, C. G., & Andrykowski, M. A. (2008). Beliefs about cancer causation and prevention as a function of personal and family history of cancer: A national, population-based study. *Psychooncology, 17*, 967–974.

Mao, J. J., Armstrong, K., Bowman, M. A., Xie, S. X., Kadakia, R., & Farrar, J. T. (2007). Symptom burden among cancer survivors: Impact of age and comorbidity. *Journal of the American Board of Family Medicine, 20*, 434–443.

Mao, J. J., Bowman, M. A., Stricker, C. T., DeMichele, A., Jacobs, L., Chan, D., & Armstrong, K. (2009). Delivery of survivorship care by primary care physicians: The perspective of breast cancer patients. *Journal of Clinical Oncology, 27*, 933–938.

Mariotto, A. B., Rowland, J. H., Ries, L. A., Scoppa, S., & Feuer, E. J. (2007). Multiple cancer prevalence: A growing challenge in long-term survivorship. *Cancer Epidemiology, Biomarkers and Prevention 16*, 566–571.

Martini, N., Bains, M. S., Burt, M. E., Zakowski, M. F., McCormack, P., Rusch, V. W., & Ginsberg, R. J. (1995). Incidence of local recurrence and second primary tumors in resected stage I lung cancer. *Journal of Thoracic and Cardiovascular Surgery, 109*, 120–129.

Mayer, D. K., Terrin, N. C., Menon, U., Kreps, G. L., McCance, K., Parsons, S. K., & Mooney, K. H. (2007). Screening practices in cancer survivors. *Journal of Cancer Survivorship, 1*, 17–26.

McCausland, J. & Pakenham, K. I. (2003). Investigation of the benefits of HIV/AIDS caregiving and relations among caregiving adjustment, benefit finding, and stress and coping variables. *AIDS Care, 15*, 853–869.

Meyerhardt, J. A., Heseltine, D., Niedzwiecki, D., Hollis, D., Saltz, L. B., Mayer, R. J., . . . Fuchs, C. S. (2006). Impact of physical activity on cancer recurrence and survival in patients with stage III colon cancer: Findings from CALGB 89803. *Journal of Clinical Oncology, 24*, 3535–3541.

Meyerhardt, J. A., Niedzwiecki, D., Hollis, D., Saltz, L. B., Hu, F. B., Mayer, R. J., . . . Fuchs, C. S. (2007). Association of dietary patterns with cancer recurrence and survival in patients with stage III colon cancer. *Journal of the American Medical Association, 298*, 754–764.

Moran, M. S., Yang, Q., Harris, L. N., Jones, B., Tuck, D. P., & Haffty, B. G. (2008). Long-term outcomes and clinicopathologic differences of African-American versus White patients treated with breast conservation therapy for early-stage breast cancer. *Cancer, 113*, 2565–2574.

Mullan, F. (1985). Seasons of survival: Reflections of a physician with cancer. *New England Journal of Medicine, 313*, 270–273.

Mustian, K. M., Morrow, G. R., Carroll, J. K., Figueroa-Moseley, C. D., Jean-Pierre, P., & Williams, G. C. (2007). Integrative nonpharmacologic behavioral interventions for the management of cancer-related fatigue. *Oncologist, 12*(Suppl 1), 52–67.

National Alliance in Caregiving & AARP. (2009). *Caregiving in the U.S.* Bethesda, MD: Author. Retrieved from http://www.caregiving.org/data/CaregivingUSAllAgesExecSum.pdf

National Cancer Institute. (2010). *Follow-up care after cancer treatment*. Bethesda, MD: Author. Retrieved from http://www.cancer.gov/cancertopics/factsheet/therapy/followup

Ng, A. K., Li, S., Recklitis, C., Diller, L. R., Neuberg, D., Silver, B., & Mauch, P. M. (2008). Health practice in long-term survivors of Hodgkin's lymphoma. *International Journal of Radiation Oncology, Biology, Physics, 71*, 468–476.

Nijboer, C., Tempelaar, R., Sanderman, R., Triemstra, M., Spruijt, R. J., & van den Bos, G. A. (1998). Cancer and caregiving: The impact on the caregiver's health. *Psychooncology, 7*, 3–13.

Nissen, M. J., Beran, M. S., Lee, M. W., Mehta, S. R., Pine, D. A., & Swenson, K. K. (2007). Views of primary care providers on follow-up care of cancer patients. *Family Medicine, 39*, 477–482.

Oeffinger, K. C. & McCabe, M. S. (2006). Models for delivering survivorship care. *Journal of Clinical Oncology, 24*, 5117–5124.

Ok, H., Marks, R., & Allegrante, J. P. (2008). Perceptions of health care provider communication activity among American cancer survivors and adults without cancer histories: An analysis of the 2003 Health Information Trends Survey (HINTS) data. *Journal of Health Communication, 13*, 637–653.

Richardson, A., & Ream, E. (1996). The experience of fatigue and other symptoms in patients receiving chemotherapy. *European Journal of Cancer Care (England), 5*, 24–30.

Royak-Schaler, R., Passmore, S. R., Gadalla, S., Hoy, M. K., Zhan, M., Tkaczuk, K., . . . Hutchison, A. P. (2008). Exploring patient–physician communication in breast cancer care for African American women following primary treatment. *Oncology Nursing Forum, 35*, 836–843.

Sabatino, S. A., Coates, R. J., Uhler, R. J., Alley, L. G., & Pollack, L. A. (2006). Health insurance coverage and cost barriers to needed medical care among U.S. adult cancer survivors age <65 years. *Cancer, 106*, 2466–2475.

Satia, J. A., Walsh, J. F., & Pruthi, R. S. (2009). Health behavior changes in White and African American prostate cancer survivors. *Cancer Nursing, 32*, 107–117.

Schootman, M., Deshpande, A. D., Pruitt, S. L., Aft, R., & Jeffe, D. B. (2010). National estimates of racial disparities in health status and behavioral risk factors among long-term cancer survivors and non-cancer controls. *Cancer Causes and Control, 21*, 1387–1395.

Schover, L. R. (2005). Sexuality and fertility after cancer. *Hematology (American Society of Hematology Education Program)*, 523–527.

Schultz, P. N., Stava, C., Beck, M. L., & Vassilopoulou-Sellin, R. (2004). Ethnic/racial influences on the physiologic health of cancer survivors. *Cancer, 100,* 156–164.

SEER. (2006). *New malignancies among cancer survivors: SEER cancer registries, 1973–2000.* Bethesda, MD: National Cancer Institute. Retrieved from http://seer.cancer.gov/publications/mpmono

SEER. (2010). *SEER Cancer statistics review, 1973–2000.* Bethesda, MD: National Cancer Institute. Retrieved from http://seer.cancer.gov/csr/1975_2007

Short, P. F., & Mallonee, E. L. (2006). Income disparities in the quality of life of cancer survivors. *Medical Care, 44*(1): 16–23.

Smith, T., Crammer, C., & Stefanek, M. (2010). *Health behaviors and beliefs among cancer survivors, family members, and the general population: The HINTS perspective.* Oral presentation at the 31st Meeting of the Society for Behavioral Medicine, Seattle, WA.

Smith, T., Kaw, C., & Love-Ghaffari, M. (2010). Employment experiences in the first year after diagnosis with cancer employment outcomes in a population-based sample of 1-year cancer survivors. *Manuscript submitted for publication.*

Smith, T., Stein, K., Mehta, C., Kaw, C., Kepner, J., Buskirk, T., . . . Baker, F. (2007). The rationale, design, and implementation of the American Cancer Society's studies of cancer survivors. *Cancer, 109*(1), 1–12.

Snyder, C. F., Earle, C. C., Herbert, R. J., Neville, B. A., Blackford, A. L., & Frick, K. D. (2008). Preventive care for colorectal cancer survivors: A 5-year longitudinal study. *Journal of Clinical Oncology, 26,* 1073–1079.

Snyder, C. F., Frick, K. D., Peairs, K. S., Kantsiper, M. E., Herbert, R. J., Blackford, A. L., . . . Earler, C. C. (2009). Comparing care for breast cancer survivors to non-cancer controls: A five-year longitudinal study. *Journal of General Internal Medicine, 24,* 469–474.

Son, K. Y., Park, S. M., Lee, C. H., Choi, G. J., Lee, D., Jo, S., . . . Cho, B. (2010). Behavioral risk factors and use of preventive screening services among spousal caregivers of cancer patients. *Supportive Care in Cancer, 19*(7), 919–927.

Stein, K. D., Smith, T., Sharpe, K., Zhao, L., & Kirch, R. (2010). *Prevalence and correlates of barriers to pain management among cancer survivors: Results of the American Cancer Society's Studies of Cancer Survivors (SCS).* Oral presentation at the 31st Meeting of the Society for Behavioral Medicine, Seattle, WA.

Stein, K. D., Syrjala, K. L., & Andrykowski, M. A. (2008). Physical and psychological long-term and late effects of cancer. *Cancer, 112,* 2577–2592.

Stolley, M. R., Sharp, L. K., Wells, A. M., Simon, N., & Schiffer, L. (2006). Health behaviors and breast cancer: Experiences of urban African American women. *Health Education and Behavior, 33,* 604–624.

Stone, P., Richards, M., A'Hern, R., & Hardy, J. (2000). A study to investigate the prevalence, severity and correlates of fatigue among patients with cancer in comparison with a control group of volunteers without cancer. *Annals of Oncology, 11,* 561–567.

Tomich, P. L., Helgeson, V. S., & Nowak Vache, E. J. (2005). Perceived growth and decline following breast cancer: A comparison to age-matched controls 5-years later. *Psychooncology, 14,* 1018–1029.

U.S. Census Bureau. (2008). *Annual estimates of the population by sex, race, and Hispanic origin for the United States: April 1, 2000 to July, 2007.* Washington, DC: Population Division, U.S. Census Bureau. Retrieved from http://www.census.gov/popest/national/asrh/NC-EST2007/NC-EST2007-03.xls

USA Today, Henry J. Kaiser Family Foundation, & Harvard School of Public Health. (2006). *National survey of households affected by cancer*. Menlo Park, CA: Henry J. Kaiser Family Foundation. Retrieved from http://www.kff.org/kaiserpolls/upload/7591.pdf

van den Beuken-van Everdingen, M. H., de Rijke, J. M., Kessels, A. G., Schouten, H. C., van Kleef, M., & Patijn, J. (2007). Prevalence of pain in patients with cancer: A systematic review of the past 40 years. *Annals of Oncology, 18*, 1437–1449.

Vicini, F., Jones, P., Rivers, A., Wallace, M., Mitchell, C., Kestin, L., . . . Martinez, A. (2010). Differences in disease presentation, management techniques, treatment outcome, and toxicities in African-American women with early stage breast cancer treated with breast-conserving therapy. *Cancer, 116*, 3485–3492.

Weitzner, M. A., McMillan, S. C., & Jacobsen, P. B. (1999). Family caregiver quality of life: Differences between curative and palliative cancer treatment settings. *Journal of Pain and Symptom Management, 17*, 418–428.

Williamson, G. M., Shaffer, D. R., & Schulz, R. (1998). Activity restriction and prior relationship history as contributors to mental health outcomes among middle-aged and older spousal caregivers. *Health Psychology, 17*, 152–162.

Yabroff, K. R., & Kim, Y. (2009). Time costs associated with informal caregiving for cancer survivors. *Cancer, 115*, 4362–4373.

Yoon, J., Malin, J. L., Tisnado, D. M., Tao, M. L., Adams, J. L., Timmer, M. J., . . . Kahn, K. L. (2008). Symptom management after breast cancer treatment: Is it influenced by patient characteristics? *Breast Cancer Research and Treatment, 108*, 69–77.

6

The Geography of Cancer and Its Risk Factors: Implications of Neighborhood Disparities for Cancer Disparities[1]

Hope Landrine, Irma Corral, Yongping Hao, Chiewkwei Kaw, Joy L. King, and Julia C. Fondren

There is now widespread interest in the role of neighborhoods in cancer and cancer disparities (Baker, Hoel, Mohr, Lipsitz, & Lackland, 2000; Krieger et al., 2002; Singh, Miller, Hankey, & Edwards, 2003). This new focus on the *geography of cancer and its risk factors* reflects mounting evidence that both are unequally distributed across neighborhoods that differ in poverty, ethnicity, and rurality (Campbell et al., 2002; Coughlin, Leadbetter, Richards, & Sabatino, 2008; Coughlin et al., 2006; Hsu, Jacobson, & Soto Mas, 2004; Onega et al., 2008). Neighborhoods contribute to disparities in cancer and its risk factors and, hence, understanding the nature of that contribution can highlight new community-level approaches to reducing cancer disparities (Kawachi & Berkman, 2003).

This chapter provides a brief overview of the geography of cancer and its risk factors. Due to space limitations, we focus only on Blacks and Whites, and exclude data on other ethnic-minority groups. Likewise, we focus on the role of geographic variables in only three of many cancer risk factors (i.e., smoking, obesity, cancer screening), to devote more attention to the role of such variables in cancer incidence, stage at diagnosis, treatment, mortality, and survival. The geographic (area-level) variables of focus are neighborhood socioeconomic status (SES), residential segregation, and rurality, the three most often examined in research. First, we define these area variables and strategies for measuring them. Next, we examine their association with the

---

[1]The findings and conclusions in this chapter are those of the author(s) and do not necessarily represent the views of the Centers for Disease Control and Prevention.

three cancer risk factors. This is followed by a summary of their associations with cancer incidence, treatment, stage at diagnosis, mortality, and survival. Finally, we discuss the possible mechanisms of area-level influences.

AREA-LEVEL VARIABLES

Neighborhood-SES

Neighborhood-SES refers to the level of poverty, economic deprivation, or affluence of an area, and can be measured at a variety of area levels, including state, county, zip code, and census tract (Krieger et al., 2002; Krieger, Chen, Waterman, Rehkpof, & Subramanian, 2003, 2005). In general, the smaller the area in which area-SES is assessed, the stronger is the association between area-SES and health. This is because large areas (e.g., states, zip codes) contain the entire range of smaller SES-areas within them—that is, both poor and affluent neighborhoods (Krieger et al., 2002, 2003, 2005). Consequently, significant area-SES differences are more often found within large areas than between them. Hence, measuring area-SES in small areas (i.e., census tract) is widely regarded as superior to measurement at larger area levels, with census-tract (CT) level measurement most predictive of health disparities (Krieger et al., 2005). This is because, unlike zip codes (mean N = 30,000) and Metropolitan Statistical Areas (MSA) such as Los Angeles–Long Beach, CA (N = several million), CTs are small (mean N = 4,000) areas that are largely homogenous in ethnicity, living conditions (e.g., amenities), life circumstances (e.g., owning vs. renting), and area-SES (e.g., property values).

Area-SES can be measured in many ways, including median price of homes, percentage of residents below the poverty line (% BPL), median household income, and the Townsend (deprivation) Index (Krieger et al., 2003, 2005). Clearly, some of these measures are simply aggregates of the individual-level SES of the area's residents (e.g., median household income), whereas others are more contextual (e.g., median price of homes, average rent paid). Hence, the correlation between individual- and area-level SES can be large when aggregate measures are used. Irrespective of whether aggregate or contextual measures are used, however, the correlation between individual- and area-SES is larger for Whites than for Blacks, because Blacks—irrespective of individual-level SES (e.g., household income)—tend to live in poorer neighborhoods than Whites of matched individual-level SES (Krieger et al., 2005; Krieger, Williams, & Moss, 1997). Nonetheless, as will be shown, individual- and area-level SES have independent associations with cancer and cancer risk factors.

Segregation

Residential segregation refers to the geographic separation of ethnic minorities (Blacks in this chapter) from Whites in residential areas (Iceland, Weinberg, & Steinmetz, 2002; Johnston, Poulsen, & Forrest, 2007). Segregation can be measured at any area level, with measurement at smaller (e.g., CT) levels preferred. Again, this is because large areas (e.g., states, counties) contain both highly segregated and integrated smaller areas within them, such that segregation differences are larger within than between large areas. Hence, like area-SES, measuring segregation at the CT level—or at the MSA level, with MSA-segregation calculated from CT data—is psychometrically superior and preferred (Iceland et al., 2002; Johnston et al., 2007).

Segregation can be measured in many ways. These include dissimilarity (the uneven distribution of Blacks and Whites in a residential area), Isolation (the probability that Blacks will encounter only other Blacks in their residential area), concentration (the population density of Black neighborhoods), clustering (the extent to which Black neighborhoods are surrounded by other Black neighborhoods), centralization (the degree to which Black neighborhoods are in a city's urban center vs. the suburbs), and hypersegregation, the simultaneous occurrence of all of these (Massey & Denton, 1988; Massey, White, & Phua, 1996; Wilkes & Iceland, 2004). Of these well-accepted measures, the Isolation Index exhibits greater psychometric integrity (i.e., validity, interpretability) than the others (Acevedo-Garcia, Lochner, Osypuk, & Subramanian, 2003; Chang, Hillier, & Mehta, 2009). Crude measures with questionable validity (e.g., percentage of Blacks in an area) often are used in research as well (Kramer & Hogue, 2009).

The correlation between segregation and area-SES is small (i.e., $r = .10-.20$), that is, there are both affluent and poor, mostly Black, neighborhoods. Likewise, the correlation between individual-SES and segregation is small; this is because, as a result of housing discrimination, most Blacks (65%) live in mostly Black (segregated) neighborhoods irrespective of their individual-SES and their preference to live in integrated areas (Adelman, 2004; Alba, Logan, & Stults, 2000; Farley, 2005; Landrine & Corral, 2009).

Rurality

The definition of rural versus urban areas is constantly changing (Probst, Moore, Glover, & Samuels, 2004), but generally refers to area population density. As of 2000, the U.S. Census Bureau defines urban areas as those with populations of 250,000 to >1 million, rural areas as those with populations of <2,500, and suburban areas as those adjacent to but outside of urban areas, with residents commuting to the urban area for work (http://www.census.gov).

AREA-LEVEL VARIABLES AND CANCER RISK FACTORS

Smoking

Area-SES

Numerous studies have examined the role of neighborhood-SES in cigarette smoking. A few of these are summarized in Table 6.1, where all studies controlled for individual-level SES. As shown, as area-SES decreases, smoking prevalence generally increases among adult women and men alike, even when controlling for age, education, and income. For example, in their study of 41,726 Black women, Datta, Subramanian et al. (2006), found an overall smoking prevalence rate of 16.2%. Smoking prevalence was nearly twice as high in high-poverty CTs (defined as ≥20% BPL) than in low-poverty CTs (≤5% BPL), after controlling for individual-level demographic factors. Likewise, a study of the 39,695 (multiethnic) participants in the Third National Health and Nutrition Examination Survey (NHANES-III) found that the percentage of smokers increased significantly with increasing neighborhood deprivation, the latter defined as the percentage of households without telephones or plumbing, median rent paid, and other variables; this effect held even after controlling for gender, age, marital status, race/ethnicity, and education and income (Stimpson, Ju, Raji, & Eschback, 2007).

Rurality and Segregation

Studies consistently have found a higher prevalence of smoking in rural than in urban areas (among men in particular), with cigarette smoking often combined with use of smokeless tobacco among rural men (e.g., Bell et al., 2009; Doescher, Jackson, Jerant, & Hart, 2006; Nelson et al., 2006). Studies of residential segregation and smoking among African Americans have yielded less consistent results (Bell, Zimmerman, Mayer, Almgren, & Huebner, 2007; Datta, Subramanian et al., 2006; Dell, Whitman, Shah, Silva, & Ansell, 2005; Northridge et al., 1998). One study found no relationship (Datta, Subramanian et al., 2006), two found smoking rates higher among Blacks in segregated-Black than in integrated areas (Dell et al., 2005; Northridge et al., 1998), and one found a U-shaped relationship between segregation and smoking during pregnancy among Black women (Bell et al., 2007). These inconsistencies may reflect sample differences in gender (women only vs. women and men), as well as differences in the measure of segregation used, as noted below.

Obesity

Area-SES

Numerous studies have found strong relationships between area-SES and obesity, that is, body mass index (BMI) ≥ 30 (e.g., Black & Macinko, 2008; Boardman, Saint Onge, Rogers, & Denney, 2005; Drewnowski, Rehm, & Solet,

TABLE 6.1 Selected Studies on the Role of Area Variables in Cancer Risk Factors

Cigarette Smoking

Author	Participants	Area-SES Measures	Low Area-SES Associated With
Datta et al. (2006)	$N = 41,726$ U.S. Black women	Census tract (CT) residents, % BPL	Increased smoking prevalence
Diez-Roux et al. (1997)	$N = 12,601$ U.S. adults	Census block (CB) median housing price, education, occupation	Increased smoking prevalence
Diez-Roux et al. (2003)	$N = 3,472$ U.S. women and men, Blacks and Whites, ages 18–30 years	CT and CB income, education, and occupation	Increased smoking prevalence among Whites only
Ross (2000)	$N = 2,482$ Illinois adults, 59% women, 84% White	CT poverty and education	Increased smoking prevalence among men only
Tseng et al. (2001)	$N = 648$ North Carolina women, 42% Black	CB poverty, unemployment, home and car ownership	Increased smoking prevalence

Obesity/BMI

Author	Participants	Area-level SES Measures	Low Area-SES Associated With
Drewnowski et al. (2007)	$N = 8,803$ adults from 74 zip codes	Zip code % BPL, median value of homes, etc.	Increased prevalence of obesity
Stimpson et al. (2007)	$N = 39,695$ adults in the NHANES III	CT % BPL, percentage without phones and other measures	Increased prevalence of obesity
Wang et al. (2007)	$N = 7,595$ California adults	CT and CB median housing values, percentage unemployed and other indices	Higher BMI and higher rates of obesity

(continued)

TABLE 6.1 *(continued)*

Author	Participants	Segregation Measure	High Segregation Associated With
Boardman et al. (2005)	National sample of N = 402,154 adults	CB proportion of Blacks	Increased obesity prevalence
Chang (2006)	National sample of N = 46,881 adults	Metropolitan statistical area (MSA) Black Isolation averaged from CT Isolation	Increased prevalence of over-weight and obesity
Chang et al. (2009)	N = 6,608 Philadelphia women	CT-level Black Isolation Index	Increased BMI and obesity prevalence
Mobley et al. (2006)	N = 2,692 women	Zip code and county-level Black Isolation Index	No significant association
Robert and Reither (2004)	N = 3,617 adults	CT-level percent Blacks	No significant association

Cancer Screening

Author	Participants	Area-SES Measure	Low Area-SES Associated With
Jackson et al. (2009)	Breast; N = 33,938 California women, ages 40–84 years	CT-level income	Lower rates of breast cancer screening
Harper et al. (2009)	Breast; women in SEER and NHIS 1987–2005	County-level % BPL	Lower rates of breast cancer screening
Coughlin et al. (2006)	Cervical; N = 49,231 women in 2000 and 2002 BRFSS	County income and education	Lower rates of PAP testing within the last 3 years

Author	Participants	Area-SES Measure	Low Area-SES Associated With
Pruitt et al. (2009)	Breast, cervical, and colorectal; review of 19 studies	Varied from CT to MSAs and county level, and from area-income/education to % BPL	Lower rates of all three types of cancer screening, largely irrespective of area-level and area-SES measures
Schootman et al. (2006)	Breast, cervical, and colorectal; $N = 118,000$ adults in 98 MSAs and 740 counties	MSA % BPL, calculated from CT data	Lower rates of all three types of screening, and higher rates of never-screening

Author	Participants	Segregation Measure	High Segregation Associated With
Dai (2010)	Breast; 12,413 women with diag-nosed breast cancer	Zip code Black Isolation Index	Increased diagnosis of late- (vs. early-) stage breast cancer
Mobley et al. (2008)	Breast; $N = 224,585$ women with breast cancer, from 11 states, SEER data	Zip code Black Isolation Index	Lower and higher screening depending on state

2007; Glass, Rasmussen, & Schwartz, 2006; Robert & Reither, 2004; Stimpson et al., 2007; Wang, Soowan, Gonzalez, MacLeod, & Winkleby, 2007). A few of these are summarized in Table 6.1, where all studies controlled for individual-level SES. As shown, as area deprivation or poverty increases, BMI increases among women and men, even when controlling for individual-level SES and other variables.

For example, a study of a random sample of 1,140 U.S. adults found that residents of hazardous neighborhoods were nearly 2 times more likely than residents of nonhazardous neighborhoods to be obese (53% vs. 27%, respectively). Neighborhood hazard was defined by the Townsend Index (housing quality, unemployment, crowding, etc.), as well as by the number of liquor stores and violent crimes (Glass et al., 2006). Likewise, in their study of the 39,695 participants in the NHANES III, Stimpson et al. (2007) found that BMI increased with increasing neighborhood deprivation, even when controlling for age, gender, income, physical activity levels, alcohol use, smoking, race/ethnicity, and education. On the whole, such findings are stronger for women than for men, suggesting that gender may mediate the relationships between neighborhood-SES and BMI (Black & Macinko, 2008; Do et al., 2007).

Rurality and Segregation

Only a few studies have examined the role of residential segregation in obesity among Black adults; these are summarized in Table 6.1 (i.e., Boardman et al., 2005; Chang, 2006; Chang et al., 2009; Mobley et al., 2006; Robert & Reither, 2004). As shown, results are mixed, with three studies finding positive relationships and two finding none. For example, Chang (2006) found a strong association between segregation and obesity among Black (but not White) adults, in which each 1 standard-deviation increase in segregation (Black Isolation) was associated with a 0.423 increase in Black BMI, and a 14% increase in Blacks' odds of being overweight—even when controlling for individual-level SES, physical activity, age, gender, and diet. Boardman et al. (2005) found nearly identical results. Alternatively, Mobley et al. (2006) and Robert and Reither (2004) found no effect. These inconsistencies probably reflect differences in the area-level and segregation measures used. Indeed, the inconsistent findings for segregation and smoking, and for segregation and obesity, may both reflect the null results obtained when using either a crude measure of segregation (percent Black) or a very large (zip code, county) area (Kramer & Hogue, 2009).

Unlike the inconsistent results for segregation and BMI, studies consistently have found that the prevalence of overweight (BMI $\geq$ 25) and obesity (BMI $\geq$ 30) are higher in urban than in rural areas among women and men, children, and adolescents (Bodor, Rice, Farley, Swalm, & Rose, 2010; Drewnowski et al., 2007; Dunton, Kaplan, Wolch, Jerrett, & Reynolds, 2009; Ford & Mokdad, 2008; Mascie-Taylor & Goto, 2007).

Cancer Screening

Area-SES

Numerous studies have found a strong association between area-SES and cancer screening. As shown by the examples in Table 6.1, the majority found that cancer screening increases with increasing area-SES (e.g., Coughlin, King, Richards, & Ekwueme, 2006; Harper et al., 2009; Jackson et al., 2009; Pruitt, Shim, Mullen, Vernon, & Amick, 2009; Schootman, Jeffe, Baker, & Walker, 2006). The few negative findings are likely to reflect differences in the area level used, with null findings generally emerging in studies that used large area levels.

Rurality and Segregation

One of the most clearly established geographic relationships is the strong association between rural residence and lower cancer screening prevalence. Consistently across a variety of types of studies and types of cancer screening, researchers have found that those who reside in rural areas are significantly less likely to have been screened for cancers, and likewise are more likely to be diagnosed at a later cancer stage than nonrural residents (Coughlin, Leadbetter, Richards, & Sabatino, 2008; Coughlin, Uhler, Bobo, & Caplan, 2004; Huang, Dignan, Han, & Johnson, 2009; Jackson et al., 2009).

Only a handful of studies have examined the association between cancer screening and residential segregation, with contradictory findings obtained (Dai, 2010; DeChello, Gregorio, & Samociuk, 2006; Haas et al., 2008; Mobley, Kuo, Driscoll, Clayton, & Ansell, 2008). Moreover, many studies did not assess cancer screening but, instead, examined cancer stage at diagnosis, with late versus early stage interpreted as a proxy for low versus high screening, respectively. For example, Dai (2010) found that as segregation (Black Isolation at the zip code level) increased, the likelihood of being diagnosed with later-stage cancers increased, this being interpreted as implying a lack of early detection. Similarly, Mobley et al. (2008) found that as Black segregation increased, the probability of cancer screening decreased in some states; in other states, increasing Black segregation (Isolation) was associated with increased screening. Such findings suggest that segregation plays a role in cancer screening, but that role varies with the type of screening (e.g., breast vs. cervical) and the region of the United States (Mobley et al., 2008).

AREA-LEVEL VARIABLES AND CANCER

Cancer Incidence

Area-SES

Numerous studies have examined the relationship between area-SES and cancer incidence, and found that results vary by cancer site/type (Singh et al., 2003; Yin et al., 2010). For example, low area-SES is associated with elevated incidence for cancers of the stomach, lung, and cervix among Blacks and Whites alike (Baquet, Horm, Gibbs, & Greenwald, 1991; Gorey & Vena, 1994; Krieger et al., 2002). Alternatively, high area-SES consistently has been found to be related to increased incidence for cancers of the female breast, prostate, and colon (Whites only—Cheng et al., 2009; Reynolds et al., 2005; Robert et al., 2004). All of the above studies adjusted for individual-level characteristics; a few are summarized in Table 6.2.

Rurality and Segregation

The association of rurality with cancer incidence generally is consistent across studies, with higher incidence in urban than in rural communities (e.g., Reynolds et al., 2005; Robert et al., 2004; Sung, Blumenthal, Alema-Mensah, & McGrady, 1997). For example, a study on urban/rural differences in cervical cancer in Georgia Medicaid recipients (N = 111,208 women, 1988–1992) found a higher incidence of cervical cancer in metropolitan Atlanta (vs. rural areas), among Black women in particular (Sung et al., 1997). Data on segregation and cancer incidence are limited. High segregation is related to increased cancer incidence associated with ambient air toxics, with Black–White disparities in cancer incidence widening with increasing segregation (Morello-Frosch & Jesdale, 2006).

Cancer Mortality and Stage at Diagnosis

Area-SES

Although the role of area-SES in cancer incidence varies by cancer type, its association with stage at diagnosis and with cancer mortality is by and large consistent across cancer types. Lower area-SES is associated with late-stage diagnosis and higher mortality for both Blacks and Whites, above and beyond individual-level demographics (Cheng et al., 2009; Echeverria, Borrell, Brown, & Rhoads, 2009; Greenlee & Howe, 2009; MacKinnon et al., 2007; Yabroff & Gordis, 2003). However, because Blacks are overrepresented in low-SES areas, they are more likely to be diagnosed with late-stage disease (e.g., Campbell et al., 2009) and exhibit higher mortality than Whites (e.g., Gerend & Pai, 2008). For example, Yabroff and Gordis (2003) examined county-level SES

TABLE 6.2 Selected Studies on the Role of Area Variables in Cancer

Association of Area-SES and Cancer Incidence, Mortality, Stage at Diagnosis, Treatment, and Survival

Author	Participants	Area-SES Measures	Low Area-SES Associated With
Yin et al. (2010)	CA statewide national sample of breast, prostate, colorectal, cervical, and lung cancer survivors diagnosed between 1998 and 2002 ($n = 376,158$)	CT and CB SES (occupation, unemployment, median household income, % BPL, median gross rent, median value of owner-occupied houses, etc.	Decreased cervical, lung, and colorectal cancer incidence (especially White); increased breast and prostate cancer incidence (Blacks and Whites)
Cheng et al. (2009)	CA statewide sample of prostate survivors diagnosed between 1998 and 2002 ($n = 98,484$)	CB SES (education, income, and occupation)	Decreased prostate cancer incidence; increased mortality
Yabroff and Gordis (2003)	National sample of breast cancer cases from SEER	County-level SES (median family income, % BPL, education, unemployment)	Decreased localized breast cancer incidence; increased distant breast cancer incidence; increased case-fatality rate
Zell et al. (2007)	CA statewide sample of pancreatic cancer cases diagnosed between 1989 and 2003 ($n = 24,735$)	CB SES (education, median household income, % BPL, median house value, median rent, occupation, employment)	Poor survival
Ward et al. (2004)	National sample from SEER diagnosed between 1975 and 2000	CT % BPL	13% higher death rates from cancer in men and 3% higher rates in women; 10% points lower in survival

(continued)

TABLE 6.2 (*continued*)

Association of Urbanicity and Cancer Incidence, Mortality, Stage at Diagnosis, Treatment, and Survival

Author	Participants	Rural-Urban Measures	High Urbanicity Associated With
Robert et al. (2004)	Population-based Wisconsin breast cancer survivors and control (*n* = 14,667)	CT and zip-code Census Bureau-defined rural and urban categories	Increased breast cancer incidence
McLafferty and Wang (2009)	IL statewide sample of breast, prostate, colorectal, and lung cancer cases diagnosed between 1998 and 2002	Zip-code level RUCA (Rural-Urban Continuum/Commuting codes from the Department of Agriculture)	Increased cancer risk, following a J-shaped progression (with small upturn in the most isolated rural areas)
Hao et al. (2010)	GA statewide colorectal survivors diagnosed between 2000 and 2004 (*n* = 4,748)	RUCA classification	Increased odds of receiving chemotherapy, but urban Blacks were less likely to receive the treatment than Whites

Author	Participants	Segregation Measures	**High Segregation Associated With**
Morello-Frosch and Jesdale (2006)	45,710 census tracts in 309 U.S. metropolitan areas	MSA Dissimilarity Index	Increased estimated cancer risk associated with ambient air toxics
Dai (2010)	Detroit breast cancer cases in 156 zip codes	Zip-code level Isolation Index	Increased risk of late stage breast cancer diagnosis
Haas et al. (2008)	SEER breast cancer senior survivors diagnosed between 1992 and 2002 (*n* = 47,866)	CT Isolation Index	Decreased odds of receiving adequate breast cancer care

and breast cancer stage at diagnosis and mortality among Blacks and Whites ages ≥ 55 years. They found that lower area-SES was associated with higher late-stage breast cancer incidence and death rates. Similarly, Echeverria et al. (2009) investigated 4,589 New Jersey urban Black and White breast cancer cases, and found that the odds of late-stage disease for women living in low-SES neighborhoods were 1.6 times higher than that of women living in more advantaged neighborhoods, even when controlling for age and race/ethnicity. Likewise, the Cheng et al. (2009) study of 8,997 California prostate cancer deaths found that higher area-SES was associated with lower prostate cancer death rates; moreover, Blacks had a twofold to fivefold increased risk of prostate cancer deaths compared to Whites across all levels of area-SES.

Rurality and Segregation

Unlike the consistent, inverse relationship between rurality and cancer incidence, studies of rurality and late-stage diagnosis and cancer mortality have yielded mixed results. Some have found late-stage diagnosis to be associated with rural residence (e.g., Jemal et al., 2005) among Blacks in particular (Amey, Miller, & Albrecht, 1997); alternatively, others have found late-stage cancers (of the female breast, colorectal, lung, and prostate) to be highest in the most highly urbanized areas and to decrease as rurality increases, with a small increase in isolated rural areas (McLafferty & Wang, 2009). Such differences may reflect use of different definitions of rural versus urban.

There are only a few studies of residential segregation and stage at diagnosis and cancer mortality. Dai (2010) found a significant association between Black segregation and late-stage diagnosis among breast cancer patients in Detroit, but Haas et al. (2008) reported no such association between segregation and breast cancer mortality, even though increased segregation is strongly associated with increased all-cause mortality (Jackson, Anderson, Johnson, & Sorlie, 2000). Again, these studies controlled for individual-level demographics.

Cancer Treatment and Survival

Area-SES

Lower area-SES is associated with a lower probability of early detection, preferred treatment, and survival of cancers for Blacks and Whites (Campbell et al., 2002; Singh et al., 2003; Tewari et al., 2005; Ward et al., 2004; Zell, Rhee, Ziogas, Lipkin, & Anton-Culver, 2007). However, the Black–White disparity in receipt of adequate cancer treatment and in survival remains irrespective of area-SES (Singh et al., 2003; Tewari et al., 2005; Ward et al., 2004). For example, Singh et al. (2003) found that the percentage of Black patients, diagnosed with localized or regional prostate cancer, receiving radical prostatectomy was lower than the percentage of Whites within each area-poverty group (CT % BPL = >10%, 10% to < 20%, 20% +). Similarly, Tewari et al. (2005) found that surgical treatment rate for clinically localized prostate cancer (diagnosed between 1980 and 1997) was 17% for Blacks versus 28% for Whites; survival rates were lower for Blacks than for Whites among patients treated conservatively or by radiation therapy, while survival rates did not differ for Blacks and Whites among those undergoing surgery. Likewise, Ward et al. (2004) found that even when CT poverty was accounted for, Blacks still had a lower 5-year survival than Whites. This pattern has been found for many other cancer sites as well (e.g., Singh et al., 2003; Zell et al., 2007).

Rurality and Segregation

Studies of the association between rurality and cancer treatment are generally consistent, with rural residence associated with underuse of surgical, radiation, and chemotherapy (Esnaola, Knott, Finney, Gebregziabher, & Ford, 2008; Hao et al., 2010; Sankaranarayanan et al., 2010). In urban areas however, a Black–White disparity in receipt of cancer treatment consistently has been found (Esnaola et al., 2008; Hao et al., 2010). For example, Hao et al. (2010) reported a rural disadvantage in receipt of chemotherapy for stage III colon and stages II/III rectum cancer patients in Georgia (n = 4,748 diagnosed during 2000–2004), after controlling for area-SES and other relevant factors (e.g., comorbidities); a Black–White disparity in receipt of adjuvant chemotherapy was observed only for patients residing in urban (vs. suburban and rural) areas. Similarly, being Black is independently associated with underuse of surgery among urban patients with nonmetastatic breast cancer in South Carolina, whereas rural residence is associated with underuse of surgery irrespective of patient race (Esnaola et al., 2008).

Studies of residential segregation and cancer treatment are less consistent. Haas et al. (2008) found that high Black segregation was associated with inadequate cancer care among 47,866 senior Black and White breast cancer survivors diagnosed during 1992–2002. However, no significant association was found between segregation and the receipt of adjuvant chemotherapy among patients with colorectal cancer in Georgia (Hao et al., 2010).

POSSIBLE MECHANISMS OF AREA-LEVEL INFLUENCES

Researchers have identified a variety of neighborhood-level resources, hazards, and barriers that play a role in the higher prevalence of cancer and cancer risk factors in urban, low-SES (i.e., inner-city), and urban Black-segregated (i.e., inner-city Black) neighborhoods, and in rural communities as well. These specific neighborhood disparities have been highlighted as contextual contributors to and social–contextual determinants of cancer disparities.

Smoking

Inner-city and inner-city Black neighborhoods contribute to high smoking among their residents through at least four pathways. The first is the significantly higher exposure to tobacco advertising—outdoors, on store windows, and at the point of purchase—in inner-city areas, with such exposure known to play a role in increased tobacco use (Barbeau, Wolin, Naumova, & Balbach, 2005; Diez-Roux, Merkin, Hannan, Jacobs, & Kiefe, 2003; Hackbarth et al., 2001; Luke, Esmundo, & Bloom, 2000). Moreover, the tobacco industry sponsors music and sporting events in inner-city Black neighborhoods, with this including displays of tobacco advertisements and logos at the events, and on the free t-shirts, hats, bags, and other items distributed (Lee, Cutler, & Burns, 2004; Yerger, Przewoznik, & Malone, 2007). Such exposure contributes to higher smoking rates among inner-city Blacks (59% of men, 41% of women) relative to their suburban cohorts and to Whites (19–25%; Delva et al., 2005).

A second mechanism is the significantly higher availability of tobacco in inner-city neighborhoods, that is, the greater number and density of convenience stores and tobacco shops, both strongly associated with increased tobacco use (Chuang, Cubbin, Ahn, & Winkleby, 2005; Siahpush, Jones, Singh, Timsina, & Martin, 2010). In addition, sales of single cigarettes—removed from the pack and sold individually for pennies—are higher in inner-city areas irrespective of area ethnicity, and in inner-city Black neighborhoods in particular; access to this cheap form of tobacco facilitates smoking among adults and youth who may be unable to afford a pack due to rising prices secondary to increasing excise taxes (Klonoff, Fritz, Landrine, Riddle, & Tully-Payne, 1994; Landrine, Klonoff, & Alcaraz, 1998; Smith et al., 2007).

A third mechanism is the high levels of stress associated with life in inner-city neighborhoods (Elliot, 2000), with smoking used as a (stress-reducing) coping mechanism for many (Bennett, Wolin, Robinson, Fowler, & Edwards, 2005; Janzon et al., 2005). Finally, the fourth mechanism is the well-known failure of inner-city physicians to advise patients—Blacks in particular—to quit smoking (Ashford et al., 2000; Bach, Pham, Schrag, Tate, & Hargraves, 2004; Gemson, Elinson, & Messeri, 1988; van Ryn, 2002). Alternatively, in rural communities, lack of access to smoking prevention and cessation play a role in excess tobacco use, along with community norms (e.g., Cox et al., 2008).

Obesity

At least six neighborhood disparities have been demonstrated to contribute to (i.e., mediate) the high rates of obesity in inner-city and inner-city Black-segregated neighborhoods. These are: (1) the failure of inner-city physicians to advise dietary modification and weight loss, especially to Blacks (Ashford et al., 2000; Bach et al., 2004; van Ryn, 2002); (2) the significantly lower access to healthy foods, supermarkets, and fresh fruits and vegetables in inner-city areas (Morland & Filomena, 2007; Morland, Wing, Diez-Roux, & Poole, 2002; Powell, Chaloupka, & Bao, 2007; Powell, Slater, Mirtcheva, Bao, & Chaloupka, 2007); (3) the significantly higher access to high-calorie, high-fat, fast-food outlets (Block, Scribner, & DeSalvo, 2004; Kwate, 2008; Powell et al., 2007); (4) the significantly lower access to exercise and other recreational facilities (Mobley et al., 2006; Moore, Diez-Roux, Evenson, McGinn, & Brines, 2008; Powell, Slater, Chaloupka, & Harper, 2006); (5) the significantly lower levels of outdoor activity and walking due to fear of crime and to absence of sidewalks, lighting, and green space (Boardman et al., 2005; Chang et al., 2009; Massey, 2001); and (6) the high stress of such neighborhoods (Elliot, 2000; Glass et al., 2006).

Specifically, inner-city and inner-city Black neighborhoods contain 2–4 times more fast-food outlets and convenience stores (Block et al., 2004; Kwate, 2008), 3 times fewer large supermarkets (Morland & Filomena, 2007; Morland et al., 2002), and are 3–8 times more likely to lack recreational facilities than other neighborhoods (Moore et al., 2008; Powell et al., 2006). Indeed, more than 30 studies have documented the paucity of healthy food choices in inner-city areas, with such neighborhoods now referred to as "food deserts," known to partially mediate poor diet and high BMI among residents (Black & Macinko, 2008; Mehta & Chang, 2008; Walker, Keane, & Burke, 2010; Wang et al., 2007). Similarly, the absence of recreational facilities has been shown to partially mediate low levels of physical activity and high BMI in inner-city neighborhoods; 70% of Black versus 38% of White neighborhoods have no recreational facilities (Gordon-Larsen, Nelson, Page, & Popkin, 2006; Mobley et al., 2006; Moore et al., 2008).

Equally important is the high level of ongoing, chronic stress associated with residing in inner-city neighborhoods. Stressful neighborhood features include garbage-filled vacant lots, abandoned and boarded buildings, graffiti, trash, constant noise, stray dogs, and other signs of neighborhood danger and deterioration (Accordino & Gary, 2000; Cohen et al., 2000; Glass et al., 2006; Massey, 2001). These features are strongly associated with chronic stress, vigilance, and poor physical and mental health (Cohen et al., 2003; Glass et al., 2006). Indeed, neighborhood danger has been shown to cause increased cortisol production, with ensuing high BMI and central adiposity irrespective of diet and physical activity (Glass et al., 2006). Likewise, chronic stress causes increased production of pro-inflammatory factors (e.g., tumor necrosis factor alpha, C-reactive protein), and other forms of physiological "wear and tear" known to be predictive of obesity and central adiposity (Black, 2002; Geronimus, Hicken, Keene, & Bound, 2006; Glass et al., 2006; Miller, Cohen, & Ritchey, 2002; Segerstrom & Miller, 2004).

Cancer Screening

Similarly, low rates of cancer screening in inner-city and inner-city Black neighborhoods in part reflect low access to health care and to cancer screening in those communities—and play a role in subsequent diagnosis of late-stage cancers as well (Coughlin et al., 2006, 2008; Dai, 2010; Datta et al., 2006; Onega et al., 2008; Schootman et al., 2006; Zenk, Tarlov, & Sun, 2006). For example, Zenk et al. (2006) found that the distance from Black neighborhoods to low- or no-cost cancer screening facilities in Chicago was significantly further than from White neighborhoods—by more than a mile. For rural populations, low access to cancer screening facilities and high barriers to transportation to such facilities are significant contributors to low screening rates (Coughlin et al., 2006, 2008; Larson & Fleishman, 2003; Probst et al., 2004). For example, Huang et al. (2009) found that the farther a woman had to travel to receive a mammogram, the greater her chances were of being diagnosed with a late-stage breast cancer. Rurality interacts with segregation to yield extremely low access to screening and to cancer care among rural Blacks (Probst, Laditka, Wang, & Johnson, 2007).

Cancer Incidence

Where cancer incidence is concerned, the higher rates of smoking in rural and in inner-city areas no doubt contribute, along with the higher rates of obesity in inner-city and inner-city Black neighborhoods, detailed above. Differences between segregated Black versus White neighborhoods in environmental exposures likewise appear to contribute to Blacks' higher incidence of certain cancers (Olden & White, 2005). National and regional studies consistently have found that environmental exposures in minority neighborhoods are 5–20 times higher than those in White neighborhoods (even after controlling for area-SES) as a result of the deliberate placement of air-polluting factories and toxic waste dumps in minority neighborhoods (Centers for Disease Control, 2005; Morello-Frosch & Jesdale, 2006; Morello-Frosch & Lopez, 2006; Olden & White, 2005). Segregated Black neighborhoods are characterized by significantly higher exposure to air toxins and persistent organic pollutants (e.g., dioxins, pesticides), as well as by significantly higher exposure to mercury, arsenic, lead, sulfur dioxide, and a myriad of known carcinogens (Centers for Disease Control, 2005; Morello-Frosch & Jesdale, 2006; Morello-Frosch & Lopez, 2006). Such higher environmental exposures have been implicated in Blacks' higher incidence of some cancers (Morello-Frosch & Jesdale, 2006).

Cancer Treatment, Mortality, and Survival

Racial and rural disparities in cancer treatment, mortality, and survival at least in part reflect the low access to high-quality, cancer treatment facilities and to oncologists in segregated Black and rural communities—resulting in under-use of surgical, radiation, and chemotherapy in those communities even when cancer is diagnosed at an early or treatable stage (Esnaola et al., 2008; Haas et al., 2008; Hao et al., 2010; Sankaranarayanan et al., 2010). Such disadvantages in the receipt of cancer treatment (particularly when coupled with late-stage diagnosis) in part explain poorer cancer survival and higher cancer death rates in those segregated Black and rural communities (Ward et al., 2004).

CONCLUSIONS

The numerous studies reviewed here reveal that residence in rural—and in inner-city and inner-city Black—neighborhoods is associated with higher rates of smoking and obesity, lower rates of cancer screening, higher cancer incidence and mortality, and lower-quality cancer treatment—irrespective of individual-level SES (personal education and income), and in some cases, irrespective of race as well. Such data imply the need to focus perhaps not so much on Black or poor people, but instead on these problematic geographic areas—in other words, on neighborhood disparities—in the effort to reduce cancer disparities.

REFERENCES

Accordino, J. J., & Gary, T. (2000). Addressing the abandoned and vacant property problem. *Journal of Urban Affairs, 22*, 301–315.

Acevedo-Garcia, D., Lochner, K., Osypuk, T., & Subramanian, S. V. (2003). Future directions in residential segregation and health research. *American Journal of Public Health, 93*, 215–220.

Adelman, R. M. (2004). Neighborhood opportunities, race, and class: The Black middle-class and residential segregation. *City & Community, 3*, 43–63.

Alba, R. D., Logan, J. R., & Stults, B. J. (2000). How segregated are middle-class African-Americans? *Social Problems, 47*, 43–58.

Amey, C. H., Miller, M. K., & Albrecht, S. L. (1997). The role of race and residence in determining stage at diagnosis of breast cancer. *Journal of Rural Health, 13*(2), 99–108.

Ashford, A., Gemson, D., Sheinfeld Gorin, S. N., Bloch, S., Lantigua, R., Ahsan, H., & Neugut, A. I. (2000). Cancer screening and prevention practices of inner-city physicians. *American Journal of Preventive Medicine, 19*, 59–62.

Bach, P. B., Pham, H. H., Schrag, D., Tate, R. C., & Hargraves, J. L. (2004). Primary care physicians who treat Blacks and Whites. *New England Journal of Medicine, 351*, 575–584.

Baker, P., Hoel, D., Mohr, L., Lipsitz, S., & Lackland, D. (2000). Racial, age, and rural/urban disparity in cervical cancer incidence. *Annals of Epidemiology, 10*(7), 466–467.

Baquet, C. R., Horm, J. W., Gibbs, T., & Greenwald, P. (1991). Socioeconomic factors and cancer incidence among blacks and whites. *Journal of the National Cancer Institute, 83*(8), 551–557.

Barbeau, E., Wolin, K., Naumova, E., & Balbach, E. (2005). Tobacco advertising in communities: Associations with race and class. *Preventive Medicine, 40*, 16–22.

Bell, J. F., Zimmerman, F. J., Mayer, J. D., Almgren, G. R., & Huebner, C. E. (2007). Associations between residential segregation and smoking during pregnancy among urban African-American women. *Journal of Urban Health, 84*, 372–388.

Bell, R. A., Arcury, T. A., Chen, H., Anderson, A. M., Savoca, M. R., Kohrman, T., . . . Quandt, S. A. (2009). Use of tobacco products among rural, older adults. *Addictive Behaviors, 34*, 662–667.

Bennett, G., Wolin, K., Robinson, E., Fowler, S., & Edwards, C. (2005). Perceived racial/ethnic harassment and tobacco use among African-American young adults. *American Journal of Public Health, 95*, 238–240.

Black, J. L., & Macinko, J. (2008). Neighborhoods and obesity. *Nutrition Reviews, 66*(1), 2–20.

Black, P. H. (2002). Stress and the inflammatory response: A review of neurogenic inflammation. *Brain, Behavior, and Immunity, 16*(6), 622–653.

Block, J., Scribner, R., & DeSalvo, K. (2004). Fast food, race/ethnicity, and income: A geographic analysis. *American Journal of Preventive Medicine, 27*(3), 211–217.

Boardman, J. D., Saint Onge, J. M., Rogers, R. G., & Denney, J. T. (2005). Race differentials in obesity: The impact of place. *Journal of Health and Social Behavior, 46*, 229–243.

Bodor, J. N., Rice, J. C., Farley, T. A., Swalm, C. M., & Rose, D. (2010). The association between obesity and urban food environments. *Journal of Urban Health, 87*(5), 771–781.

Campbell, N., Elliott, A., Sharp, L., Ritchie, L., Cassidy, J., & Little, J. (2002). Impact of deprivation and rural residence on treatment of colorectal and lung cancer. *British Journal of Cancer, 87*(6), 585–590.

Campbell, R. T., Li, X., Dolecek, T. A., Barrett, R. E., Weaver, K. E., & Warnecke, R. B. (2009). Economic, racial and ethnic disparities in breast cancer in the US: Towards a more comprehensive model. *Health & Place, 15*(3), 855–864.

Centers for Disease Control. (2005). *Third national report on human exposure to environmental chemicals* (NCEH Pub. No. 05-0570). Atlanta, GA: Author.

Chang, V. W. (2006). Racial residential segregation and weight status among U.S. adults. *Social Science & Medicine, 63*, 1289–1303.

Chang, V. W., Hillier, A. E., & Mehta, N. K. (2009). Neighborhood racial isolation, disorder and obesity. *Social Forces, 87*, 2063–2092.

Cheng, I., Witte, J. S., McClure, L. A., Shema, S. J., Cockburn, M. G., John, E. M., & Clarke, C. A. (2009). Socioeconomic status and prostate cancer incidence and mortality rates among the diverse population of California. *Cancer Causes & Control, 20*(8), 1431–1440.

Chuang, Y.-C., Cubbin, C., Ahn, D., & Winkleby, M. A. (2005). Effects of neighborhood socioeconomic status and convenience store concentration on individual-level smoking. *Journal of Epidemiology & Community Health, 59*, 568–573.

Cohen, D. A., Mason, K., Bedimo, A., Scribner, R., Basolo, V., & Farley, T. A. (2003). Neighborhood physical conditions and health. *American Journal of Public Health, 93*, 467–471.

Cohen, D., Spear, S., Scribner, R., Kissinger, P., Mason, K., & Wildgen, J. (2000). Broken windows and the risk of gonorrhea. *American Journal of Public Health, 90*(2), 230–236.

Coughlin, S. S., King, J., Richards, T. B., & Ekwueme, D. U. (2006). Cervical cancer screening among women in metropolitan areas of the United States by individual-level and area-based measures of socioeconomic status, 2000 to 2002. *Cancer Epidemiology, Biomarkers, and Prevention, 15*, 2154–2159.

Coughlin, S. S., Leadbetter, S., Richards, T. B., & Sabatino, S. A. (2008). Contextual analysis of breast and cervical cancer screening and factors associated with health care access among United States women, 2002. *Social Science & Medicine, 66*(2), 260–275.

Coughlin, S. S., Richards, T. B., Thompson, T., Miller, B. A., VanEenwyk, J., Goodman, M. T., & Sherman, R. L. (2006). Rural/nonrural differences in colorectal cancer incidence in the United States, 1998–2001. *Cancer, 107*(5 Suppl.), 1181–1188.

Coughlin, S. S., Uhler, R. J., Bobo, J. K., & Caplan, L. (2004). Breast cancer screening practices among women in the United States, 2000. *Cancer Causes & Control, 15*, 159–170.

Cox, L. S., Cupertino, A. P., Mussulman, L. M., Nazir, N., Greiner, K. A., Mahnken, J. D., . . . Ellerbeck, E. F. (2008). Design and baseline characteristics from the KAN-QUIT disease management intervention for rural smokers in primary care. *Preventive Medicine, 47*, 200–205.

Dai, D. (2010). Black residential segregation, disparities in spatial access to health care facilities, and late-stage breast cancer diagnosis in metropolitan Detroit. *Health & Place, 16*, 1038–1052.

Datta, G. D., Colditz, G. A., Kawachi, I., Subramanian, S. V., Palmer, J. R., & Rosenberg, L. (2006). Individual-, neighborhood-, and state-level socioeconomic predictors of cervical carcinoma screening among U.S. Black women. *Cancer, 106*, 664–669.

Datta, G. D., Subramanian, S. V., Colditz, G. A., Kawachi, I., Palmer, J. R., & Rosenberg, L. (2006). Individual, neighborhood, and state-level predictors of smoking among U.S. Black women: A multi-level analysis. *Social Science & Medicine, 63*, 1034–1044.

DeChello, L. M., Gregorio, D. I., & Samociuk, H. (2006). Race-specific geography of prostate cancer incidence. *International Journal of Health Geographics, 5*, 59–67.

Dell, J. L., Whitman, S., Shah, A. M., Silva, A., & Ansell, D. (2005). Smoking in 6 diverse Chicago communities. *American Journal of Public Health, 95*, 1036–1042.

Delva, J., Tellez, M., Finlayson, T. L., Gretebeck, K. A., Siefert, K., Williams, D. R., & Ismail, A. I. (2005). Cigarette smoking among low-income African-Americans. *American Journal of Preventive Medicine, 29*, 218–221.

Diez-Roux, A. V., Merkin, S. S., Hannan, P., Jacobs, D. R., & Kiefe, C. I. (2003). Area characteristics, individual-level socioeconomic indicators, and smoking in adults. *American Journal of Epidemiology, 157*, 315–326.

Diez-Roux, A. V., Nieto, F., Muntaner, C., Tyroler, H., Comstock, G., Shahar, E., . . . Szklo, M. (1997). Neighborhood environments and coronary heart disease. *American Journal of Epidemiology, 146*, 48–63.

Do, D. P., Dubowitz, T., Bird, C. E., Lurie, N., Escarce, J. J., & Finch, B. K. (2007). Neighborhood context and ethnic differences in BMI. *Economics & Human Biology, 5,* 179–203.

Doescher, M. P., Jackson, E. J., Jerant, A., & Hart, G. L. (2006). Prevalence and trends in smoking: A national rural study. *Journal of Rural Health, 22,* 112–118.

Drewnowski, A., Rehm, C. D., & Solet, D. (2007). Disparities in obesity rates: Analysis by ZIP code area. *Social Science & Medicine, 65,* 2458–2463.

Dunton, G. F., Kaplan, J., Wolch, J., Jerrett, M., & Reynolds, K. D. (2009). Physical environmental correlates of childhood obesity. *Obesity Reviews, 10,* 393–402.

Echeverría, S. E., Borrell, L. N., Brown, D., & Rhoads, G. (2009). A local area analysis of racial, ethnic, and neighborhood disparities in breast cancer staging. *Cancer Epidemiology, Biomarkers and Prevention, 18*(11), 3024–3029.

Elliot, M. (2000). The stress process in neighborhood context. *Health & Place, 6,* 287–299.

Esnaola, N. F., Knott, K., Finney, C., Gebregziabher, M., & Ford, M. E. (2008). Urban/rural residence moderates effect of race on receipt of surgery in patients with nonmetastatic breast cancer. *Annals of Surgical Oncology, 15*(7), 1828–1836.

Farley, J. E. (2005). Race not class: Explaining racial housing segregation in the St. Louis metropolitan area. *Sociological Forces, 38,* 133–150.

Ford, E. S., & Mokdad, A. H. (2008). Epidemiology of obesity in the Western hemisphere. *Journal of Clinical Endocrinology & Metabolism, 93,* S1–S8.

Gemson, D. H., Elinson, J., & Messeri, P. (1988). Differences in physician preventive practice patterns for White and minority patients. *Journal of Community Health, 13,* 53–64.

Gerend, M. A., & Pai, M. (2008). Social determinants of Black–White disparities in breast cancer mortality: A review. *Cancer Epidemiology, Biomarkers and Prevention, 17*(11), 2913–2923.

Geronimus, A. T., Hicken, M., Keene, D., & Bound, J. (2006). "Weathering" and age patterns of allostatic load scores among Blacks and Whites in the United States. *American Journal of Public Health, 96,* 826–833.

Glass, T. A., Rasmussen, M. D., & Schwartz, B. A. (2006). Neighborhoods and obesity in older adults. *American Journal of Preventive Medicine, 31,* 455–463.

Gordon-Larsen, P., Nelson, M. C., Page, P., & Popkin, B. M. (2006). Inequality in the built environment underlies key health disparities in physical activity and obesity. *Pediatrics, 117,* 417–424.

Gorey, K. M., & Vena, J. E. (1994). Cancer differentials among US blacks and whites: Quantitative estimates of socioeconomic-related risks. *Journal of the National Medical Association, 86,* 209–215.

Greenlee, R. T., & Howe, H. L. (2009). County-level poverty and distant stage cancer in the United States. *Cancer Causes & Control, 20*(6), 989–1000.

Haas, J. S., Earle, C. C., Orav, J. E., Brawarsky, P., Neville, B. A., & Williams, D. R. (2008). Racial segregation and disparities in cancer stage for seniors. *Cancer, 113*(8), 2166–2172.

Hackbarth, D., Scnopp-Wyatt, D., Katz, D., Williams, J., Silvestri, B., & Pfleger, M. (2001). Collaborative research and action to control geographic placement of outdoor advertising of alcohol and tobacco products in Chicago. *Public Health Reports, 116,* 213–230.

Hao, Y., Landrine, H., Jemal, A., Ward, K. C., Bayakly, A. R., Young, J. L., Jr., Ward, E. M. (2010). Race, neighbourhood characteristics and disparities in chemotherapy for colorectal cancer. *Journal of Epidemiology & Community Health, 65*(3), 211–217. doi:10.1136/jech.2009.096008

Harper, S., Lynch, J., Meersman, S. C., Breen, N., Davis, W. W., & Reichman, M. C. (2009). Trends in area-socioeconomic and race-ethnic disparities in breast cancer incidence, stage at diagnosis, screening, mortality, and survival among women ages 50 years and over (1987–2005). *Cancer Epidemiology, Biomarkers & Prevention, 18*, 121–131.

Hsu, C. E., Jacobson, H. E., & Soto Mas, F. (2004). Evaluating the disparity of female breast cancer mortality among racial groups: A spatiotemporal analysis. *International Journal of Health Geographics, 3*(4), 1–11. Retrieved from http://ij-healthgeographics.com

Huang, B., Dignan, M., Han, D., & Johnson, O. (2009). Does distance matter? Distance to mammography facilities and stage at diagnosis of breast cancer in Kentucky. *Journal of Rural Health, 25*, 366–371.

Iceland, J., Weinberg, D. H., & Steinmetz, E. (2002). *Racial and ethnic segregation in the United States, 1980–2000.* Washington, DC: U.S. Government Printing Office.

Jackson, M. C., Davis, W. W., Waldron, W., McNeel, T. S., Pfeiffer, R., & Breen, N. (2009). Impact of geography on mammography use in California. *Cancer Causes & Control, 20*, 1339–1353.

Jackson, S. A., Anderson, R. T., Johnson, N. J., & Sorlie, P. D. (2000). The relation of residential segregation to all-cause mortality. *American Journal of Public Health, 90*, 616–617.

Janzon, E., Engstrom, G., Lindstrom, M., Berglund, G., Hedblad, B., & Janzon, L. (2005). Who are the "quitters"? A cross-sectional study of circumstances associated with women giving up smoking. *Scandinavian Journal of Public Health, 33*, 175–182.

Jemal, A., Ward, E., Wu, X., Martin, H. J., McLaughlin, C. C., & Thun, M. J. (2005). Geographic patterns of prostate cancer mortality and variations in access to medical care in the United States. *Cancer Epidemiology, Biomarkers and Prevention, 14*(3), 590–595.

Johnston, R., Poulsen, M., & Forrest, J. (2007). Ethnic and racial segregation in U.S. metropolitan areas, 1980–2000. *Urban Affairs Review, 42*(4), 479–504.

Kawachi, I., & Berkman, L. (2003). *Neighborhoods and health.* New York: Oxford University Press.

Klonoff, E. A., Fritz, J. M., Landrine, H., Riddle, R., & Tully-Payne, L. (1994). The problem and sociocultural context of single cigarette sales. *Journal of the American Medical Association, 27*, 618–620.

Kramer, M. R., & Hogue, C. R. (2009). Is segregation bad for your health? *Epidemiologic Reviews, 31*, 178–194.

Krieger, N., Chen, J. T., Waterman, P. D., Rehkopf, D. H., & Subramanian, S. V. (2003). Race/ethnicity, gender, and monitoring socioeconomic gradients in health: A comparison of area-based socioeconomic measures. *American Journal of Public Health, 93*, 1655–1671.

Krieger, N., Chen, J. T., Waterman, P. D., Rehkopf, D. H., & Subramanian, S. V. (2005). Painting a truer picture of U.S. socioeconomic and racial/ethnic health inequalities: The Public Health Disparities Geocoding Project. *American Journal of Public Health, 95*, 312–323.

Krieger, N., Chen, J. T., Waterman, P. D., Soobader, M. J., Subramanian, S. V., & Carson, R. (2002). Geocoding and monitoring US socioeconomic inequalities in mortality and cancer incidence: Does choice of area-based measure and geographic level matter? *American Journal of Epidemiology, 156,* 471–482.

Krieger, N., Williams, D. R., & Moss, N. E. (1997). Measuring social class in US public health research. *Annual Review of Public Health, 18,* 341–378.

Kwate, N. O. (2008). Fried chicken and fresh apples: Racial segregation as a fundamental cause of fast food density in Black neighborhoods. *Health & Place, 14*(1), 32–44.

Landrine, H., & Corral, I. (2009). Separate and unequal: Residential segregation and Black health disparities. *Ethnicity & Disease, 19*(2), 179–184.

Landrine, H., Klonoff, E. A., & Alcaraz, R. (1998). Minors' access to single cigarettes in California. *Preventive Medicine, 27,* 503–505.

Larson, S., & Fleishman, J. (2003). Rural–urban differences in usual source of care and ambulatory service use. *Medical Care, 41*(7 Suppl.), iii65–iii74.

Lee, D., Cutler, B. D., & Burns, J. (2004). The marketing and de-marketing of tobacco products to low-income African-Americans. *Health Marketing Quarterly, 22,* 51–68.

Luke, D., Esmundo, E., & Bloom, Y. (2000). Smoke signs: Patterns of tobacco billboard advertising in a metropolitan region. *Tobacco Control, 9,* 16–23.

MacKinnon, J. A., Duncan, R. C., Huang, Y., Lee, D. J., Fleming, L. E., Voti, L., . . . Wilkinson, J. D. (2007). Detecting an association between socioeconomic status and late stage breast cancer using spatial analysis and area-based measures. *Cancer Epidemiology, Biomarkers and Prevention, 16*(4), 756–762.

Mascie-Taylor, C. G., & Goto, R. (2007). Human variation and body mass index: A review of the universality of BMI cut-offs, gender and urban–rural differences, and secular changes. *Journal of Physical Anthropology, 26,* 109–112.

Massey, D. S. (2001). Residential segregation and neighborhood conditions in US metropolitan areas. In N. J. Smelser, W. Wilson, & F. Mitchell (Eds.), *America becoming: Racial trends and their consequences* (pp. 391–434). Washington, DC: National Academies Press.

Massey, D. S., & Denton, N. A. (1988). The dimensions of residential segregation. *Social Forces, 67*(2), 281–315.

Massey, D. S., White, M. J., & Phua, V. C. (1996). The dimensions of segregation revisited. *Sociological Methods & Research, 25,* 172–206.

McLafferty, S., & Wang, F. (2009). Rural reversal? Rural–urban disparities in late-stage cancer risk in Illinois. *Cancer, 115*(12), 2755–2764.

Mehta, N. K., & Chang, V. W. (2008). Weight status and restaurant availability. *American Journal of Preventive Medicine, 34*(2), 127–133.

Miller, G. E., Cohen, S., & Ritchey, A. K. (2002). Chronic psychological stress and the regulation of pro-inflammatory cytokines. *Health Psychology, 21,* 531–541.

Mobley, L. R., Kuo, T. M., Driscoll, D., Clayton, L., & Anselin, L. (2008). Heterogeneity in mammography use across the nation: Separating evidence of disparities from the disproportionate effects of geography. *International Journal of Health Geographics, 7,* 32–50.

Mobley, L. R., Root, E. D., Finklestein, E. A., Khavjou, O., Farris, R. P., and Will, J. C. (2006). Environment, obesity, and cardiovascular disease risk in low-income women. *American Journal of Preventive Medicine, 30,* 327–332.

Moore, L. V., Diez-Roux, A. V., Evenson, K. R., McGinn, A. P., & Brines, S. J. (2008). Availability of recreational resources in minority and low socioeconomic status areas. *American Journal of Preventive Medicine, 34*(1), 16–22.

Morello-Frosch, R., & Jesdale, B. M. (2006). Separate and unequal: Residential segregation and estimated cancer risks associated with ambient air toxics in U.S. metropolitan areas. *Environmental Health Perspective, 114*(3), 386–393.

Morello-Frosch, R., & Lopez, R. (2006). The riskscape and the color line: Examining the role of segregation in environmental health disparities. *Environmental Research, 102,* 181–196.

Morland, K., & Filomena, S. (2007). Disparities in availability of fruits and vegetables between racially segregated urban neighborhoods. *Public Health Nutrition, 10,* 1481–1489.

Morland, K., Wing, S., Diez-Roux, A., & Poole, C. (2002). Neighborhood characteristics associated with the location of food stores and food service places. *American Journal of Preventive Medicine, 22,* 23–29.

Nelson, D. E., Mowery, P., Tomar, S., Marcus, S., Giovino, G., & Zhao, L. (2006). Smokeless tobacco use among adults and adolescents in the U.S. *American Journal of Public Health, 96,* 897–905.

Northridge, M. E., Morabia, A., Ganz, M. L., Bassett, M. T., Gemson, D., Andrews, H., & McCord, C. (1998). Contribution of smoking to excess mortality in Harlem. *American Journal of Epidemiology, 147,* 250–258.

Olden, K., & White, S. L. (2005). Health-related disparities: Influence of environmental factors. *Medical Clinics of North America, 89,* 721–738.

Onega, T., Duell, E., Shi, X., Wang, D., Demidenko, E., & Goodman, D. (2008). Geographic access to cancer care in the U.S. *Cancer, 112*(4), 909–918.

Powell, L. M., Chaloupka, F. J., & Bao, Y. (2007). The availability of fast food and full-service restaurants in the United States: Associations with neighborhood characteristics. *American Journal of Preventive Medicine, 33*(S4), S240–S245.

Powell, L. M., Slater, S., Chaloupka, F. J., & Harper, D. (2006). Availability of physical-activity-related facilities and neighborhood demographic and socioeconomic characteristics: A national study. *American Journal of Public Health, 96,* 1676–1680.

Powell, L. M., Slater, S., Mirtcheva, D., Bao, Y., & Chaloupka, F. J. (2007). Food store availability and neighborhood characteristics in the United States. *Preventive Medicine, 44,* 189–195.

Probst, J., Laditka, S., Wang, J., & Johnson, A. (2007). Effects of residence and race on burden of travel for care. *BMC Health Services Research, 7*(1), 40.

Probst, J., Moore, C., Glover, S., & Samuels, M. (2004). Person and place: The compounding effects of race/ethnicity and rurality on health. *American Journal of Public Health, 94,* 1695–1703.

Pruitt, S. L., Shim, M. J., Mullen, P. D., Vernon, S. W., & Amick, B. C. (2009). Association of area socioeconomic status and breast, cervical, and colorectal cancer screening: A systematic review. *Cancer Epidemiology and Biomarkers, 18,* 2579–2599.

Reynolds, P., Hurley, S. E., Quach, A. T., Rosen, H., Von Behren, J., Hertz, A., & Smith, D. (2005). Regional variations in breast cancer incidence among California women, 1988–1997. *Cancer Causes & Control, 16*(2), 139–150.

Robert, S. A., & Reither, E. N. (2004). A multilevel analysis of race, community disadvantage, and body mass index among adults in the U.S. *Social Science & Medicine, 59,* 2421–2434.

Robert, S. A., Strombom, I., Trentham-Dietz, A., Hampton, J. M., McElroy, J. A., Newcomb, P. A., & Remington, P. L. (2004). Socioeconomic risk factors for breast cancer: Distinguishing individual- and community-level effects. *Epidemiology, 15*(4), 442–450.

Ross, C. (2000). Walking, exercising, and smoking: Does neighborhood matter? *Social Science & Medicine, 51,* 265–274.

Sankaranarayanan, J., Watanabe-Galloway, S., Sun, J., Qiu, F., Boilesen, E. C., & Thorson, A. G. (2010). Age and rural residence effects on accessing colorectal cancer treatments: A registry study. *American Journal of Managed Care, 16*(4), 265–273.

Schootman, M., Jeffe, D. B., Baker, E. A., & Walker, M. S. (2006). Effect of area poverty rate on cancer screening across U.S. communities. *Journal of Epidemiology & Community Health, 60,* 202–207.

Segerstrom, S. C., & Miller, G. E. (2004). Psychological stress and the human immune system: A meta-analytic study of 30 years of inquiry. *Psychological Bulletin, 130,* 601–630.

Siahpush, M., Jones, P. R., Singh, G. K., Timsina, L. R., & Martin, J. (2010). Association of availability of tobacco products with socioeconomic and racial/ethnic characteristics of neighborhoods. *Public Health, 124*(9), 525–529.

Singh, G. K., Miller, B. A., Hankey, B. F., & Edwards, B. K. (2003). *Area socioeconomic variations in U.S. cancer incidence, mortality, stage, treatment, and survival, 1975–1999* (NIH Pub. No. 03-5417). Bethesda, MD: National Cancer Institute.

Smith, K. C., Stillman, F., Bone, L., Yancey, N., Price, E., Belin, P., & Kromm, E. E. (2007). Buying and selling "loosies" in Baltimore. *Journal of Urban Health, 84,* 494–507.

Stimpson, J. P., Ju, H., Raji, M. A., & Eschbach, K. (2007). Neighborhood deprivation and health risk behaviors in NHANES III. *American Journal of Health Behavior, 31,* 215–222.

Sung, J. F., Blumenthal, D. S., Alema-Mensah, E., & McGrady, G. A. (1997). Racial and urban/rural differences in cervical carcinoma in Georgia Medicaid recipients. *Cancer, 80,* 231–236.

Tewari, A., Horninger, W., Pelzer, A. E., Demers, R., Crawford, E. D., Gamito, E. J., . . . Menon, M. (2005). Factors contributing to the racial differences in prostate cancer mortality. *British Journal of Urology International, 96*(9), 1247–1252.

Tseng, M., Yeatts, K., Millikan, R., & Newman, B. (2001). Area-level characteristics and smoking in women. *American Journal of Public Health, 91,* 1847–1859.

van Ryn, M. (2002). Research on the provider contribution to race/ethnic disparities in medical care. *Medical Care, 40*(Suppl.), I140–I151.

Walker, R. E., Keane, C. R., & Burke, J. G. (2010). Disparities and access to health food in the United States: A review of food deserts literature. *Health & Place, 16,* 876–884.

Wang, M. C., Soowan, K., Gonzalez, A. A., MacLeod, K. E., & Winkleby, M. A. (2007). Socioeconomic and food-related physical characteristics of the neighborhood environment are associated with body mass index. *Journal of Epidemiology & Community Health, 61,* 491–498.

Ward, E., Jemal, A., Cokkinides, V., Singh, G. K., Cardinez, C., Ghafoor, A., & Thun, M. (2004). Cancer disparities by race/ethnicity and socioeconomic status. *CA: A Cancer Journal for Clinicians, 54*(2), 78–93. Retrieved from http://caonline .amcancersoc.org/cgi/reprint/54/2/78

Wilkes, R., & Iceland, J. (2004). Hypersegregation in the 21st century. *Demography, 41,* 23–36.

Yabroff, K. R., & Gordis, L. (2003). Does stage at diagnosis influence the observed relationship between socioeconomic status and breast cancer incidence, case-fatality, and mortality? *Social Science & Medicine, 57*(12), 2265–2279.

Yerger, V. B., Przewoznik, J., & Malone, R. E. (2007). Racialized geography, corporate activity, and health disparities: Tobacco industry targeting of inner cities. *Journal of Health Care for the Poor and Underserved, 18,* 10–38.

Yin, D., Morris, C., Allen, M., Cress, R., Bates, J., & Liu, L. (2010). Does socioeconomic disparity in cancer incidence vary across racial/ethnic groups? *Cancer Causes & Control, 21*(10), 1721–1730.

Zell, J. A., Rhee, J. M., Ziogas, A., Lipkin, S. M., & Anton-Culver, H. (2007). Race, socioeconomic status, treatment, and survival time among pancreatic cancer cases in California. *Cancer Epidemiology, Biomarkers and Prevention, 16*(3), 546–552.

Zenk, S. N., Tarlov, E., & Sun, J. (2006). Spatial equity in facilities providing low- or no-fee screening mammography in Chicago neighborhoods. *Journal of Urban Health, 83*(2), 195–210.

II

INTERVENTIONS FOR ELIMINATING CANCER DISPARITIES

7

5-a-Day and Fit-for-Life Badge Programs for Cancer Prevention in Boy Scouts[1]

Amy Shirong Lu, Janice Baranowski, Debbe Thompson,
Karen W. Cullen, Tom Baranowski, Russ Jago, and Richard Buday

Overweight children are at increased risk of becoming overweight adults, and this risk increases throughout childhood (Whitaker, Wright, Pepe, Seidel, & Dietz, 1997). The odds ratio of becoming an obese adult is 1.3 for overweight 1- to 2-year-olds, 4.1 for overweight 3- to 5-year-olds, and up to 28.3 for overweight 10- to 14-year-olds (Whitaker et al., 1997). Parental obesity is a strong predictor of adult obesity among children less than 10 years old; but among children 10 years old or greater, the child's weight status is the stronger predictor of adult obesity (Whitaker et al., 1997). Adult obesity is associated with an increased incidence of several cancers, including colon (Murphy, Calle, Rodriguez, Khan, & Thurn, 2000), breast (Carmichael & Bates, 2004; Harvie, Hooper, & Howell, 2003), and endometrial (Kaaks, Lukanova, & Kurzer, 2002) cancers. Insulin-like growth factor 1 (IGF-1), a polypeptide thatenhances tumor development by stimulating cell proliferation and inhibiting apoptosis (Kaaks & Lukanova, 2001), is associated with increased adiposity in both children (Ong, Kratzsch, Keiss, & Dunger, 2002; Wabitsch et al., 1996), and adults (Nam et al., 1997; Voskuil et al., 2001). Elevated levels of IGF-1 have been associated with an increased risk of colon (Giovannucci, 2001), prostrate (Chan, Rimm, Colditz, Stampfer, & Willett, 1994), and breast cancer (Hankinson et al., 1997). Increased levels of certain cytokines such as adiponectin (Mantzoros et al., 2004; Miyoshi et al., 2003) and IL-6 (Fontanini

[1]This research was largely funded by a grant from the American Cancer Society (TURSG-3 04). This work is also a publication of the United States Department of Agriculture (USDA/ARS) Children's Nutrition Research Center, Department of Pediatrics, Baylor College of Medicine, Houston, Texas, and had been funded in part with federal funds from the USDA/ARS under Cooperative Agreement No. 58-6250-6001. The contents of this publication do not necessarily reflect the views or policies of the USDA, nor does mention of trade names, commercial products, or organizations imply endorsement from the U.S. government.

169

et al., 1999; Onuma, Bub, Rummel, & Iwamoto, 2003; Schneider et al., 2000), and the cytokine-like protein leptin (Hardwick, Van Den Brink, Offerhaus, Van Deventer, & Pepelenbosch, 2001), are elevated with adiposity and increased cancer risk. Elevated insulin levels, as in obesity-related metabolic syndrome and type 2 diabetes, are also a risk for cancer mortality (Borugian et al., 2004). Some breast cancers likely initiated during puberty, with the rapid growth in breast tissue (Colditz & Frazier, 1995). Obese girls may be at greater risk of breast cancer, due to the earlier development (Freedman et al., 2002) and the larger accumulation of breast tissue (Freedman et al., 2003). Thus, childhood obesity increases the risk of a number of cancers.

Disparities in mortality and health outcomes have been established by socioeconomic status and ethnicity both worldwide and in the United States (Kumanyika et al., 2008). Among the many factors contributing to these health disparities in obesity and cancer risks are differences in lifestyle practices, including diet (Kranz et al., 2009) and physical activity (Kumanyika & Yancey, 2009), and the increased adiposity resulting from energy unbalance (Kumanyika et al., 2008). Fruit and vegetable (FV) intake within the context of lower caloric intake (Ledoux, Hingle, & Baranowski, 2010) and physical activity are behaviors directly related to childhood obesity prevention (Roblin, 2007). Helping children to eat more fruits and vegetables and to participate in more physical activity should have long-term health benefits (Baranowski et al., 2000).

Commonly, children consume well below the recommended minimum of five servings of fruits and vegetables per day (Baranowski, Smith, et al., 1997; Domel et al., 1993) and perform physical activity for much less than the recommended 60 minutes per day standard (Troiano et al., 2008). Of particular concern are minority populations with lower income (Taylor, Baranowski, & Young, 1998), who are more sedentary (Taylor, Beech, & Cummings, 1997) and more likely to develop chronic diseases related to sedentary lifestyles than the general population (U.S. Department of Health and Human Services, 1990). Black adolescents and females also report lower preferences for vegetables than their White counterparts (Granner et al., 2004). Since lifestyle interventions have generally not worked among ethnic-minority children (Whitt-Glover & Kumanyika, 2009), effective interventions are needed for low-income and minority populations (Taylor et al., 1998). Since dietary and physical activity habits form in early childhood and are usually maintained into adulthood (Kelder, Perry, Klepp, & Lytle, 1994; Malina, 2008), early intervention should help to reduce multiple health risks. An important related issue is whether interventions initially designed to meet the needs of one specific ethnic minority can be employed across a wider audience.

Behavioral interventions induce changes in mediating variables (i.e., factors that causally influence the behavior, such as the home environment or self-efficacy to perform behavior). Changes in the mediating variables change the behavior (Baranowski et al., 1997). Behavioral interventions need to identify and work in channels appropriate to specific kinds of children to optimize their effect on the mediating variables. Previous research has shown that a badge program could change behaviors among Girl Scouts (Cullen, Bartholomew, & Parcel, 1997). Almost 3 million boys were involved in scouting in the United States in 2008 (Boy Scouts of America, 2008). Scouts are encouraged to take responsibility for developing good health habits, a component of physical fitness (Cullen et al., 1998). "Urban Boy Scouts" provides a promising opportunity to reach inner-city ethnic-minority children (Cullen et al., 1998). Boy Scouts thus provide a promising channel to enable boys to adopt a healthier lifestyle. In light of this opportunity, we built a relationship with the Urban Boy Scout program of the Sam Houston Council in 1998, to enhance their fitness badge programs. The leaders of Urban Scouting were interested in providing meaningful experiences for their scouts, who were at high risk for obesity and consequent cancer. They participated in the program design.

GOAL AND HYPOTHESIS

The goal of this project was to enable Boy Scouts to eat five or more servings of FV and engage in 30 minutes or more of moderate to vigorous physical activity per day. The hypothesis was that a behavior-change program based on social cognitive theory principles and change procedures would help scouts make changes toward these goals.

CONCEPTUAL FOUNDATION

Behaviors are under the influence of multiple factors, making them difficult to change (Baranowski, Lin, et al., 1997). Most identified behavioral influences (candidate mediators for intervention programs) had low predictiveness (Baranowski, Cullen, & Baranowski, 1999) and only a few significantly predicted behavior (Barrios & Costell, 2004). Most childhood obesity prevention programs do not have the desired effect (Brown, Kelly, & Summerbell, 2007). Thus, a challenge is how to design and implement behavioral change procedures among targeted populations through appropriate implementation channels (Kalakanis & Moulton, 2006; O'Connor, Jago, & Baranowski, 2009).

Simply providing children with the knowledge that eating fruits and vegetables and being physically active will prevent obesity, cancer, heart disease, and diabetes does not necessarily motivate them to actively make healthier choices (Contento, 2008). Thus, providing some knowledge of what behaviors to change and how to change them may be necessary, but not sufficient, for behavior change. Health behavior interventions are most likely to be effective if guided by relevant behavioral theories (Contento, Manning, & Shannon, 1992). Using the mediating/moderating variable model as the conceptual framework, interventions need to target variables that influence the behavior (Baranowski, Lin, et al., 1997).

Bandura's social cognitive theory (SCT) (Bandura, 1986) described a system of triadic reciprocal determinism of cognitive, environmental, and behavioral factors, that has been a commonly used theoretical foundation for behavior change programs. Observational learning, or the vicarious acquisition of knowledge and skills from watching others, is a primary source of information that promotes both cognitive and behavioral development. By observing other people's behavior, people may acquire information about many challenges, and about the skills needed to overcome them. Self-efficacy is the belief in one's ability to perform specific behaviors (Bandura, 1977) and mediates the application of knowledge and skills to behavior change (Maibach & Cotton, 1995). Outcome expectancy is the expectation that certain behaviors produce outcomes (Bandura, 1994). People act on their beliefs about what they are capable of doing and about the outcome of their behavior. Linking healthy behaviors to attaining something that kids want (i.e., rewards), such as achievement badges for Boy Scouts, and delivering the message in a fun, interactive way, such as logging into an interactive website to read comics and play online games, should motivate them to improve their diet and physical activity (Baranowski et al., 2002; Jago et al., 2006).

THE INITIAL PROGRAM

The 5-a-Day achievement badge for Urban Boy Scouts was a preliminary intervention designed to help African American Boy Scouts to increase their fruit and vegetable consumption. To ensure that the intervention materials were culturally sensitive (Resnicow, Baranowski, Ahluwalia, & Braithwaite, 1999), focus group discussions were conducted (Cullen et al., 1998). The focus groups (Cullen et al., 1998) found that the urban Boy Scouts' preference for vegetables was low; their FV-preparation skills were limited; and they did not purchase FV for snacks. Although FV were available at home, they were not in easily accessible forms, and the boys reported low participation in food preparation. They reported setting only global goals (e.g., general aims such as getting good grades or being popular at school) and did not understand self-monitoring their progress toward achieving their goals. Although African American (AA) boys were likely to consume FV as often as corresponding European American boys, there were ethnic differences regarding the type of FV consumption. For example, African American boys were more likely to have eaten potato salad, whereas European American boys were more likely to have consumed bananas, strawberries, watermelon, other white potatoes, corn, salsa, and vegetable soups.

A pilot test (Baranowski et al., 2002) was conducted with Boy Scouts and their families to assure clarity of message, relevance, and acceptance by the target group. Although the pilot test resulted in a 0.8 FV serving increase (Baranowski et al., 2002) among African American Boy Scout troops in Houston, Texas, the research team learned that the 1-hour educational session during every week's troop meeting conflicted excessively with other troop responsibilities. As a result, many of the in-troop behavioral components were transferred online, so as to minimize troop time.

Two innovative Boy Scout badge programs were developed, each with 9-session in-troop activities, plus corresponding weekly Internet activities. Troop leaders led the weekly in-troop sessions, which focused on fun (as an outcome expectation) and interactive skill-building activities that taught the scouts related functional knowledge and skills to enhance the scouts' self-efficacy, and allowed them to achieve their behavior change goals. The online components incorporated fun and interactive role modeling, goal-setting, goal review, and problem-solving elements that allowed the scouts to set and review their behavioral change goals, and solve potential problems throughout that process. Each week, the in-troop interactive activities took about 20–30 minutes, and the online program activities took about 10–20 minutes to complete, giving a total of about 30–50 minutes of program activities. The completion of goals took additional time at home during the week, depending on the goals that the scouts set, for which the scouts received goal points toward earning their respective badges (5-a-Day or Fit-for-Life).

THE 5-A-DAY BADGE PROGRAM

The goal of the 5-a-Day badge program was to help scouts learn to eat at least five servings of FV a day, by setting weekly goals to eat FV at a specific meal or snack, and establishing skills and an environment supportive of that. Each week during the troop meeting, the scouts participated in the 5-a-Day badge skill-building activities, which were focused on learning FV preparation skills (by preparing meal-specific, quick, and easy FV recipes that had been taste tested with boys prior to the program). Such in-troop preparation of simple recipes taught scouts recipe preparation skills, and the tasting should have enhanced their preference for FV (Birch, McPhee, Shoba, Pirok, & Steinberg, 1987). The scouts received a 5-a-Day recipe book with all the troop recipes, and additional ones to prepare later at home.

Week 1 in-troop activities: At the initial troop meeting, troop leaders announced the new 5-a-Day achievement badge and explained the requirements for earning the badge, including attending meetings, preparing FV recipes, logging onto the badge website, and completing goal-setting and monitoring tasks. The scouts were given rules and safety tips to follow during recipe preparation, including always to wash their hands before handling or eating food, the fundamentals of collecting ingredients, and cooking utensils, knife, and other kitchen equipment safety information; they were instructed to always have an adult present to supervise them, since most boys around 10–14 years old do not have enough experience to prepare recipes by themselves. The weekly recipe preparation assignment chart and the rotation of duties were explained and the scouts were given their first recipe to prepare for tasting. The food preparation process was completed solely by the scouts, but was closely supervised by the troop leader. The scouts were given a "My Way to 5-a-Day" motto, to help them remember how to find and prepare FV they liked to eat. At the end of each session, the troop leader reminded the scouts to go to the badge website that evening or the next day, to set their badge goal to eat FV for an after-school snack.

Week 2 in-troop activities: At the beginning of each subsequent week, the troop leader met with each scout, prior to the formal troop meeting, to review his web log-in and goal achievement. This week, the scouts played a "SOLVE IT" game (based on the TV game show *Family Feud*) to problem-solve ways to overcome barriers to meeting their badge goal. The game scenarios included common problems that scouts have in meeting their goal to eat FV for a meal or snack. Then the scouts discussed the next week's goal, to eat a fruit or drink a 100% fruit juice for breakfast, and prepared two breakfast fruit smoothie recipes to taste.

Week 3 in-troop activities: The scouts talked about what they usually ate for an after-school snack and how they could incorporate FV snacks into their usual routine. They discussed the next week's goal, to eat FV for an after-school snack, and prepared two fruit snack recipes to taste.

Week 4 in-troop activities: The scouts talked about what they usually ate for school lunch and how they could incorporate a vegetable snack into their usual lunch. They discussed the next week's goal—to eat a vegetable at school lunch—and prepared two vegetable lunch recipes to taste.

Week 5 in-troop activities: The scouts talked about what vegetable they usually ate for dinner. Since increased availability and accessibility of FV at home has been correlated with intake (Jago, Baranowski, Baranowski, Cullen, & Thompson, 2007), scouts used role-playing activities to learn asking and negotiating skills so that they could ask for FV at home. This prepared them for setting their next week's goal, to eat a vegetable at dinner. The scouts then prepared two vegetable dinner recipes to taste.

Week 6 in-troop activities: The scouts talked about what they usually ate at their favorite fast-food restaurant and how they could incorporate FV into their selections, using real fast-food restaurant menus to find appropriate choices. They also discussed the next week's goal, to eat FV at a fast-food restaurant. Next the scouts prepared two 100% fruit juice drink recipes to taste.

Week 7 in-troop activities: The scouts reviewed what they learned about eating FV for meals and snacks, and completed a worksheet to create their own "My Way to 5-a-Day" plan for their goal to eat five servings of FV on Saturday and Sunday during the upcoming weekend. Next, the scouts prepared two vegetable snack recipes to taste.

Week 8 in-troop activities: The scouts reviewed what they had learned about eating FV for meals and snacks while working on the 5-a-Day badge. They played a "Top 10" game to help them create their own "My Way to 5-a-Day" plan to meet next week's goal, to eat five servings of FV every day after they received their 5-a-Day badge. Next, the scouts prepared their own combination of vegetables in a "That's a Wrap" sandwich recipe to eat.

Week 9 in-troop activities: The 5-a-Day achievement badge award ceremony was held. Troop leaders repeated the purpose of the badge program, then congratulated and recognized all scouts who had successfully completed the 5-a-Day achievement badge requirements and earned their badge. Each scout's name was called as he was presented with the 5-a-Day achievement badge, given a handshake, and told that he should wear it with pride, knowing that he had achieved the goal of learning how to eat five servings of FV a day, every day. The troop leader ended the ceremony by reminding the scouts to continue to eat five servings of FV every day.

In addition to the weekly troop meeting activities, scouts logged onto the badge website each week, where they set their badge requirement goals to eat FV and make FV recipes at home. To ensure that the badge goals only included FV, scouts played video games on the website to learn what foods counted as FV, and what food items—such as juice drinks, Kool-aid, apple pie, French fries, and so on—were excluded, either because they did not have enough FV or because they were too high in fat and sugar. To be counted, a FV goal must include at least a full serving of FV and must be cooked without fat. The goals on the badge website had the scouts clearly state what behavior they would do, as well as when and how they would do it (i.e., action implementation intentions). Scouts had one week in which to complete each badge requirement goal. The troop leader monitored the scouts' weekly log-ons and accumulated points.

The welcome page featured four cartoon images of the "Troop 5 Alive" scouts of different racial and ethnic groups, with a black background color. Each participating scout had his own username and password to log into the website, and was encouraged to log in at least twice a week. The initial log-in was to set their goal, and the second was to record achievement of their goal before the next week's troop meeting. Once logged in, the badge website page contained three sections. At the top was a "5-a-Day" bar, showing the scout's progression across the week's goals. On the left navigation panel there were different tabs, containing the various games and goal sections for the 5-a-Day badge.

The scouts set their 5-a-Day badge goal by clicking on "Go for the Goal" button on the left. That week's goal (e.g., after-school veggie snack for 3 days plus prepare 5-a-Day badge recipe at home) and goal statement (e.g., this week, your goal is to eat one more serving of veggies than you usually eat for an after-school snack on three different days) would appear in the middle of the screen. By clicking on the "start" button, the scouts were directed to "Go for the Goal," where they selected the dates and the targeted FV for each week's goals. At the end, the scouts would see a summary page with the days and FV that they had chosen to meet those goals. Next, they set the Snack Down Recipe Goal by clicking on the recipe that they wanted to prepare at home for their family for the goal. They could also view recipes before making the selection. After selecting the day on which they wanted to make the recipe, they could print their detailed goal to post on the refrigerator, as a reminder of what they needed to do for the week.

When the scouts had completed their goals, before they came back to the troop meetings next week, they logged onto the website to review their goals, and to indicate the completion of the goals by checking the boxes under each goal. Those who did not meet their weekly goals participated in online and in-person problem-solving (i.e., coping implementation intentions). The in-person problem-solving session would be conducted by the troop leader just prior to the weekly meetings.

In addition to the goal-setting component, the badge website contained a number of activities (Real Times 5, Make Your Mark, Add 'Em Up, Snack Down Recipe, Are You Game? and SOLVE IT) with which the scouts could interact during the week.

Real Times 5 was a weekly comic strip about how the "Troop 5 Alive" scouts, Jason, Jamal, Carlos, and David, met their weekly goals to earn their 5-a-Day badge. Each weekly comic described how these scouts achieved goals similar to those of the real scouts, as well as overcoming problems through self-regulatory and asking skills. Self-monitoring and problem-solving elements were included for the real scouts, to enhance their self-regulatory skills. Each episode ended with a cliff-hanger, or an unresolved problem likely to keep one of the scouts from achieving his dietary goal (e.g., a scout told his friends that he wanted to drop out of the program because his mother did not keep fruits and vegetables at home). As in a soap opera, this was intended to attract the real scout to return to the website, to find out what happened next.

Make Your Mark was a weekly problem-solving poll that asked scouts how they would solve the cliff-hanger to the problem that "Troop 5 Alive" encountered in meeting their badge requirements. The scouts read the problem and chose what they thought was the best solution for the comic character to meet the 5-a-Day badge goal. The poll provided various solutions, including both good and bad ones. After selecting a solution, a scout was given feedback on whether or not the selected solution would likely work, and why.

In the Add 'Em Up section, a scoreboard displayed each scout's current total of 5-a-Day badge points toward receiving their badge.

Snack Down Recipes was the online archive that stored the weekly troop and web recipes as part of the 5-a-Day badge.

In the Are You Game? section, scouts used the FV skills and knowledge learned during troop meetings to play games for additional knowledge points toward their badge. The scouts competed against other scouts in their troop in this section, and could earn "Elite 5" status if they obtained one of the top five scores on a particular game. Due to the competition factor, this was one of most visited sections of the badge website.

SOLVE IT helped a scout who experienced problems meeting his goals to find a workable solution to meet his next goal. A tailored step-by-step plan to identify the barriers and ways to overcome the barriers was created. The scout was able to print the solutions to help meet his goals. Scouts received points for completing the SOLVE IT activity. To make the process easy to remember and interesting, a SOLVE IT Rap was included:

"S" Solvin' problems / won't take long
"O" Once I know / what went wrong
"L" Look at ways / write them down
"V" Vote for one / works all round
"E" Eager to try / my new plan

In the event that the troop members needed to contact the troop leader or had some problems with the website, they could click the "Contact Us" button and type in the message through an online form. The intervention staff answered questions within 24 hours.

Each week, the scouts earned points toward the 5-a-Day badge for participating in the in-troop activities, logging onto the badge website, setting their behavioral goals, and completing their weekly goals. Scouts had to earn at least 10,200 of the total 17,600 possible points, to earn the 5-a-Day achievement badge. Scouts earned 100 points per week by attending weekly troop meetings, and participating in the badge activities during the troop meetings; 100 points per week by logging onto the website to set the weekly goals; 100 points per week by viewing the online comics; 100 points per week by participating in problem-solving polls; 100 points per week by recording how they did on their goals at the end of the week; 1,000 points per week by achieving the 5-a-Day goal; and 500 points per week by preparing a 5-a-Day web recipe for their families. The participants could also earn an extra 100 points by returning completed problem solutions to help meet their 5-a-Day goals, and an additional 100 points by cleaning up after the troop meetings each week.

THE FIT-FOR-LIFE ACHIEVEMENT BADGE PROGRAM

The goal of the Fit-for-Life badge program was to increase the scouts' moderate to vigorous physical activity (PA) levels to 30 minutes a day, 5 times per week by setting weekly goals to do PA while wearing a pedometer to track their steps. Like the 5-a-Day badge program, the Fit-for-Life program combined offline weekly troop meetings with online sessions.

Each week during the troop meeting, the scouts participated in the Fit-for-Life badge skill-building activities to promote PA skills such as flexibility, strengthening, and cardiovascular fitness through sports such as basketball, football, baseball, and soccer, played during troop meetings and later at home, using a pedometer to record their steps during these activities.

Week 1 in-troop activities: At the initial troop meeting, troop leaders announced the new Fit-for-Life achievement badge, which would help scouts learn to be more physically active by doing PA drills to improve their skills in some sports, doing PA five times a week, and knowing the different components of fitness. Troop leaders explained that PA referred to an activity that kept a person moving continuously, and that doctors usually recommended that everyone do at least 30 minutes of PA a day, 5 days a week. Each scout received a pedometer to record his steps during PA. The scouts were instructed to wear the pedometer during the 8-week badge program, to track the number of steps taken during their PA. They were also instructed how to use the reset button before starting the PA each day. They were encouraged to reach a minimum of 5,000 counts for each activity goal, and to record their pedometer counts on the badge website each week as part of their goal achievement. If a scout lost the pedometer, he would only be able to record what activities he had done for the weekly goal.

Since boys of this age generally are interested in sports (Cardon et al., 2005), troop leaders organized a series of PA drill exercises to build skills to play sports. One scout was chosen to lead the stretches and one scout was chosen to be in charge of the equipment. Each drill lasted around 15–17 minutes. These sport-related drills included baseball stretches, ultimate football, baseball drills, football strengthening drills, soccer strengthening drills, a basketball knockout game, and a soccer drill game, and varied from week to week. The scouts also received a PA drills booklet to help them set and achieve their PA goals. Each of the booklets listed the information about their PA drill requirements and instructions. It also listed the required activities from each section of the intervention website, as a to-do list. At the end of each troop meeting, the troop leader reminded the scouts to go to the badge website that evening or the next day, to set their badge goal to do 30 minutes (or 5,000 pedometer steps) of PA twice in the next week.

Week 2 in-troop activities: At the beginning of each subsequent week, the troop leader met with each scout, prior to the formal troop meeting, to review his web log-in and goal achievement. This week, the scouts played SOLVE IT (designed to resemble the TV program *Family Feud*), but with a PA and health focus that reinforced problem-solving and helped the scouts identify solutions to barriers to meeting their PA badge goal. The game scenarios included common problems that scouts have in meeting their PA or pedometer goal. It echoed the SOLVE IT component on the website, which helped the scouts to identify reasons why they did not meet the goal, and gave step-by-step solutions to overcome the problems. Then the scouts discussed the different types of fitness (flexibility, strengthening, and aerobic activity). Next, the scouts participated in baseball flexibility drills.

Week 3 in-troop activities: The scouts discussed PA levels and heart rates, and participated in the ultimate football game.

Week 4 in-troop activities: The scouts discussed safety guidelines for a variety of sports and activities, and participated in baseball drills.

Week 5 in-troop activities: The scouts discussed safety guidelines for weight lifting, and participated in football strengthening drills.

Week 6 in-troop activities: The scouts participated in soccer strengthening drills and a soccer game.

Week 7 in-troop activities: The scouts participated in role-playing activities to learn asking and negotiation skills, so that they could ask their parents for help in meeting their PA goals, and participated in the basketball knock-out game.

Week 8 in-troop activities: The scouts reviewed what they had learned about PA while working on the Fit-for-Life badge. They played a "Top 10" game to help them create their own plan to continue to do PA every day after they received their Fit-for-Life badge, and participated in an indoor soccer skills game.

Week 9 in-troop activities: After 8 weeks of intervention, the scouts were awarded their Fit-for-Life badges during a special badge ceremony. The troop leaders repeated the purpose of the badge program, then congratulated and recognized all scouts who had successfully completed the Fit-for-Life achievement badge requirements and earned their badge. Each scout's name was called as they were presented with the Fit-for-Life achievement badge, given a handshake, and told he should wear it with pride, knowing that he had achieved the goal of learning how to be PA every day. The troop leader ended the ceremony by reminding the scouts to continue to be PA every day.

Like the 5-a-Day badge, scouts logged onto the Fit-for-Life badge website each week, where they set their badge requirement goals to do 30 minutes of PA for a varying number of days each week, and to record the resulting pedometer step counts during those PA.

The welcome page featured the same four "Troop 5 Alive" scouts, but with the Fit-for-Life title. The Fit-for-Life website gave each scout his unique username and password for logging-in purposes, and they were encouraged to log in at least twice a week. The initial log-in was to set their goal, and the second was to record the achievement of their goal before the next week's troop meeting. The Fit-for-Life website's navigation areas and screens were similar to those of the 5-a-Day site, but were related to PA.

The scouts' first log-on was to click on Challenge Yourself, to set their badge requirement goals to do PA for at least 30 minutes for the week. Then they would click "Go set goal," to move to the next section of the page, where they could select the day, PA, and time of day to do their PA for their first day's goal from drop-down boxes (e.g., Thursday, February 20, 2003, After School, Bicycling). They could earn extra points for the week by choosing stretches or strengthening moves in addition to the 30-minute daily PA. After they had set their goal for each day to do PA, they would see a summary page with the days, the PA, and the time of day they had chosen to meet the goals. After that, the scouts could print the page to remind them of the goals that they had set.

Scouts had one week to complete the goals. Before returning to the next weekly troop meeting, the scouts were to log on a second time to record completion of their goals. By clicking on the Challenge Yourself page, the scouts were able to see all of the goals they had selected plus three more forms to fill: the time of the activity, the pedometer counts, and whether they had met the goal (check mark). Once they had entered the information, they clicked the "update goal" button to report that to the system.

The participants were to set progressively more difficult PA goals each week. When a scout experienced problems meeting his goals for the week, he would click a button called SOLVE IT, so that he could meet his goals the next week. Like 5-a-Day, the scouts were asked to identify the barriers and ways to overcome them. Similarly, a tailored step-by-step solution to the problem would be created for the scout. He was instructed to print out the final solution to help with achieving the goals. A scout received points toward his badge for completing the SOLVE IT activity. The same SOLVE IT Rap was also placed in the center of the page.

In addition, the badge website contained a number of activities (Real Times 5, Make Your Mark, Add 'Em Up, What Moves You? Are You Game? and SOLVE IT) that the scouts could complete during the week.

Real Times 5 was the weekly animated role-modeling comic book story, that modeled how the same four Boy Scouts, Jason, Jamal, Carlos, and David, were able to meet their weekly goals to earn their Fit-for-Life badge, as well as overcome problems in meeting their goals. Each session ended with a cliff-hanger designed to attract the scouts to come back next time.

The Make Your Mark was the weekly poll that asked scouts to help solve the problems that the scouts in the comic series were facing in meeting their badge requirements. The problems were ones that the scouts were likely to face themselves when working toward their Fit-for-Life badge goals. The poll provided various possible solutions: some were good, whereas others were not. After the scouts had selected a solution, they were given feedback and suggestions on whether or not that solution would work. If the scouts did not make a good choice, they were prompted to choose another one.

In addition to the web games, What Moves You? was a timed fitness game that challenged the scouts to do timed PA—for example, jumping jacks, running and touching the stove in the kitchen—in front of the computer. The activities encouraged body movement, and the scouts could replay as many times as they liked to beat their time. They could also compete against their fellow scouts to see who got the best score.

To increase log-on rates, there was another, different PA knowledge game, Are You Game? on the website each week. Scouts needed to use their PA knowledge and the skills learned during troop meetings and on the website to play a game each week (e.g., How much do you know about PA, stretching, and strengthening?). If they made a wrong answer, they would lose points. The scouts competed against other scouts in their troop in this section, and could earn "Elite 5" status if they obtained one of the top 5 scores on a particular game.

The scouts could also update their emails by updating their profiles or contact the program leaders via the online forms.

Each week, the scouts earned points toward the Fit-for-Life badge for attending the troop meetings, participating in weekly PA drills or games at their troop meetings, logging onto the Fit-for-Life website and setting their behavioral goals, and completing their weekly goals. To earn the Fit-for-Life achievement badge, scouts had to earn at least 7,900 out of the total 13,600 possible points. Scouts earned 100 points per week by attending weekly troop meetings, and participating in the PA during the troop meetings; 100 points per week by logging onto the website to set the weekly goals; 100 points per week by viewing the online comics; 100 points per week by participating in problem-solving polls; 100 points per week by recording how they did on their goals at the end of the week; 1,000 points per week by achieving the Fit-for-Life goals; and 100 points per week by achieving their Fit-for-Life extra point goals. The participants could also earn an extra 100 points by returning completed problem solutions to help meet their Fit-for-Life goals.

Representing Baylor College of Medicine, each troop leader was asked to abide by the dress code by wearing "professional" (for 5-a-Day badge) or "professional athletic" outfits (for Fit-for-Life badge), to ensure appropriate personal appearance. All project staff signed a confidentiality statement stating that they would respect scouts' confidentiality during data collection. To minimize troop behavior problems, staff were given tip sheets about child behavior management. Staff were required to have each entire lesson well rehearsed and completely organized, moving quickly between activities. They were encouraged to meet the regular troop leaders to establish rapport and to finalize their troop schedule for implementation of the intervention. At the beginning of the meeting, they were instructed to be friendly, introduce themselves, and engage in small talk about their troop and/or lives as the scouts were checked in for the first time. They were asked to practice the behavioral objectives and expectations before the sessions, and given specific information about communication styles (e.g., use short, goal-directed sentences, and use both verbal and nonverbal gestures to give the scouts instruction and assist them in achieving the goals). Specific instructions were also given to staff regarding common situations and disruptive forms of behavior.

SUPPORT FROM THE BOY SCOUTS ORGANIZATION

The Sam Houston Council of Boy Scouts of America was very receptive and facilitated contacts to recruit troop leaders in several districts. As an efficacy trial, all program staffing was provided by the research grant.

OUTCOME EVALUATION

Design: An experiment (treatment vs. control) was conducted with Boy Scout troops in Houston, Texas. One group participated in 5-a-Day badge, which targeted increasing Boy Scouts' consumption of FV to five servings a day. The other group received a "mirror image" PA intervention, the Fit-for-Life badge, which targeted increasing Boy Scouts' PA levels to 30 minutes or more per day for 5 or more times a week. The intervention was conducted in two waves in the spring (16 troops) or fall (26 troops) of 2003 as a randomized trial, with troops assigned to intervention or control conditions after baseline data collection.

Sample size and power: The study was powered to detect a difference of 0.5 FV servings a day. A conservative estimate for sample size was calculated (Cohen, 1988) for the two-way analysis of variance (ANOVA), with the change from baseline to post-1 representing the dependent variable and with group and wave as factors (Cohen, 1988). With an alpha of .01 and a moderate effect size ($d = .50$), 204 participants were needed to achieve 80% power. This number was doubled to include the change from baseline to post-2, and multiplied by a variance inflation factor (Donner & Klar, 1996) to account for the nesting of subjects within troops. Given an intra-class correlation of .01 associated with troop (Baranowski et al., 2002) and approximately 10 scouts per troop, the minimum number of participants needed was 445.

Inclusionary criteria: The troop inclusionary criterion was a high likelihood of scouts having a home computer with Internet access. Scout inclusionary criteria included participating troop membership, a home computer with Internet access, and written consent/assent.

Recruitment: Permission to conduct the study was obtained from Sam Houston Area Council of Boy Scouts of America. Presentations were then made to troop leaders; scouts were recruited from troops expressing interest in the study. The 5-a-Day and Fit-for-Life badge interventions included 473 10- to 14-year-old Boy Scouts, recruited from 42 troops. The Urban Scouting Program, which served the needs of inner-city boys, was defunct at the time of this badge program evaluation and so could provide no inner-city troops to participate.

MEASURES

Demographics: Scouts' ethnicity and the highest household educational attainment were obtained by parental self-report at the time of consent.

Anthropometrics: Anthropometric data (height, weight, and BMI) were collected using standardized protocols, a stadiometer, and an electric scale (Jago et al., 2006).

FV consumption: Fruit and vegetable consumption were measured using a modified Food Frequency Questionnaire validated against 24-hours dietary recalls ($r = .92$) with Urban Boy Scouts (Cullen, Baranowski, Baranowski, Hebert, & de Moor, 1999). It included four 100% juice, 17 fruits, and 17 vegetables. The response scale represented the nonaveraged number of servings consumed in the previous 7 days. Fruit juice (FJ) and low-fat vegetables (LV) were analyzed separately. FJ consumption was computed by summing servings of the 4 juice and 17 fruit. LV consumption was determined by removing three high-fat vegetables (i.e., French fries, potato salad, and other potatoes) and computing the servings of the remaining 14 lower-fat items (e.g., carrots, broccoli).

Social desirability: Social desirability of response was assessed using the 9-item "Lie Scale" from the Revised Children's Manifest Anxiety Scale (Reynolds & Paget, 1983). The scale has a 5-item response format ("never" to "always"). The "lie" score was determined by summing the responses. The instrument has shown good reliability and validity in children across a variety of ethnic groups (Dadds, Perrin, & Yule, 1998).

Physical activity: Physical activity was monitored for three consecutive days at each assessment, using the MTI accelerometer (Manufacturing Technologies Inc., Fort Walton Beach, Florida). The MTI has been shown to be a valid measure of physical activity in adolescents (Puyau, Adolph, Vohra, & Butte, 2002). Each monitor was programmed to begin recording at midnight, after the measurement meeting. The monitors were removed on the fourth morning after data collection. Two hypothesized mediators, self-efficacy and preferences, were measured at each time period, using validated questionnaires (Sherwood et al., 2004).

Accelerometry data for a day were included if the scout met a previously developed MTI inclusion criterion of at least 800 minutes between 6 a.m. and midnight (Treuth et al., 2004). In accordance with previous studies (Jago, Anderson, Baranowski, & Watson, 2005; Treuth et al., 2004), a Statistical Package for the Social Sciences (SPSS) program identified minutes in which the monitor was not worn, using a criterion of 20 or more continuous minutes of zeros. Days with less than 800 minutes of recorded data were considered invalid (Treuth et al., 2004). To maximize the sample size, participants were included in the analysis if they possessed at least one complete day during each measurement period. There were 240 (82.4%) of the participants at baseline who possessed three valid days of data, with 240 (68.2%) and 197 (70.6%) at post-1 and post-2. Forty-four (15.2%), 75 (21.2%), and 43 (15.4%) of participants possessed two valid days at baseline, post-1, and post-2. Seven (2.4%), 37 (10.5%), and 39 (14.0%) participants possessed one valid day at baseline, post-1, and post-2.

Adolescent-specific cutpoints (Puyau et al., 2002) were used to categorize the physical activity in each minute as sedentary ($<$ 800 counts), light (800–3,199 counts), or moderate to vigorous intensity ($\geq$ 3,200 counts). To account for differences in the times for which the monitors were worn, mean minutes of activity at each level were weighted by the inverse of the proportion of time for which the monitor was worn. Mean minutes in each category per day were then calculated. The mean number of counts per minute, an indicator of the total volume of activity in which the participant engaged, was also calculated. There were no significant ($P < .05$) differences in minutes of sedentary, light, or moderate to vigorous physical activity or counts per minute when 1, 2, or 3 valid days were used as inclusion criteria for accelerometer data.

Incentives for participation: Troop leaders received a $1,000 incentive for use for their troop following post-2 data collection. Participating scouts received graduated incentives of $25, $30, and $35 for participating in each of the three assessments. A sewn-cloth badge was awarded to scouts who had accumulated enough points.

Statistical analyses: Repeated measures analyses were completed using the Proc Mixed (Little, Milliken, Stroup,& Wolfinger, 1996) procedure in

SAS 9.1, to detect differences in diet or physical activity over time between the intervention and control groups. Main effects for treatment groups (intervention, control), visit time (baseline, post-1, and post-2), wave (spring, fall), and the interactions within groups, visit time, and wave main effects were treated as fixed effects. Scouts were nested within troops and the troop treated as a random effect. Separate analyses were run for each dependent variable. Models were then rerun controlling for BMI, ethnicity, and parental education. Alpha was set at .05.

RESULTS

Four-hundred seventy-three 10- to 14-year-olds were recruited from 42 Houston-area troops. Participants were 13 years of age in the average, and predominantly Anglo-American (72%) or Hispanic (13%). Approximately 36% of the sample was college graduates; 64% of the eligible sample was enrolled. Parental education, group, and wave were significantly related ($P = .007$), with more participants from the control group in the fall wave living in households in which at least one parent had a college or postgraduate degree (Jago et al., 2006). Average troop attendance was 81%; 76% (78% 5-a-Day and 75% Fit-for-Life) logged onto the study website at least once a week.

Both of the nine-session troop-plus-Internet interventions resulted in behavior change. Baseline FV consumption was approximately 2.5 servings per day (Thompson et al., 2009). Average baseline FJ and LV consumption did not significantly differ between groups. A significant group × time interaction was observed for FJ consumption ($P = .003$). Regression estimates representing the change at post-1 yielded significant group differences in FJ consumption ($P = .028$). FJ consumption at post-1 increased by nearly one serving, with a mean increase (and standard error) of 0.94 (0.0) servings in the 5-a-Day group, compared to a mean increase of 0.56 (0.0) servings in the control group. The post-1 changes translated into a positive effect (effect size, 0.4 servings) for the 5-a-Day group. However, the improvement was not maintained. Although not significant, the changes at post-2 from baseline translated into a positive effect (effect size, 0.4 servings) for the control group. There was a significant group × time × wave interaction for LV consumption ($P = .014$). Regression estimates yielded a significant ($P = .005$) group difference in LV consumption between baseline and post-2 in the spring wave, with the control group reporting a mean increase of 0.85 (0.1) servings and the 5-a-Day reporting a slight mean decrease of −0.14 (0.1) servings. Although not significant, the changes at post-1 translated to a positive effect (effect size, 0.2 servings) for the 5-a-Day group, whereas changes at post-2 translated into a positive effect (effect size, 0.5 servings) for the control group.

The baseline MVPA (moderate to vigorous physical activity) was approximately 25 minutes per day (Jago et al., 2006). There was a three-way interaction term (treatment group × time × wave), indicating a significant ($t = 2.54$, $df = 498$, $p = .011$) increase in light intensity physical activity from baseline to post-1 in the spring intervention group (143.6 at baseline to 155.9 at post-1). There were no significant differences between baseline and post-2 minutes of light intensity physical activity, and no other significant main or interaction terms. There were no significant main effects or interaction terms in the moderate to vigorous or counts per minute models. Rerunning the models controlling for demographics did not significantly change the results. Seventy-nine percent of the participants obtained the Fit-for-Life badge, but there were no significant group (badge vs. no badge) or group by time interactions.

DISCUSSION

The Boy Scout badge programs offered a unique opportunity to reach boys and their families with a behavioral change intervention which was consistent with the mission of the Boy Scouts of America. The institutionalization of such a permanent badge requirement could provide a stable structure to deliver health activities to youth around the country.

The curriculum was developed through extensive focus-group discussions with African American scouts and their parents. This ensured that the intervention would fit the participants' ethnic and cultural background at both the surface and deeper structures (Resnicow et al., 1999). The lack of ethnic group differences in program outcomes indicated that the programs initially targeted to meet the needs of African American Boy Scouts were effective with a broader group of scouts.

The Boy Scout badge programs were theory-based. Interventions to improve Boy Scouts'dietary and PA behaviors help to address the issue of childhood obesity and early cancer prevention among children, especially ethnic minorities. Due to the difficulties associated with changing dietary and PA behaviors, all possible health education communication channels should be utilized under theoretical guidance. The combination of in-person and Internet-based scouting programs was an effective method of childhood obesity and cancer-prevention–related behavior change.

Editor's Note: This program was designed to help Boy Scouts from multiple ethnic groups increase fruit and vegetable consumption and increase vigorous exercise. Deliberate efforts were put into creating a culturally sensitive program, including holding focus groups with African American scouts and their parents, as well as pilot testing of the program among African American troops. Due to strong support from the area Council of Boy Scouts, 470 scouts in 42 troops across several districts were recruited for the evaluation phase of this study. Regrettably and unexpectedly, the Urban

Scouting Program, which served inner-city boys (primarily African American), closed down during this period. As a result, the efficacy of this program was evaluated only among Anglo-American and Hispanic youth. Despite this serious setback, we chose to include this chapter for several reasons: (a) the efficacy of this program, developed for African American youths, was illustrated in youth from other ethnic groups; (b) we hope that these findings will stimulate future research, in which the efficacy of this program in multiple ethnic groups will be tested; (c) as the program was developed with input from, and pilot testing with, African American youth, it can be tried in other African American communities; and (d) it is an illustration of what can happen in the real world—despite all the best intentions, careful, well thought out preparations, and appropriate pilot testing, just as you are ready to implement the program, life gets in the way. All of us will face similar challenges along the way; the key, of course, is not to give up, but find ways to overcome them or develop new strategies. *R.E.*

REFERENCES

Bandura, A. (1977). Self-efficacy: Toward a unifying theory of behavior change. *Psychological Review, 84*(2), 191–215.

Bandura, A. (1986). *Social foundations for thought and action: A social cognitive theory.* Englewood Cliffs, NJ: Prentice Hall.

Bandura, A. (1994). Self-efficacy. In V. S. Ramachaudran (Ed.), *Encyclopedia of human behavior* (Vol. 4, pp. 71–81). New York, NY: Academic Press.

Baranowski, T., Baranowski, J., Cullen, K. W., deMoor, C., Rittenberry, L., Hebert, D., & Jones, L. (2002). 5 a Day achievement badge for African-American Boy Scouts: pilot outcome results. *Preventive Medicine, 34*(3), 353–363.

Baranowski, T., Cullen, K. W., & Baranowski, J. (1999). Psychosocial correlates of dietary intake: Advancing dietary intervention. *Annual Review of Nutrition, 19,* 17–40.

Baranowski, T., Lin, L. S., Wetter, D. W., Resnicow, K., & Hearn, M. D. (1997). Theory as mediating variables: Why aren't community interventions working as desired? *Annals of Epidemiology, 7*(7, Suppl. 1), S89–S95.

Baranowski, T., Mendlein, J., Resnicow, K., Frank, E., Cullen, K. W., & Baranowski, J. (2000). Physical activity and nutrition (PAN) in children and youth: Behavior, genes, and tracking in obesity prevention. *Preventive Medicine, 31,* S1–S10.

Baranowski, T., Smith, M., Hearn, M. D., Lin, L. S., Baranowski, J., Doyle, C., . . . Wang, D. T. (1997). Patterns in children's fruit and vegetable consumption by meal and day of the week. *Journal of the American College of Nutrition, 16,* 216–223.

Barrios, E. X., & Costell, E. (2004). Review: Use of methods of research into consumers' opinions and attitudes in food research. *Food Science and Technology International, 10,* 359–371.

Birch, L. L., McPhee, L., Shoba, B. C., Pirok, E., & Steinberg, L. (1987). What kind of exposure reduces children's food neophobia? Looking vs. tasting. *Appetite, 9*(3), 171–178.

Borugian, M. J., Sheps, S. B., Kim-Sing, C., Van Patten, C., Potter, J. D., Dunn, B., . . . Hislop, T. G. (2004). Insulin, macronutrient intake, and physical activity: Are potential indicators of insulin resistance associated with mortality from breast cancer? *Cancer Epidemiology, Biomarkers &Prevention, 13*(7), 1163–1172.

Boy Scouts of America. (2008). Facts about scouting. Retrieved May 4, 2010, from http://www.scouting.org/About/FactSheets/ScoutingFacts.aspx

Brown, T., Kelly, S., & Summerbell, C. (2007). Prevention of obesity: A review of interventions. *Obesity Reviews, 8*(Suppl. 1), 127–130.

Cardon, G., Philippaerts, R., Lefevre, J., Matton, L., Wijndaele, K., Balduck, A., & De Bourdeaudhuij, I. (2005). Physical activity levels in 10- to 11-year-olds: Clustering of psychosocial correlates. *Public Health Nutrition, 8*(7), 896–903.

Carmichael, A. R., & Bates, T. (2004). Obesity and breast cancer: A review of the literature. *Breast, 13*, 85–92.

Chan, J. M., Rimm, E. B., Colditz, G. A., Stampfer, M. J., & Willett, W. C. (1994). Obesity, fat distribution, and weight gain as risk factors for clinical diabetes in men. *Diabetes Care, 17*(9), 961–969.

Cohen, J. (1988). *Statistical power analysis for the behavioral sciences.* Hillsdale, NJ: Lawrence Erlbaum.

Colditz, G. A., & Frazier, A. L. (1995). Models of breast cancer show that risk is set by events of early life: Prevention efforts must shift focus. *Cancer Epidemiology, Biomarkers & Prevention, 4*(5), 567–571.

Contento, I. R. (2008). Nutrition education: Linking research, theory, and practice. *Asia Pacific Journal of Clinical Nutrition, 17*(Suppl. 1), 176–179.

Contento, I. R., Manning, A., & Shannon, B. (1992). Research perspective on school-based nutrition education. *Journal of Nutrition Education, 24*, 247–260.

Cullen, K. W., Baranowski, T., Baranowski, J., Hebert, D., & de Moor, C. (1999). Pilot study of the validity and reliability of brief fruit, juice and vegetable screeners among inner city African-American boys and 17–20 year old adults. *Journal of the American College of Nutrition, 18*(5), 442–450.

Cullen, K. W., Baranowski, T., Baranowski, J., Warnecke, C., de Moor, C., Nwachokor, A., . . . Jones, L. A. (1998). "5 A Day" achievement badge for Urban Boy Scouts: Formative evaluation results. *Journal of Cancer Education, 13*(3), 162–168.

Cullen, K. W., Bartholomew, L. K., & Parcel, G. S. (1997). Girl scouting: An effective channel for nutrition education. *Journal of Nutrition Education, 29*, 86–91.

Dadds, M. R., Perrin, S., & Yule, W. (1998). Social desirability and self-reported anxiety in children: An analysis of the RCMAS Lie scale. *Journal of Abnormal Child Psychology, 26*(4), 311–317.

Domel, S., Baranowski, T., Davis, H., Thompson, W. O., Leonard, S. B., Riley, P., . . . Smyth, M. (1993). Development and evaluation of a school intervention to increase fruit and vegetable consumption among 4th and 5th grade students. *Journal of Nutrition Education, 25*, 345–349.

Donner, A., & Klar, N. (1996). Statistical considerations in the design and analysis of community intervention trials. *Journal of Clinical Epidemiology, 49*(4), 435–439.

Fontanini, G., Campani, D., Roncella, M., Cecchetti, D., Calvo, S., Toniolo, A., & Basolo, F. (1999). Expression of interleukin 6 (IL-6) correlates with oestrogen receptor in human breast carcinoma. *British Journal of Cancer, 80*, 579–584.

Freedman, D. S., Khan, L. K., Serdula, M. K., Dietz, W. H., Srinivasan, S. R., & Berenson, G. S. (2002). Relation of age at menarche to race, time period, and anthropometric dimensions: The Bogalusa Heart Study. *Pediatrics, 110*(4), e43.

Freedman, D. S., Khan, L. K., Serdula, M. K., Dietz, W. H., Srinivasan, S. R., & Berenson, G. S. (2003). The relation of menarcheal age to obesity in childhood and adulthood: The Bogalusa Heart Study. *BMC Pediatrics, 3*(1), 3.

Giovannucci, E. (2001). Insulin, insulin-like growth factors and colon cancer: A review of the evidence. *Journal of Nutrition, 131*, 3109s–3120s.

Granner, M. L., Sargent, R. G., Calderon, K. S., Hussey, J. R., Evans, A. E., & Watkins, K. W. (2004). Factors of fruit and vegetable intake by race, gender, and age among young adolescents. *Journal of Nutrition Education and Behavior, 36*(4), 173–180.

Hankinson, S. E., Willett, W. C., Colditz, G. A., Hunter, D. J., Michaud, D. S., Deroo, B., . . . Pollak, M. (1997). Circulating concentrations of insulin-like growth factor-I and risk of breast cancer. *Lancet, 351*, 1393–1396.

Hardwick, J. C., Van Den Brink, G. R., Offerhaus, G. J., Van Deventer, S. J., & Pepelenbosch, M. P. (2001). Leptin is a growth factor for colonic epithelial cells. *Gastroenterology, 121*, 79–90.

Harvie, M., Hooper, L., & Howell, A. H. (2003). Central obesity and breast cancer risk: A systematic review. *Obesity Reviews, 4*, 157–173.

Jago, R., Anderson, C. B., Baranowski, T., & Watson, K. (2005). Adolescent patterns of physical activity differences by gender, day, and time of day. *American Journal of Preventive Medicine, 28*(5), 447–452.

Jago, R., Baranowski, T., Baranowski, J., Cullen, K. W., & Thompson, D. (2007). Distance to food stores & adolescent male fruit and vegetable consumption: Mediation effects. *International Journal of Behavioral Nutrition and Physical Activity, 4*(1), 35.

Jago, R., Baranowski, T., Baranowski, J., Thompson, D., Cullen, K. W., Watson, K., & Liu, Y. (2006). Fit For Life Boy Scout badge: Outcome evaluation of a troop & Internet intervention. *Preventive Medicine, 42*(3), 181–187.

Kaaks, R., & Lukanova, A. (2001). Energy balance and cancer: The role of insulin and insulin-like growth factor-I. *Proceedings of the Nutrition Society, 60*, 91–106.

Kaaks, R., Lukanova, A., & Kurzer, M. S. (2002). Obesity, endogenous hormones, and endometrial cancer risk: A synthetic review. *Cancer Epidemiology, Biomarkers & Prevention, 11*, 1531–1543.

Kalakanis, L., & Moulton, B. (2006). School-based interventions for childhood obesity. *Texas Legislative Council Research Division: Facts at a Glance*. Retrieved June 29, 2011, from http://www.tlc.state.tx.us/pubspol/childobesity.pdf

Kelder, S. H., Perry, C. L., Klepp, K. I., & Lytle, L. L. (1994). Longitudinal tracking of adolescent smoking, physical activity, and food choice behaviors. *American Journal of Public Health, 84*(7), 1121–1126.

Kranz, S., Mitchell, D. C., Smiciklas-Wright, H., Huang, S. H., Kumanyika, S. K., & Stettler, N. (2009). Consumption of recommended food groups among children from medically underserved communities. *Journal of the American Dietetic Association, 109*(4), 702–707.

Kumanyika, S. K., Obarzanek, E., Stettler, N., Bell, R., Field, A. E., Fortmann, S. P., . . . Hong, Y. (2008). Population-based prevention of obesity: The need for comprehensive promotion of healthful eating, physical activity, and energy balance: A scientific statement from American Heart Association Council on Epidemiology and Prevention, Interdisciplinary Committee for Prevention (formerly the Expert Panel on Population and Prevention Science). *Circulation, 118*(4), 428–464.

Kumanyika, S. K., & Yancey, A. K. (2009). Physical activity and health equity: Evolving the science. *American Jornal of Health Promotion, 23*(6), S4–S7.

Ledoux, T. A., Hingle, M. D., & Baranowski, T. (2010). Relationship of fruit and vegetable intake with adiposity: A systematic review. *Obesity Reviews, 12*(5), e143–e150.

Little, R. C., Milliken, G. A., Stroup, W. W., & Wolfinger, R. D. (1996). *SAS system for mixed models*. Cary, NC: SAS Institute, Inc.

Maibach, E., & Cotton, D. (1995). Moving people to behavior change: A staged social cognitive approach to message design. In E. Maibach & R. Parrott (Eds.), *Designing health messages: Approaches from communication theory and public health practice* (pp. 41–64). Thousand Oaks, CA: Sage Publications.

Malina, R. M. (2008). Promoting physical activity in children and adolescents: A review. *Clinical Journal of Sport Medicine, 18*(6), 549–550.

Mantzoros, E., Petridou, E., Dessypris, N., Chavelas, C., Dalamaga, M., Alexe, D. M., . . . Trichopoulos, D. (2004). Adiponectin and breast cancer risk. *Journal of Clinical Endocrinology and Metabolism, 89*, 1102–1107.

Miyoshi, Y., Funahashi, T., Kihara, S., Taguchi, T., Tamaki, Y., Matsuzawa, Y., & Noguchi, S. (2003). Association of serum adiponectin levels with breast cancer risk. *Clinical Cancer Research, 9*, 5699–5704.

Murphy, T.K., Calle, E.E., Rodriguez, C., Khan, H.S., & Thurn, M. J. (2000). Body mass index and colon cancer mortality in a large prospective study. *American Journal of Epidemiology, 152*, 847–854.

Nam, S.Y., Lee, E. J., Kim, K. R., Cha, B. S., Song, Y. D., Lim, S. K., . . . Huh, K. B. (1997). Effect of obesity on total and free insulin-like growth factor (IGF)-1, and their relationship to IGF-binding protein (BP)-1 IGFBP-2, IGFBP-3, insulin and growth hormone. *International Journal of Obesity Related Metabolic Disorders, 21*, 355–359.

O'Connor, T. M., Jago, R., & Baranowski, T. (2009). Engaging parents to increase youth physical activity: A systematic review. *American Journal of Preventive Medicine, 37*, 141–149.

Ong, K., Kratzsch, J., Keiss, W., & Dunger, D. (2002). Circulating IGF-1 levels in childhood are related to both current body composition and early postnatal growth. *Journal of Clinical Endocrinology and Metabolism, 87*, 1041–1044.

Onuma, M., Bub, J. D., Rummel, T. L., & Iwamoto, Y. (2003). Prostrate cancer cell-adipocyte interaction: Leptin mediates androgen-independent prostate cancer cell proliferation through c-Jun NH@-terminal kinase. *Journal of Biology and Chemistry, 43*, 42660–42667.

Puyau, M. R., Adolph, A. L., Vohra, F. A., & Butte, N. F. (2002). Validation and calibration of physical activity monitors in children. *Obesity Research, 10*(3), 150–157.

Resnicow, K., Baranowski, T., Ahluwalia, J. S., & Braithwaite, R. L. (1999). Cultural sensitivity in public health: Defined and demystified. *Ethnicity & Disease, 9*(1), 10–21.

Reynolds, C. R., & Paget, K. O. (1983). National normative and reliability data for the Revised Children's Manifest Anxiety Scale. *School Psychology Review, 12*, 324–336.

Roblin, L. (2007). Childhood obesity: Food, nutrient, and eating-habit trends and influences. *Applied Physiology, Nutrition, and Metabolism, 32*(4), 635–645.

Schneider, M. R., Hoeflich, A., Fischer, J. R., Wolf, E., Sordat, B., & Lahm, H. (2000). Interleukin-6 stimulates clonogenic growth of primary and metastatic human colon carcinoma cells. *Cancer Letters, 151*, 31–38.

Sherwood, N. E., Taylor, W. C., Treuth, M., Klesges, L. M., Baranowski, T., Zhou, A., . . . Miller, W. (2004). Measurement characteristics of activity-related psychosocial measures in 8- to 10-year-old African-American girls in the Girls Health Enrichment Multisite Study (GEMS). *Preventive Medicine, 38*(Suppl.), S60–S68.

Taylor, W. C., Baranowski, T., & Young, D. R. (1998). Physical activity interventions in low-income, ethnic minority, and populations with disability. *American Journal of Preventive Medicine, 15*(4), 334–343.

Taylor, W. C., Beech, B. M., & Cummings, S. S. (1997). Increasing physical activity levels among youth: A public health challenge. In D. K. Wilson, J. R. Rodriguez, & W. C. Taylor (Eds.), *Health-promoting and health-compromising behaviors among minority adolesents.* Washington, DC: American Psychological Association.

Thompson, D., Baranowski, T., Baranowski, J., Cullen, K. W., Jago, R., Watson, K., & Liu, Y. (2009). Boy Scout 5-A-Day badge: Outcome results of a troop and Internet intervention. *Preventive Medicine, 49,* 518–526.

Treuth, M. S., Sherwood, N., Baranowski, T., Butte, N. F., Jacobs, D. R., McClanahan, B., ... Obarzanek, E. (2004). Physical activity self report and accelerometry measures from the Girls health Enrichment Multi-site Studies (GEMS). *Preventive Medicine, 38,* S43–S49.

Troiano, R. P., Berrigan, D., Dodd, K. W., Masse, L. C., Tilert, T., & McDowell, M. (2008). Physical activity in the United States measured by accelerometer. *Medicine and Science in Sports and Exercise, 40*(1), 181–188.

U.S. Department of Health and Human Services. (1990). *Healthy People 2000: National health promotion and disease prevention objectives.* Washington, DC: U.S. Government Printing Office.

Voskuil, D. W., Mesquita, H. B. B., Kaaks, R., van Noord, P. A. H., Rinaldi, S., Riboli, E., ... Peeters, P. H. (2001). Determinants of circulating insulin-like growth factor (IGF) I and IGF binding proteins 1–3 in premenopausal women: Physical activity and anthropometry (Netherlands). *Cancer Causes & Control, 12,* 951–958.

Wabitsch, M., Blum, W. F., Muche, R., Heinze, E., Haug, C., Mayer, H., & Teller, W. (1996). Insulin-like growth factors and their binding proteins before and after weight loss and their associations with hormonal and metabolic parameters in obese adolescent girls. *International Journal of Obesity, 20,* 1073–1080.

What Moves You? (n.d.). Retrieved from http://www.kidnetic.com

Whitaker, R. C., Wright, J. A., Pepe, M. S., Seidel, K. D., & Dietz, W. H. (1997). Predicting obesity in young adulthood from childhood and parental obesity. *New England Journal of Medicine, 337*(13), 869–873.

Whitt-Glover, M. C., & Kumanyika, S. K. (2009). Systematic review of interventions to increase physical activity and physical fitness in African-Americans. *American Journal of Health Promotion, 23*(6), S33–S56.

8

A Systematic Approach to Developing Contextually, Culturally, and Gender-Sensitive Interventions for African American Men: The Example of *Men 4 Health*

Derek M. Griffith, Katie Gunter, and Julie Ober Allen

Research on racial and ethnic health disparities has continued to grow over the past decade, but disparities in cancer morbidity and mortality between racial and ethnic groups (Frohlich & Potvin, 2008; Geiger, 2006; Griffith, Moy, Reischl, & Dayton, 2006; Sankar et al., 2004) and between men and women continue to persist and, in some cases, widen (American Cancer Society, 2009). While there has been progress in our understanding of racial differences in health status, there remains considerable disagreement on why disparities persist and what should be done to eliminate them. More research is needed that helps to identify how and where to intervene to eliminate racial and ethnic disparities in health, particularly for cancer disparities (Adler, 2006).

The health behaviors and disparate health outcomes that are of primary interest to social scientists are rooted in historical and contemporary inequalities in education, justice, social and political power, and economics (Griffith et al., 2006). These factors not only directly affect health behaviors and health outcomes, but the ecological contexts in which these outcomes occur. Investigators, however, tend to examine health disparities by fragmenting contributing factors into separate contextual and individual-level components (Williams & Jackson, 2005). While this yields needed information on unique relationships and disease pathways, it provides an incomplete picture. Achieving the goal of eliminating racial health disparities in the United States requires research that synthesizes available knowledge and provides a more comprehensive understanding of racial differences in health outcomes (Adler, 2006; Moy, Arispe, Holmes, & Andrews, 2005). Health disparities are created and maintained through multiple and varied pathways that must be understood and addressed holistically.

Increasingly, health behavior interventions and the theories that inform them have considered how multiple levels and dimensions of the social ecological contexts of health may influence risk, behaviors, and outcomes (McLeroy, Bibeau, Steckler, & Glanz, 1988). Although these approaches have become more systematic in considering the influences of race and ethnicity on health, few have considered how race and ethnicity intersect with gender, particularly male gender.

While it is critical to continue focusing on eliminating racial and ethnic disparities in cancer, it is not clear that race and ethnicity are the most important characteristics affecting cancer risk behavior. Men are more likely than women to engage in over 30 behaviors that have been known to increase the risk of injury, morbidity, and mortality, many of which are behavioral risk factors for cancer (Courtenay, 2000); this suggests that there is a potential benefit of examining gender, particularly male gender, in combination with other risk factors for understanding and addressing cancer disparities. While sex refers to biologically determined factors, gender refers to differences between men and women that stem from social and cultural origins (Payne, 2006). While cultural sensitivity is generally recognized as a necessary component for effective health promotion programs, it has typically been utilized to address racial and ethnic differences, and in a way that has been consistently more successful at engaging women (Resnicow, Baranowski, Ahluwalia, & Braithwaite, 1999). Incorporating the gendered nature of culture, particularly for men, may be essential for interventions focused on reducing men's health risk behaviors to be successful. Gender influences health and intersects with other known determinants of health to play an important role in health behavior, particularly in exacerbating and mitigating men's health behaviors and cancer outcomes.

In this chapter, we argue that attending to male gender in addition to race and ethnicity in population-based interventions is vital to improving health and eliminating cancer disparities. We will briefly review the cancer epidemiology of African American men. We will then provide an overview of an existing culturally sensitive, research-tested intervention, *Body and Soul*, which we are adapting to more effectively engage and change the behavior of African American men. We chose to adapt *Body and Soul* as it has demonstrated success in improving our behaviors of interest—healthier eating and physical activity—in multiple efficacy and effectiveness trials with African Americans, albeit primarily with women (Resnicow et al., 2004). The remainder of the chapter describes the process that we developed and are currently employing to adapt the core components of *Body and Soul* into a more male-gender–sensitive intervention called *Men 4 Health* (*M4H*). We conclude with a brief discussion of lessons learned and recommendations for adapting interventions to be more male-gender sensitive.

THE CANCER EPIDEMIOLOGY OF AFRICAN AMERICAN MEN

Men in the United States have slightly less than a 1 in 2 lifetime risk of developing cancer, and that risk is dramatically higher for African American men (American Cancer Society, 2004). African American men have approximately a 37% higher death rate from cancer than White men (Powe et al., 2009). For African American men aged 45 and older, cancer is the first or second leading cause of death (American Cancer Society, 2009; Taylor et al., 2001). Between 1975 and the early 1990s, the disparity in cancer death rates between African American and White males widened, and today it remains larger than it was in 1975 (Ward et al., 2004). In addition, African American and White disparities in cancer mortality rates are greater for African American men than African American women (American Cancer Society, 2009).

Of all cancers, prostate, lung, and colon cancers have both the highest incidence and mortality rates for African American men (American Cancer Society, 2009). Together, these three cancers comprised 60% of all cancer incidence and 54% of all cancer mortality for African American males in 2009. For these cancers, African American men are less likely than White men to undergo screening tests, have their cancer diagnosed at early or localized stages, and have access to appropriate and timely cancer treatment (American Cancer Society, 2009). When compared to White men, African American men have higher incidence and mortality rates for prostate, lung, and colon cancer, and lower 5-year survival rates (American Cancer Society, 2009).

The health behaviors of African American men seem to contribute to their high rates of colon, lung, and possibly prostate cancer (Koh, Massin-Short, & Elqura, 2009). The evidence linking physical activity and cancer is strong for colon cancer and suggestive for many other types of cancer including lung and prostate cancers (Friedenreich & Orenstein, 2002; Gotay, 2005). Consumption of foods that are high in fat from animal sources, red meat, and processed meats and low consumption of fruits and vegetables also tend to increase colorectal cancer risk, as does obesity (Schneider, 2009). Approximately half of African American men in the United States report no leisure time physical activity (Ward et al., 2004). African American men aged between 35 and 50 years eat, on average, only 3.5 of the 9 recommended daily servings of fruits and vegetables, fewer than any other racial or ethnic group (National Cancer Institute, 2002). Approximately one fourth (24.4%) of African American men are obese, which is second only to the obesity rate for American Indian/Alaska Native men (Ward et al., 2004). These patterns of disease suggest that race and gender play an essential role in cancer morbidity and mortality of African American men, and need to be more effectively considered to eliminate racial and gender disparities in cancer.

AN OVERVIEW OF *BODY AND SOUL*

Although several studies have examined factors associated with obesity among African Americans in general and African American men in particular, little is currently known about how to effectively intervene to improve dietary practices and rates of physical activity of African American men. *Body and Soul* is one of only two community-based, research-tested intervention programs recognized by the National Cancer Institute (NCI) has been found to be efficacious with African American populations, and that is available on the NCI's Cancer Control Planet. The *Body and Soul* intervention was developed by combining methods from previous evidenced-based research on dietary behavior change in African Americans with theory-based research identifying social and cognitive variables associated with health behaviors (Resnicow et al., 2004). Despite the success of *Body and Soul* at improving healthy eating and physical activity, it has thus far failed to enroll and retain significant numbers of African American men: over 70% of each sample has been female.

The Theoretical Foundations of *Body and Soul*

Body and Soul utilizes constructs from social support theory (Israel, 1985; Israel & McLeroy, 1985), social cognitive theory (Bandura, 2001), and self-determination theory (Ryan & Deci, 2000). Social support theory emphasizes the importance of social influence and social support in shaping and maintaining health behavior, and several studies have found that behavior-specific social support is related to healthy dietary practices (Ammerman, Lindquist, Lohr, & Hersey, 2002). Social cognitive theory incorporates both psychosocial factors influencing health behavior and strategies for promoting behavior change. Social cognitive theory posits that behavioral capability (i.e., knowledge and skill to perform a given behavior) and self-efficacy (i.e., the belief that one is capable of performing a behavior) are important causal factors related to healthy eating and physical activity (Steptoe et al., 2003). Self-determination theory focuses on social and contextual conditions that facilitate self-motivation and healthy psychological development (Ryan & Deci, 2000). Ryan and colleagues (1997) found evidence of a relationship between intrinsic motivation and long-term changes in physical activity; specifically, the people who reported higher intrinsic motivation were more likely to sustain higher rates of physical activity than those with lower rates of intrinsic motivation (Ryan, Frederick, Lepes, Rubio, & Sheldon, 1997). Trudeau and colleagues found evidence of a relationship between intrinsic motivation and fruit and vegetable intake in a cross-sectional study (Trudeau, Kristal, Li, & Patterson, 1998).

Intervention Components of *Body and Soul*

Body and Soul includes four basic components: church-wide activities, organizational policy change, motivational interviewing, and self-help materials. As a condition for participating in the project, individual churches agree to carry out several core components, including holding a kickoff event, establishing a project committee, hosting at least three church-wide nutrition events, and having at least one additional event involving the pastor. The churches also agree to make at least one policy change (e.g., offer healthy food in addition to traditional options at church-wide events). All individuals enrolling in *Body and Soul* receive the *Eat for Life (EFL)* cookbook as well as several American Cancer Society educational pamphlets. Finally, peer counselors are trained in motivational interviewing, which is a counseling approach that helps individuals work through their ambivalence about behavior change, overcome their own barriers, and explore potential untapped sources of motivation. In our efforts to adapt *Body and Soul* to more effectively engage men, we examined the setting (faith-based organizations vs. other organizations), contextual and psychosocial factors, and motivations to engage in healthy eating and physical activity.

FOUNDATIONS OF THE INTERVENTION ADAPTATION AND DEVELOPMENT PROCESS

While there is consensus that health promotion programs should be culturally sensitive, there has been surprisingly little conceptual work defining cultural sensitivity and testing the effectiveness of culturally sensitive interventions (Resnicow et al., 1999). Cultural sensitivity is the extent to which health promotion materials and programs incorporate ethnic/cultural characteristics, experiences, norms, values, behavior patterns, consumer preferences, and beliefs of a focus population as well as relevant historical, environmental, and social forces in design, delivery, and evaluation (Resnicow et al., 1999).

Developing Culturally Sensitive Health Promotion Interventions

According to Resnicow and colleagues (1999, 2004), cultural sensitivity is composed of two dimensions: surface structure and deep structure. Surface structure involves matching intervention materials, messages, and events to observable, "superficial" (although nonetheless important) characteristics of a focus population. Surface structure may involve using people, places, language, music, food, locations, product brands, and clothing style familiar to, representative of, and preferred by, the target audience. Surface structure also includes identifying what channels (e.g., media) and settings (e.g., churches, schools) are most appropriate for delivery of messages and programs. With regard to cultural competence, or interpersonal sensitivity, this generally entails using ethnically matched staff to recruit participants as well as deliver and evaluate programs (Resnicow et al., 1999). In effect, surface structure refers to the extent to which interventions appear to fit within a culture. Surface structure is generally achievable through expert and community participation, as well as the involvement of the focus population in the intervention development process.

The second dimension, deep structure, has received less attention and can be more elusive, yet is an essential aspect of determining relevance and effectiveness. Deep structure refers to the cultural, social, historical, and psychological forces that influence the target health behavior in the proposed focus population, as well as the population's unique environmental and psychological barriers and enabling factors. Whereas surface structure generally increases the receptivity or acceptance of messages, deep structure conveys salience. Surface structure is a prerequisite for feasibility, whereas deep structure determines efficacy. Deep structure involves understanding how particular sociodemographic and ethnic populations differ from other groups, as well as how ethnic, cultural, social, environmental, and historical factors may influence specific health behaviors within that population (Airhihenbuwa, DiClemente, Wingood, & Lowe, 1992). This entails understanding how members of the focus population perceive the etiology and treatment of a particular illness or behavioral risk factor (Airhihenbuwa et al., 1992). Culturally tailored interventions need to address and accommodate cultural values and historical beliefs to have credibility.

One strategy that has been used to tap into deep structural elements of interventions is ethnic mapping (Resnicow et al., 1999; Resnicow, Soler, Braithwaite, Ahluwalia, & Butler, 2000). This process has been used to provide valuable information for tailoring interventions by asking focus groups of the population of interest to classify aspects of the target behavior along a continuum. Most often, because cultural sensitivity has been operationalized as ethnic or racial sensitivity, participants have been asked to rate foods or types of physical activity on a continuum of race and ethnicity (e.g., mostly for Blacks; equally for Blacks and Whites; mostly for Whites).

Limitations of Cultural Sensitivity

While using a culturally sensitive approach to developing interventions is considered an important aspect of health behavior interventions, there is little agreement on how we might operationally define cultural sensitivity. What constitutes aspects of surface and deep structure, for example, and how should other aspects of identity (e.g., age, gender) be considered? The process of ethnic mapping provides a useful example of this challenge.

Ethnic mapping implicitly assumes that race and ethnicity are the most salient aspects of identity that are relevant to behavior change. We, however, posit that gender is an equally important aspect of identity that may influence health behavior. Consequently, the challenge becomes: How do we adapt the mapping process for use with African American men? Do we first ask men to rate items or activities along a racial/ethnic continuum, and then ask them to do the same along a gender continuum (e.g., mostly a male thing; equally a male and female thing; mostly a female thing)? Do we challenge men further by inviting them to rate items in a more complex matrix, maybe crossing race/ethnicity and gender (e.g., mostly for Black males; mostly for White females; equally for Black males and Black females)? This conundrum highlights a few critical challenges in adapting and developing behavioral interventions:

- How do we decide what aspects of identity (and other factors) are most relevant to health behavior?
- Who is best positioned to determine how aspects of identity intersect?
- Are psychosocial factors (i.e., social support, cultural norms, stressors) equally relevant for different behaviors, such as eating behavior and physical activity?

Toward an Intersectional Approach to Developing Behavioral Interventions

A broad conception of health that incorporates social relations and institutions and situates health within communities and families is becoming more prevalent in the social sciences (Weber & Parra-Medina, 2003). This approach calls for research that simultaneously addresses the intersection of several key aspects of identity that affect health and health behavior: race/ethnicity, gender, class, socioeconomic status (SES), sexual identity, age, rural–urban, address, and region (of country, state, and city), among others. Because these dimensions are all socially constructed, they simultaneously and more accurately reflect the complex array of factors that influence health and health behavior. The goal of this approach is to consider how individual agency and choice, contextual and environmental influences, and physiological and biologic factors combine to impact health (Rieker & Bird, 2005). An intersectional approach helps us to consider how the multiple levels of influence included in a social ecological model (individual, interpersonal/social network, organizational, community, and environmental and policy) combine with critical aspects of identity (race, ethnicity, gender) to influence health and health behavior.

The intersectional perspective to research on health behavior remains in its infancy (Mullings & Schulz, 2006), and it has rarely, if ever, been used with African American men. Health promotion interventions have remained focused on the aspects of identity that are most congruent with the disease epidemiology (i.e., we should focus on ethnic identity because people's health outcomes vary significantly by ethnicity), rather than considering personal characteristics that also may influence the behavior of interest (i.e., gender, age, religiosity). Research in health behavior has recognized that these factors influence health behavior, but they have yet to be incorporated effectively into more comprehensive and complex theoretical, conceptual, or framework approaches to understanding the multilevel factors that influence how and where we intervene to address health behavior.

In the remainder of this chapter, we outline the strategy we have used to disentangle the complex array of factors that influence the eating behavior and physical activity of African American men. We argue that we can use health behavior theory and other scientific literature to guide this work, but that critical first steps are: (1) Marshalling a team that can help us to see blind spots and assumptions we may unintentionally make about the determinants of health behavior and the most important and plausible places to intervene; and (2) Conducting exploratory research to gain the perspectives of our population of interest, urban African American men, and those who know them best on what factors influence their health behaviors and their relative importance compared to other life priorities.

THE FOUNDATIONS OF *MEN 4 HEALTH*

Step 1: Use a CBPR Approach

Our approach to systematically adapting and developing interventions begins with a community-based participatory research (CBPR) approach (Israel, Eng, Schulz, & Parker, 2005; Minkler & Wallerstein, 2003; Viswanathan et al., 2004). CBPR is a collaborative research approach that is designed to ensure and organize the participation of communities affected by the issue being studied, representatives of organizations, and researchers in all phases of the research (Bowman, 1989, 2006; Geertz, 1973; Griffith et al., 2007, 2008; Johnson et al., 2009; Zimmerman et al., 2004). CBPR can enhance the capacity of a project to: bring together diverse partners with multiple skills, expertise, and sensitivities to examine and address complex problems in culturally appropriate ways (Butterfoss, Goodman, & Wandersman, 1993; Israel, Schulz, Parker, & Becker, 1998; Minkler, 2004); increase the relevance, usefulness, and applicability of intervention research (Israel et al., 1998; Schulz et al., 1998); and enhance the quality and validity of intervention research by integrating the knowledge and theory of the local partners involved and tailoring interventions to the local community context (Israel et al., 1998; Kerner, Dusenbury, & Mandelblatt, 1993). Kerner, Trock, and Mandelblatt assert that "only efforts to involve these high-risk populations as partners in cutting-edge cancer research can ensure that the research findings will be accepted by the community and that the interventions tested have a reasonable chance of proving themselves cost effective and sustainable after the research funding has ended" (Kerner, Trock, & Mandelblatt, 2004).

The participation of community members is integral to our approach. To ensure community participation and oversight, we created and regularly convene with a Community Steering Committee that guides, reviews, and provides insight on *M4H* activities throughout the research process. The Community Steering Committee is composed of community leaders, representatives of community-based organizations, project personnel, and university researchers, but led by one of our community outreach staff members. *M4H's* outreach staff is composed of African American men who are from, and currently live in, the cities of interest. They also have experience and reputations of being actively involved in addressing men's health issues in these communities. They strategically attend events and utilize their interpersonal skills, membership in social and faith-based organizations, and informal social networks to raise awareness about the study, distribute flyers, and recruit a diverse sample of men and women in the focus population of the study. Their local knowledge and ability to build upon existing interpersonal relationships help to gauge community needs and interests while assessing issues that are meaningful in the lives of African American men.

Step 2: Conduct and Analyze Focus Groups

In addition to engaging key community members, we conducted exploratory focus groups to examine individual and collective perspectives on the broad social, cultural, and environmental barriers and facilitators to African American men's healthy eating and physical activity. Of particular interest was how intersections of race/ethnicity, gender, life stage, and social and environmental contexts influence these men's health behaviors. Focus groups provided the ideal strategy for examining how individual skills, motivation, and knowledge intersect with social and environmental factors to influence physical activity and eating among African American men. Qualitative methods are effective for capturing emergent and unanticipated responses, providing participants with an opportunity to voice their perspectives, and understanding interactions and relationships between variables for theory development and intervention planning (Banyard & Miller, 1998; Geertz, 1973; Zimmerman et al., 2004). Women were included as focus group participants to examine the barriers and facilitators that they perceived for men, to gain their perspective on the stressors that influenced men's health and health behavior, and to capture the role they saw themselves playing in promoting men's healthy eating and physical activity.

Focus group participants were recruited by snowball sampling via word of mouth, fliers, and the extensive social networks of the project's outreach staff and Community Steering Committee partner organizations. The focus population for the male focus groups was African American men, ages 35 years and older, living in the Flint, Ypsilanti, and Detroit metropolitan areas of Southeast Michigan. The participants in the female focus groups were women who had close relationships with men meeting the criteria for the male focus groups and included men's spouses, sisters, daughters, and friends. Focus groups were conducted separately with men and women. One hundred fifty-four African American men participated in 18 focus groups: 10 groups with a total of 63 men from Flint; 4 groups with a total of 42 men from Ypsilanti; and 4 groups with a total of 49 men in Detroit. Half of the men's focus groups concentrated on eating behavior and half on physical activity. Seventy-seven women took part in 8 focus groups: 5 groups with a total of 50 women in Flint; and 3 groups with a total of 27 women in Ypsilanti. Our data organization process of chunking and assigning codes to text was similar to the methods used by Griffith and colleagues (Griffith et al., 2007, 2008). We sought to confirm the accuracy of our findings and interpretations by conducting three member checking groups—two with men and one with women. These groups also helped us to consider environmental and historical contextual issues relevant to the geographic locations.

Step 3: Interpret Focus Group Findings Using a CBPR Approach

In this section, we briefly discuss selected but key findings that describe the factors that our population of interest suggested influenced their behavior. We juxtapose what we anticipated to find based on the literature with what we found from the data. We also discuss what we learned from our Community Steering Committee and Community Outreach team.

Barriers to Healthy Eating and Physical Activity

One of the major barriers to African American men's consistent and sustained healthy eating and physical activity appears to have more to do with competing priorities in their lives, and less with issues of masculinity or health. While the literature on men's health highlights how men's gender socialization and resultant beliefs and attitudes about masculinity are major factors that influence behaviors associated with increased cancer risk (e.g., overeating, consuming fatty foods and few fruit and vegetables, physical

inactivity) (Courtenay, 2000), African American men participating in our focus groups articulated "competing priorities" or a "hierarchy of responsibilities" that pose barriers to them prioritizing their own health and health
practices. These African American men described how their roles as providers, parents, spouses, and community members were more important than
taking care of their personal health. This prioritization also was reinforced
by spouses, extended family members, and employers, who expected men to
attend to work, family, and community roles and responsibilities, even if it
meant taking time away from engaging in regular physical activity, preparing or purchasing healthier food, and engaging in other health behavior (e.g.,
sleeping or seeking medical care). Health is often considered a low priority
for men until poor health impairs some aspect of their lives (e.g., sexual relationships, job) or roles (e.g., provider, father, spouse) that is considered a
higher priority (Bowman, 1989, 2006).

Social Support from Peers and Spouses

Focus group feedback improved our consideration of the potential role
of peer support to address dietary and physical activity behaviors among
African American men. Initially, we expected male peer support to be of primary importance for addressing both eating behavior and physical activity among African American men, and spousal support to be an important,
yet secondary, source of support. We are finding that these sources of social
support vary by health behavior, however. Preliminary focus group data
analysis suggests that peer support from other men may be a critical part of
changing physical activity behaviors, but may be less influential for addressing changes in dietary behaviors. Women, particularly spouses, seem to be
key, if not the most important, sources of influencing married men's dietary
behaviors, but are far less influential in engaging men in physical activity
behavior changes. Our preliminary qualitative data suggest that women
are central figures who may have the capacity to support the behaviors of
African American men, particularly as they relate to diet.

Our focus group data suggest that spouses play considerable roles in
influencing the health of older African American men (Griffith, Johnson,
Allen, & Hill, 2009; Johnson et al., 2009). Men in this study articulated less on
the role of supportive female family members as facilitating linkage to care,
but did describe the role of their spouses in helping them to make healthy
lifestyle changes related to physical activity and eating. While men received
medical advice or instruction from physicians about behavior changes that
they needed to make, spouses provided support to attempt the first steps
toward healthy diet or physical activity. One of the biggest barriers voiced
by men in the focus groups concerned men simply not knowing how to
make behavioral and lifestyle changes prescribed by physicians. Another

critical barrier was if the prescribed changes conflicted with deep-seated norms and behaviors that seemed to have positive outcomes for men over their lives.

Faith-Based Organizations Versus Other Organizational Settings

African American faith-based organizations have historically figured prominently in serving as a setting for social activities, a tool for organizing in the community, a vehicle for sharing information, and a means of providing social services (Billingsley, 1999). However, faith-based, worksite, and other community-based studies of diet and physical activity have consistently enrolled more women in their studies and reported more robust findings for women than men (Resnicow et al., 2002, 2004, 2005; Sorensen et al., 1998, 1999, 2002, 2003). In prior studies it has been noted that African American women attend religious services more frequently, are more likely to be church members, and express higher levels of religiosity than African American men (Taylor, 1988; Victor et al., 2004). While the role of spirituality and religion among African American men remains important, we decided to explore and consider other organizations that men may frequent more than faith-based organizations.

Initially, we attempted to reach African American men through men's civic, social, and fraternal organizations. Whether founded to support African Americans in urban areas or to provide social and educational support to aspiring college and graduate students on college campuses, fraternal organizations have been an important institution within African American communities, and particularly among African American men. The African American Greek letter organizations, which were originally founded for college students, quickly grew to also support African American men who have graduated and moved on to a new phase of life. Many of these fraternal and civic organizations have national and international graduate chapters, connecting men of African descent around the world beyond their college years. These organizations serve as spaces to help convene and support African American men, and they are potential settings to intervene to improve the eating and physical activity of African American men. In these settings, we aimed to build on the values, support, and camaraderie of organizations influential in the lives of African American men.

In addition to civic and fraternal organizations, we also considered barbershops. Barbershops are important institutions for African American men. In addition to grooming services, barbershops often provide a safe space for men to connect and communicate about issues most salient to them. While some have utilized these spaces to provide health information, we sought to indentify alternative sites for reaching men and for influencing their health behavior, in an attempt to explore a variety of organizations that are central to the lives and relationships of Black men.

In our experience, fraternities and lodges present some challenges for intervention activities and may not be the ideal organizational contexts for interventions to improve the health of African American men. However, these settings may pose fewer challenges in other communities, populations, or economic contexts. In our experience, in an economically challenged community or among an economically challenged population, less time and money is allocated for recreational activities that may be associated with social or fraternal organizations, and an economically struggling community undermines the viability of these institutions and organizations. In an economically challenged setting, fraternities, lodges, and social organizations may not be as financially stable, strong, or supported; and if men are not regularly participating in these organizations, then these settings do not have significant influence in men's lives. Additionally, the confidential nature of membership to these organizations poses barriers for intervention activities or community presentations and does not allow for an open setting for intervention.

TOWARD *MEN 4 HEALTH*: A CULTURALLY AND GENDER-SENSITIVE HEALTH PROMOTION INTERVENION

The process that we outline in this chapter is a model that others may use to adapt existing interventions to new populations and health issues or use to develop new interventions that consider both race/ethnicity and gender. Through the process we are using to develop *M4H*, we are examining the factors that influence African American men's eating and physical activity, and the contextual factors that help and hinder their ability to maintain healthy behaviors over time. Our approach suggests that future interventions with African American men should expand notions of cultural sensitivity to include gender sensitivity and the myriad factors that affect health behavior.

The intersectional approach we propose is, admittedly, complex and may yield more immediate questions than specific directions for where and how to intervene to improve health behavior. On the other hand, an intersectional approach considers a broader array of factors from the perspective of the population of interest. It also provides a lens that helps intervention researchers consider how people in the populations of interest view the multilevel factors that influence health behavior—elements of the social ecology of people's lived experiences that rarely can be factored into health behavior interventions. These contextual and environmental factors may be the key to understanding not only how to change behavior but also to maintain behavior change, since often it is the intersection of health with other nonhealth aspects of people's lives that impedes their ability to maintain recommended levels of health behavior. If viewed through the lens of how members of the population view their challenges, we believe that interventions can give people the needed information, tap into the necessary motivation, and train them to have the essential behavioral skills to adapt to unhealthy environments and life stressors, and sustain healthy behavior change. As technology continues to progress, individually tailored materials, not just print materials, seem to be a promising vehicle through which highly efficacious, high-reach, low-cost interventions can be delivered in a way that is most relevant to the aspects of people's identity that influence their health behavior.

ACKNOWLEDGMENTS

This chapter was supported in part by grants from the American Cancer Society (Mentored Research Scholar Grant, number MRSGT-07-167-01-CPPB), the Michigan Center for Urban African American Aging Research, and the Cancer Research Fund of the University of Michigan Comprehensive Cancer Center, and by two centers at the University of Michigan School of Public Health: the Center on Men's Health Disparities and the Center for Research on Ethnicity, Culture and Health.

REFERENCES

Adler, N. (2006). Overview of health disparities. In G. E. Thompson, F. Mitchell, & M. B. Williams (Eds.), *Examining the health disparities research plan of the National Institutes of Health: Unfinished business* (pp. 121–174). Washington, DC: National Academies Press.

Airhihenbuwa, C. O., DiClemente, R. J., Wingood, G. M., & Lowe, A. (1992). HIV/AIDS education and prevention among African-Americans: A focus on culture. *AIDS Education and Prevention, 4*(3), 267–276.

American Cancer Society. (2004). *Cancer facts & figures: 2004.* Atlanta, GA: Author.

American Cancer Society. (2009). *Cancer facts & figures for African Americans 2009–2010.* Atlanta, GA: Author.

Ammerman, A. S., Lindquist, C. H., Lohr, K. N., & Hersey, J. (2002). The efficacy of behavioral interventions to modify dietary fat and fruit and vegetable intake: A review of the evidence. *Preventive Medicine, 35*(1), 25–41.

Bandura, A. (2001). Social cognitive theory: An agentic perspective. *Annual Review of Psychology, 52*, 1–26.

Banyard, V. L., & Miller, K. E. (1998). The powerful potential of qualitative research for community psychology. *American Journal of Community Psychology, 26*(4), 485–506.

Billingsley, A. (1999). *Mighty like a river: The Black church and social reform.* New York, NY: Oxford University Press.

Bowman, P. J. (1989). Research perspectives on Black men: Role strain and adaptation across the adult life cycle. In R. L. Jones (Ed.), *Black adult development and aging* (pp. 117–150). Berkeley, CA: Cobb & Henry.

Bowman, P. J. (2006). Role strain and adaptation issues in the strength-based model: Diversity, multilevel, and life-span considerations. *Counseling Psychologist, 34*(1), 118–133.

Butterfoss, F. D., Goodman, R. M., & Wandersman, A. (1993). Community coalitions for prevention and health promotion. *Health Education Research, 8*(3), 315–330.

Courtenay, W. H. (2000). Constructions of masculinity and their influence on men's well-being: A theory of gender and health. *Social Science & Medicine, 50*(10), 1385–1401.

Friedenreich, C. M., & Orenstein, M. R. (2002). Physical activity and cancer prevention: Etiologic evidence and biological mechanisms. *Journal of Nutrition, 132*(11 Suppl.), 3456–3464.

Frohlich, K. L., & Potvin, L. (2008). The inequality paradox: The population approach to vulnerable populations. *American Journal of Public Health, 98*(2), 216–221.

Geertz, C. (1973). *The interpretation of cultures.* New York, NY: Basic Books.

Geiger, H. J. (2006). Health disparties: What do we know? What do we need to know? What should we do? In A. J. Schulz & L. Mullings (Eds.), *Gender, race, class and health: Intersectoral approaches* (pp. 261–288). San Francisco, CA: Jossey-Bass.

Gotay, C. C. (2005). Behavior and cancer prevention. *Journal of Clinical Oncology, 23*(2), 301–310.

Griffith, D. M., Allen, J. O., Zimmerman, M. A., Morrel-Samuels, S., Reischl, T. M., Cohen, S. E., & Campbell, K. A. (2008). Organizational empowerment in community mobilization to address youth violence. *American Journal of Preventive Medicine, 34*(3 Suppl.), S89–S99.

Griffith, D. M., Johnson, J. L., Allen, J. O., & Hill, G. (2009, July). *Two sides of African American men's health: Perspectives on the role of women in men's health from the* Men 4 Health *study.* Poster presentation at the American Cancer Society's 2009 conference, Health Equity: Through the Cancer Lens, Las Vegas, NV.

Griffith, D. M., Mason, M., Rodela, M., Matthews, D. D., Tran, A., Royster, M., . . . Eng, E. (2007). A structural approach to examining prostate cancer risk for rural southern African American men. *Journal of Health Care for the Poor and Underserved, 18*(Suppl.), 73–101.

Griffith, D. M., Moy, E., Reischl, T. M., & Dayton, E. (2006). National data for monitoring and evaluating racial and ethnic health inequities: Where do we go from here? *Health Education & Behavior, 33*(4), 470–487.

Israel, B. A. (1985). Social networks and social support: Implications for natural helper and community level interventions. *Health Educucation Quarterly, 12*(1), 65–80.

Israel, B. A., Eng, E., Schulz, A. J., & Parker, E. A. (2005). Introduction. In B. A. Israel, E. Eng, A. J. Schulz, & E. A. Parker (Eds.), *Methods in community-based participatory research for health* (pp. 3–26). San Francisco, CA: Jossey-Bass.

Israel, B. A., & McLeroy, K. R. (1985). Introduction. Special issue on social networks and social support: Implications for health education. *Health Educucation Quarterly, 12*(1), 1–4.

Israel, B. A., Schulz, A. J., Parker, E. A., & Becker, A. B. (1998). Review of community-based research: Assessing partnership approaches to improve public health. *Annual Review of Public Health, 19,* 173–202.

Johnson, J. L., Griffith, D. M., Allen, J. O., Herbert, K., Hill, G., & Gaines, H. (2009, November). *Close to home: Women's perspectives on African American men's eating and physical activity*. Paper presented at the annual meeting of the American Public Health Association, Philadelphia, PA.

Kerner, J. F., Dusenbury, L., & Mandelblatt, J. S. (1993). Poverty and cultural diversity: Challenges for health promotion among the medically underserved. *Annual Review of Public Health, 14*, 355–377.

Kerner, J. F., Trock, B. J., & Mandelblatt, J. S. (2004). Breast cancer in minority women. In J. R. Harris, M. E. Lippman, M. Morrow, & C. K. Osborne (Eds.), *Diseases of the breast* (p. 1358). Philadelphia, PA: Lippincott Williams & Wilkins.

Koh, H. K., Massin-Short, S., & Elqura, L. (2009). Disparities in tobacco use and lung cancer. In H. K. Koh (Ed.), *Toward the elimination of cancer disparities* (pp. 109–135). New York, NY: Springer.

McLeroy, K. R., Bibeau, D., Steckler, A., & Glanz, K. (1988). An ecological perspective on health promotion programs. *Health Education Quarterly, 15*(4), 351–377.

Minkler, M. (2004). Ethical challenges for the "outside" researcher in community-based participatory research. *Health Education & Behavior, 31*(6), 684–697.

Minkler, M., & Wallerstein, N. (Eds.). (2003). *Community based participatory research for health*. San Francisco, CA: Jossey-Bass.

Moy, E., Arispe, I. E., Holmes, J. S., & Andrews, R. M. (2005). Preparing the national healthcare disparities report: Gaps in data for assessing racial, ethnic, and socioeconomic disparities in health care. *Medical Care, 43*(3 Suppl.), I9–I16.

Mullings, L., & Schulz, A. J. (2006). Intersectionality and health: An introduction. In A. J. Schulz & L. Mullings (Eds.), *Gender, race, class and health: Intersectional approaches* (pp. 3–20). San Francisco, CA: Jossey-Bass.

National Cancer Institute. (2002). *How diet affects African-American men's health*. Bethesda, MD: Author.

Payne, S. (2006). *The health of men and women*. Malden, MA: Polity Press.

Powe, B. D., Cooper, D. L., Harmond, L., Ross, L., Mercado, F. E., & Faulkenberry, R. (2009). Comparing knowledge of colorectal and prostate cancer among African American and Hispanic men. *Cancer Nursing, 32*(5), 412–417.

Resnicow, K., Baranowski, T., Ahluwalia, J. S., & Braithwaite, R. L. (1999). Cultural sensitivity in public health: Defined and demystified. *Ethnicity & Disease, 9*(1), 10–21.

Resnicow, K., Campbell, M. K., Carr, C., McCarty, F., Wang, T., Periasamy, S., . . . Stables, G. (2004). *Body and soul*: A dietary intervention conducted through African-American churches. *American Journal of Preventive Medicine, 27*(2), 97–105.

Resnicow, K., Jackson, A., Blissett, D., Wang, T., McCarty, F., Rahotep, S., & Periasamy, S. (2005). Results of the *Healthy Body Healthy Spirit* trial. *Health Psychology, 24*(4), 339–348.

Resnicow, K., Jackson, A., Braithwaite, R., DiIorio, C., Blissett, D., Rahotep, S., & Periasamy, S. (2002). *Healthy Body Healthy Spirit*: A church-based nutrition and physical activity intervention. *Health Education Research, 17*(5), 562–573.

Resnicow, K., Soler, R., Braithwaite, R. L., Ahluwalia, J. S., & Butler, J. (2000). Cultural sensitivity in substance use prevention. *Journal of Community Psychology, 28*(3), 271–290.

Rieker, P. P., & Bird, C. E. (2005). Rethinking gender differences in health: Why we need to integrate social and biological perspectives. *Journals of Gerontology: Series B, 60*(Suppl. 2), 40–47.

Ryan, R. M., & Deci, E. L. (2000). Self-determination theory and the facilitation of intrinsic motivation, social development, and well-being. *American Psychologist, 55*(1), 68–78.

Ryan, R. M., Frederick, C. M., Lepes, D., Rubio, N., & Sheldon, K. M. (1997). Intrinsic motivation and exercise adherence. *International Journal of Sport Psychology, 28,* 335.

Sankar, P., Cho, M. K., Condit, C. M., Hunt, L. M., Koenig, B., Marshall, P., . . . Spicer, P. (2004). Genetic research and health disparities. *Journal of the American Medical Association, 291*(24), 2985–2989.

Schneider, E. C. (2009). Disparities and colorectal cancer. In H. K. Koh (Ed.), *Toward the elimination of cancer disparities* (pp. 161–178). New York, NY: Springer.

Schulz, A. J., Parker, E. A., Israel, B. A., Becker, A. B., Maciak, B. J., & Hollis, R. (1998). Conducting a participatory community-based survey: Collecting and interpreting data for a community health intervention on Detroit's east side. *Journal of Public Health Management and Practice, 4*(2), 10–24.

Sorensen, G., Hunt, M. K., Cohen, N., Stoddard, A., Stein, E., Phillips, J., . . . Palombo, R. (1998). Worksite and family education for dietary change: The Treatwell 5-a-Day program. *Health Education Research, 13*(4), 577–591.

Sorensen, G., Stoddard, A., Peterson, K., Cohen, N., Hunt, M. K., Stein, E., . . . Lederman, R. (1999). Increasing fruit and vegetable consumption through worksites and families in the Treatwell 5-a-Day study. *American Journal of Public Health, 89*(1), 54–60.

Sorensen, G., Stoddard, A. M., LaMontagne, A. D., Emmons, K., Hunt, M. K., Youngstrom, R., . . . Christiani, D. C. (2002). A comprehensive worksite cancer prevention intervention: Behavior change results from a randomized controlled trial (United States). *Cancer Causes Control, 13*(6), 493–502.

Sorensen, G., Stoddard, A. M., LaMontagne, A. D., Emmons, K., Hunt, M. K., Youngstrom, R., . . . Christiani, D. C. (2003). A comprehensive worksite cancer prevention intervention: Behavior change results from a randomized controlled trial (United States). *Journal of Public Health Policy, 24*(1), 5–25.

Steptoe, A., Perkins-Porras, L., McKay, C., Rink, E., Hilton, S., & Cappuccio, F. P. (2003). Psychological factors associated with fruit and vegetable intake and with biomarkers in adults from a low-income neighborhood. *Health Psychology, 22*(2), 148–155.

Taylor, K. L., Turner, R. O., Davis, J. L., 3rd, Johnson, L., Schwartz, M. D., Kerner, J., & Leak, C. (2001). Improving knowledge of the prostate cancer screening dilemma among African American men: An academic-community partnership in Washington, DC. *Public Health Reports, 116*(6), 590–598.

Taylor, R. J. (1988). Structural determinants of religious participation among Black Americans. *Review of Religious Research, 30,* 114–125.

Trudeau, E., Kristal, A. R., Li, S., & Patterson, R. E. (1998). Demographic and psychosocial predictors of fruit and vegetable intakes differ: Implications for dietary interventions. *Journal of the American Dietetic Association, 98*(12), 1412–1417.

Victor, R. G., Haley, R. W., Willett, D. L., Peshock, R. M., Vaeth, P. C., Leonard, D., . . . Dallas Heart Study Investigators. (2004). The Dallas Heart Study: A population-based probability sample for the multidisciplinary study of ethnic differences in cardiovascular health. *American Journal of Cardiology, 93*(12), 1473–1480.

Viswanathan, M., Ammerman, A., Eng, E., Gartlehner, G., Lohr, K. N., Griffith, D. M., . . . Whitener, L. (2004). *Community-based participatory research: Assessing the evidence.* Rockville, MD: Agency for Healthcare Research and Quality.

Ward, E., Jemal, A., Cokkinides, V., Singh, G. K., Cardinez, C., Ghafoor, A., & Thun, M. (2004). Cancer disparities by race/ethnicity and socioeconomic status. *CA: A Cancer Journal for Clinicians, 54*(2), 78–93.

Weber, L., & Parra-Medina, D. (2003). Intersectionality and women's health: Charting a path to eliminating health disparities. In V. Demos & M. T. Segal (Eds.), *Advances in gender research: Gender perspectives on health and medicine* (pp. 181–230). Amsterdam, The Netherlands: Elsevier.

Williams, D. R., & Jackson, P. B. (2005). Social sources of racial disparities in health. *Health Affairs, 24*(2), 325–334.

Zimmerman, M. A., Morrel-Samuels, S., Wong, N., Tarver, D., Rabiah, D., & White, S. (2004). Guns, gangs, and gossip: An analysis of student essays on youth violence. *Journal of Early Adolescence, 24*, 385–411.

9

The North Carolina BEAUTY and Health Project: Preventing Cancer in African American Beauty Salons

*Laura A. Linnan, Cherise B. Harrington, John M. Rose,
Veronica Carlisle, and Morris Boswell*

Approximately 30% of cancer deaths annually are attributable to diet (American Institute for Cancer Research, 2007; National Cancer Institute, 2005; North Carolina Central Cancer Registry, 2004) and, when combined with physical inactivity, are second only to tobacco as the leading causes of preventable cancer deaths (Mokdad, Marks, Stroup, & Gerberding, 2004). Because cancer remains the second leading cause of death nationally, and in North Carolina, intervening to reduce known modifiable behavioral risks to cancer is imperative (North Carolina Advisory Committee on Cancer Coordination and Control, 2001). Modifiable behavioral risks for cancer include overweight/obesity, physical inactivity, diet high in fat, and inadequate intake of fruits/vegetables (American Cancer Society, 2005; National Cancer Institute, 2005). Adults in North Carolina rank poorly among all states on eating at least five servings of fruits and vegetables a day (35th), engaging in regular physical activity (25th) (America's Health Rankings & United Health Foundation, 2009), and obesity (38th) (Levi & Trust for America's Health, 2009). African American (AA) women in North Carolina experience a strikingly disproportionate share of the cancer incidence and mortality burden (North Carolina Advisory Committee on Cancer Coordination and Control, 2001; North Carolina Central Cancer Registry, 2004). For example, the overall age-adjusted cancer mortality for African American women (per 100,000) was 24.1 (compared with 16.8 for White women). Thus, cancer disparities warrant powerful, effective primary prevention intervention strategies that can reach large numbers of African American women.

Churches are an important venue (Fox, Pitkin, Paul, Carson, & Duan, 1998) and to maximize exposure to lifesaving health interventions identifying additional key community settings is needed. In an effort to explore alternative but promising settings for reaching AA women, we focused on beauty salons. This chapter will describe a 10-year collaborative partnership between a research team at the University of North Carolina Chapel Hill School of Public Health and Lineberger Comprehensive Cancer Center, and North Carolina beauty salon owners, stylists, and their customers, to promote health and address cancer disparities. Beauty salons are located in communities of all sizes, rural and urban. North Carolina has over 11,304 licensed beauty salons, and more than 60,000 licensed cosmetologists. Nationally, U.S. beauty salons employ approximately 1,123,151 licensed cosmetologists (Rudner, 2003); and the numbers of salons and cosmetologists increase every year (U.S. Department of Labor, 2004). Beauty salons are one of the primary businesses owned by African American women. Beauty salons are a unique and historically important "safe place" for African Americans to congregate and share information (Linnan & Ferguson, 2007). Not only are beauty salons a potentially excellent place to reach African American women, but this setting benefits from the fact that licensed cosmetologists have a unique and trusted relationship with their customers. Specifically, licensed cosmetologists serve as "natural helpers," who represent "individuals [within communities] whom others spontaneously seek out for advice, support, and assistance" (Earp & Flax, 1999). Public health interventions with natural helpers have proven particularly successful with women and minority groups (Campbell et al., 1999, 2000; Keyserling et al., 2000; Kleindorfer et al., 2008; Linnan et al., 2001; Tessaro, 1997; Tessaro et al., 2000). For all of these reasons, we contend that beauty salons represent a promising setting for sharing lifesaving cancer prevention information with African American women who suffer disparities in health. This chapter will describe how community-based participatory research principles guided the development of a beauty-salon–based intervention (North Carolina BEAUTY [Bringing Education And Understanding To You] and Health research study) that was culturally and contextually appropriate, and then was rigorously tested within a large group randomized trial funded by the American Cancer Society as part of the Targeted Research Scholar Funds for Underserved Populations (TURSG-02–190–01-PBP). A brief history, a description of the intervention development process, selected results from the research study, lessons learned, and implications for practice and research will be addressed.

A COMMUNITY-BASED PARTICIPATORY RESEARCH APPROACH TO DEVELOPING A BEAUTY-SALON–BASED INTERVENTION

Community-based participatory research (CBPR) is a collaborative process between researchers and community partners to investigate issues relevant to the community, and to work toward achieving change within that community. The CBPR approach, if done well, should build trust (Linnan, Carlisle et al., 2005) and is believed to increase the likelihood that the intervention will be sustained over time (Minkler, 2000; Minkler, & Wallerstein, 2003; Viswanathan et al., 2004). We began with the question: "Is it a good idea to try and promote health in beauty salons?" First, we convened a BEAUTY Advisory Board to help educate our research team about how the beauty salon industry works, and guide the process for answering that overall question. Members first met in January 2000, and they are still working with the research team 10 years later. Members included two individuals who directed beauty schools in area community colleges, and one who was the marketing director for a private beauty school; as well as the President of the North Carolina Cosmetology Association, three licensed cosmetologists and salon owners, a beauty product distributor, a health educator from the county health department, representatives from the American Cancer Society and from Cancer Information Service outreach programs, as well as members of the research team (see Table 9.1). We met monthly in the early stages of our work together, in the local community, with meeting space supported by the Chamber of Commerce. Board members first advised us

TABLE 9.1 The BEAUTY (and Barbershop) Advisory Board Committee (2000 to Present)

Member	Affiliation
Morris Boswell[a]	Guilford Technical College, Cosmetology and Barbering State Board of Cosmetic Art
Roxana Murfree-Alston[a]	Dudley Beauty School (Sales)
Clastine Pool-Covington[a]	Dudley Beauty School (Training)
Jerry Head, Jr.	Cancer survivor
Donna Hooker Sharon Martin[a]	Donna's Hair Salon
B. Levitas Becky Hartt Minor Laura Krajewski[a]	Cancer Information Service
Ed Hooker	E-Style Barbershop
Al Richmond[a]	North Carolina Institute for Minority Economic Development North Carolina Minority Prostate Cancer Awareness Action Team
Joyce Thomasa	Central Carolina Community College, Cosmetology and Barbering, State Board of Cosmetic Art (ret.)
Cornell Wright	Center for Health and Healing

[a]These individuals were original members of the BEAUTY Advisory Board.

to survey licensed cosmetologists to find out if they were interested in working with researchers to promote health in the salons. The complete results of that survey are published elsewhere (Linnan et al., 2001), but briefly, we learned that licensed stylists were highly interested in working with us to promote health in the salons, that they talk about health often with their customers, and that they are most comfortable talking about diet, physical activity, and weight issues. They also told us about preferred ways to get training/information about health. Additionally, it was found that the top two ways in which stylists preferred to share information with their clients included distributing print materials (69%) and talking with clients during appointments (61%) (Linnan et al., 2001). These results were critical to our thinking about intervention development, as well as convincing the research team and Advisory Board members that licensed stylists were willing partners, that we should focus efforts on diet and physical activity as topics where stylists had the greatest interest/comfort, and that a variety of intervention opportunities would be suitable for the salons.

After the initial stylist survey results, we conducted several additional formative research studies to further develop both the methods and the approach to how best to intervene in the beauty salons. At each step, we developed our plans and shared data/results with help and direction from the Advisory Board members. After the stylist survey, we conducted an observational study in 10 salons to assess the quality, amount, and type of health discussions that take place within the context of a typical stylist–customer visit, as a way of looking for intervention leverage points (Solomon et al., 2004). While there were many similarities in the type of conversations held in different salons, on average, customers in the African American salons spent nearly 20 minutes more than did customers in the White salons. We also learned that nearly 20% of conversations were health related, and those conversations were initiated equally by stylists and customers. Observational results revealed many options for creating a health-supportive salon environment by introducing healthy snacks, and using available media channels in the salons.

Using these results, combined with stylist survey data and feedback from our Advisory Board members, we next conducted a feasibility study testing our ability to recruit and intervene by training cosmetologists to deliver key messages to their clients, develop in-salon educational displays to stimulate conversations about health, and to assess results. The pilot study results are summarized elsewhere (Linnan, Ferguson et al., 2005). Briefly, we successfully recruited salons/stylists, developed and trained stylists to deliver three key health messages, and then evaluated the effects of those efforts on stylists and customers immediately post-intervention and at a 12-month follow-up. The results revealed significant increases in stylist self-efficacy to deliver key messages, and positive customer self-reported changes in behaviors (i.e., fruit/vegetable intake, physical activity, and using the 1–800–4–CANCER information line) among those who received the intervention sustained at a 12-month follow-up (Linnan, Ferguson et al., 2005). This pilot study provided encouraging evidence that stylists shared information that they learned in training, and that customers heard, understood, and reported acting upon the information that they received from stylists. In fact, customers who reported more talk with stylists were associated with more positive health changes (Linnan, Ferguson et al., 2005). With a highly collaborative approach in partnership with owners, stylists, and their customers, the successes and lessons learned during these initial studies prepared us to propose a larger trial to test several different salon-based intervention approaches.

THE NORTH CAROLINA BEAUTY AND HEALTH PROJECT

Design and Background

We secured funding from the American Cancer Society to conduct a large, group randomized intervention trial in beauty salons to test the effects of two promising intervention strategies on eating at least five servings of fruits/ vegetables per day, reducing calories from fat, and increasing moderate physical activity among customers. Six evidence- and theory-guided campaigns were developed. Each campaign included a theme focused on one of the health outcomes and 3 to 5 key messages that were included in the targeted health magazines, stylist training workshops, and the educational displays placed in each salon. Table 9.2 summarizes the themes and key messages of each of the six campaigns. Using the formative research results, advice from the Advisory Board members, and results from a series of focus groups we conducted with customers of various ages (Kim et al., 2007), one campaign was delivered to each salon each quarter over the 2-year intervention period.

A 2 (stylist training workshops—Y/N) × 2 (targeted health magazine— Y/N) factorial design was used to test the effects of the two intervention strategies. Thus, each salon (and all the customers enrolled from that salon) were randomly assigned into one of four intervention arms: targeted health magazine (TM), stylist training workshops (STW), targeted health magazine plus stylist training workshops (BOTH), or neither (CONTROL). ALL salons (TM, STW, BOTH, CONTROL) received educational displays for the salon. The CONTROL salons received educational displays with campaign themes and messages that did not focus on the primary outcomes (see Table 9.2). Customers in salons randomized to the TM arm got the campaign messages via targeted health magazines sent to them at home; customers in salons randomized to the STW arm got the campaign messages from stylists who had attended one of the stylist training workshops; and customers in BOTH got a targeted health magazine sent to the home, plus messages delivered from the stylists who attended stylist training workshops.

TABLE 9.2 BEAUTY Campaigns and Key Health Messages

Campaign Name/Theme	Primary and Secondary Outcomes	Key Campaign Health Messages	"Control" Campaigns
Campaign 1 The Good News About Cancer Prevention (January–March)	• Fruit and vegetable consumption • Dietary fat intake • Physical activity • Cancer screening (mammogram, Pap test, colonoscopy) • Weight	1. African American women (compared with White women) are diagnosed with cancer more often and are more likely to die with they are diagnosed with cancer! 2. Good news: More than 50% of cancers can be prevented by making changes in our lifestyle . . . especially, eating at least 5–9 servings of fruits and vegetables a day, being physically active for at least 30 minutes most days of the week, and limiting exposure to smoke. 3. Talk with your doctors and get recommended cancer screening tests so that if you have cancer, it can be found at an early stage when it is easier to treat. 4. Use the 1-800-4-CANCER phone number to get more information about cancer, and how to reduce your risk.	• Foot care
Campaign 2 Get Movin'– Every Little Move Counts for BEAUTY and Health (April–June)	• Physical activity • Weight	1. Fit physical activity into your day, every day. Every little move counts! 2. Get 30-10–5! That's 30 minutes of physical activity, in as short as 10 minutes at a time, for at least 5 days of the week. 3. Maintain a healthy weight with physical activity and you will reduce your risk of cancer! 4. Find one or more activity buddies. A buddy is a person who will do physical activity with you! Different buddies for different days of the week or different types of activities are okay.	• Financial health
Campaign 3 Healthy Eating! Healthy Weight! Healthy You! (July–September)	• Fruit and vegetable consumption • Weight	1. Eat at least 5 but up to 9 servings of fruits and vegetables a day! 2. Having an unhealthy weight puts you at risk for many health problems. 3. If you are overweight or obese, start to lose weight now! 4. Eat fewer high-fat foods to maintain a healthy weight. 5. Keep your portion sizes small.	• Adult immunization

Campaign Name/Theme	Primary and Secondary Outcomes	Key Campaign Health Messages	"Control" Campaigns
Campaign 4 The BEAUTY in Knowing ... and Acting on Your Knowledge (October–December)	• Cancer screening (breast, cervical, and colorectal cancers)	1. Talk to your doctor about getting the correct cancer screening tests for your age and family history. 2. Get screened to help find cancer early when it can be treated most successfully. 3. Getting screened and treating cancer at an early stage could help you live longer and have more time with loved ones.	• Substance abuse
Campaign 5 New Year, New You! (January–March)	• Dietary fat intake • Weight	1. Read your labels! Knowing what's in the foods you eat can help you make healthier choices about what you buy and eat. 2. Use fat sparingly! Try herbs and spices to season your food, or less fattening meats to prepare vegetables. And if you must use butter and oils—cut back on the usual amount you use! 3. Keep portions small! Portion sizes at home and while eating out have increased over the last 20 years. Try to reduce your portion size if you want to eat healthier, and either maintain a healthy weight, avoid gaining weight with age, or lose weight. 4. Set achievable goals, and stick with them. Whether it's starting a new habit or eliminating an old habit, make a commitment to take a small step every day. 5. Slips don't mean stops! Every day is a new day to reach your goal. It's okay if you get off track every now and then. Don't give up— just try again. You can do it!	• Time management
Campaign 6 Walk for Beauty and Health (April–June)	• Physical activity • Weight	1. WALK at least 30–10–5 to get the health benefits of physical activity; walk more if your goal is to lose weight. 2. Ask a friend or family member to walk with you! 3. Live a physically active life—you'll feel better. 4. Keep a daily record of your weight, walking time and distance to watch your progress.	• Sickle cell anemia

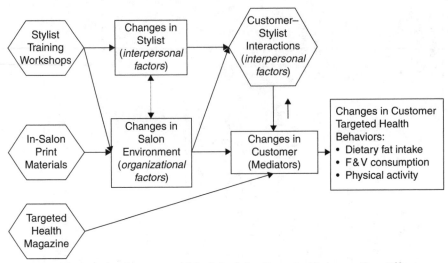

FIGURE 9.1   The Conceptual Model of the Expected Intervention Effects
for the BEAUTY Project

Intervention Development—Theoretical Foundations

The social ecological framework (SEF) (Stokols, 1992; Stokols, Pelletier, & Fielding, 1996) was a helpful heuristic for conceptualizing the multi-level intervention that was developed and tested in the BEAUTY study. According to the SEF, there are multiple levels of influence on each targeted customer behavior (i.e., increasing fruit/vegetable intake, reducing fat intake, and increasing physical activity). For this trial, we focused on three (of five) levels of influence within the SEF (see Figure 9.1): *intrapersonal* (e.g., stylist and customer knowledge, attitudes, self-efficacy, motivations); *interpersonal* (e.g., interactions between the stylist and customer about health messages); and *organizational* (e.g., access and/or support within the salon environment). According to the SEF, behavior change will be more likely if one is able to engage multiple levels of influence. We utilized constructs from both social cognitive theory (SCT) (Bandura, 2000) and the transtheoretical model of behavior change (TTM) (Prochaska, Redding, & Evers, 1997).

At the *intrapersonal* level, we focused on characteristics within the individual (customer or stylist); specifically, readiness to change (TTM construct) and self-efficacy to change the targeted behavior (SCT construct). Intervention strategies to move the individual along the stages of readiness to change, and to improve self-efficacy to make the change, were embedded in several components of the stylist training workshops (e.g., discussions on separating fact from fiction and "how to" sessions for making health changes) and the targeted health magazines (e.g., features on participating stylists who had made positive health changes).

At the *interpersonal* level, we focused on the interactions between the stylist and customer. In the stylist training workshops, we used demonstrations and role plays to increase the self-efficacy of stylists to include the key messages in conversations with customers during a typical salon visit. We did not demand that stylists deliver all messages at each visit. Instead, we told stylists that they were the "experts" about each customer, and encouraged them to assess the "readiness" of each customer to accept one or more messages on a typical visit. In the targeted health magazines, we included spotlights on successful stylists and customers as role models for success—consistent with the observational learning construct of SCT as a way of building the self-efficacy of the customer for the desired behaviors as well as building the self-efficacy of the stylist to talk with the customers. At the *organizational* level, we focused on the SCT construct of "reciprocal determinism," where a customer's health behavior influences (and is influenced by) the salon environment. Thus, each campaign included a display where the key messages were highlighted in an interactive, attractive way that would allow customers to view the display while waiting in the salon, or where stylists could refer customers to pick up materials and information as they were leaving the salon.

In addition to key theoretical foundations, social marketing principles guided the development of each campaign by including themes, simple/clear health messages, and attractive, eye-catching materials for the salon, stylist, and customer that were customer focused and pretested before each quarterly campaign launch. All materials in the displays, stylist training workshops, and targeted health magazines were designed with a similar BEAUTY Project "look," including consistent colors, font style, and logo.

This intervention study did not test a single theoretical model; instead, we were conceptually organized using the social ecological framework, and responsive to calls for more theory-driven intervention studies that had speci-fied (a priori) key theoretical constructs. This multilevel intervention reinforced cancer prevention messages through a variety of educational methods expected to influence customers, stylists, owners, interactions between customers and stylists, and the salon environment itself. The conceptual model depicting how the intervention strategies at each level of the SEF work to influence study outcomes is depicted in Figure 9.1. Additional details are provided about the specific components/features of the targeted health magazines and stylist training workshops included in each campaign, as well as the intent of the educational displays.

Stylist Training Workshops

Stylists and owners in salons randomized to the STW or BOTH conditions were invited to attend a 4-hour training workshop for each of the six quarterly campaigns. The workshops were held at local public libraries and on Mondays, when salons were typically closed for stylist convenience. The workshops were organized and conducted by the research team, with assistance from Advisory Board members (stylists, owners who were credible sources of information for participating stylists), with occasional outside experts (nurses or physicians), and/or cancer survivors. The workshops were designed to increase stylist/owner knowledge about the core health messages, and help them develop ways to share the health messages with their clients during normal hairstyling appointments. The workshops covered the same key components for every campaign, including: (1) an update on BEAUTY Project timeline and upcoming events; (2) sharing success stories from past campaigns; (3) a review of the targeted health messages specific to the campaign, along with an expert presentation on the topic addressed by the health messages (e.g., nutrition, exercise, cancer screening); (4) the introduction of new in-salon display materials; (5) role-playing on initiating conversations and delivering targeted health messages; (6) a problem-solving session, including a group discussion around barriers and facilitators; and (7) making personal promises as a goal-setting exercise. The stylists/owners were provided with written training materials covering the information they needed for each campaign, along with a three-ring binder in which to store the materials. If a salon did not have at least one stylist at a workshop, then a project staff member would conduct a make-up training session with participating stylists from that salon within 2 weeks of the missed workshop. Stylists attending the workshops (but not those who received make-up trainings) received stipends to cover their time and travel costs, and were provided lunch.

Targeted Health Magazines

Enrolled customers of salons randomized to the TM and BOTH conditions received six quarterly, targeted health magazines, delivered to their homes. In addition, a copy of the magazine was delivered to the salons randomized to the TM and BOTH conditions, so that customers, stylists, and owners would be able to read and discuss the magazine contents in the salons. The topical content of the quarterly magazines corresponded to the six health campaigns of the BEAUTY Project. Each eight-page magazine featured educational articles, interactive quizzes, and photographic images of African American women who were actual participating customers and stylists. Similar to the in-salon displays, the magazines had an overall

BEAUTY Project design and format, as well as a consistent structure across the six campaigns, including: (1) a project update; (2) a customer success/ feature story; (3) "Ask Your Stylist" BEAUTY and health tips; (4) a feature story on one health behavior/screening guideline; (5) an interactive game, puzzle, or trial skill (e.g., a healthy recipe); (6) community resources—where to go for more information; (7) a personal promise pledge; and (8) a medical disclaimer. A new targeted "Beauty From the Inside Out" magazine was delivered to each participating customer in the TM or BOTH arm, on the same timetable as each stylist training workshop that was held for the campaign launch.

In-Salon Educational Displays

All participating salons received a tri-fold educational display with key messages highlighted for the six health campaigns. Salons in the CONTROL arm received displays with the same format and design, but with information unrelated to the primary study outcomes. The displays included the following components for every campaign: (1) a set of targeted health messages specific to the campaign; (2) print materials or handouts; (3) an interactive quiz, or "try it out" tips, related to the targeted health messages; (4) suggestions for getting more information or related resources; and (5) an "Ask Your Stylist" cue to action, with at least one picture of an enrolled stylist. Depending on the campaign, additional print materials were provided to the salons, such as brochures, flyers, or stickers for the booth mirrors with the targeted health messages (another cue to action for stylist–customer interaction). Project staff delivered materials and set up displays in the salons at the beginning of each campaign. A total of six displays with associated print materials were offered quarterly over the intervention period, in all study conditions.

Salon Recruitment

Salons were eligible to participate in the study if they: (1) were located within a 75-mile radius of Chapel Hill; (2) were not part of a franchise; (3) served primarily African American customers; and (4) served at least 75 customers. Once salons were approached, eligibility was verified, and an initial interest in participating was established, a project team member brought a 13-minute recruitment video that included extensive interviews with Advisory Board members, who extolled the benefits of joining the study and encouraged salon owners and stylists to enroll. Interested salons that were able to achieve customer recruitment standards (at least 55) were enrolled.

CUSTOMER RECRUITMENT

Salon customers were recruited for the BEAUTY Project during enroll-ment events held in the enrolled salons. As described above, each salon was required to recruit at least 55 customers during these events to par-ticipate in the project, and only those salons that met this requirement were eventually enrolled. A customer was eligible to join the study if she was an African American woman, at least aged 18, and she was a regu-lar customer of the salon (e.g., had visited the salon more than twice). If she met these initial criteria, then she was asked to sign an informed consent agreement form and complete a Physical Activity Readiness Questionnaire (PAR-Q). If she answered "Yes" to any of the PAR-Q ques-tions, she was asked to have a physician provide medical consent for her to participate in the study. Eligible customers were asked to complete the baseline BEAUTY and Health survey (BHS) questionnaire, and return it either in a postage-paid envelope to the research team or drop it off back at the salon, in a sealed envelope; telephone surveys were made available to participants unable to return the paper version of the questionnaire. Once the completed BHS questionnaire was returned and received, then the customer was considered fully enrolled in the study. The initial 40 salons recruited a total of 1,209 customers, while 1,123 customers were enrolled from the 37 salons that remained in the study. Figure 9.2 shows study participation at the salon and customer levels over time.

Measurement Schedule

To evaluate the primary (percentage of calories from fat, servings of fruits/vegetables, physical activity) and secondary (weight and screening beha-viors) outcomes at the customer level, we compared baseline and fol-low-up responses to the BEAUTY and Health customer survey. The 19-page BHS was distributed to each enrolled customer. Dietary habi-ts were measured at baseline and follow-up using the 60-item version of the NCI Health Habits and History Questionnaire (Block et al., 1986), which has been validated with a low-income Black population (Coates et al., 1991). From this measure, we calculated daily fruit and vegetable servings and the percentage of calories from fat at both time points for each cus-tomer. We measured physical activity using a single item, "I currently en-gage in regular physical activity," with respondents answering either "Yes" or "No." Prior to this item, the questionnaire included an explanation of what constitutes physical activity and what it means for physical activity to be "regular." Body mass index (BMI) was calculated using self-reported estimates of height and weight. In determining adherence to cancer screen-ing guidelines, we used recommendations by the American Cancer Society

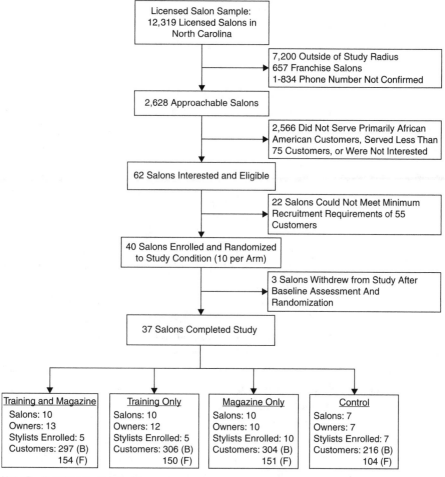

Note: B = Baseline; F = Follow-up.

FIGURE 9.2   The BEAUTY CONSORT Diagram

(ACS) for breast, cervical, and colorectal cancer (American Cancer Society, 2001). For breast cancer, we classified women as adherent if they reported a mammogram within the past year at follow-up (among women 40 years of age and older). Women reporting a Pap smear test within the past 3 years at follow-up were considered adherent. For colorectal cancer, we considered women age 50 years and older adherent if they reported a fecal occult blood test (FOBT) in the past year or a flexible sigmoidoscopy or colonoscopy within the past 5 years (note that data were not available for colonoscopy tests within the past 10 years). We also collected information on customer demographics, health status, and salon behavior.

To evaluate interactions between customers and stylists, we assessed changes from baseline to follow-up from customer self-report of health talk on the BHS. In addition, we recorded conversations (20) during the salon observations at multiple time points during the intervention period, using established protocols. A 2-hour observation was conducted in each salon by a trained female African American observer on a "busy" day as determined by the salon owners, with "conversation" as the unit of analysis. Stylist "reach" was defined as the proportion of all licensed cosmetologists per participating salon that enrolled in the BEAUTY Project, calculated as the total number of enrolled stylists divided by the total number of licensed stylists working at the salon (as reported by the owner).

RESULTS

Participating Salons

Of the 12,319 licensed salons in the state, a total of 5,119 were found to be located within a 75-mile radius of Chapel Hill. Salons known to be part of franchises and those whose telephone numbers could not be confirmed were excluded. Staff identified 2,628 salons and they were assessed for eligibility: that they catered mostly to African American customers; had more than 75 "regular" customers; and had at least one stylist willing to sign on to the study. From those approached, 62 salons were interested and eligible to participate (see the CONSORT diagram; Figure 9.2). Of those 62 salons, 40 were ultimately able to meet the customer recruitment goals and were randomized into one of the four intervention arms. However, following randomization, three salons that were randomized into the CONTROL arm withdrew from the study, making the final number of participating salons 37. Forty-two owners (several salons had more than one owner) and an additional 27 licensed stylists were enrolled from the 37 participating salons.

From interviews with all participating salon owners at baseline (100% response rate, $n = 40$), we learned that the typical salon in our study was open for 10.3 years; had an average of three employees who worked in the salon for an average of 5.9 years; and most owners (63%) reported being in the salon daily. Sixty-seven percent of owners believed that participation in the BEAUTY Project would improve the reputation of the salon in the community; and 92.5% would recommend participation in a study like the BEAUTY Project to other salon owners.

Customer Description

Overall, 1,123 customers enrolled in the study from the 37 participating beauty salons and completed a baseline survey, and 559 (49.8%) completed the follow-up survey. Retention patterns overall and by study arm from baseline to follow-up are summarized in Figure 9.2. At baseline, the average customer age was 38.4 years, 55% were single, 47% were college graduates or higher, 34% had a yearly household income between $24,999 and $49,999, and 34% had a yearly household income of $50,000 or more. Among enrolled customers, 73% were overweight/obese, 36% reported getting moderate, regular physical activity (PA), 86% consumed more than 30% of their total calories per day from fat, and 20% reported eating at least five servings of fruits and vegetables per day (Table 9.3). At baseline, there were significant group differences by education level ($x^2 = 14.73$, $p < .05$) and age ($F_{(3,1056)} = 4.91$, $p < .01$), which were adjusted for in the final modeling efforts.

Most customers (88%) reported attending the salon at least once every 7 weeks; 57% visited every 2–4 weeks; and 18% visited at least once weekly. Nearly all (98%) tried to see the same stylist at each visit; 69.7% reported spending between 1.5 and 3 hours per visit, and 18% spent more than 3 hours per visit (Linnan et al., 2007). On average at baseline, customers reported talking with their stylists "very much/a lot" about health; and only 11% reported their health as "excellent."

Approximately half of the customers at baseline completed the follow-up survey ($n = 559/1,123$) and those who were retained were more educated ($x^2 = 12.92$, $p < .01$; HS: 15.6 vs. 14.9, some college: 28.8 vs. 37.5, college graduate: 55.7 vs. 47.6); had a higher income ($x^2 = 6.27$, $p < .05$; < 24.9K: 18.4 vs. 23.5, 25–49.9K: 38.7 vs. 38.4, 50K+: 43.0 vs. 38.0); were more likely to be overweight/obese as measured by BMI ($x^2 = 8.03$, $p < .05$; normal: 19.6 vs. 25.3, overweight: 31.5 vs. 28.9, obese: 48.3 vs. 44.5); and were less likely to self-report more favorable general health status ($x^2 = 203.51$, $p < .001$; poor/fair: 42.4 vs. 11.3, good/excellent: 57.6 vs. 88.7) compared to the initial group at baseline.

Primary Outcomes

As shown in Table 9.4, there were no significant differences between intervention groups on our primary or secondary outcomes (i.e., daily percentage of calories from fat, daily fruits and vegetables, BMI, and regular PA). However, there were some promising modest improvements in health behaviors among participants overall. On average, the daily percentage calories from fat decreased for all respondents ($F_{(1,422)} = 9.22$, $p < .01$), with minimal (but nonsignificant) differences between the treatment arms. Increased consumption of daily fruit and vegetable servings were reported by all respondents, regardless of treatment condition. Additionally, while the majority of respondents did not report engaging in regular physical activity at either time point, there was an increase in the overall number of participants

TABLE 9.3 Customer Characteristics at Baseline (N = 1,123)

Demographic Characteristics	All N = 1,123		Control N = 216		Magazine N = 304		Training N = 306		Both N = 297	
Age (years)[a]	N	m (SD)	n	m (SD)	n	m (SD)	n	m (SD)	n	m (SD)
	1,060	38.5 (12.0)	205	36.8 (11.9)	290	37.3 (12.6)	287	39.1 (11.8)	278	40.3 (11.5)
	Freq	%	Freq	%	Freq	%	Freq	%	Freq	%
Weight status										
Normal	275	26.6	47	23.3	75	27.1	75	26.6	65	23.8
Overweight	299	28.9	60	29.7	86	31.0	79	28.0	74	27.1
Obese	460	44.5	90	44.6	114	41.2	125	44.3	131	48.0
Education level[a]										
High school or less	163	14.9	23	11.0	40	13.4	56	18.7	44	15.4
Some college	410	37.5	94	44.8	107	35.9	116	38.8	93	32.5
College graduate or more	520	47.6	93	44.3	151	50.7	127	42.5	149	52.1
Household income ($)										
< 25k	240	21.4	41	20.8	67	23.7	74	27.3	58	21.6
25–49.9k	392	34.9	83	42.1	106	37.5	87	32.1	116	43.1
≥ 50k	388	34.6	73	37.1	110	38.9	110	40.6	95	35.3
Marital status										
Married	489	45.0	92	44.2	137	46.0	137	43.5	123	45.0
Single	598	55.0	116	55.8	161	54.0	161	56.5	160	55.0

Health Characteristics	N	m (SD)	n	m (SD)	n	m (SD)	n	m (SD)	n	m (SD)
	Freq	%	Freq	%	Freq	%	Freq	%	Freq	%
General health										
Poor/Fair	119	11.3	27	13.2	36	12.5	29	10.2	27	9.7
Good/Excellent	936	88.7	177	86.8	251	87.5	256	89.8	252	90.3
Current regular PA										
No	695	64.1	136	64.8	190	68.1	183	61.6	186	65.0
Yes	390	35.9	74	35.2	102	34.9	114	38.4	100	35.0
Daily percentage from fat										
< 30	134	13.9	28	14.8	29	11.3	37	14.0	40	15.7
> 30	831	86.1	161	85.2	228	88.7	228	86.0	214	84.3
Five daily fruits and vegetables										
No	878	79.8	167	78.8	241	81.4	246	81.7	224	77.0
Yes	222	20.2	45	21.2	55	18.6	55	18.3	67	23.0

[a]Significant group differences. Totals may be less than the stated sample size due to missing data. m = mean, SD = standard deviation.

TABLE 9.4 Customer Baseline/Follow-up on Primary and Secondary Outcomes, by Arm

	All N = 559		Control N = 106		Magazine N = 151		Training N = 148		BOTH N = 154	
	n	m (SD)	n	m (SD)	n	m (SD)	n	m (SD)	n	m (SD)
Daily percentage of calories from fat[a]										
Baseline	429	35.9 (5.5)	83	36 (5.5)	122	35.9 (5.1)	111	35.8 (5.1)	110	35.9 (5.4)
Follow-up	426	35.1 (5.9)	83	35.4 (5.7)	122	34.6 (5.3)	111	35.2 (5.6)	110	35.4 (6.6)
Difference	426	−0.8 (5.1)	83	−0.5 (5.6)	122	−1.3 (4.5)	111	−0.6 (4.8)	110	−0.6 (5.5)
Daily servings of fruits and vegetables										
Baseline	490	3.6 (1.9)	92	3.9 (1.7)	127	3.6 (1.9)	130	3.2 (1.8)	141	3.8 (1.9)
Follow-up	490	3.7 (1.8)	92	3.8 (1.8)	127	3.7 (1.7)	130	3.6 (1.9)	141	3.7 (1.8)
Difference	490	0.1 (1.9)	92	−0.8 (1.7)	127	0.1 (2.0)	130	0.3 (1.9)	141	−0.1 (1.9)
BMI										
Baseline	497	30.2 (7.1)	97	30.0 (6.8)	130	29.8 (6.8)	134	30.2 (7.5)	136	30.7 (7.1)
Follow-up	497	30.6 (6.9)	97	29.5 (6.9)	130	30.0 (6.7)	134	31.1 (7.4)	136	31.9 (11.2)
Difference	497	0.4 (3.6)	97	.4 (2.6)	130	.2 (3.3)	134	0.9 (4.3)	136	0.2 (3.7)
	Freq	%	Freq	%	Freq	%	Freq	%	Freq	%
Number who reported engaging in regular PA										
Baseline	390	35.4	74	35.2	102	34.9	114	38.4	100	35.0
Follow-up	238	43.0	42	40.0	63	42.3	62	42.5	71	46.4

[a]Significant differences from baseline to follow-up. Totals may be less than the stated sample size due to missing data. m = mean, SD = standard deviation.

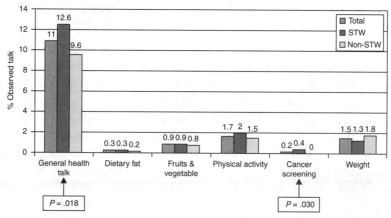

FIGURE 9.3   Observed Health Talk in Salons: Salons With
Stylist Training Workshops (STW) Versus Salons With No Stylist Training
Workshops (Non-STW)

who reported being moderately physically active at follow-up, regardless of treatment condition. And at follow-up, the majority of respondents reported being adherent to age-appropriate cancer screening guidelines for breast, cervical, and colorectal cancer.

Secondary Outcomes—Interactions Between Stylists and Customers

At baseline, observations in salons/environmental scans for a minimum of 2 hours on a "busy" day revealed that 17% of all conversations that occurred in salons were health related. Slightly more than half (56%) of health conversations were initiated by stylists and the most common topics discussed were diet, exercise, and weight or body appearance. At follow-up, as seen in Figure 9.3, the amount of general health talk observed in the salons that received stylists training workshops (STW=salons in the ST and BOTH arms) was significantly higher than was the general health talk observed in non-STW salons (TM or CONTROL salons) ($p < .05$). Although we did not observe increases in health talk about specific risk factors, the number of conversations about cancer screenings increased in the salons with some type of stylist training workshop compared to the salons with no stylist training ($p < .05$). We also compared customer-reported talk with stylists from baseline to follow-up and by study arm. Overall, the amount of customer-reported health talk increased between baseline and follow-up ($F_{(1,535)} = 25.39$, $p < .001$); however, the amount of customer-reported health talk did not differ significantly by intervention arm.

SUMMARY, LESSONS LEARNED, AND IMPLICATIONS FOR FUTURE SALON-BASED RESEARCH AND PRACTICE

The North Carolina BEAUTY and Health Project has a 10-year history of working in partnership with beauty salon owners, licensed stylists, and their customers to promote health and address cancer disparities with salon-based interventions. The results of this large, ACS-funded randomized trial demonstrated that it is feasible to recruit large numbers of salons (40), stylists/owners (more than 70), and their customers (over 1,000) to participate in a research study held within beauty salons. This is an important finding, because places where large numbers of African American women can be successfully reached and engaged in health promotion research, outside of churches, are limited. We attribute part of this success to the use of CBPR approaches that engaged all key stakeholders in this partnership approach to research. While it was challenging to retain customers in the study over the 18-month intervention period (e.g., only 50% completed the follow-up surveys), we learned a lot in this study about how to improve our measurement protocols, as well as our data collection instruments, that will enhance future research efforts. Specifically, we expect that brief questionnaires, the use of telephone and in-person interviews (vs. paper surveys), and in-salon survey events should improve future retention efforts. As evidence of these improvements, our most recent barbershop-based customer retention rates approached nearly 70% due to lessons learned from this salon-based study (Linnan, Rose, Li, & Carlisle, 2009).

In addition to our successful recruitment efforts, our results suggests that African American women—owners, stylists, and customers—were very pleased with the idea of offering health and cancer prevention information in the beauty salons. Participating owners were receptive to joining future studies, participating stylists were eager to attend future training workshops, and customers were highly satisfied with the targeted health magazines and displays. In other words, the empirically based answer to our question "Is it a good idea to promote health in beauty salons?" was a resounding "YES!" from our key partners. However, given the lack of a main (significant) effect on the primary outcomes at the customer level, the challenge ahead is to figure out the best study designs, the most appropriate intervention strategies, and the right dose of intervention required to produce desired changes among stylists and customers. Here, several important lessons were learned that can benefit future research and practice. First, the intervention dose delivered to any given customer will need to be increased in future studies—in our study, the dose was too weak to produce change in desired behavioral outcomes. Thus, instead of a 2 × 2 factorial design testing different intervention strategies (e.g., targeted magazines vs. stylist training), we probably should have thrown a "kitchen sink" intervention strategy (e.g., a larger dose of intervention-targeted magazines plus stylist training plus more intensive, personal behavior change interventions) into this first large effectiveness trial in the beauty salon, rather than splitting up individual intervention approaches. Changing the design and increasing the "dose" of intervention delivered to customers (e.g., including more than information by providing access to behavior change programs or screening services in the salon) would also be a desirable improvement. A two-group design of a more intensive, multicomponent intervention should be the next intervention tested in beauty salons, and we should be especially mindful of including more than just information, but also skill-building activities and/or contests.

Second, we will reconsider the role of the stylist in future salon-based intervention research studies and practice-based work. Our results suggest that stylists are ready and eager to help promote health in the salons. Stylists care about their customers, are generally good communicators, and they work in settings where they reach a lot of women, can reinforce information over time, and are passionate about the community they serve. However, we also learned that stylists are extremely busy. They work long hours and the job is physically and emotionally demanding. While they were eager to participate in our study, they often found it challenging to attend the training workshop offered quarterly, since it was held on the only day they had off (Mondays) and it was a day when many other tasks had to be done. Although our observed salon-based study results demonstrated that "general health talk" significantly increased in the salons where stylists were assigned to one of the stylist training arms (STW or BOTH), we also learned from our stylists that we could improve our future training efforts. Specifically, we will spend more time working with the stylists to assess and address their personal health behaviors before we ask them to talk with customers about health behavior changes. Given formative research results, we assumed that all stylists were good communicators and equally "ready" to talk with their customers about making health changes in diet and physical activity. Unfortunately, we attempted to intervene simultaneously with both stylists and customers in the large trial. However, many of the stylists really needed time to focus on their own health before they were comfortable encouraging their customers to make changes. Thus, we first intend to identify "healthy" stylists who are interested and able to serve as role models and peer educators in future studies. Specifically, we plan to spend 6–12 months working with stylists, who then can be selected out as healthy role models in the salons to help encourage customer changes. Another lesson about stylists is that we need to be very selective about the time and travel demands that we place on them. More in-salon, personalized training opportunities versus group workshops are likely to increase attendance and sustain stylist interest and participation in the project over time. Further, we should not assume all that stylists are equally comfortable or interested in talking with their customers about health. There are more "ready and able" stylists and some "less ready and less able" stylists, so we need to avoid assumptions and make sure that we engage with stylists who are able to take on and embrace this new role.

In addition to a more intensive intervention dose, and more up-front time spent focused on stylists as "role models" of healthy behaviors, we also probably need to "keep it simple" and focus on a single (or two) risk factors as opposed to trying to work on three primary outcomes and two secondary outcomes in the same study. Any single message or behavior change target in our BEAUTY Project intervention was likely to be "lost" amid the overload of information about dietary fat, fruits and vegetables, physical activity, cancer screening behaviors, and weight. Combined with a lack of opportunity to really "try out" and/or "get tangible support" for any given behavioral change strategy, it is likely that we further diluted the intervention dose by spreading our messages too thinly. A single risk factor focus is likely where our next study will aim. Consistent with CBPR principles, we will continue to be mindful of the interests of our partners, and addressing overweight/obesity is the likely "next" behavioral focus for our beauty salon intervention work. In addition, we will work to maximize the type of social support we believe is possible with salon-based interventions, by having activities, assessments, and support meetings in the salons as opposed to relying on just reaching women in the salons and hoping that they will make the changes on their own.

We were encouraged by the small, but important, effects on several dietary outcomes that we observed from the targeted magazines we sent to customers at home. We will be sure to include some version of these targeted magazines in future studies. Targeted magazines have been effective in church-based and worksite-based interventions with African American women (Campbell et al., 2000; Resnicow et al., 2000). The stylist training workshops helped to increase observed general health talk, but we may need to rethink the way in which we utilize the stylist in future salon-based research studies. It may be helpful to focus the role of the stylist on support, encouragement, and/or referral, as opposed to trying to train stylists to deliver key health messages. Thus, we may engage stylists to convene and encourage customers to participate in research, to sponsor in-salon events, and to act as role models for encouraging customer behavior change. A more engaged beauty salon is a worthy goal, and while customers spend a lot of time in the salon, they are typically in the salon at very different days and times. Thus, "after-hour" salon events, contests, and/or the use of new technologies (kiosks, web-based programs) to enhance intervention effects will be considered for future studies.

Every study has both strengths and limitations. Several key strengths of the North Carolina BEAUTY and Health Project included: the fact that the research team utilized CBPR principles in the development of all aspects of the study; the fact that the intervention was guided by theory and built upon 2 years of formative research results (e.g., stylist survey, salon observational studies, customer focus groups, and a pilot intervention study); that we adapted an evidence-based intervention (targeted health magazines) for the beauty salon environment; and that we evaluated the effects of these interventions using a very rigorous study design. Despite the care taken in both the intervention and the evaluation, we did not achieve the intended outcomes at the customer level. However, there were a number of noteworthy limitations to this study as well. First, despite a great deal of interest among beauty salons and stylists in participating in this study, there was loss to follow-up at both the salon and customer levels that limited power and ability to detect differences. Second, although we did a lot of careful work to develop new measures and data collection procedures for this new setting/ population, we had limited success getting data from stylists. We worked with our Advisory Board members to strategize several approaches to gathering data from stylists, but in the end, it was clear that interviews were preferable to written surveys. Unfortunately, this was a lesson learned too late to affect the study data collection effort, and thus it limited our ability to explain the study outcomes. As mentioned previously, we believe that there were many intervention challenges related to working in a new setting and due to being a little over-ambitious in our study design and intervention test. Despite this, our study results and work with the Advisory Board members have laid the foundations for a number of important next research and practice-based programs in beauty salons.

We are convinced that beauty salons (and barbershops) remain a terrific setting for reaching and intervening with women (and men) on a number of health issues. Our BEAUTY Project helped us learn lessons that will improve our future studies and help inform the growing evidence base that exists in these settings. We recently examined published research articles describing interventions, formative research, and recruitment studies involving beauty salons and barbershops. We found 18 articles describing intervention study results that were conducted in 14 different states. Most interventions were implemented in one location; however, one study had programs in 19 cities in 6 states. Half of the interventions were located in barbershops alone, 35% in salons alone, and the remainder were based in both barbershop and salon locations. Half of the interventions were collaborative, while 35% were researcher delivered, and 15% were stylist or barber delivered. The majority of programs were targeted at African American or Afro-Caribbean customers (80%), and 45% targeted males, whereas 35% targeted females. Customers were participants in 17 interventions and the number of customers ranged from 20 to 14,000.

Stylists and/or barbers or owners were participants in 10 studies and the number of stylists/barbers/owners ranged from 5 to 700, with the majority (80%) of studies having between 5 and 40 participating. Almost half of all interventions (45%) gave an incentive to the stylist/barber, customer, or both for participation. The interventions focused on cancers (55%), hypertension (15%), diabetes, kidney or cardiovascular disease (10%), nutrition and physical activity (5%), smoking (5%), stroke (5%), and general health (5%). Most study designs were nonexperimental (60%), including 6 of the 7 researcher-delivered interventions. CBPR was used to inform half of all interventions. Education was the objective of half of the interventions, whereas the remainder focused on health behavior change, including screening behaviors (40%), or training stylists/barbers to deliver interventions (10%). Outcomes were measured in the majority of studies (85%). The BEAUTY Project was among the largest of these studies and one of the few that were rigorously evaluated.

In summary, our results indicate that beauty salons were effective in reaching African American women with lifesaving information and resources to address cancer disparities. Based on critically valuable lessons learned in this study, we have new insights and strategies for how to best work in partnership with salon owners, stylists, and their customers to create powerful interventions that are both contextually and culturally appropriate. There are interesting challenges to working within beauty salons, particularly when done in partnership with the owners, stylists, and customers. Given the opportunities for reach and reinforcement of information in the salons, we intend to increase the dose of intervention and rethink how best to work with stylists to benefit from the unique stylist–customer relationship and, ultimately, to maximize the effects of future beauty-salon–based interventions. Given that beauty salons are an important historical "safe haven" for the African American community, we are optimistic that—in these important community settings—we can reach, and begin to address or eliminate, disparities among African American women who suffer disproportionately high rates of cancer and other leading causes of death.

REFERENCES

American Cancer Society. (2001). *Cancer prevention and early detection facts and figures 2001*. Atlanta, GA: Author.

American Cancer Society. (2005). *Cancer facts and figures 2005* (Vol. 2005). Atlanta, GA: Author.

America's Health Rankings & United Health Foundation. (2009). *North Carolina (2009)*. Retrieved February 9, 2010, from http://www.americashealthrankings.org/yearcompare/ 2008/2009/NC.aspx

American Institute for Cancer Research. (2007). *Food, nutrition, physical activity, and the prevention of cancer: A global perspective.* World Cancer Research Fund. Washington, DC: Author.

Bandura, A. (2000). *Social foundations of thought and action.* Englewood Cliffs, NJ: Prentice Hall.

Block, G., Hartman, A. M., Dresser, C. M., Carroll, M. D., Gannon, J., & Gardner, L. (1986). A data-based approach to diet questionnaire design and testing. *American Journal of Epidemiology, 124*(3), 453–469.

Campbell, M. K., Demark-Wahnefried, W., Symons, M., Kalsbeek, W. D., Dodds, J., Cowan, A., . . . McClelland, J. W. (1999). Fruit and vegetable consumption and prevention of cancer: The Black Churches United for Better Health project. *American Journal of Public Health, 89*(9), 1390–1396.

Campbell, M. K., Motsinger, B. M., Ingram, A., Jewell, D., Makarushka, C., Beatty, B., . . . Demark-Wahnefried, W. (2000). The North Carolina Black Churches United for Better Health project: Intervention and process evaluation. *Health Education & Behavior, 27*(2), 241–253.

Coates, R. J., Eley, J. W., Block, G., Gunter, E. W., Sowell, A. L., Grossman, C., & Greenberg, R. S. (1991). An evaluation of a food frequency questionnaire for assessing dietary intake of specific carotenoids and vitamin E among low-income black women. *American Journal of Epidemiology, 134*(6), 658–671.

Earp, J. A., & Flax, V. L. (1999). What lay health advisors do: An evaluation of advisors' activities. *Cancer Practice, 7*(1), 16–21.

Fox, S., Pitkin, K., Paul, C., Carson, S., & Duan, N. (1998). Breast cancer screening adherence: Does church attendance matter? *Health Education & Behavior, 25*, 742–758.

Keyserling, T. C., Ammerman, A. S., Samuel-Hodge, C. D., Ingram, A. F., Skelly, A. H., Elasy, T. A., . . . Henríquez-Roldán, C. F. (2000). A diabetes management program for African American women with type 2 diabetes. *Diabetes Educator, 26*(5), 796–805.

Kim, K., Linnan, L., Kulik, N., Carlisle, C., Enga, Z., & Bentley, M. (2007). Linking beauty and health among African American women: Using focus group results to build culturally and contextually appropriate interventions. *Journal of Social and Behavioral Health Sciences, 1*(1), 41–59.

Kleindorfer, D., Miller, R., Sailor-Smith, S., Moomaw, C., Khoury, J., & Frankel, M. (2008). The challenges of community-based research: The beauty shop stroke education project. *Stroke, 39*(8), 2331–2335.

Levi, J., & Trust for America's Health. (2009). Section 1: Obesity rates and related trends. In *F as in Fat: How obesity polices are failing America.* Washington, DC: Trust for America's Health.

Linnan, L., Carlisle, V., Hanson, K., Ammerman, A., Evenson, K., & Rose, J. (2005, April 21–22). *Building trust by building relationships: Evolution of the North Carolina BEAUTY and Health Project.* Paper presented at the Exploring Models to Eliminate Cancer Disparities among African American and Latino Populations: Research and Community Solutions; American Cancer Society, Atlanta, GA.

Linnan, L., & Ferguson, Y. (2007). Beauty salons: A promising health promotion setting for reaching and promoting health among African American women. *Health Education & Behavior, 6*(37), 517–530.

Linnan, L., Ferguson, Y., Wasilewski, Y., Lee, A. M., Yang, J., & Katz, M. (2005). Results of the North Carolina BEAUTY and Health Pilot Project. *Health Promotion Practice, 6*(2), 164–173.

Linnan, L., Kim, A. E., Wasilewski, Y., Lee, A. M., Yang, J., & Solomon, F. (2001). Working with licensed cosmetologists to promote health: Results from the North Carolina BEAUTY and Health Pilot Study. *Preventive Medicine, 33*(6), 606–612.

Linnan, L., Rose, J., Carlisle, V., Evenson, K., Mangum, A., Hooten, E., . . . Biddle, A. (2007). The North Carolina BEAUTY and Health Project: Overview and baseline results. *Community Psychologist, 40*(2), 61–66.

Linnan, L., Rose, J., Li, J., & Carlisle, V. (2009). *Reaching and engaging Black men in barbershops: Results of the Cancer Understanding Today Study (CUTS)*. Society for Behavioral Medicine Annual Meeting. Montreal, Canada.

Minkler, M. (2000). Using participatory action research to build healthy communities. *Public Health Reports, 115*(2–3), 191–197.

Minkler, M., & Wallerstein, N. (2003). *Community based participatory research for health* (1st ed.). San Francisco, CA: Jossey-Bass.

Mokdad, A. H., Marks, J. S., Stroup, D. F., & Gerberding, J. L. (2004). Actual causes of death in the United States, 2000. *Journal of the American Medical Association, 291*(10), 1238–1245.

National Cancer Institute. (2005). *State cancer profiles*. Bethesda, MD: Author.

North Carolina Advisory Committee on Cancer Coordination and Control. (2011). *The North Carolina Cancer Control Plan, 2001–2006*. Raliegh, NC: North Carolina Department of Environment, Health and Natural Resources.

North Carolina Central Cancer Registry. (2004). *North Carolina facts and figures, 2004*. Raleigh, NC: Author.

Prochaska, J. O., Redding, C. A., &Evers, K.E. (1997). The transtheoretical model and stages of change. In K. Glanz, F. M. Lewis, & B. K. Rimer (Eds.), *Health behavior and health education: Theory, research, and practice* (2nd ed., pp. 60–84). San Francisco, CA: Jossey-Bass.

Resnicow, K., Odom, E., Wang, T., Dudley, W. N., Mitchell, D., Vaughan, R., . . . Baranowski, T. (2000). Validation of three food frequency questionnaires and 24-hour recalls with serum carotenoid levels in a sample of African-American adults. *American Journal of Epidemiology, 152*, 1072–1080.

Rudner, L. M. (2003). *Cosmetology job demand survey*. Alexandria, VA: National Accrediting Commission of Cosmetology Arts and Sciences.

Solomon, F. M., Linnan, L. A., Wasilewski, Y., Lee, A. M., Katz, M. L., & Yang, J. (2004). Observational study in ten beauty salons: Results informing development of the North Carolina BEAUTY and Health Project. *Health Education & Behavior, 31*(6), 790–807.

Stokols, D. (1992). Establishing and maintaining healthy environments. Toward a social ecology of health promotion. *American Psychologist, 47*(1), 6–22.

Stokols, D., Pelletier, K. R., & Fielding, J. E. (1996). The ecology of work and health: Research and policy directions for the promotion of employee health. *Health Education Quarterly, 23*(2), 137–158.

Tessaro, I. (1997). The natural helping role of nurses in promoting healthy behaviors in communities. *Advanced Practice Nursing Quarterly, 2*(4), 73–78.

Tessaro, I. A., Taylor, S., Belton, L., Campbell, M. K., Benedict, S., Kelsey, K., & DeVellis, B. (2000). Adapting a natural (lay) helpers model of change for worksite health promotion for women. *Health Education Research, 15*(5), 603–614.

U.S. Department of Labor. (2004). *Occupational outlook handbook, 2004–05 edition— Barbers, cosmetologists, and other personal appearance workers*. Washington, DC: U.S. Department of Labor, Bureau of Labor Statistics.

Viswanathan, M., Ammerman, A., Eng, E., Gartlehner, G., Lohr, K. N., Griffith, D., . . . Whitener, L. (2004). *Community-based participatory research: Assessing the evidence. Evidence Report/Technology Assessment No.99* (No. AHRQ Pub. No. 04-E022–2). Rockville, MD: Agency for Healthcare Research and Quality.

10

Promoting Healthy Eating by Strengthening Family Relations: Design and Implementation of the *Entre Familia: Reflejos de Salud* Intervention

Guadalupe X. Ayala, Leticia Ibarra, Elva Arredondo, Lucy Horton, Erika Hernandez, Humberto Parada, Donald Slymen, Cheryl Rock, Moshe Engelberg, and John P. Elder

One of several health behaviors linked to cancer is diet (American Cancer Society, 2009; Miller, Lesko, Muscat, Lazarus, & Hartman, 2010). Diet, and specifically the consumption of fruits and vegetables, is associated with reduced cancer risk (Hung et al., 2004). Few Latino/Hispanic women and men consume fruits and vegetables five or more times per day (28% and 20%, respectively; Blanck, Gillespie, Kimmons, Seymour, & Serdula, 2008). In addition, Latinos consume fewer fruits and vegetables the longer they live in the United States and with a greater degree of acculturation (as manifested by English language use) (Ayala, Baquero, & Klinger, 2008; Satia-Abouta, Patterson, Neuhouser, & Elder, 2002). Thus, cancer preventive behaviors such as healthy eating exhibited upon arrival in the United States appear to diminish over time spent in this country. In addition, there is a growing body of evidence that more recent immigrants to the United States no longer exhibit such healthy dietary patterns and, instead, exhibit greater risk patterns and morbidity than observed in previous generations of immigrants, such as a greater prevalence of obesity and diabetes (Satia-Abouta, 2010). There is a need for interventions to ameliorate this deterioration in health behaviors associated with obesity. One approach to build on is the implementation of family-based interventions to promote behaviors such as the intake of sufficient amounts of fruits and vegetables. Family-based interventions are consistent with the cultural norms and practices of Mexican immigrants/Mexican Americans (Elder, Ayala, Parra-Medina, & Talavera, 2009). Moreover, these types of interventions have the potential to impact multiple family members simultaneously, thus increasing the reach of our interventions (Kitzman-Ulrich et al., 2010).

Family-based interventions are promising, as they highlight the potential for child and family change (Haire-Joshu et al., 2008). An important consideration in family-based research is who is involved. Family-based interventions to promote healthy eating have involved the parents alone (parenting studies: Golan & Crow, 2004) or the parents and children together (typically dyad or family studies: Rodearmel et al., 2006). However, in most published research, the parent involved is the mother (Pearson, Atkin, Biddle, & Gorely, 2010). Examining the role of fathers has received far less attention in the field, and is only now being examined as an important influence on children's diet (Morgan et al., 2010). The *Entre Familia: Reflejos de Salud* (In the Family: Reflections on Health) study attempts to fill this gap.

THE PRESENT STUDY

Most family-based research to promote healthy eating has centered on the mother. To fill a gap in family-based interventions, we designed an intervention to involve multiple family members, including fathers. The *Entre Familia* study is a randomized controlled trial that is testing a 4-month, 10-session family-based intervention to promote fruit and vegetable consumption and other dimensions of healthy eating. The control condition is a delayed treatment condition in which families receive the intervention materials after all assessments are completed. Outcomes are being assessed on 360 mothers, 360 children, and a 25% ($n = 90$) subsample of fathers at 3 time-points (baseline, 4 months posttest, and 12-month follow-up).

This chapter describes how the intervention was developed with input from community residents, community partners, and investigators. In addition, we share baseline data from a subsample of recruited mothers and fathers ($n = 69$ dyads) to illustrate ways in which their parenting styles, related to their children's diets, are concordant or discordant. This information is useful for designing interventions that capitalize on the strengths of each parent to create the healthiest home environment possible.

METHODS

Study Setting

Entre Familia is being conducted in Imperial County, California. This county, located on the United States/Mexico border, has an estimated population of >160,000, with >122,000 (76%) of the population being Latino. Estimates from the 2006–2008 American Community Survey suggest that 31% of the residents of Imperial County were born in a foreign country (compared to 27% in California), 63% completed high school education or higher compared to 80% in California, and 53% were in the labor force compared to 65% in California. The median household income in 2008 was estimated at $37,492, compared to $61,154 in California (U.S. Census Bureau, 2010). In 2009 and again in 2010, Imperial County had the highest unemployment rates in the United States. Study activities are occurring in nearly all cities in Imperial County, though predominantly in Brawley, El Centro, and Calexico, given their size. These cities are similar demographically, but they differ in their proximity to the United States/Mexico border, with Brawley being the furthest from the border.

This study involves a partnership between the Institute for Behavioral and Community Health (IBACH) at San Diego State University Research Foundation and *Clínicas de Salud Del Pueblo*, Inc. (CDSDP), a private, non-profit corporation, providing comprehensive primary care services to residents throughout Imperial and Riverside Counties. All intervention activities are organized from CDSDP; evaluation activities are organized from a study office approximately 30 miles from the clinic offices.

Recruitment of Families

Research assistants were hired to carry out family recruitment and administer study surveys. Three bilingual, bicultural research assistants are carrying out these efforts; all of them live within the study area, are a part of the local community, and have prior research experience. Project staff developed a training manual to assist the training process. Topics covered in training included: the role of a research assistant, a study overview and timeline, building rapport with potential study families, confidentiality and professionalism, procedures for the accurate and consistent collection of anthropometric data, consent procedures for adults and children, review and practice of all study surveys, general interviewing principles, participant folder management and data storage, and protocols for managing study incentives. A competency test was administered at the end of training to ensure that the research assistants were ready to work with families. This included assessing accuracy and reliability of anthropometric measurements within and between research assistants.

Families involved in the *Entre Familia* study represent a convenience sample. Research assistants and CDSDP staff are conducting presentations to local organizations and schools, meeting face to face with community residents at local events (i.e., health fairs and community walks), and distributing fliers/posters in targeted places in Imperial County (i.e., clinics, schools, family resource centers, other community outlets). A project announcement was placed in a free community periodical for 4 weeks. Currently, CDSDP is mailing informational letters to potentially eligible families. Research assistants then telephone these families to determine their eligibility and interest in the program.

After an interested family is identified, one research assistant assesses eligibility. This assessment is usually conducted by telephone; however, screening is done in person if both the research assistant and mother are present (e.g., at a recruitment event). The research assistant assesses family eligibility by completing a three-page screener with the mother. To qualify, the mother has to meet the following inclusion criteria: be at least 18 years of age, be a resident of Imperial County, have at least one child between the ages of 7 and 13, self-identify as Latino, be able to read and speak Spanish, and live in the same household as her child and husband/partner for at least 4 days of the week. Reasons for exclusion include having a family member being on a medically prescribed diet and the family having plans to move outside of Imperial County during the study time frame of 10 months.

If the family is deemed eligible and wishes to participate in the program, an appointment is scheduled to complete the baseline assessment. A second three-page screener is completed with the interested father if he is present during this process, or at the first appointment. Each family is assigned an identification number to protect confidentiality. Each identification number consists of four digits: the first indicates which region of the county the family resides in (north, central, or south), and the last three are unique family identifiers. After completing the baseline assessment (described further below), families are randomized to the intervention condition or the delayed treatment control condition.

Intervention

Intervention Development

The research team is composed of investigators with expertise in health promotion, psychology, nutrition, and communication, plus community-based health care providers and experienced *promotoras*. This team worked together to develop a comprehensive *promotora* training manual, a *promotora* toolkit, a nine-part DVD series, and an accompanying family workbook. In addition, formative research methods, including focus groups and a card sort task, were implemented with members of the target audience to inform intervention development. The focus groups were structured using a panel series design. Panel series focus groups involve convening a group of individuals to participate in a series of consecutive focus groups (three meetings, scheduled a week apart) that build on each other (Ayala et al., 2006). This allows the researcher to obtain in-depth information on a particular topic.

The topic of the first focus group centered on identifying the interpersonal interactions that occur between family members related to their food habits and physical activity. The second group involved determining the appropriate message framing for the intervention. The third group examined how to structure the intervention to involve the entire family. Two panel series were conducted, with a total of 19 adults participating. One series was conducted in El Centro and the other in Calexico. The vast majority of adult participants were women (90%; $n = 17$); only two were men. The average age of participants was 40.4 years ($SD = 12.6$), 58% were married, 47% were employed either full- or part-time, 68% spoke mainly Spanish, and 11% were on a restricted diet (for hypertension or hypercholesterolemia). The mean years living in the United States was 17.7 ($SD = 12.3$).

Because so few fathers attended the focus groups, men were recruited to participate in a card-sort task and complete a one-time interview on their parenting style and demographic information, including hours worked per week and when they generally arrived home from work. Card-sort tasks are a relatively common form of assessing attitudes, though not used as frequently in public health. The fathers participated in a 10-minute card-sort task to identify the top roles they played in their family's lives, using a set of 15 cards with images and words representing various father roles. The men were then asked to use the same cards to identify the top challenges or barriers they faced as fathers. Following the card-sort task, the fathers answered a brief survey of parenting and demographic questions. A total of 562 men were approached in a mall and outside several large supermarkets; 16% were ineligible, 6% were not interested, 15% did not have time, and 51% did not live in the target communities. A total of 68 (12%) men completed the card sort task. Most of the men were married (94%; $n = 64$) and working (90%; $n = 61$). Fathers reported the following top five roles that they played in their families: *El proveedor* (the financial provider), *El protector* (the protector), *El cariñoso* (the one who gives affection), *El motivador de estudios* (the education promoter), and *El motivador de deportes* (the promoter of sports/ activity). The top five challenges that the fathers faced included: *El sr. decisiones* (Mr. decision-maker), *El arbitro* (the referee/arbitrator), *El tranquilo* (the one who keeps things calm), *El niñero* (the babysitter), and *El promotor de diversión* (Provider of fun/diversion). Information from the focus groups plus the card sort task—along with feedback from the investigators, health care providers, and *promotoras*—was instrumental in designing the materials described below.

The *promotora* training manual consists of 13 sections. The first section introduces the *promotora* to the organization, the goals of the *Entre Familia* study, the study timeline, what it means to be an *Entre Familia promotora*, operational definitions of social support, and the importance of healthy eating for cancer prevention. The second section provides in-depth training on nutrition for cancer prevention, how to use our R-*MESA* strategy for dietary change, and the opportunity to practice their portion estimation skills. The R-*MESA* strategy was designed by the first author in a previous study (Elder, Ayala, Slymen, Arredondo, & Campbell, 2009); the acronym is easy to remember, given that "*mesa*" translates into "table," which is where most food is consumed in the home. It teaches the importance of dietary behaviors including reducing portion sizes of high-fat foods, modifying existing dishes, eliminating unhealthy foods, substituting healthier options for less healthy options, and adding more fruits and vegetables to snacks and meals. The third session provides an overview of the family intervention strategies, including the overall structure, what a home visit looks like, and how to monitor intervention delivery. The remaining 10 sections are designed to model the family home visit for the *promotora*. During this part of the training, *promotoras* are also given a toolkit to use during the home visits, including a DVD player, several games designed by the program and accompanying game pieces, business cards, food models, and various office supplies.

Using data from our formative research and working with a professional production company, we produced a nine-episode situation comedy (sitcom). The sitcom depicts a typical Mexican family struggling to change its eating habits. Each episode includes a 12-minute storyline, followed by a female narrator describing the three main points of the episode. Each episode is designed to capture the attention of all family members by depicting characters that are very similar to the target population. To accompany the sitcom, we produced a 10-part family workbook. Each part of the workbook includes the following elements: (1) a cover page with three main objectives; (2) a page with the main points of the sitcom, along with a written script of the female narrator's comments (see Figure 10.1); (3) a family session information page, which provides the primary didactic content for the session; (4) a goal-setting page; (5) a skill-building page; (6) a fun activity page; and (7) a homework assignment. The family workbook is in the Spanish langauge only, is written at a sixth- to eighth-grade reading level, and is spiral bound.

Promotora Selection and Training

The *promotoras* implementing the program were identified from among promotoras involved with other projects at CDSDP plus referrals and self-identification from flyers distributed in various community settings and through various networks. All interested promotoras completed an application form and participated in an interview with the CDSDP project coordinator and the research project manager. Promotoras with the following

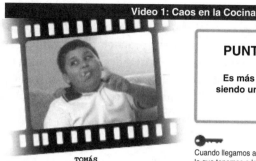

Video 1: Caos en la Cocina

TOMÁS
Mamá, mamá, ¡ya llegué de la escula:

ESPERANZA
¡Tomás García: Espero que no hayas
llegado con tu show de aventar cosas,
tirarte al sillón y llenarte de
fritangas. ¡¿Me oistes?¡

PUNTO CLAVE #1:

**Es más fácil ser saludable
siendo una familia organizada**

Cuando llegamos a casa, es más fácil comer
lo que tenemos a la mano. Si no preparamos
meriendas saludables y los tenemos
disponibles, es más probable que comamos
comida chatarra.

Nutrición: ¿Cómo pueden ayudar a los niños para
que tengan y coman meriendas saludables para
evitar el consumo de comida chatarra?

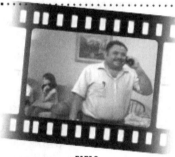

PABLO
¿Si, bueno, nablo con Mas-A Pizza?
Si quiero la espcial de martes, a
ja, la pizza de león extra grande...
ehmm, la que lleva todas los cortes de
carne....si, póngale más queso...no,
no necesito la ensalada--:somos leones
no conejos!

PUNTO CLAVE #2:

**Cada miembro de la familia juega
un papel importante con respecto
a la salud de la familia**

Todos contribuimos a la salud de nuestra
familia. Las actitudes y acciones de todos sobre
la comida tienen consecuencias en el presente
y en el futuro, Inculcar comer más frutas y
verduras a nuestro niños los ayudará a tener
un porvenir más saludable.

Nutricion: ¿Quién es el campeón de comer frutas y
verduras en su familia y cómo puede motivar a los
demás a comer más frutas y verduras?

(continuar)

**FIGURE 10.1   A Sample of a Family Manual With Main Teaching Points,
From the DVD**

qualities were selected to become involved in the *Entre Familia* study: good
communication skills, good organizational skills, an interest in promoting
healthy eating, comfortable conducting home visits, with access to transportation, and available to work on evenings and weekends.

Six promotoras participated in 80 hours of training with two members of
the research team. The first part of the training (45 hours) was conducted over
a 3-week period, with *promotoras* and trainers meeting three times a week, for
5 hours in each training session. The first three training sessions were designed to introduce the promotora to the program, the promotion of healthy
eating, and the intervention materials. The remaining six training sessions

were meant to model the actual home visits and telephone calls with the families, thus allowing the promotoras to experience the program themselves. The remaining 35 hours were spent practicing the training sessions and preparing for a written competency examination. After passing the competency examination, the promotoras were ready to deliver the intervention. Currently, five promotoras are delivering the intervention; one promotora transferred to a different program in the clinic.

Intervention Implementation

Our approach to intervention implementation is to promote behavior change through humor, fun activities, and family interactions. The *Entre Familia* intervention consists of 10 promotora-facilitated sessions, held over a 4-month period. *Promotoras* facilitate the first seven sessions in the family's home consecutively, and the last four sessions alternate between telephone calls and home visits to ensure that the family takes ownership of the knowledge and skills acquired, and does not depend on the promotoras for continued accountability. Each home visit lasts for 1.5–2.0 hours and telephone calls are approximately 15–30 minutes long.

A total of six cycles of the intervention are being completed, with 30 families participating in each cycle. During each cycle, five *promotoras* working 20 hours a week are assigned five or six families each. Once families are randomized into the intervention, the field project coordinator assigns them to a *promotora*. The *promotora* is provided with the family's ID number, mother's name, address, and telephone number. The promotora then sends the mother a letter of introduction, to identify herself and inform her that she will be contacting her soon to schedule the first visit. The expectation is to conduct the first visit within 1 week of assignment. Once the promotora arrives at the family's home, the sessions follow a standard protocol as outlined in the manual: (1) review homework from the previous session; (2) watch, rate, and discuss the sitcom episode; (3) present a mini-lecture; (4) have the families complete the promise of the week (a form of goal-setting); (5) engage in a fun activity; and (6) review the homework assignment. Telephone calls follow a different format, with the promotoras checking in with the mother to determine her family's progress with completing their goals and homework assignments. Once all sessions are completed, families are given a certificate of completion and congratulated on their dedication and effort.

Promotoras collect family engagement data by completing a home visit log that tracks dose delivered, fidelity to the standard home visit protocol, family readiness for the visit, and family engagement during the visit. In addition, *promotoras* attend weekly meetings with the field project coordinator, and periodically with the principal investigator and director of programs at CDSDP, to share accomplishments and discuss concerns.

Evaluation

Procedures

Data collection is primarily conducted in the families' homes. If the mother wishes to meet in a different location, the meeting is planned at CDSDP or at the *Entre Familia* study offices. The research assistant starts the visit by reading and explaining the consent form to the mother and father. After each parent signs a separate form, the research assistant then explains the assent form to the child, and asks him or her to sign. The research assistant then administers the surveys with each participant individually and reads through each question (in the order of mother, father, child). Response cards appropriate to each survey are used to show the participant answer choices to each question.

    Mother surveys are always conducted in Spanish; however, the research assistant gives the father and child the option of completing the survey in either English or Spanish. The average time (including breaks) to complete a mother survey is 90 minutes, and 15 minutes for a father survey. Older children (10–13 years) need 20 minutes to complete a survey and younger children (7–9 years) usually need 40 minutes. The visit is concluded with height and weight measurements on the mother and child. This procedure is followed for the baseline, 4 months posttest, and 12-month follow-up assessments.

Measures

Family relations are measured using three subscales from the Family Functioning Scale (Bloom & Naar, 2004), which itself was derived from the Family Environment Scale (Moos & Moos, 1994). These subscales are cohesion, expressiveness, and disengagement, and each contains five items. Responses are made on a 4-point Likert-type scale from 1 = very untrue to 4 = very true. Where needed, responses are reverse-coded and then a mean score is computed, with higher scores reflecting stronger family relations for the cohesion (α = .63) and expressiveness (α = .74) subscales, and less strong for the disengagement scale (α = .47). All alpha coefficients are based on the 275 mothers recruited to date (see the Results section).

    Parenting practices are measured using a modified version of the 26-item PEAS scale (Larios, Ayala, Arredondo, Baquero, & Elder, 2009). We modified the PEAS scale to focus exclusively on diet by cutting the 10 parenting practices related to physical activity, adding nine statements to augment the diet-related Reinforcement and Discipline subscales, and adding a new subscale titled Diet-Related Parental Permissiveness. With only two exceptions, the factor analysis confirmed the additions of these items in their hypothesized subscales. After removing two items related to parenting on fruits and vegetables that did not load at .40 or above on any factor, the 23-item, diet-modified PEAS scale assesses the following constructs: Monitoring (5 items, $\alpha = .86$), Reinforcement (4 items, $\alpha = .65$), Permissiveness (4 items, $\alpha = .78$), Limit setting (2 items, $\alpha = .62$), Control (5 items, $\alpha = .74$), and Discipline (3 items, $\alpha = .74$). As on the original PEAS scale, responses are made on a 5-point Likert-type scale from 1 = never to 5 = very often, with higher scores denoting more frequent use of this parenting practice.

The concept of spousal interference was developed for this study, based on our formative research. A 6-item scale was created to assess whether the spouse or partner engaged in unsupportive behaviors related to diet, such as purchasing unhealthy food against their partner's wishes and eating too many snacks in front of the family. Responses are made on a 5-point scale from 1 = never to 5 = very often. A mean score is computed such that a higher score reflects greater spousal interference for making healthy changes in the home ($\alpha = .88$). Table 10.1 presents selected items from measured constructs.

Data Analyses

Data management and statistical analyses for the quantitative portion of this study were performed using the Statistical Package for the Social Sciences (SPSS) Version 18 and Statistical Analysis Software (SAS) Version 9.2.

TABLE 10.1   Selected Items From Measured Constructs

Family functioning	*Cohesiveness*: Family members really helped and supported one another.
	Expressiveness: In our family, it was important for everyone to express their opinion.
	Disengagement: Family members did not check with each other when making decisions.
Parenting practices	*Monitoring*: How often did you keep track of sweet snacks (candy, ice cream, cake) that your children ate?
	Reinforcement: How often did you encourage your children to try new fruits and vegetables?
	Permission: How often did your children have to ask permission before getting a second helping?
	Limit setting: How often did you limit the number of high-fat snacks your children ate?
	Control: How often did you tell your children to eat everything on their plates?
	Discipline: How often did you discipline your children for eating a snack without your permission?
Spousal interference	How often did your spouse/partner bring home unhealthy foods for the family to eat?

Descriptive analyses were first conducted to assess the distribution and normality of the variables, as well as the reliability of scales. Univariate analyses were then conducted, followed by a series of Wilcoxon signed-rank tests to compare mother and father responses on parenting and family relations. All significance tests used an alpha level of .05.

RESULTS

Participants

This intervention trial aims to recruit 360 families, including a 25% subsample ($n = 90$) that includes fathers. As of November 2010, 275 mother and child pairs had been recruited, 69 of which included fathers. Therefore, 69 mother–father dyads were used in the present analyses. Of these families, 33% ($n = 23$) were recruited through letters sent by CDSDP and 66% ($n = 46$) were recruited through community recruitment efforts.

Maternal and paternal demographic information are presented in Table 10.2. The fathers are on average about 4 years older than the mothers, with the mean age of mothers being 37.9 ($SD = 7.6$, range = 25– 55) and the mean age of fathers being 41.7 ($SD = 8.8$, range = 25–61). About 55% (54) of the study participants are married (or living as married) and have an average of two children under the age of 18 in the home. Of the 69 mothers, 53% (36) have a high school education or greater, 35% are employed, and 77% were born in Mexico. On the other hand, of the 69 fathers recruited to date, 53% (39) have a high school education or greater, 73% (49) are employed, and 83% (57) were born in Mexico. Answers ascertained from the mothers only on family income and food assistance indicate that 57% (37) of these families are below the

TABLE 10.2 Demographic Characteristics of Participating Families ($N = 69$)

	Mothers Mean (*SD*) or % (*n*)	Fathers Mean (*SD*) or % (*n*)
Mean age (*SD*)	37.9 (7.6)	41.7 (8.8)
% married or living as married	78.3% (54)	81.2% (56)
Mean number of children in the home (*SD*)	2.32 (1.11)	n/a
% completed high school or GED	52.9% (36)	58.2% (39)
% employed	34.8% (24)	73.1% (49)
% poverty	56.9% (37)	n/a
% on food assistance	52.2% (36)	n/a
% own a home	50.7% (35)	n/a
% foreign born	76.8% (53)	82.6% (57)

n/a = not asked.

U.S. Census Bureau's 2009 poverty threshold and 52% (36) receive assistance from the Women, Infants, and Children Program, the Supplemental Nutrition Assistance Program (formerly Food Stamps), or both.

Assessment of Scales

Scale properties were examined by looking at each scale's histogram. Normality was determined if the histograms appeared symmetrical and using the Kolmogorov–Smirnov D statistic of the goodness-of-fit tests. For mothers, only the Control ($D = 0.23, p > .15$, skewness $= -0.17$), Monitoring ($D = 0.10, p = .12$, skewness $= -0.28$), and Permissiveness ($D = 0.10, p = .10$, skewness $= 0.09$) subscales met the criteria for normality. For fathers, only the Permissiveness subscale ($D = 0.10, p = .11$, skewness $= 0.06$) met the criteria for normality. Because only 4 of the 20 scales appeared to be normally distributed, nonparametric tests were used to examine for similarities and differences in mothers' and fathers' reported family relations, parenting practices, and spousal interference behaviors.

Wilcoxon Signed-Rank Tests

The results of the Wilcoxon signed-rank tests are summarized in Table 10.3. For the three family relations scales, mothers and fathers both reported high levels of family cohesion, high levels of family expressiveness, and low levels

TABLE 10.3   Results of the Wilcoxon Signed-Rank Tests Between Mothers and Fathers on Selected Variables[a]

Variable	Possible Scores	Mother Median Score	Father Median Score	Z	p-Value
Family functioning					
Cohesion	1.0–4.0	3.8	3.6	−0.9	.371
Expressiveness	1.0–4.0	3.8	3.6	−1.9	.061
Disengagement	1.0–4.0	1.6	1.6	−0.4	.716
Parenting practices					
Monitoring	1.0–5.0	3.0	2.6	−3.1	.002
Limit Setting	1.0–5.0	4.0	3.0	−3.4	.001
Reinforcement	1.0–5.0	3.8	3.5	−2.9	.003
Permissiveness	1.0–5.0	2.8	2.8	−0.6	.539
Control	1.0–5.0	2.8	3.2	−0.6	.573
Discipline	1.0–5.0	2.0	2.3	−1.2	.230
Spousal interference	1.0–5.0	1.7	1.2	−2.3	.019

[a]Higher scores indicate higher family cohesion, higher family expressiveness, higher family disengagement, higher control, higher limit setting, higher reinforcement, higher monitoring, higher permissiveness, higher discipline, and higher spousal interference.

of family disengagement. Furthermore, mothers reported no significant difference in levels of family cohesion, family expressiveness, and family disengagement compared with fathers. In terms of parenting practices, both mothers and fathers reported similar moderate levels of control, permissiveness, and discipline. However, mothers reported significantly higher levels of limit setting, reinforcement, and monitoring of their children's dietary intake than did fathers. Spousal interference, assessed by a project-developed 6-item scale, revealed that although mothers and fathers reported low levels of spousal interference, mothers reported significantly higher levels of interference by the fathers than did fathers by mothers.

CONCLUSIONS

This study examined differences between mothers and fathers in terms of their perceptions of their family's functioning, their own parenting practices, and the extent to which they believed that their spouse engaged in interference behaviors. Similarities and differences were sought to help shed light on how to design more effective methods for engaging both parents in creating a healthy home environment.

Few differences were observed in the mothers' and fathers' perceptions of the family's functioning, suggesting that there may be few disagreements on how the family is doing (Ohannessian, Lerner, Lerner, & von Eye, 1995). In terms of parenting practices, higher levels of monitoring, limit setting, and reinforcement of children's diets were reported by the mothers than the fathers. This difference is important, given that results from a previous cross-sectional study conducted in San Diego suggested that Latina mothers who engaged in higher levels of monitoring had children who ate healthier diets (Arredondo et al., 2006). These findings may be explained by cultural influences on the differential involvement of Latina mothers in these activities compared to fathers (Hofferth, 2003). Gender role differences have been found to be greater among less- versus more-acculturated families (Hofferth, 2003), a population that is similar to those involved in *Entre Familia*.

No differences were observed in permissiveness, control, or discipline. Both mothers and fathers reported a moderate to high level of permissiveness, control, and discipline in their children's eating habits, important findings given the association of these variables with healthy and unhealthy eating habits among children (Ventura & Birch, 2008). For example, a modest number of studies have found an association between stricter parenting styles and children's health status. Using a nationally representative Australian sample, Wake and colleagues examined the association between children's body mass index (BMI) and mothers' and fathers' parenting styles (Wake, Nicholson, Hardy, & Smith, 2007). Adjusting for parental BMI status, their findings suggest an inverse association between paternal control and children's BMI (more father control associated with a lower BMI). Similarly, Lytle et al. (2003) found that the children of fathers who were less authoritative (setting appropriate limits while being supportive) ate more fruits and vegetables. Considering our findings on parenting practices, questions remain as to whether children are at lesser or greater health risk depending on the parenting practices of both parents. Finally, mothers, to a greater extent than fathers, reported that their spouses interfered with their efforts to promote healthy eating in the home. Spousal interference is a new concept that we developed given consistent evidence from our formative research that it is a significant barrier to family change. Overall, however, the frequency of interference was fairly low, suggesting that it may not be as prevalent as previously thought.

Limitations

Although the present study adds important new findings on how mothers and fathers are similar and different on dimensions associated with children's risk for obesity and cancer, certain limitations are recognized. The quantitative data are from a subsample of mothers and fathers involved in *Entre Familia*. Their data may not reflect the full sample and, as such, we must exercise caution in drawing conclusions from these findings. The study took place among Mexican American and Mexican immigrant families in well-established but geographically isolated border communities, just minutes away from a much larger Mexican community (Mexicali, Mexico). The results may not be generalized to other Latino subgroups and to individuals not living in rural border communities.

Implications

The *Entre Familia* study holds promise for identifying methods for promoting healthy eating using a whole-family approach. Future studies should consider evaluating the impact that mothers and fathers have on each other in relation to their children's diets and health practices. Little is known about the dynamic that occurs between mothers and fathers and how this influences their children's health practices. Community-based programs that aim to promote healthy eating should consider involving fathers. Fathers are likely to directly and indirectly influence their children's health practices through their wives' parenting practices. Few intervention studies have evaluated the impact that fathers have on their children's health practices and outcomes. Stein and colleagues suggest that involving fathers in health promotion efforts can lead to positive health behaviors among children, including a decrease in children's adiposity (2005). Future studies may want to consider whether parental influence varies depending on the child's age. Mothers and fathers may have different degrees of influence over their children at different ages and stage of development. Finally, future studies should explore the potential influencing role of older siblings within the family unit, and whether there are effects on the parenting styles of parents toward their younger children.

ACKNOWLEDGMENTS

This research was supported by a grant to Dr. Ayala from the American Cancer Society (RSGPB 113653). Additional support was provided to Drs. Ayala, Arredondo, and Elder from the Centers for Disease Control and Prevention (U48DP001917-01) and to Dr. Elder from UCSD's Moore's Cancer Center Disparities Program (P30 CA23100). The authors wish to thank the *promotoras*, who provided critical feedback in the development of the intervention, and the families for their participation in the study.

REFERENCES

American Cancer Society. (2009). *Diet and physical activity: What's the cancer connection?* Atlanta, GA: Author. Retrieved March 21, 2010, from http://www .cancer.org/docroot/PED/content/PED_3_1x_Link_Between_Lifestyle_and_ CancerMarch03.asp

Arredondo, E. M., Elder, J. P., Ayala, G. X., Campbell, N., Baquero, B., & Duerksen, S. (2006). Is parenting style related to children's healthy eating and physical activity in Latino families? *Health Education and Research, 21*(6), 862–871.

Ayala, G. X., Baquero, B., & Klinger, S. (2008). A systematic review of the relationship between acculturation and diet among Latinos in the United States: Implications for future research. *Journal of the American Dietetic Association, 108*(8), 1330–1344.

Ayala, G. X., Miller, D., King, D., Riddle, C., Zagami, E., & Willis, S. (2006). Asthma in middle schools: What students want in a program. *Journal of School Health, 76*, 208–214.

Blanck, H. M., Gillespie, C., Kimmons, J. E., Seymour, J. D., & Serdula, M. K. (2008). Trends in fruit and vegetable consumption among U. S. men and women, 1994–2005. *Preventing Chronic Disease, 5*(2), A35. Retrieved November 12, 2010, from http://www.cdc.gov/pcd/issues/2008/apr/07_0049.htm

Bloom, B. L.,& Naar, S. (2004). Self-report measures of family functioning: Extensions of a factorial analysis. *Family Process, 33*(2), 203–216.

Elder, J. P., Ayala, G. X., Parra-Medina, D., & Talavera, G. A. (2009). Health communication in the Latino community: Issues and approaches. *Annual Review of Public Health, 30*, 227–251.

Elder, J.P., Ayala, G. X., Slymen, D. J., Arredondo, E. M., & Campbell, N. R. (2009). Evaluating psychosocial and behavioral mechanisms of change in a tailored communication intervention. *Health Education and Behavior, 36*(2), 366–380.

Golan, M., & Crow, S. (2004). Targeting parents exclusively in the treatment of childhood obesity: Long-term results. *Obesity Research,12*(2), 357–361.

Haire-Joshu, D., Elliott, M. B., Caito, N. M., Hessler, K., Nanney, M. S., Hale, N., . . . Brownson, R. C. (2008). High 5 for Kids: The impact of a home visiting program on fruit and vegetable intake of parents and their preschool children. *Preventive Medicine, 47*(1), 77–82.

Hofferth, S. L. (2003). Race/ethnic differences in father involvement in two-parent families: Culture, context, or economy? *Journal of Family Issues, 24*(2), 185–216.

Hung, H. C., Joshipura, K. J., Jiang, R., Hu, F. B., Hunter, D., Smith-Warner, S. A., . . . Willett, W. C. (2004). Fruit and vegetable intake and risk of major chronic disease. *Journal of the National Cancer Institute, 96*(21), 1577–1584.

Kitzman-Ulrich, H., Wilson, D. K., St. George, S. M., Lawman, H., Segal, M., & Fairchild, A. (2010). The integration of a family systems approach for understanding youth obesity, physical activity, and dietary programs. *Clinical Child Family Psychology Review, 13*, 231–253.

Larios, S. E., Ayala, G. X., Arredondo, E. M., Baquero, B., & Elder, J. P. (2009). Development and validation of a scale to measure Latino parenting strategies related to children's obesigenic behaviors: The Parenting strategies for Eating and Activity Scale (PEAS). *Appetite, 52*(1), 166–172.

Lytle, L. A., Varnell, S., Murray, D., Story, M., Perry, C., Birnbaum, A. S., & Kubik, M. Y. (2003). Predicting adolescents' intake of fruits and vegetables. *Journal of Nutrition Education and Behavior, 35*, 170–178.

Miller, P. E., Lesko, S. M., Muscat, J. E., Lazarus, P. & Hartman, T. J. (2010). Dietary patterns and colorectal adenoma and cancer risk: A review of the epidemiological evidence. *Nutrition and Cancer, 62*(4), 413–424.

Moos, R., & Moos, B. (1994). *Family environment scale manual: Development, applications, research* (3rd Ed.). Palo Alto, CA: Consulting Psychologist Press.

Morgan, P. J., Lubans, D. R., Callister, R., Okely, A. D., Burrows, T. L., Fletcher, R., & Collins, C. E. (2010). The "Healthy Dads, Healthy Kids" randomized controlled trial: Efficacy of a healthy lifestyle program for overweight fathers and their children. *International Journal of Obesity, 35*, 436–447.

Ohannessian, C. M., Lerner, R. M., Lerner, J. V., & von Eye, A. (1995). Discrepancies in adolescents' and parents' perceptions of family functioning and adolescent emotional adjustment. *Journal of Early Adolescence, 15*, 490–516.

Pearson, N., Atkin, A.J., Biddle, S.J.H., & Gorely,R. (2010). A family-based intervention to increase fruit and vegetable consumption in adolescents: A pilot study. *Public Health Nutrition, 13*(6), 876–885.

Rodearmel, S. J., Wyatt, H. R., Barry, M. J., Dong, F., Pan, D., Israel, R. G., . . . Hill, J. O. (2006). A family-based approach to preventing excessive weight gain. *Obesity, 14*(8), 1392–1401.

Satia, J.A. (2010). Dietary acculturation and the nutrition transition: An overview. *Applied Physiology Nutrition and Metabolism, 35*(2), 219–223.

Satia-Abouta, J., Patterson, R. E., Neuhouser, M. L., & Elder, J. (2002). Dietary acculturation: Applications to nutrition research and dietetics. *Journal of the American Dietetic Association, 102*(8), 1105–1118.

Stein, R. I., Epstein, L. H., Raynor, H. A., Kilanowski, C. K., & Paluch, R. A. (2005). The influence of parenting change on pediatric weight control. *Obesity Research, 13*, 1749–1755.

U. S. Census Bureau. (2010). 2006–2008 American Community Survey 3-year estimates. Washington, DC: Author. Retrieved November 3, 2010, from http://factfinder.census.gov

Ventura, A. K., & Birch, L. L. (2008). Does parenting affect children's eating and weight status? *International Journal of Behavioral Nutrition and Physical Activity, 5*, 15.

Wake, M., Nicholson, J. M., Hardy, P., & Smith, K. (2007). Preschooler obesity and parenting styles of mothers and fathers: Australian National Population Study. *Pediatrics, 120*, 1520–1527.

11

Racial Disparities in Breast and Cervical Cancer: Can Legislative Action Work?

E. Kathleen Adams and Li-Nien Chien

Despite overall progress in the detection and early treatment of many cancers, disparities persist. While Black non-Hispanic women have a lower incidence of breast cancer across all ages than White non-Hispanics, their mortality rate from this cancer is higher than that for non-Hispanic Whites, and both their incidence and mortality rates for cervical cancer are higher than that experienced by non-Hispanic Whites (American Cancer Society, 2009). An important reason for disparities in mortality is that minority and other disadvantaged women are more likely to be diagnosed at advanced stages of disease, with those uninsured or Medicaid-insured consistently more likely to present with advanced stages of cancer (Chen, Schrag, Halpern, Stewart, & Ward, 2007; Elmore et al., 2005; Gwyn et al., 2004).

Breast cancer is the most common site of a new cancer among women and is second only to lung cancer in terms of deaths among women. Since many risk factors for breast cancer are not easily amenable to change, public policy has focused on early detection through screening and effective treatment of diagnosed cases (Pamuk, Makuc, Heck, Reuben, & Lochner, 1998). While studies point to continued underutilization of screening (Burns et al., 1996; Shavers & Brown, 2002; Smith-Bindman et al., 2006), the gap in mammography between non-Hispanic Blacks and Whites has narrowed, equal to about 2–3 percentage points in more recent years (Adams, Breen, & Joski, 2007; American Cancer Society, 2009). Yet, studies continue to indicate that non-Hispanic Black and Hispanic patients have an increased risk of advanced stages at diagnosis for breast and other cancers, even after controlling for insurance and other demographics (Halpern, Bian, Ward, Schrag, & Chen, 2007).

Cervical cancer is less prevalent and is preventable through early detection and treatment of precancerous conditions. With respect to invasive cervical cancer, the incidence and mortality has declined dramatically since the mid-1940s due to wide use of Papanicolaou (Pap) smear tests and detection/treatment of cervical intraepithelial neoplasia (CIN) (Casper & Clarke, 1998; Devesa et al., 1987; Schoell, Janicek, & Mirhashemi, 1999). Yet, lower income, less education, and lack of insurance (Akers, Newmann, & Smith, 2007; Bradley, Given, & Roberts, 2004) are all factors associated with higher incidence and mortality from cervical cancer, largely due to failure to detect the cancer at an early stage and the unavailability of treatment when detected (Breen, Wagener, Brown, Davis, & Ballard-Barbash, 2001; Harlan et al., 2005; Hewitt, Devesa, & Breen, 2004; Rodriguez, Ward, & Perez-Stable, 2005; Roetzheim et al., 1999; Sung, Alema-Mensah, & Blumenthal, 2002; Thorpe & Howard, 2003).

For the United States to reach the Healthy People 2020 (HP2020) goal of eliminating health disparities (U.S. Department of Health & Human Services, 2009) in breast cancer mortality and other diseases, we need more information regarding the types of interventions and/or policies that can be used to affect access to early detection and treatment for women with cancers, regardless of their racial/ethnic backgrounds.

BACKGROUND ON LEGISLATION

To help reduce disparities in breast and cervical cancer, the U.S. government began to invest in the National Breast and Cervical Cancer Early Detection Program (NBCCEDP) in 1991. Under the NBCCEDP, states received federal funding channeled through the Centers for Disease Control and Prevention (CDC) and had the option of providing supplemental funds to reach more women (Centers for Disease Control and Prevention Division of Cancer Prevention and Control, 2010). The NBCCEDP targeted racial/ethnic minorities, and during the 1991–1995 time period, the women tested were disproportionately non-Hispanic African American and Hispanic (Koh & Francis, 1990). National data have confirmed relatively greater increases in mammography use among non-Hispanic African Americans than among White women aged 40–64 in the early years of the program, from 1991 to 1994 (Makuc, Breen, & Freid, 1999). As the NBCCEDP matured, research indicated that the longevity of the program within a state was associated with significantly increased rates of both mammography and Pap tests for non-Hispanic Whites, but the data and analysis could not confirm this effect for Black, non-Hispanic women (Adams et al., 2007). However, public insurance was found to have an equal effect to that of private insurance in promoting increased testing for non-Hispanic Blacks and Hispanics, but not for White non-Hispanics, in this study. Hence, multiple public policies are likely needed to reduce disparities in screening.

Since the NBCCEDP did not cover all needed diagnostic services, nor any treatment costs, it inadvertently created a "treatment gap" for low-income and minority women (Lantz et al., 1999). Providers reported limiting the number of women screened because of the burden of finding treatment resources in this situation (Lantz et al., 2000). Such delays in treatment can be critical, as the literature suggests that initiation of treatment more than 90 days after an abnormal mammogram might be associated with decreased survival rates (Richards, Westcombe, Love, Littlejohns, & Ramirez, 1999). Subsequent legislation tried to address these concerns, and the outlook for early/appropriate treatment among poor (generally <250% Federal Poverty Level [FPL]) minority women diagnosed with breast and/or cervical cancer changed significantly on October 24, 2000 with the passage of the Breast and Cervical Cancer Prevention and Treatment Act (BCCPTA). The BCCPTA established a new Medicaid coverage option that permitted states to extend Medicaid to any uninsured woman under 65 diagnosed with breast or cervical cancer or pre-invasive cervical disease when screened through the NBCCEDP. States could also designate women as having been "screened under the Program" even if they were screened by other providers; 12 states adopted this option (Centers for Medicare & Medicaid Services, 2010). States also differed with respect to the recertification process used for BCCPTA women, provider payment rates, and delivery systems.

The BCCPTA legislation has the potential to reduce long-standing disparities across income groups and race. Even when policies reduce such gaps overall, however, disparities may continue if policies affect utilization of health care services differently across racial/ethnic groups (Koh & Francis, 1990). It is important, then, to gauge not only the overall effect of legislation such as BCCPTA but also its effects by race/ethnicity and, if possible, by geographic area. Due to its relative newness, there have been few national or state-specific studies. We discuss in this chapter the findings of available studies of BCCPTA and our earlier analysis of Georgia's BCCPTA program, called the Women's Health Medicaid Program (WHMP). We add a new analysis of the effects of BCCPTA by race in Georgia. We also discuss the general challenges that researchers face when designing and completing analysis of legislation, so as to inform policy makers in a timely manner.

ESTIMATED EFFECTS OF BCCPTA LEGISLATION

The only national study of the effects of BCCPTA used a pre–post analysis of time to definitive diagnosis and treatment over all women and by race/ethnicity (Lantz & Soliman, 2009). The results indicated both a positive effect—a decrease in time to definitive diagnosis for cervical cancer—and a negative effect—a delay in time to definitive diagnosis for breast cancer cases. Moreover, both the positive and negative effects of BCCPTA held only for White non-Hispanics. While White women were more likely to have a delay in the time to definitive breast cancer diagnosis, this delay was not sufficient in length to indicate that BCCPTA changed the proportion of women who initiated treatment within a 30- or 60-day time period after diagnosis. Another negative effect of BCCPTA—an increase in time to treatment initiation (7–15 days) for cervical cancer—found in this study, held only for non-Hispanic Blacks and Hispanics. This delay was sufficient in length for there to be a significant reduction in the probability of treatment initiation within 60 days of diagnosis. These types of delays reduce the ability of the system to achieve quality benchmarks for these racial/ethnic groups. The authors noted that these delays might be due to a lack of access to Medicaid-participating providers or, as noted in another study, delays in making and keeping appointments among disadvantaged and immigrant women (Ogilvie, Shaw, Lusk, Zazulak, & Kaczorowski, 2004). Lantz and Soliman (2009) also noted that women of color had longer mean times (days) to: (1) definitive diagnosis after an abnormal screening test, and (2) treatment initiation in both the pre- and post-BCCPTA periods, which is a cause for concern.

One of the few state-specific studies of BCCPTA used Massachusetts (MA) data to analyze two legislative policy changes. The first was the initiation of targeted funding for case managers through the NBCCEDP (Public Law 105–340) in 1998 and, subsequently, the implementation of BCCPTA in 2004 (it was delayed in MA). Their results indicated that low-income women (<250% FPL) in Massachusetts experienced a decrease in the probability of a delayed diagnosis (>60 days from an abnormal mammography to a diagnostic resolution) after the introduction of NBCCEDP case management, but that there was no additional improvement in this outcome from the implementation of BCCPTA (Lobb, Allen, Emmons, & Ayanian, 2010). Important to our focus on disparities, the reduction in the percentage of women with a delayed diagnosis, from 33% to 23% of those with an abnormal mammogram, did not differ by race or ethnicity. However, neither the case management nor BCCPTA policy implementation was associated with decreases in treatment delay (>90 days after abnormal mammogram) for any racial/ethnic group.

BCCPTA in Georgia

Given the latitude that states had to implement BCCPTA, as well as the wide variation observed in states' sociodemographics and Medicaid eligibility rules that affected women with these cancers prior to BCCPTA, it is likely that the impact of this legislation on the timing of women's enrollment, treatment, and patterns of treatment varied from state to state. To date, we know of no state-specific studies of BCCPTA other than the Massachusetts and earlier Georgia studies. The Georgia analysis used a quasi-experimental analytic design, with treatment and control groups, to better identify the effect of BCCPTA separate from other changes occurring over time that could affect access to cancer care for all low-income women. The specific statistical analysis used to examine outcomes of BCCPTA (time to enrollment, probability of enrollment while at an early stage, and disenrollment and treatment patterns) are described in later sections of this chapter, along with the results on each outcome.

The Georgia analysis was possible due to the creation of a unique database. Specifically, the Georgia Comprehensive Cancer Registry (GCCR) incident cases from January 1, 1999 through December 31, 2004 were linked to Medicaid enrollment files from January 1998 through December 2005. The GCCR has been a statewide, population-based cancer registry in Georgia since 1999. After linking with patients' encrypted social security numbers, female Medicaid enrollees diagnosed with breast, cervical, and one of five control cancers (bladder, colorectal, melanomas of the skin, non-Hodgkin lymphoma, and thyroid), and enrolled in Medicaid either prior to or after their cancer diagnosis, were identified using both the GCCR and diagnosis codes on claims. Women ever enrolled under the BCCPTA, were also identified using just enrollment data, since women with pre-invasive cervical disease or *in situ* stage cervical cancer were omitted from the GCCR and, yet, newly eligible for Medicaid under BCCPTA. Georgia's Medicaid program provided monthly enrollment records as well as all inpatient, outpatient, and drug claims detail through June 2006. Thus, we could observe treatments through June 2006 for incident cases enrolled by December 2005. Using this linked file, we were able to: (1) document the timing of both Medicaid enrollment and disenrollment in relation to a woman's cancer diagnosis; (2) identify the progression of the disease by the time of enrollment; and (3) examine the receipt of alternative treatments over the period of time she was enrolled in Medicaid.

Analysis of the effects of BCCPTA on enrollment indicated that out of 1,000 women diagnosed with breast or cervical cancer in Georgia from 1999 through 2004, the implementation of BCCPTA, or the WHMP in Georgia, led to an additional two or three more cases enrolling in Medicaid per month (Adams, Chien, Florence, & Raskind-Hood, 2009). It also resulted in these women getting enrolled in Medicaid more quickly; analysis indicated that the time between initial cancer diagnosis as reported in the GCCR and eventual Medicaid enrollment was shortened by between 7 and 8 months. Once enrolled, Georgia's BCCPTA recertification process was easier than for other Medicaid eligibility groups (e.g., self-report, no income verification) and, hence, created a situation in which coverage was more stable. Relative to women with one of the control cancers, the rates of disenrollment from Georgia Medicaid declined over 50% for women with either breast or cervical cancer from the pre- to the post-BCCPTA period (Chien & Adams, 2010).

In this chapter, we have extended the Georgia analysis by first examining whether the enrollment effects seen for the overall sample differed by race for either breast or cervical cancer cases and, in turn, whether there were differences in the rate at which Blacks versus Whites disenrolled from Medicaid. A key reason to enroll women more quickly was to allow them to start treatment while at an early stage of their cancer and, in turn, potentially reduce morbidity and mortality. An important outcome would be that women diagnosed at an early stage enrolled in Medicaid while still at an early stage of disease. We completed analysis of disease progression by time of enrollment for breast cancer cases using the stage at diagnosis as found in the GCCR data. We note that, throughout this analysis, we analyzed differences only between Blacks and Whites, and not between other races. To categorize women by race as completely as possible, we used our two sources of information, the GCCR and Medicaid enrollment files, with the registry being the "gold" standard. Both data sources contained a Hispanic category and where this was denoted, we identified these women and omitted them from the analysis. Hence, our groups are largely non-Hispanic Blacks and Whites; hereafter, we refer to them as Blacks and Whites.

BCCPTA by Race in Georgia

The sample for our analyses of the enrollment outcomes by race began with the 31,825 breast, cervical (local or later stage), and control cancer incident cases as found in the GCCR from 1999 through 2004. This population was predominately White at 74%, with 22% Black, and 4% of other racial/ethnic groups. After we excluded those aged under 19 at the time of diagnosis ($n = 44$), those who had enrolled after December 2005 ($n = 54$)—since only part of the sample could be followed after 2005—and those for whom this cancer was not their first ($n = 3,431$), the sample for the enrollment analysis by race was 28,296. Of these, a total of 3,404 enrolled in Georgia Medicaid in the month of, or sometime after, their diagnosis. Among these women, 49% were White and 46% were Black; the remaining 5% of other or unknown race/ethnicity were omitted from the analysis. The final sample sizes were 27,103 for analysis of enrollment rates and 3,227 for analysis of the duration between cancer diagnosis and Medicaid enrollment. We discuss later the samples used for analysis of stage at time of Medicaid disenrollment and treatment patterns for those with breast and cervical cancer and enrolled in Medicaid.

Enrollment in BCCPTA in Georgia by Race

To examine the effects of BCCPTA on enrollment among women with breast and cervical cancers in Georgia, we performed a time-to-event (here, enrollment) model. This model estimated the likelihood of the event at a given time for the woman who was not enrolled before her cancer diagnosis. The likelihood function of enrollment by time (*t*) is as follows:

$$h(t)_i = exp(\beta_0 + \beta_1 Cancer + \beta_2 BCCPTA + \beta_3 Cancer \\ \times BCCPTA + \gamma X_i + \delta T_t + \eta C_t + \varepsilon_i) \qquad (1)$$

where the hazard (*h*) is enrollment in Medicaid in month *t* after their cancer diagnosis; *Cancer* is a dummy variable denoting the primary cancer site; *BCCPTA* is a dummy indicating the pre-/post-policy implementation periods; *Cancer* $\times$ *BCCPTA* is a dummy variable denoting the interaction of the pre-/post-BCCPTA period with the primary cancer site; X_i is a vector of individual covariates; T_t is a year dummy; and C_t is a vector of county covariates that could affect the probability that a woman was uninsured. The effect of BCCPTA was derived by using difference-in-difference analysis. That is, we estimated the effect of BCCPTA by using our control cancers to "difference" out the effects of other factors that changed pre- and post-BCCPTA that could affect the probability that any woman with cancer, not just those affected by BCCPTA, enrolled in Medicaid. This was estimated using the interaction term in Equation 1.

While the widely used Cox proportional hazard rate model (nonparametric model) is more flexible for big datasets, our data failed to meet the assumption of proportional hazards for several subgroups. Hence, we tested and reported results of the parametric model with a Weibull distribution. The Weibull had the highest likelihood ratio across alternative functional forms and the results were robust across functions.

The data in Table 11.1 provided summary statistics on the estimated effects of BCCPTA on the numbers of women enrolling in Medicaid by race. This type of analysis was reported earlier, for our full sample (Adams et al., 2009). As these data showed, in the pre-BCCPTA period, Black women in Georgia with either breast or invasive cervical cancers were more likely to enroll in Medicaid than White women. For example, the rates of enrollment among Blacks were 5–8 per 1,000 person–months for breast and invasive cervical cancer cases, respectively, versus only 2–4 for White women with these

TABLE 11.1 Unadjusted and Adjusted Enrollment Rates (per 1,000 Person–Months) for Treatment (Breast and Cervical) and Control Cancers Pre– Versus Post-BCCPTA by Race

	Pre-BCCPTA				Post-BCCPTA				Percentage Change (Post − Pre)/Pre	
	Unadjusted		Adjusted[a]		Unadjusted		Adjusted[a]		Unadjusted	Adjusted[a]
	Mean	95% CI	Mean	95% CI	Mean	95% CI	Mean	95% CI	(%)	(%)
White										
Breast	1.20	1.09–1.33	2.04	1.94–2.13	2.77	2.57–2.99	3.37	3.22–3.53	129.95	65.66
Cervical	4.63	3.78–5.66	3.87	3.58–4.16	11.90	10.15–13.95	6.39	5.93–6.84	157.22	64.93
Control	1.24	1.07–1.45	—	—	1.65	1.43–1.89	—	—	32.65	
Black										
Breast	5.29	4.81–5.83	5.43	5.23–5.62	10.11	9.37–10.90	7.43	7.17–7.68	90.93	36.86
Cervical	10.28	8.03–13.15	8.36	7.79–8.94	23.07	19.07–27.91	12.06	11.26–12.85	124.53	44.18
Control	5.16	4.33–6.14			7.74	6.67–8.98			49.96	

BCCPTA indicates the Breast and Cervical Cancer Prevention and Treatment Act; CI = confidence interval.
Pre-BCCPTA, January 1999 through June 2001; post-BCCPTA, July 2001 through December 2004.
Sample size = 27,103.
[a]The adjusted enrollment rate is predicted from difference-in-difference estimation of the parametric hazard model with Weibull distribution. Covariates included age at diagnosis, marital status, cancer stage at diagnosis, urban/rural, resident county's health resources, and socioeconomic status in resident county (county has a teaching hospital, percentage of service employment, percentage of small-firm [<10 employees] employment, unemployment rate).

same cancers prior to BCCPTA. The effect of the implementation of BCCPTA, or Georgia's WHMP, was to increase the rate of enrollment for women with both cancers and for the racial groups within them. Although the rates per 1,000 person–months increased more (increases of 2–4 women per month) for Blacks than for Whites (increases of 1–2 women per month), the percentage increase was actually higher for Whites (almost 65%) than for Blacks (37% for breast, and 44% for cervical cancer cases) due to the relatively lower baseline rates of enrollment among Whites.

We also used the data to examine time to enrollment in Medicaid pre- and post-BCCPTA, as shown in Table 11.2. Since we had data on the actual date of diagnosis but we only had the month of enrollment, we assigned each date of diagnosis to the appropriate month and then counted the months from diagnosis to Medicaid entry or date of death. Women enrolled in the month of diagnosis were assigned a time of 0.5 months. To estimate our models on time to enrollment, we used ordinary least square (OLS) models with log transformation:

$$Log \text{ (Time to Enrollment}_i) = \alpha + \beta_1 Cancer + \beta_2 BCCPTA$$
$$+ \beta X_3 Cancer \times BCCPTA + \gamma X_i + \delta T_t + \eta C_t + \varepsilon_i \ldots \quad (2)$$

Again, the difference-in-differences was derived from the interaction term in the estimated equation.

The results in Table 11.2 were of special importance, as they indicated striking delays between the time of cancer diagnosis and eventual Medicaid enrollment prior to BCCPTA. Based on the descriptive (unadjusted) data in Table 11.2, women with breast cancer experienced delays in time to enrollment equal to 15 months for Blacks and up to 18 months for Whites during this period. While time to enrollment was shorter for women in both treatment and control groups after BCCPTA implementation, the delay *decreased* by 9, to almost 14, months for women with breast or cervical cancer (see unadjusted difference pre-BCCPTA vs. post-BCCPTA, in Table 11.2) versus a decline of only around 4 months for women with cancers in the control group.

After we controlled for other covariates that could affect the time to enrollment, the reduction in these delays was statistically significant, and greater for women in the treatment versus control group of cancers, indicating an "effect" of the BCCPTA. Moreover, the reduction in delays to enrollment was greater for Blacks with breast cancer (9 months) than for Whites (around 8 months), so that Blacks enrolled somewhat more quickly (around 4 months) than Whites (4.5 months) in the post-BCCPTA period. Patterns for women with cervical cancer (local or later stage) were different in that the reductions in time to enrollment were slightly greater for Whites (8.5 vs. 8 months for Blacks), so that White women enrolled within 3 months while Blacks took just a little over 3 months.

TABLE 11.2 Unadjusted and Adjusted Time (Months) From Initial Cancer Diagnosis to Eventual Medicaid Enrollment for Women With Treatment (Breast and Cervical) Versus Control Cancers Pre-BCCPTA Versus Post-BCCPTA, by Race

| | Pre-BCCPTA | | | | Post-BCCPTA | | | | Difference (Post − Pre) | |
| | Unadjusted | | Adjusted[a] | | Unadjusted | | Adjusted[a] | | Unadjusted | Adjusted[a] |
	Mean	95% CI	Mean	95% CI	Mean	95% CI	Mean	95% CI	Mean	Mean
White										
Breast	18.31	16.32–20.31	12.79	12.42–13.16	4.46	3.79–5.14	4.58	4.44–4.71	−13.85	−8.21
Cervical	14.46	11.27–17.66	11.02	10.65–11.40	2.82	1.86–3.78	2.56	2.48–2.65	−11.64	−8.46
Control	13.49	10.93–16.06	—		8.98	7.47–10.49	—		−4.51	
Black										
Breast	14.92	13.20–16.64	13.38	12.96–13.81	4.34	3.74–4.94	3.98	3.85–4.11	−10.58	−9.40
Cervical	11.56	7.27–15.85	10.89	10.51–11.27	2.54	1.46–3.63	3.03	2.92–3.14	−9.02	−7.97
Control	10.39	7.56–13.22	—		7.00	5.66–8.33	—		−3.39	

BCCPTA indicates the Breast and Cervical Cancer Prevention and Treatment Act; CI = confidence interval. Pre-BCCPTA, January 1999 through June 2001; post-BCCPTA, July 2001 through December 2004. Sample size = 3,227.

[a]The adjusted time from initial cancer diagnosis to eventual Medicaid enrollment is predicted from the difference-in-difference estimation of the regression model with log-linear distribution. Covariates included age at diagnosis, marital status, cancer stage at diagnosis, urban/rural, resident county's health resources, and socioeconomic status in resident county (county has a teaching hospital, percentage of service employment, percentage of small-firm [<10 employees] employment, unemployment rate).

Stage, Enrollment, and Treatment Patterns by Race

We next used the Georgia data to examine stage at time of enrollment, disenrollment of those women who had enrolled in Medicaid with treatment and control cancers, and treatment patterns for those enrolled within the BCCPTA eligibility category and whom we could observe for up to 2 years within the Medicaid claims. These are discussed, in turn, in the following sections.

Stage at Enrollment by Race

As noted, earlier enrollment could mean that women enter into Medicaid and, in turn, receive treatment while still at an early stage of disease. To derive our dependent variable, we first used stage as reported in the GCCR for women entering Medicaid within 6 months of their cancer diagnosis, regardless of what stage was reported. For those who enrolled in Medicaid more than 6 months after diagnosis, we also derived a measure of stage based on Medicaid claims. To do this, we applied the ICD-9-CM codes from the Disease Staging: Coded Criteria, v. 5.24 (The MEDSTAT Group, Inc., Ann Arbor, MI) and worked in conjunction with GCCR staff to match the staging from this Disease Staging algorithm into the scheme of *in situ*, local, regional, or distant, as reported in the GCCR (the full list of codes for breast and our control cancers are available upon request). For those diagnosed "early" in the GCCR and enrolled in Medicaid more than 6 months after their diagnosis, we indicated a change in their stage if, using the Disease Staging algorithm and claims data, there was an indication of disease progression to regional or distant.

We only completed the stage analysis for breast cancer cases, since the registry does not include early stage or pre-invasive cervical disease cases. The sample of women enrolled pre- and post-BCCPTA for whom we had both race and stage data was 2,668 (see Table 11.3). In multivariate analysis of the full sample (Chien, Adams, & Yang, in press) we found effects of BCCPTA on preventing disease progression by the time of Medicaid enrollment. However, that analysis was limited by the relatively small sample of cancers in our control group with stage data, and the sample was further limited when divided by race. Indeed, the small sample size precluded multivariate analysis within racial groups.

Due to the importance of this issue, however, we have presented descriptive data in Table 11.3 on the percentage of breast cancer cases for which there was evidence of "disease progression" between their time of diagnosis and Medicaid enrollment in the pre- versus post-BCCPTA period, by race. For both Blacks and Whites, there was some indication that BCCPTA improved prospects for treatment at early stage. Whereas 40% of Whites were diagnosed at an early stage of breast cancer in the pre-BCCPTA period, only

TABLE 11.3 Percentage of Early Stage[a] at Cancer Diagnosis and at Medicaid Enrollment for Women With Treatment (Breast) and Control Cancers Pre-BCCPTA Versus Post-BCCPTA, by Race

	Pre-BCCPTA			Post-BCCPTA			Difference (Post – Pre)	Difference-in-difference estimation
	Cancer diagnosis (%)	Medicaid enrollment (%)	Tumor progression[b] (%)	Cancer diagnosis (%)	Medicaid enrollment (%)	Tumor progression[b] (%)		
White								
Breast	40.07	36.03	–4.04	49.83	49.30	–0.53	3.51	
Control	25.00	22.32	–2.68	28.36	26.87	–1.49	1.19	2.32
Black								
Breast	36.22	32.20	–4.02	44.46	43.61	–0.85	3.17	
Control	19.59	18.56	–1.03	19.40	19.40	0.00	1.03	2.14

BCCPTA indicates the Breast and Cervical Cancer Prevention and Treatment Act.
Pre-BCCPTA, January 1999 through June 2001; post-BCCPTA, July 2001 through December 2004.
Sample size = 2,668.
[a]Early stage included *in situ* and local using SEER summary-stage methodology.
[b]Tumor progression denoted evidence of a change from early-stage cancer diagnosis in registry to stage as measured after 6 months of Medicaid enrollment.

36% enrolled in Medicaid without disease progression. After BCCPTA, 50% were both diagnosed and enrolled while at an early stage. Hence, there was about a 3.5 percentage point increase in the percentage of White women with breast cancer whose tumor did *not* progress by the time of Medicaid enrollment. For Blacks, the percentage diagnosed at an early stage pre-BCCPTA was lower than for Whites, at 36%, and only 32% enrolled without evidence of "disease progression" in this pre-BCCPTA period. In the post-BCCPTA period, the percentage of Blacks diagnosed and enrolled at an early stage was equal, almost 44%—indicating progress, but still lower than the 50% observed for Whites in the post-BCCPTA period.

Disenrollment Patterns by Race

We completed multivariate analysis of those enrolled in Medicaid using the same statistical methods as described above for the probability of enrollment. We noted that once women were enrolled with breast or cervical cancers in Georgia's WHMP, they were more likely to stay enrolled post-BCCPTA (see Table 11.4). In the overall sample, we found that relative to women with one of the control cancers, women with breast or cervical cancer were 50% less likely to disenroll post- versus pre-BCCPTA (Chien & Adams, 2010). When this analysis was repeated by race (see Table 11.4), there was a comparable gain for both Blacks and Whites with breast cancer; the rate of disenrollment declined due to the BCCPTA by 55–56% for both races. There was, however, an important differential seen for Blacks with cervical cancer; the BCCPTA was associated with a reduced disenrollment rate of 48% for Whites but a 65% reduction for Blacks with this cancer. For both races with these cancers, these changes translated into almost six more months of enrollment—although, as noted, there was a slightly greater increase for Blacks versus Whites with cervical cancer. This longer enrollment period should increase the probability that women have continuity of care and complete their cancer treatment regimen while under Medicaid coverage.

Treatment Patterns by Race

In Table 11.5, we have presented data on the patterns of cancer treatment that women received once they were enrolled in Medicaid under Georgia's WHMP. In this analysis, we limited our sample to those who enrolled in Medicaid under the BCCPTA eligibility category. In this analysis, we additionally included those who were diagnosed with pre-invasive cervical disease through Medicaid enrollment files and tested for differences by race in the receipt of treatments appropriate to this disease. We estimated logistic regression models on the odds of receipt of specific forms of cancer treatment and used White patients as the reference group. We have

TABLE 11.4 The Unadjusted and Adjusted Disenrollment Rates (per 100 Person–Months) of Treatment (Breast and Cervical) Pre- Versus Post-BCCPTA by Race

| | Pre-BCCPTA | | | | Post-BCCPTA | | | | Percent change (Post – Pre)/pre | |
| | Unadjusted | | Adjusted[a] | | Unadjusted | | Adjusted[a] | | Unadjusted | Adjusted[a] |
	Mean	95% CI	Mean	95% CI	Mean	95% CI	Mean	95% CI	(%)	(%)
White										
Breast	2.72	2.38–3.10	3.61	3.50–3.72	1.25	1.09–1.44	1.61	1.56–1.66	−53.94	−55.46
Cervical	5.22	4.19–6.50	6.47	6.24–6.69	2.35	1.87–2.96	3.30	3.19–3.42	−55.00	−48.94
Control	5.81	4.89–6.90	—		6.49	5.43–7.76	—		11.76	
Black										
Breast	2.91	2.59–3.28	3.73	3.64–3.82	1.52	1.33–1.74	1.64	1.60–1.68	−47.71	−56.03
Cervical	5.05	3.85–6.63	6.12	5.92–6.32	2.49	1.89–3.28	2.13	2.06–2.20	−50.63	−65.22
Control	4.17	3.41–5.09	—		6.82	5.65–8.22	—		63.50	

BCCPTA indicates the Breast and Cervical Cancer Prevention and Treatment Act; CI = confidence interval.
Pre-BCCPTA, January 1999 through June 2001; post-BCCPTA, July 2001 through December 2004.
Sample size = 3,227.
[a]The adjusted disenrollment rate is predicted from the difference-in-difference of the parametric hazard model with Weibull distribution. Covariates included age at diagnosis, marital status, cancer stage at diagnosis, urban/rural, resident county's resident county's health resources, and socioeconomic status (county has a teaching hospital, percentage of service employment in county, percentage of county employment in small firms [<10 employees], percentage Medicaid recipients in county).

TABLE 11.5   Multiple Regression Analysis of the Receipt of Treatment Among (Breast and Cervical) Cancer Cases, Odds Ratios for Blacks Versus Whites by Type or Treatment

	Adjusted[a]		
	OR	95% CI	p-Value
Breast Cancer Cases			
Any treatment	0.718	0.296–1.741	0.463
Any drug regimen	1.035	0.662–1.617	0.880
Any radiation	1.179	0.879–1.581	0.272
Any surgery	0.942	0.655–1.356	0.749
Last/definitive surgery (either lumpectomy or mastectomy)	0.928	0.650–1.326	0.683
Lumpectomy vs. mastectomy	0.991	0.711–1.382	0.957
Lumpectomy with vs. without radiation	1.091	0.621–1.919	0.762
Mastectomy and follow-up One vs. none	**2.681**	**1.220–5.894**	**0.014**
Two and more vs. none	1.726	0.807–3.692	0.160
Cervical cancer cases			
Pre-invasive			
Cancer work-up	0.832	0.624–1.110	0.211
Pre-invasive treatment	**1.885**	**1.259–2.822**	**0.002**
Simple hysterectomy	**0.494**	**0.311–0.783**	**0.003**
Invasive			
Cancer work-up	0.700	0.231–2.118	0.528
Invasive surgical treatment	**0.417**	**0.203–0.857**	**0.017**
Radiation	2.145	0.941–4.893	0.070
Chemotherapy	1.035	0.530–2.022	0.919

Sample sizes: N = 979 for breast cancer cases; N = 1,580 for cervical cancer cases.
Time period of study: July 2001 through July 2006.
[a]White is reference group, covariates included age at Medicaid enrollment, cancer stage at diagnosis, Charlson comorbidity index, enrolled in Medicaid prior to month of diagnosis, continuous enrollment of over 24 months, urban/rural percentage of resident county population with income less than $15,000, resident county's health resources (county has hospital with oncology services, has at least one Commission on Cancer approved hospital, number of obstetricians/gynecologists per 1,000 women)
Bold data denote that the outcomes were significantly different between blacks and whites at p value <= .05.

presented the relative odds of Black patients receiving cancer treatment as identified from Medicaid claims (the treatment codes are available upon request from the authors).

We noted that BCCPTA women differed from other Medicaid enrollees in that they were of relatively higher income and were linked more closely to their providers due to the structure of the WHMP and its recertification process. In this analysis, then, we examined differences in treatment patterns for Black versus White women all of whom were enrolled in BCCPTA. Their BCCPTA eligibility category denoted that, while of different racial backgrounds, they were: (1) similar in terms of socioeconomic status; and (2) were being treated largely within the same health care delivery system.

In the analysis presented in Table 11.5, we looked for significant differences by race after controlling for following variables: age at Medicaid enrollment; cancer stage at diagnosis; the Charlson comorbidity index; whether enrolled in Medicaid prior to cancer diagnosis; whether enrolled over 24 months; county of residence (urban/rural); percentage of resident county population with income less than $15,000; resident county's health resources (the county has at least one hospital with oncology services and at least one Commission on Cancer approved hospital, and the number of obstetricians/gynecologists per 1,000 women). We tested for a wide array of treatments over the 24 months after enrollment, including any drug, radiation, or surgical treatment. For breast cancer, we also tested for the probability of lumpectomy versus mastectomy as the "definitive" surgery among those with any surgery. If multiple surgeries were found in the claims data, the "definitive" surgery was assigned as the last one observed. As these analyses showed, there were no significant differences for Blacks versus Whites, with one exception. Black women receiving a mastectomy were more likely to receive at least one follow-up (chemotherapy, hormonal, or other drug regimen) than their White counterparts within the Medicaid WHMP.

In Table 11.5, we also showed the patterns of treatment in WHMP for pre-invasive cervical disease or invasive cervical cancer. Here, there were differences by race. Blacks were almost twice as likely as Whites within the WHMP to receive some treatment for pre-invasive (CIN II or CIN III) cervical disease. There was also a stark difference in the rate of hysterectomy among the races. Black women were less than half as likely to have a simple hysterectomy if their disease was pre-invasive, and to have any invasive surgery (simple or radical hysterectomy, pelvic lymph node dissection, paraaortic lymph node sampling, radical trachelectomy, removal of cervical stump, and pelvic exenteration [or] pelvic evisceration) if their cervical cancer was invasive. These differences were significant even after controlling for the covariates as noted earlier.

DISCUSSION

The strength of legislative action is that it can compel entities such as states, employers, or other geopolitical jurisdictions to provide or enhance programs that are available to all those identified as eligible within the legislative language. While the BCCPTA language left it up to state option to provide the new program, a majority of states had adopted the BCCPTA and Georgia was among the first to do so, increasing its Medicaid cancer caseload by almost one third in 2003 alone (Adams et al., 2007). Although one of the mandates under the BCCPTA was that women were eligible if they were screened for breast or cervical cancer by another legislated program, the NBCCEDP, states also had "Screening Options" to designate women as having been "screened under the Program" even if their screening provider was not funded through the NBCCEDP (Centers for Medicare & Medicaid Services, 2010). This flexibility essentially allowed states to determine availability/accessibility to the new eligibility category. States that selected only to include NBCCEDP-funded providers may have inadvertently limited women's access to the BCCPTA (Carreyrou, 2007). However, Georgia was one of 12 states that expanded its provider network beyond the NBCCEDP to any provider in the state, thereby providing greater potential access. The data indicated that in 2003, nearly 75% of the women in Georgia coming into the BCCPTA entered through non-NBCCEDP-funded providers (Adams et al., 2007).

Although the BCCPTA legislation should have had a strong effect across all states, the one national study of the BCCPTA presented troubling results in the form of increased time to treatment initiation (7–15 days) for Blacks and Hispanics with cervical cancer. This effect resulted in a significant reduction in the probability of treatment initiation within 60 days of treatment. If such effects held in other evaluations of BCCPTA nationally and within each state, this would indicate that the potential of this legislation to improve the system's ability to achieve quality benchmarks for all racial/ethnic groups was less than optimal. State-specific studies can shed insight on the particular effects of BCCPTA as it was implemented and managed within each state's provider and public health systems.

The findings presented here for the state of Georgia largely showed an improvement in access to Medicaid and its providers for both Blacks and Whites. While differences were somewhat nuanced, the Georgia BCCPTA, WHMP, was associated with effects that may address long-standing disparities in breast and cervical cancer across the races. For example, the number of Black women with breast or cervical cancer enrolling in Medicaid was greater in both the pre- and post-BCCPTA periods, and the increases associated with BCCPTA meant that even more Black women enrolled per 1,000 person–months observed in the post-BCCPTA period. Given the lower incidence of breast cancer among Black women, the higher enrollment rates for Blacks might just reflect a higher likelihood that they were otherwise uninsured or that they fell under the NBCCEDP income eligibility criteria. In Georgia, it appears that the WHMP helped Black women experience a 1-month gain in time to enrollment relative to Whites and, in turn, an increase in the percentage entering Medicaid while still at an early stage of disease. Once in treatment for breast cancer, the data indicated that Blacks received similar treatment—and if there were any differences, it was more follow-up for Black women who received mastectomies.

With respect to cervical cancer cases, the effects of BCCPTA in Georgia also appeared positive. There was again an increase in enrollment, with the number of Black incident cases enrolling in the post-BCCPTA period being twice that for Whites. While the drop in time to enrollment with WHMP was not as large for Blacks as for Whites, there was a greater reduction in the rate at which Blacks subsequently disenrolled from Medicaid. This might be associated with the significantly higher probability of treatment for Blacks versus White with pre-invasive cervical cancer in the WHMP. The only remaining significant difference in treatment patterns seen for Blacks versus Whites with cervical cancer was the markedly lower probability of surgical treatment. This difference held for both pre-invasive and invasive cervical cases and was consistent with the small literature on disparities in cervical cancer treatment. One study indicated that African Americans above age 35 were less likely to receive a hysterectomy (del Carmen et al., 1999) and another indicated that among women with stage IB cervical cancer, Black women were less likely than White women to be treated with surgery or combined therapy (Thoms et al., 1998). Both of these differentials could be related to the higher mortality rates observed for Black women with cervical cancer, and could diminish the ability of the WHMP or other insurance programs to lower the mortality rate of Blacks with this cancer.

CHALLENGES AND LIMITATIONS

Analysis of the effects of legislation poses challenges with respect to the study design and data needs as well as administrative, and even political, issues. When legislation is passed, it is of great importance for both the political leaders and the parties affected by the legislation to discern whether it has its intended effects. Yet, researchers cannot rely on randomization of persons into groups affected and not affected by the legislation in order to detect true "effects." The second-best solution is to use a quasi-experimental design, or one in which the researcher identifies the "targeted" group—those affected by the change inherent in the legislation—and a "control" group—similar to the targeted group, but not affected by the legislative change in policy. Once this is done, the researcher then needs data on outcomes and confounding factors for both of these groups and for periods before and after the change in policy.

Such a design creates extensive data needs, especially in the area of cancer control, where stage of cancer is a critical variable for analysis, and registry data is the "gold standard" for this measure. Since registry data provide only a part of the picture, many have stressed the importance of linking cancer registry data with other data, such as Medicaid and Medicare claims. These data are seen as providing valuable enhancements in terms of insurance coverage, treatment (e.g., chemotherapy), and outcomes over longer periods of time after a cancer diagnosis. To analyze the effects of legislative policy such as the BCCPTA, for example, we needed to know the timing of enrollment, details of the disease at that time, and other confounders or outcomes (comorbidity, length of time to treatment, disenrollment, etc.), which required data observed over a longer follow-up period than that covered by the cancer registry.

Obtaining permission to use data such as Medicaid claims requires a state-by-state effort and is really only the first step in the process. Linkage of registry and administrative data for research purposes also requires knowledge of the Medicaid program itself, the strengths and weaknesses of these data, and significant programming expertise and funding. A recent paper on the issues entailed in such efforts (Bradley, Penberthy, Devers, & Holden, 2010) noted that this type of linkage poses the following challenges: (1) understanding who "owns" the data and what this means in terms of access to it; (2) developing collaborations with these and possibly, other organizations; (3) establishing a strong case for the value of linking the data; (4) addressing the mechanics of the linkage itself; (5) assessing alternative methods of linking and finally; (6) evaluating the quality of the linkage. Our effort in Georgia entailed all of these challenges, and working out the details across multiple agencies led to significant delays in obtaining the data for analysis and, in turn, its completion.

Due to these challenges and the subsequent demands on time and resources, linkages to Medicaid data are more likely to be state-specific than national—like the linkage of Medicare and Surveillance, Epidemiology, and End Results (SEER) data. This is appropriate since Medicaid is not a uniform, national program as is Medicare and, indeed, exhibits significant variation across states. However, such studies based on linked state data will likely be limited in number and the research, as shown here, will be limited to state-specific results. This is a key limitation of our analysis. Use of only the Georgia data means that we could not generalize the results; nor could we make comparisons with the effects of BCCPTA in states with more restrictive policies. For example, we were not able to evaluate the effects of different levels of state implementation of the NBCCEDP legislation, to determine the extent to which this led to reductions in disparities in other states. If the data were linked over a longer period, we could have tested for effects of Georgia's change in its recertification process—but this remains another limitation at the present time.

Other limitations of our analysis might include the choice of control cancers. We began with women with colorectal cancer as our control group and found that not only was the group of women entering Medicaid with this cancer relatively small in number but, due in part to the structure of Medicaid eligibility, they were far more likely to be at a regional or distant stage than those with breast cancer. Early on in our analysis, then, we expanded to include other cancers in our control group. We worked closely with physicians and registry staff in choosing these cancers, with one criterion being that screening and early detection could possibly lead to more treatment options and/or better outcomes for the cancer. Such choices may be questioned by other researchers or clinicians and this, as well as the imprecision of measuring stage for women entering Medicaid more than 6 months after their diagnosis, can be seen as additional limitations of our effort.

Despite such limitations, more power would come from having ongoing linkages that allow researchers to measure effects of BCCPTA state by state and over longer periods. Linked data would also allow for analysis of other policy changes, adherence to guidelines or other quality metrics and, if linked to private claims data, comparison across payers. Such analyses must be left to future research efforts.

CONCLUSION

The quasi-experiment created by the BCCPTA legislation and its implementation showed the potential of our nation to expand access to insurance and treatment, in a very timely fashion, to low-income persons with clear medical needs. This legislation was implemented as the WHMP in Georgia and in such a way that women got into the program more quickly, received appropriate and perhaps more complete treatment. Further, in the case of cervical cancer, treatment was extended to those with pre-invasive disease in a timely manner. The latter is a highly cost-effective use of public funds, since it can prevent this disease from becoming invasive. Most important, the positive effects of BCCPTA in Georgia were shared by both Blacks and Whites, and where differences emerged, they reflected somewhat quicker enrollment, a longer time on Medicaid, and more treatment for Blacks—as seen in the case of pre-invasive cervical disease and follow-up after mammography. Another key difference seen in our data, lower hysterectomies among Blacks with cervical cancer, perhaps reflects a choice made to retain reproductive capacity. It is important, however, to assess whether these are fully informed choices and, in turn, if they are related to higher rates of mortality among Black women with this cancer. Finally, the linkage of registry and Medicaid claims data clearly enhanced our ability to look at BCCPTA, and such linkages would allow for analysis of future legislation and, indeed, measuring access for women with breast, cervical, and other cancers in the periods leading up to and following the implementation of the Patient Protection and Affordable Care Act (PPACA) in 2014.

REFERENCES

Adams, E. K., Breen, N., & Joski, P. J. (2007). Impact of the National Breast and Cervical Cancer Early Detection Program on mammography and Pap test utilization among White, Hispanic, and African American women: 1996–2000. *Cancer Supplement, 109*(2), 348–358.

Adams, E. K., Chien, L.-N., Florence, C. S., & Raskind-Hood, C. (2009). The Breast and Cervical Cancer Prevention and Treatment Act in Georgia effects on time to Medicaid enrollment. *Cancer, 115*(6), 1300–1309.

Akers, A. Y., Newmann, S. J., & Smith, J. S. (2007). Factors underlying disparities in cervical cancer incidence, screening, and treatment in the United States. *Current Problems in Cancer, 31*(3), 157–181.

American Cancer Society. (2009). *Cancer facts & figures for African Americans 2009–2010.* Atlanta, GA: Author.

Bradley, C. J., Given, C. W., & Roberts, C. R. (2004). Health care disparities and cervical cancer. *American Journal of Public Health, 94*(12), 2098–2103.

Bradley, C. J., Penberthy, L., Devers, K. J., & Holden, D. J. (2010). Health services research and data linkages: Issues, methods and directions for the future. *Health Services Research, 45*(5), 1468–1488.

Breen, N., Wagener, D. K., Brown, M. L., Davis, W. W., & Ballard-Barbash, R. (2001). Progress in cancer screening over a decade: Results of cancer screening from the 1987, 1992, and 1998 National Health Interview Surveys. *Journal of the National Cancer Institute, 93*(22), 1704–1713.

Burns, R. B., McCarthy, E. P., Freund, K. M., Marwill, S. L., Schwartz, M., Ash, A., Moskowitz, M. (1996). Black women receive less mammography even with similar use of primary care. *Annals of Internal Medicine, 125*(3), 173–182.

Carreyrou, J. (2007, September 13). Legal loophole ensnares breast-cancer patients. *Wall Street Journal*, pp. A1, A13.

Casper, M. J., & Clarke, A. E. (1998). Making the Pap smear into the "right tool" for the job: Cervical cancer screening in the USA, circa 1940–95. *Social Studies of Science, 28*(2), 255–290.

Centers for Disease Control and Prevention Division of Cancer Prevention and Control. (2010). National Breast and Cervical Cancer Early Detection Program (NBCCEDP). Retrieved September 27, 2010, from http://www.cdc.gov/cancer/nbccedp/about.htm

Centers for Medicare & Medicaid Services. (2010). Breast and cervical cancer prevention and treatment activity map. Retrieved June 29, 2011, from http://www.cms.hhs.gov/MedicaidSpecialCovCond/Downloads/BREASTand CERVICALCANCERPREVENTIONandTREATMENTACTIVITYMAP.pdf

Chen, A. Y., Schrag, N. M., Halpern, M., Stewart, A., & Ward, E. M. (2007). Health insurance and stage at diagnosis of laryngeal cancer. Does insurance type predict stage at diagnosis? *Archives of Otolaryngology—Head and Neck Surgery, 133*(8), 784–790.

Chien, L.-N., & Adams, E. K. (2010). The effect of the Breast and Cervical Cancer Prevention and Treatment Act on Medicaid disenrollment. *Women's Health Issues, 20*(4), 266–271.

Chien, L.-N., Adams, E. K., & Yang, Z. (in press). Medicaid enrollment at early stage of disease: The effects of the Breast and Cervical Prevention and Treatment Act in Georgia. *Inquiry* 48(3).

del Carmen, M. G., Montz, F. J., Bristow, R. E., Bovicelli, A., Cornelison, T., & Trimble, E. (1999). Ethnic differences in patterns of care of stage 1A1 and stage 1A2 cervical cancer: A SEER database study. *Gynecologic Oncology, 75*(1), 113–117.

Devesa, S. S., Silverman, D. T., Young, J. L., Jr., Pollack, E. S., Brown, C. C., Horm, J. W., . . . Fraumeni, J. F., Jr. (1987). Cancer incidence and mortality trends among whites in the United States, 1947–84. *Journal of the National Cancer Institute, 79*(4), 701–770.

Elmore, J. G., Nakano, C. Y., Linden, H. M., Reisch, L. M., Ayanian, J. Z., & Larson, E. B. (2005). Racial inequities in the timing of breast cancer detection, diagnosis, and initiation of treatment. *Medical Care, 43*(2), 141–148.

Gwyn, K., Bondy, M. L., Cohen, D. S., Lund, M. J., Liff, J. M., Flagg, E. W., . . . Coates, R. J. (2004). Racial differences in diagnosis, treatment, and clinical delays in a population-based study of patients with newly diagnosed breast carcinoma. *Cancer, 100*(8), 1595–1604.

Halpern, M. T., Bian, J., Ward, E. M., Schrag, N. M., & Chen, A. Y. (2007). Insurance status and stage of cancer at diagnosis among women with breast cancer. *Cancer, 110*(2), 403–411.

Harlan, L. C., Greene, A. L., Clegg, L. X., Mooney, M., Stevens, J. L., & Brown, M. L. (2005). Insurance status and the use of guideline therapy in the treatment of selected cancers. *Journal of Clinical Oncology, 23*(36), 9079–9088.

Hewitt, M., Devesa, S. S., & Breen, N. (2004). Cervical cancer screening among U.S. women: Analyses of the 2000 National Health Interview Survey. *Preventive Medicine, 39*(2), 270–278.

Koh, S. C., & Francis, B. (1990). Differences in birth outcomes between Whites and non-Whites, a switching regression model. *Journal of Economics, XVI,* 7–17.

Lantz, P. M., Richardson, L. C., Macklem, D. J., Shugarman, L. R., Knutson, D. B., & Sever, L. E. (1999). Strategies for follow-up and treatment services in state breast and cervical cancer screening programs. *Women's Health Issues, 9*(1), 42–49.

Lantz, P. M., Richardson, L. C., Sever, L. E., Macklem, D. J., Hare, M. L., Orians, C. E., & Henson, R. (2000). Mass screening in low-income populations: The challenges of securing diagnostic and treatment services in a national cancer screening program. *Journal of Health Politics, Policy and Law, 25*(3), 451–471.

Lantz, P. M., & Soliman, S. (2009). An evaluation of a Medicaid expansion for cancer care: The Breast and Cervical Cancer Prevention and Treatment Act of 2000. *Women's Health Issues, 19,* 221–231.

Lobb, R., Allen, J. D., Emmons, K. M., & Ayanian, J. Z. (2010). Timely care after an abnormal mammogram among low-income women in a public breast cancer screening program. *Archives of Internal Medicine, 170*(6), E1–E8.

Makuc, D. M., Breen, N., & Freid, V. (1999). Low income, race, and the use of mammography. *Health Services Research, 34*(1), 229–239.

Ogilvie, G. S., Shaw, E. A., Lusk, S. P., Zazulak, J., & Kaczorowski, J. A. (2004). Access to colposcopy services for high-risk Canadian women: Can we do better? *Canadian Journal of Public Health, 95*(5), 346–351.

Pamuk, E., Makuc, D., Heck, K., Reuben, C., & Lochner, K. (1998). *Socioeconomic status and health chartbook: Health, United States, 1998.* Hyattsville, MD: National Center for Health Statistics.

Richards, M. A., Westcombe, A. M., Love, S. B., Littlejohns, P., & Ramirez, A. J. (1999). Influence of delay on survival in patients with breast cancer: A systematic review. *The Lancet, 353,* 1119–1126.

Rodriguez, M. A., Ward, L. M., & Perez-Stable, E. J. (2005). Breast and cervical cancer screening: Impact of health insurace status, ethnicity, and nativity of Latinas. *Annals of Family Medicine, 3*(3), 235–241.

Roetzheim, R. G., Pal, N., Tennant, C., Voti, L., Ayanian, J. Z., Schwabe, A., & Krischer, J. P. (1999). Effects of health insurance and race on early detection of cancer. *Journal of the National Cancer Institute, 19*(16), 1409–1415.

Schoell, W. M. J., Janicek, M. F., & Mirhashemi, R. (1999). Epidemiology and biology of cervical cancer. *Seminars in Surgical Oncology, 16*(3), 203–211.

Shavers, V. L., & Brown, M. L. (2002). Racial and ethnic disparities in the receipt of cancer treatment. *Journal of the National Cancer Institute, 94*(5), 334–357.

Smith-Bindman, R., Miglioretti, D. L., Lurie, N., Abraham, L., Ballard-Barbash, R., Strzelczyk, J., . . ., Kerlikowske, K. (2006). Does utilization of screening mammography explain racial and ethnic differences in breast cancer? *Annals of Internal Medicine, 144*(8), 541–553.

Sung, J. F. C., Alema-Mensah, E., & Blumenthal, D. S. (2002). Inner-city African American women who failed to receive cancer screening following a culturally-appropriate intervention: the role of health insurance. *Cancer Detection and Prevention, 26*(1), 28–32.

Thoms, W. W., Unger, E. R., Carisio, R., Nisenbaum, R., Spann, C. O., Horowitz, I. R., & Reeves, W. C. (1998). Clinical determinants of survival from stage Ib cervical cancer in an inner-city hospital. *Journal of the National Medical Association, 90*(5), 303–308.

Thorpe, K. E., & Howard, D. (2003). Health insurance and spending among cancer patients. *Health Affairs,* hlthaff.w3.189.

U.S. Department of Health & Human Services. (2009). *Healthy people 2020 public meetings 2009 draft objectives.* Retrieved June 29, 2011, from http://pdpciowa.org/Meetings/Appendices/JanuaryMaterials2010/Appendix7_CombinedPDFHP2020Objectives.pdf

12

Messengers for Health: Apsáalooke Women Capture the Vision of Wellness

Vanessa Watts Simonds, Suzanne Christopher,
Beldine Crooked Arm Pease, Lois Jefferson, Carol Howe,
Deb LaVeaux, Myra Lefthand, Rochelle Lodgepole,
Alma McCormick, Larna Old Elk, Eleanor Pretty On Top,
Colleen Simpson, Maudine Stewart,
and Chaplain Carol Whiteman[1]

On the Crow reservation, as they have for generations, groups of women sit together and joke and chat. But it is in these woman-to-woman conversations that there is a significant change. Words once considered taboo in the tribe—"Pap," "cervical cancer," and "breast"—now are common in the mix of Crow and English discussion. This change has occurred due to the efforts of those working with the Messengers for Health program (hereafter called Messengers), a community-based program that aims to change health disparities regarding low rates of cancer screening among Apsáalooke (Crow Indian) women.

This chapter presents the development and implementation of the Messengers for Health (MFH) program. This project is a community-based participatory research (CBPR) project, in which community members and university staff and students are involved in all phases of the research process. Thus, the approach to the writing of this chapter is somewhat unique compared to usual academic writing and it is presented in a more traditional storytelling fashion. The content of this chapter came from several discussion sessions where people involved in the project shared stories about the impact of, and lessons learned from, our program. Discussions took place among lay health advisors (LHAs) of the program, board members, project staff, and past and current student staff members. Notes were taken at these meetings and everyone was invited to write anything they felt was important and send it to the first author. Board members and staff

---

[1]This chapter is dedicated in memorial to Carol Whiteman for her inspiration and passion.

met and decided on the most important sections to include in the chapter. The first author compiled and organized the quotes and stories into a rough draft. This draft was presented to board members and project staff who, in a series of meetings, went through the text line by line, editing for clarity, making sure that the chapter accurately reflected the program, and ultimately agreeing on all content. Board members wanted to make sure that the language was simple and free of jargon. The result is this chapter, in which we present our project.

THE STRENGTHS OF THE APSÁALOOKE (CROW INDIAN) PEOPLE

The Crow Tribe has approximately 11,000 members, of whom 8,000 reside on the reservation. Many tribal members speak Crow as their first language, which reveals the strength and maintenance of the culture. They are originally called "Apsáalooke," or "children of the large-beaked bird." Apsáalooke people are known for the strength of their clan system and their strong family ties. The reservation is rural and encompasses approximately 2.3 million acres in southern Montana, including the Wolf, Pryor, and Big Horn mountain ranges. As Chief Arapooish said, "The Crow Country is in exactly the right place. Everything good is to be found there. There is no country like the Crow Country."

If there is one word that could describe the culture of the Crow people, it would be *respect*. Respecting yourself, others, and the environment is the foundation of the Crow culture. Traditionally, Crow women are raised to be respectful of their bodies, in how they behave, and how they dress. The importance of modesty for Crow women is related to the concept of respecting one's body. For the Messengers project to be successful in dealing with very personal health issues, the project had to be sensitive to this important characteristic of Crow women.

The respectful ways in relating to each other not only exist in the immediate family, but also in the extended family. The Crow people are close-knit as a family. It is common for relatives to visit each other at their homes and spend quality time together. It is important to note that in the Crow culture, one's clan, immediate family, and extended family are very close and these ties are extremely important. For example, a cousin is equal to one's brother or sister, an aunt is the same as one's mother, and an uncle to one's father. These strong clan and family ties form the basis for the information networks of communication and impact all relationships. The Messengers project has utilized these networks to reach out and become set within the community.

The Crow Nation is a matrilineal tribe, so women play a very important role. Women are given much respect because they are the givers of life. They are strong spiritually, emotionally, and physically to keep the family together. Women's role in the family dynamic is that of *givers*. In our project, we often use the phrase, "Women form the backbone of the family and the tribe." When Crow women want something to get done, it gets done. Strong Crow women have formed the foundation of the Messengers project. Crow culture provides valuable resources that were used throughout the development of the Messengers project to improve the health of the people.

BEFORE MESSENGERS FOR HEALTH

There is no Crow word for cancer and before this project, saying this word out loud was to ask for it to come upon you. Women did not talk with other women about cancer screenings or share with others—including family members—when they had a cancer diagnosis. Women received cancer diagnoses alone, went through treatment alone, and often only at the end of their lives shared their diagnosis. There was a lack of communication between mother and daughter relationships regarding sex. The only time the topic of sex was mentioned in conversation was when Crow women sat around visiting and someone would tease someone else in a joking manner. It is difficult to convey the strength of these cultural taboos and the efforts it took for Messengers to break through these barriers. Not only are women now talking about cancer screenings to each other, but they are approaching project staff in public and asking for appointments to be scheduled. Cancer survivors are speaking out in public and a support group has started where people publicly show that cancer is not a death sentence.

Before Messengers, most women were unaware what a Pap test was and did not know that cervical cancer can be prevented. In our initial survey, conducted before we started the project, we found that 37% of the women had not had a Pap test in the previous year, 34% had not heard of a test to check for cervical cancer, and 71% reported not having read or heard anything about cervical cancer in the past year. Regarding risk factors, 55% of women did not know that a woman is more likely to get cervical cancer if she had sex at an early age, and 29% did not know that a woman is more likely to get cervical cancer if she had many sexual partners. Also, more than a quarter of the women surveyed responded "No" to a question asking if there are things a woman can do to prevent or control cervical cancer. These results from our initial survey showed that an important gap existed regarding cervical cancer education and screening. A second survey several years into the program showed significant changes in these statistics (see "Evaluating the Impact on the Crow Community").

BACKGROUND ON THE PARTNERSHIP—IMPLEMENTING CBPR

Messengers is filled with Crow cultural values to successfully change attitudes and behaviors surrounding cancer prevention. This was ensured through the use of a process of doing research called CBPR. CBPR enables for true partnership, collaboration, co-learning, and hence, true change (Wallerstein & Duran, 2006). Native Americans have many reasons for preferring CBPR projects as opposed to conventional research (Burhansstipanov, Christopher & Schumacher, 2005; Strickland, 2006). There are many recommendations for conducting appropriate research with Native communities, including respecting tribal diversity, building on tribal strengths, prioritizing the needs of the community, and ensuring that the community receives benefits from the research (Christopher, 2005). MFH obtained Institutional Review Board (IRB) approval from the university and also went through the Indian Health Service (IHS) Billings Area IRB. In addition, although the Crow tribe does not have a formal IRB, the project received approval from the Crow tribal chairman and the Billings Area service unit director. When working with Native communities, is it necessary to respect tribal sovereignty (Laveaux & Christopher, 2009).

Messengers is committed to following the principles of CBPR; for example, our Community Advisory Board, called the Messengers Executive Board, is closely engaged with all steps and aspects of the project. In research projects, often community members are brought in only to assist with data collection or to get *buy-in* for a researcher's ideas. With MFH, for example, all surveys are codeveloped and co-analyzed with university and community partners. Journal articles are cowritten with community and university partners. We believe that the positive results of this study were directly due to the use of a CBPR approach, such as building on community strengths, equally involving all partners in all phases of research, promoting co-learning and empowerment, and distributing findings to all partners. This project has changed public awareness of research and researchers on the reservation, opening the door for other projects that use respectful and culturally competent research approaches.

Messengers developed out of an initial partnership between Alma McCormick, a Crow community member passionate about cancer education, and Suzanne Christopher, a researcher from Montana State University (MSU). Alma McCormick works on the project in the Crow community, and prior to funding for the project was involved in a state health department project aimed at increasing awareness and prevention of cancer among tribal members. Her interest for working in cancer education comes from her own experience of having had a child who lost a battle with cancer at a very early age. Suzanne Christopher has a background that instilled in her the principles of social justice. She believes that you do not go into communities and tell people what to do; instead, you ask people what they need and how we can work together. Alma recognized Suzanne's gentle and humble nature and Suzanne recognized Alma's passion and integrity, and together they formed the basis for the partnership that resulted in Messengers. The project developed further when Alma and other community members informed Suzanne of the need for cancer education and outreach on the Crow reservation, and Suzanne shared with Alma her interest in writing a collaborative grant for a cancer project with the Crow Nation. MFH developed as a result of more than 5 years of meetings between community and university partners (Christopher, Watts, McCormick, & Young, 2008).

EXPANSION OF THE PARTNERSHIP: BUILDING TRUST IN THE COMMUNITY

Although research is a basic component of eliminating health disparities, many tribal nations have had bad experiences with researchers and with the research process. Too often, research has been conducted *on* rather than *with* tribal communities, resulting in their being labeled or stereotyped (Christopher, 2005). Thus, trust is important when working with American Indian tribes who for good reason often have a high level of distrust for outsiders (Christopher, Watts, et al., 2008). The steps our project took to gain trust in the community are as follows: First, we recognized community history, including research that had already been conducted in the community. Second, the project would directly benefit the community. Third, the community and university partners would work together on all phases of the work. Fourth, we would keep the community informed on the progress of the project. Lastly, we would do all that we could to continue the program indefinitely. We matched our words with actions. For example, on the fourth point, we have open community meetings to talk about our work and have articles in the local tribal newspaper. On the second point, instead of doing what many researchers have done in the past—that is, collecting data and then disappearing—we collected data and used it to shape the community health intervention to improve the health of Crow tribal members. The data stays in the community for community benefit.

DEVELOPMENT OF THE INTERVENTION—MESSENGERS FOR HEALTH

The program began with community meetings in 1996 and received funding beginning in 2001. Members of the Crow Nation worked with MSU researchers to codevelop an outreach program that would be most effective to educate the Crow women. It was decided in the initial meetings that implementing a one-on-one educational approach would be most successful. This approach would use many of the cultural strengths already in the Crow community; for example, the important role of respected women and their tight-knit family networks. Community members provided direct guidance in the areas of assessment, development, and implementation of the outreach intervention. In addition, the educational materials, such as brochures, teaching tools, and videos, were developed cooperatively with community members and designed specific to the Crow culture. Community members serving as advisors to the project began to formally serve as Executive Board members for the project.

The composition of the Board consists of 7–11 members. The Board has primarily been composed of Crow tribal members, with a non-Indian health care provider from the IHS serving on the Board at various times. The role of the Board members is to review and provide guidance on all aspects of the program and assist with project oversight by monitoring the pulse of the program in the community. The need for the Board to provide this level of detailed assistance explains why the Board has met approximately once per month since 2001. At times when there is greater activity (e.g., development of videos), the Board meets more often. The Board is also a link with the greater Crow community, providing information about the project to the community and bringing community ideas and suggestions to the project.

THE EDUCATIONAL APPROACH

MFH developed as a CBPR project with the aims of increasing knowledge of, positive attitudes toward, and screening for cervical cancer among Crow women on the Crow reservation. A number of studies have also focused on increasing rates of screening for cervical cancer among Native Americans and have been successful. Several effective strategies from other projects have also been used in our intervention. LHAs provide information (Dignan et al., 1998) by distributing culturally relevant educational materials and providing reminder calls for appointments (Lanier, Kelly, & Holck, 1999). Our study focuses on cultural strengths, similar to other studies with Native Americans (Hodge, Fredericks, & Rodriguez, 1996; Strickland, Squeoch, & Chrisman, 1999). A holistic approach to wellness is used in our educational messages, similar to Strickland et al.'s (1999) recommendation of promoting screening as a part of wellness. In addition, as other studies have demonstrated, working in full partnership with community members provides opportunities to enhance knowledge and skills for all those from the community who are participating, as well as providing a foundation for future research within the community (Matsunaga et al., 1996).

As mentioned, the intervention uses LHAs or women who are viewed as natural helpers in the community, and who others turn to for support and advice (Eng, 1993; Eng, Parker, & Harlan, 1997). The lay health approach portrays how community members naturally relate to one another and matches research and theory on social support and social networks. Social support is defined as resources provided by other persons (Cohen & Syme, 1985). Research indicates that social support influences both emotional and physical health (Berkman, 1984, 1995; Reblin & Uchino, 2008). LHAs in the Messengers program provide information and support to community women from a trusted network member—which is vitally important, because surveys with Apsáalooke women found that they often do not trust health professionals at the IHS (Christopher, Gidley, Letiecq, Smith, & McCormick, 2008).

In the Crow culture, values and knowledge are passed down by examples in daily experiences and through stories shared orally. This method of learning matches concepts in social cognitive theory (SCT) (Bandura, 1998), also known as social learning theory (Baranowski, Perry, & Parcel, 2002), which is a part of this intervention. The main components of SCT in this intervention are observational learning, behavioral capability, and reinforcements. For example, observational learning states that people can be influenced by role models that they trust. In our intervention, the LHAs serve as trustworthy role models by receiving Pap screenings and thus influencing others to do the same. One strength of an LHA intervention is the ability to impact change at the intrapersonal, interpersonal, community, and policy level. It has been suggested that to sustain change in communities, health programs need to be developed at broader levels than just the individual (McLeroy, Bibeau, Steckler, & Glanz, 1988).

The educational intervention of the one-on-one approach is gentle and respectful, reflecting this important Crow cultural trait. The LHAs, or Messengers as they are called in the Messengers project, were recruited based on their qualities and following the recommendations of community members. The project currently supports 22 Messengers, and has supported up to 33. They represent the seven district areas of the reservation and receive training on health issues and cancer screenings. Messengers talk with other women in the community on a daily basis and encourage them to receive cancer screening examinations. The Project Coordinator facilitates one-on-one training, and guides, motivates, and empowers each Messenger. She provides opportunities for hands-on teaching, such as during educational outreach booths and in schools. As women observe and learn from her, they become confident that they are able to do the same. Most Messengers have no formal schooling in health or in education. Many have gone from not being able to speak comfortably in a public meeting to giving presentations in communities.

MESSENGERS IN ACTION

The project has facilitated opportunities for empowering Messengers to become leaders in the community. One Messenger stated that the success of the project has been a "way to empower, to take responsibility for our own health. [We are] taking responsibility, educating, and dispelling myths [about cancer]." Messengers have shared how they value their responsibilities as educators and leaders in their communities. One Messenger commented, "We are called into a leadership role for our community, [community members] look up to us."

The Messengers program provides support for the Messengers through an initial training session and monthly meetings. Messengers also receive a monthly stipend to partially compensate them for the time and energy they devote to the project. To document that Messengers are conducting outreach with at least 15 women per month, they submit an outreach log that includes the initials of the person with whom they conducted outreach, and the date and time of the meeting. The first group of Messengers participated in training sessions before they began their outreach. The training covered a description of the Messengers program, the qualifications, duties, and responsibilities of Messengers, a volunteer agreement, record keeping, one-on-one and group outreach, and understanding cancer, cervical health, and other important health issues. This training was evaluated and found to be successful in raising cancer awareness and knowledge (Watts, Christopher, Smith, & Knows His Gun McCormick, 2005). As the program continues and new Messengers join the project, they have an initial training session with the Project Coordinator. The Messengers and project staff come together each month to share with each other, and to keep up to date with current health issues. Often, a guest is invited to provide a brief overview of a health topic of interest. Guest speakers have included IHS providers who have talked about breast cancer, cervical cancer, and human papillomavirus (HPV). Other guest speakers have discussed nutrition, smoking cessation, colon cancer, drug abuse, and many other topics. Although the project is focused on cancer screening, community members approach Messengers for many other issues and so they are supported in this through educational efforts.

Some meetings focus on enhancing outreach strategies. Messengers share their own personal outreach barriers and experiences. Several Messengers have discussed the difficulty they have when some women refuse to get a Pap test, or to even talk about getting a Pap test. Other meetings have focused on gaining leadership skills. Messengers role-play to practice outreach strategies. Often, there is time for Messengers to meet in small groups to plan community meetings. We have lead Messengers who represent the various districts of the Crow reservation. Each lead Messenger is responsible for organizing group outreach in their district. The Messengers staff encourages lead Messengers to organize community meetings in their districts. District meetings also include guest speakers and are an avenue for reaching out to community women. Messengers also host district-wide community meetings in the summer, where cancer survivors share their stories and community women have fun playing educational games.

Having cancer survivors sharing their stories in public venues is a significant accomplishment of the program. Before this project, people with cancer suffered alone and in silence. Now, Messengers provide avenues for survivors to share their stories, thus providing hope, inspiration, and encouragement to the community.

As mentioned previously, Messengers use the strengths of the Crow culture. Messengers have the liberty to use whatever method they feel is best to reach women. For example, building on the strength of close-knit family ties, Messengers provide home visits to their extensive social networks. Many Messengers speak their native tongue and provide outreach in the community, effectively communicating in the Crow language. Through the education provided by Messengers, Crow women have become empowered to take care of their cervical health. Women now know the importance of receiving a Pap test and are approaching Messengers in public, requesting to be scheduled for Pap test and mammogram appointments.

Outreach occurs on a daily basis. As a Messenger strolls through the grocery store and is greeted by her friends, relatives, and coworkers, one or more of them is likely prompted to remember that they are due for their annual examination. "Hey, can you schedule me for a Pap?" is a question that Messengers are used to hearing, even in public places. Other Messengers are out and about in the community spreading awareness and are known for their persistent promotion of the importance of early detection. On the other hand, in some cases Messengers prefer to be less noticeable. The project provides business cards with the question, "Do I need a Pap test?" A Messenger can discreetly hand the card to a woman and get the conversation started.

When Crow women, young and old, get together, you will hear lots of talking and laughter. It is during this social time that the conversation may touch on the topic of sex, usually in a joking manner. Now the conversation has become a little more serious, because women are openly discussing such issues as sexually transmitted infections and risks for cervical cancer. Although modesty is an important trait among Crow women, it no longer keeps them from having a Pap test examination. Women know they can schedule an appointment with a female provider with whom they may feel more comfortable.

Recently, Messengers took the step of developing a much needed cancer support group for the Crow Nation. Community members stated that this was something that had been needed for a very long time and that we were in a position where the community was looking to this program to take this step. The trust developed with the community by means of the program has allowed this to occur.

EVALUATING THE IMPACT ON THE CROW COMMUNITY

Messengers uses both qualitative and quantitative data to evaluate its effectiveness. We have conducted a rigorous random sample pretest and posttest to statistically assess our outcomes. In 2002, prior to the LHA intervention, we conducted a pretest survey of a random sample of 101 women, to measure knowledge, comfort, and awareness about Pap tests and cervical cancer. In 2005, we conducted a posttest survey with a separate random sample of 83 women. Participants were randomly selected from the Crow tribal roll, which includes all enrolled members of the tribe. For information about the development of the survey, see Smith, Christopher, and McCormick (2004). In this assessment, we saw statistically significant increases in knowledge about cervical cancer and in women's comfort about discussing cancer issues, and increases in women's awareness of cervical cancer and in the Messengers for Health project (Christopher, Gidley, et al., 2008). These statistics are even more meaningful because the surveys were done with random samples of women in the community as opposed to asking women who were specifically educated by women conducting outreach with the project (the Messengers). This shows that MFH has broad community impact. We used field notes, meeting minutes, and community perceptions to evaluate the project and to elicit further meaning from our survey data.

We have utilized other evaluation methods as well, including an evaluation of the training for the Messengers and an evaluation of the Advisory Board. The pre-/post-evaluation of the Messengers' training showed a statistically significant increase in cervical health knowledge. Thus, we felt that the Messengers could correctly relay information to other Crow women. The evaluation of the Advisory Board was very positive and pointed to the sense of empowerment that board members had about their role in the project, as shown in this quote: "Even though maybe she has a PhD in health, or maybe she's a doctor, or maybe she's been working in health for so many years, or [working for] the state . . . and I'm a college student . . . and everybody's different, but yet when we come to that table we're all one."

Another example of the effectiveness of the program is the positive effect that the program has had for the Messengers themselves and their role in the community. As the project has gained recognition among community members, Messengers are being called upon as a resource for cancer and aspects of other health education. During the 2008 annual Crow Fair Pow

Wow, an honor dance for cancer survivors was organized by the Messengers project. Crow women in the community recognized their friends and relatives who were participating in the dance. After this event, community women were prompted to go to the Messengers for information. As one Messenger relayed, "Crow women see us, and these women know who we are and they ask questions."Another Messenger mentioned, "[A] step at a time, the more we are out there the more we break down walls. This cancer is a preventable disease. [With this project] we are far ahead of other Native communities." The success of Messengers is also illustrated by its impact on students from both MSU and Little Big Horn College (the tribal college on the Crow reservation). Messengers has provided many unique opportunities to these students. With Messengers, exposure to CBPR goes far beyond a textbook understanding of the principles of CBPR. Students gain hands-on experience with CBPR in a tribal community. Many Native American students, the majority of them from the Crow tribe, have participated in various aspects of the Messengers for Health project. Students are certified in human subjects research and work on projects such as writing human subjects applications, developing questionnaires, conducting interviews, analyzing interviews, and ultimately becoming authors on manuscripts and traveling to national meetings to present their research. All of this experience provides excellent preparation for graduate school and for professional jobs working in health-related fields with Indian communities. Many former students have careers in health-related fields working with Native communities. Student involvement is a very important part of the program, as more Native Americans are needed as health workers and researchers, to change the health disparities that exist in tribal communities.

EXPANSION OF MESSENGERS FOR HEALTH: THE ADVOCATE PROGRAM

The accomplishments of Messengers have expanded beyond the scope of the LHA intervention. Messengers has partnered with the Crow IHS since its inception and has enjoyed a bidirectional relationship, learning and growing from each other. Examples of this include the Project Coordinator being provided with office space at the Crow Hospital, several members of the medical staff serving on our Advisory Board over the years, and regular meetings and consultations between various Messengers and IHS staff members. Our relationship with the IHS took on new dimensions in 2005, when the Advisory Board, Messengers, project staff, and community members decided in an open process to add a new component to the project that directly dealt with patient–physician relationships. Individuals felt that the project was doing a good job of outreach to women in the community, resulting in more women receiving Pap tests. However, there still existed a need to work together with the IHS to "support the IHS in providing high quality health care to our community."

Our first step was a community-developed video for non-Crow health providers at the IHS, which portrayed some of the unique Crow cultural ways, traditions, beliefs, and ceremonies with the hope of enhancing health-care providers' ability to communicate and work effectively with members of the Crow Nation. Written guidelines were developed to assist providers in how the themes from the video might impact patient care and how they could apply the information while providing care. For example, a theme of the video is "Crow people are very close-knit as a family, clan, and tribe." The guidelines stated, "Patients may bring family members to appointments and patients in the hospital may have many visitors and family who stay with them. Decisions are often not made by the individual patient. You can save time by asking 'Is everyone here?' when discussing a patient's status and treatment options."

A reconciliation ceremony was held to unveil the video and to allow the opportunity for providers and community members to talk openly about past issues and future hopes for the community and IHS working together. Dr. Ronit Elk, our Program Officer at the American Cancer Society, attended the reconciliation ceremony and offered these words: "During the film, there was complete silence in the huge auditorium. Everyone, and I mean everyone, was focused on a film that not only portrayed people who looked and sounded like themselves (probably the first ever), but also lauded their culture. Thunderous applause, wet cheeks, and stunned disbelief followed the showing, and everyone wanted a copy to take home and show others." She went on to say, "The excitement of this research program is that it will serve as a model for Native American communities and the IHS health care facilities that serve them."

We then developed our Health Advocate program, which allows health care providers and community members the opportunity to be aware of each other's unique cultural backgrounds to develop a relationship of understanding, acceptance, and trust. The primary focus is to establish one-on-one partnerships between IHS health care providers and Crow community members who serve as Advocates. The aim is for the Advocate and the healthcare provider team to meet as a pair, and also for the group of Advocates and providers to meet once a month. The Advocate invites his or her provider partner to attend community activities to gain a broader aware-ness of the Crow people and their culture. The project goal is to increase understanding and respect between providers and community members, and ultimately to develop more open and effective communication between providers and patients and improved health of the Crow people. We have faced some challenges, such as provider shortages and IHS administrative turnover, and we are still persevering to achieve our goal. We have not done a formal evaluation of the program, but informal evaluations show that some providers have seen significant improvements in their communication with patients, and that community members are supportive of the program and say this is something that has been needed for a long time. One example is a provider who misinterpreted his patients' body language (e.g., not making direct eye contact, leaning back in their chairs) as a lack of interest, or not listening to the provider. After learning from the Advocate about Crow communication styles, he learned that his patients are showing him respect and his interactions significantly improved.

WORKING TOGETHER WITH THE CROW NATION

Messengers has ongoing interactions with IHS and other community organizations. Many of the health programs, such as the Crow Meth [amphetamine] Project and the Crow Diabetes Project, have invited the Project Coordinator to speak at their awareness events. The diabetes program has involved Messengers in some of their outreach activities. The Project Coordinator is often invited to set up a booth or provide a presentation at health-related events. All of the local schools invite the Project Coordinator to speak to students about reproductive health, which shows the support and trust the community has in the Messengers project.

Messengers has also developed a strong relationship with the Crow Tribal Legislative Branch and the Crow Tribal Administration. The Legislative Branch fully supports the work of Messengers, and a Tribal Resolution (LR09–02) of approval and support is in place. The Tribal Administration is also very supportive and offers its assistance to expresses its sincere appreciation to Messengers for providing a benefit to the Crow people.

THE FUTURE OF MESSENGERS FOR HEALTH

Messengers for Health has established integrity, trust, and strong support in the Crow community. Although the funding from the American Cancer Society will eventually come to a close, project members are committed to sustaining it into the future. The project is likely to continue as a service-oriented program versus a research-focused project. In February 2010, after a year of preparation, we submitted paperwork to the Internal Revenue Service to become a 501(c)(3) nonprofit corporation and received this status in August 2010. We know of no other Native American program that started out as a research grant and has evolved into a Native nonprofit. We have purposively engaged in activities that will sustain us far into the future. For example, MFH became an Affiliate of the Seventh Generation Fund (SGF) for Indian Development. Affiliates are Native communities or organizations who come "in-house" with the SGF because they are emerging programs that do not yet have the staff or capacity to run as solo 501(c)(3) nonprofit organizations. Being an Affiliate allows a group to direct its efforts toward accomplishing its goals and objectives, whereas SGF assists with administration, technical training, fiscal management, program oversight, and organizational development (from the SGF website). The Project Coordinator and Board Chair recently went to a training with SGF on nonprofit leadership. In 2009, two staff members were accepted into the Hopa Mountain Strengthening the Circle Program. This program is a Native nonprofit leadership program that aims to build the capacities of experienced and emerging nonprofit organizations. Staff members have taken grant writing training, learned about funding agencies that support Native nonprofits, and visited with foundation executives to help plan for our future.

BEYOND CANCER AWARENESS

Messengers has not only made a major impact on the Crow Nation in the area of cancer awareness, but has also become a recognized example of effective CBPR in a Native American community. The intervention model utilized by Messengers can be a protocol applied to address the health needs and disparities of other Indian tribes and minorities. The success of Messengers for Health was used to leverage a $6.5 million Center of Excellence in Health Disparities grant from the National Institutes of Health to expand CBPR projects across the state of Montana. The Center for Native Health Partnerships (cnhp.montana.edu) began in 2007 and has provided funding for CBPR projects on all seven of Montana's reservations and in two urban Indian communities. The primary university partner for Messengers serves as the Principal Investigator for the center and the primary tribal community partner is the Chair of the Center's Steering Committee.

Messengers has developed trust with the Crow community, which was the foundational key, and we continue to build on that trust. The CBPR approach partnered community members with university staff and students in providing advice, input, and direction to the program. Messengers applied this method of utilizing community partnerships to develop an outreach program to best meet the needs of the Crow people. The effective CBPR approach of Messengers has opened the door in the Crow Nation for future research opportunities for CBPR projects to address other needs and issues.

REFERENCES

Bandura, A. (1998). Health promotion from the perspective of social cognitive theory. *Psychology & Health, 13*(4), 623–649.

Baranowski, T., Perry, C. L., & Parcel, G. S. (2002). How individuals, environments, and health behaviors interact. In K. Glanz, B. K. Rimmer, & F. M. Lewis (Eds.), *Health behavior and health education: Theory, research and Practice* (3rd ed.). San Francisco, CA: Jossey-Bass.

Berkman, L. F. (1984). Assessing the physical health effects of social networks and social support. *Annual Review of Public Health, 5,* 413–432.

Berkman, L. F. (1995). The role of social relations in health promotion. *Psychosomatic Medicine, 57*(3), 245–254.

Burhansstipanov, L., Christopher, S., & Schumacher, S. A. (2005). Lessons learned from community-based participatory research in Indian country. *Cancer Control, 12*(Suppl. 2), 70–76.

Christopher, S. (2005). Recommendations for conducting successful research with Native Americans. *Journal of Cancer Education, 20*(1 Suppl.), 47–51.

Christopher, S., Gidley, A. L., Letiecq, B., Smith, A., & McCormick, A. K. (2008). A cervical cancer community-based participatory research project in a Native American community. *Health Education & Behavior, 35*(6), 821–834.

Christopher, S., Watts, V., McCormick, A. K., & Young, S. (2008). Building and maintaining trust in a community-based participatory research partnership. *American Journal of Public Health, 98*(8), 1398–1406.

Cohen, S., & Syme, S. L. (1985). Issues in the study and application of social support. In S. Cohen & S. L. Syme (Eds.), *Social support and health.* San Francisco, CA: Academic Press.

Dignan, M. B., Michielutte, R., Wells, H. B., Sharp, P., Blinson, K., Case, L. D., . . . McQuellon, R.P. (1998). Health education to increase screening for cervical cancer among Lumbee Indian women in North Carolina. *Health Education Research, 13*(4), 545–556.

Eng, E. (1993). The Save our Sisters Project. A social network strategy for reaching rural black women. *Cancer, 72*(3 Suppl.), 1071–1077.

Eng, E., Parker, E., & Harlan, C. (1997). Lay health advisor intervention strategies: A continuum from natural helping to paraprofessional helping. *Health Education & Behavior, 24*(4), 413–417.

Hodge, F. S., Fredericks, L., & Rodriguez, B. (1996). American Indian women's talking circle. A cervical cancer screening and prevention project. *Cancer, 78*(7 Suppl.), 1592–1597.

Lanier, A. P., Kelly, J. J., & Holck, P. (1999). Pap prevalence and cervical cancer prevention among Alaska Native women. *Health Care for Women International, 20*(5), 471–486.

Laveaux, D., & Christopher, S. (2009). Contextualizing CBPR: Key principles of CBPR meet the Indigenous research context. *Pimatisiwin, 7*(1), 1.

Matsunaga, D. S., Enos, R., Gotay, C. C., Banner, R. O., DeCambra, H., Hammond, O. W.,… Tsark, J. A. (1996). Participatory research in a Native Hawaiian community. The Wai'anae Cancer Research Project. *Cancer, 78*(7 Suppl.), 1582–1586.

McLeroy, K. R., Bibeau, D., Steckler, A., & Glanz, K. (1988). An ecological perspective on health promotion programs. *Health Education Quarterly, 15*(4), 351–377.

Reblin, M., & Uchino, B. N. (2008). Social and emotional support and its implication for health. *Current Opinion in Psychiatry, 21*(2), 201–205.

Smith, A., Christopher, S., & McCormick, A. K. (2004). Development and implementation of a culturally sensitive cervical health survey: A community-based participatory approach. *Women Health, 40*(2), 67–86.

Strickland, C. J. (2006). Challenges in community-based participatory research implementation: Experiences in cancer prevention with Pacific Northwest American Indian tribes. *Cancer Control, 13*(3), 230–236.

Strickland, C. J., Squeoch, M. D., & Chrisman, N. J. (1999). Health promotion in cervical cancer prevention among the Yakama Indian women of the Wa'Shat Longhouse. *Journal of Transcultural Nursing, 10*(3), 190–196.

Wallerstein, N. B., & Duran, B. (2006). Using community-based participatory research to address health disparities. *Health Promotion Practice, 7*(3), 312–323.

Watts, V., Christopher, S., Smith, J., & Knows His Gun McCormick, A. (2005). Evaluation of a lay health advisor training for a community-based participatory research project in a Native American community. *American Indian Culture and Research Journal, 29*(3), 59–79.

13

Tools for Improving Colorectal Cancer Screening Rates: Multimedia Versus Print in an Underserved Community

Gregory Makoul, David W. Baker, Denise Scholtens, and Ann Trauscht

Colorectal cancer (CRC) is one of the most common types of cancer in the United States, exceeded only by lung and prostate cancer in men and lung and breast cancer in women (American Cancer Society, 2009; Holden et al., 2010). It is the second leading cause of cancer death among men and women: In 2009, approximately 147,000 American adults were newly diagnosed with CRC, and an estimated 50,000 died as a result of the disease (American Cancer Society, 2009; Holden et al., 2010). CRC is ideally suited for early detection strategies, since precancerous adenomas precede the development of malignancies (Levin & Murphy, 1992; Lieberman, 1995; Mandel et al., 1993; Newcomb, Norfleet, Storer, Surawicz, & Marcus, 1992; Selby, Friedman, Quesenberry, & Weiss, 1992; Simon, 1998a, 1998b; Winawer, Flehinger, Schottenfeld, & Miller, 1993; Winawer et al., 1997; Winawer et al., 1993). Surveillance, Epidemiology, and End Results (SEER) data reveal that 90% of people for whom CRC was caught early lived at least 5 years. However, only 39% of all CRC cases were caught before metastasis (Parker, Davis, Wingo, Ries, & Heath, 1998).

The U.S. Preventive Services Task Force strongly recommends that persons aged 50 and older undergo screening for CRC using standard screening technologies, with a screening frequency that varies from test to test (Pignone, Rich, Teutsch, Berg, & Lohr, 2002a, 2002b; U.S. Preventive Services Task Force, 2008). The American Cancer Society (ACS) and professional associations have issued similar guidelines (American Cancer Society, 2010; Byers, Levin, Rothenberger, Dodd, & Smith, 1997; Goldstein & Messing, 1998; Winawer et al., 2003; Winawer & Shike, 1995). Recommended screening tests include fecal occult blood test (FOBT), fecal immunochemical test (FIT), flexible sigmoidoscopy, colonoscopy, and double-contrast barium enema (American Cancer Society, 2011; Byers et al., 1997). Virtual colonoscopy is currently under study; it neither detects very small polyps nor allows removal of tissue samples or polyps during the procedure (American Cancer Society, 2011). Medicare covers annual stool-card tests as well as periodic flexible sigmoidoscopies, colonoscopies, and barium enemas (Ko, Kreuter, & Baldwin, 2002). In the absence of a single optimal test, patient preference and access play an important role in deciding which test should be used (Leard, Savides, & Ganiats, 1997). For instance, while FOBT is less sensitive than colonoscopy for detecting CRC, it is noninvasive, has a lower risk of complications, and carries lower costs.

CRC screening is among the clinical preventive services with the highest priority rankings and lowest delivery rates (Coffield et al., 2001). Despite evidence supporting CRC screening in general and clinical guidelines supporting specific procedures, only a small percentage of the screening-eligible population has been screened by any appropriate method (Anderson & May, 1995; *Behavioral Risk Factor Surveillance System Public Use Data Tape, 2004,* 2005; Coffield et al., 2001; Centers for Disease Control and Prevention (CDC), 1999). The challenge of screening may be even greater in disadvantaged communities. Safety-net clinics, which provide health care for individuals regardless of their insurance status or ability to pay, are the source of care for a disproportionately high number of African American and Hispanic/Latino patients (National Association of Community Health Centers, 2005). The African American population has the highest morbidity and mortality rate due to CRC, and the Hispanic/Latino population has been documented as having the lowest CRC screening rates, putting this group at great risk for late-stage presentation of disease (American Cancer Society, 2006).

Two significant barriers to CRC screening in primary care practice may be interrelated: (1) many patients are unaware of their risk for developing CRC and/or unaware of screening options; and (2) many physicians do an inadequate job of discussing CRC and/or appropriate screening options with their patients. Studies have noted relatively little knowledge of CRC and related screening options in the general population, as well as among poor and underserved populations (Blalock, DeVellis, Afifi, & Sandler, 1990; Box, Nichols, Lallemand, Pearson, & Vakil, 1984; Brown, Potosky, Thompson, & Kessler, 1990; Farrands, Hardcastle, Chamberlain, & Moss, 1984; Price, 1993; Wong, Nenny, Guy, & Seow-Choen, 2002). Moreover, low levels of knowledge have been linked with compromised perceptions of risk for CRC and under utilization of appropriate screening services (Brenes & Paskett, 2000; Bunn, Bosompra, Ashikaga, Flynn, & Worden, 2002; Kelly & Shank, 1992; Ling, Moskowitz, Wachs, Pearson, & Schroy, 2001; McCaffery et al., 2001; Myers, Vernon, Tilley, Lu, & Watts,

1998; Vernon, Myers, Tilley, & Li, 2001; Weller, Owen, Hiller, Willson, & Wilson, 1995; Wolf et al., 2001). Several studies investigating noncompliance with FOBT found that the primary reason for not returning the test was that the patient was asymptomatic and did not see the need to participate (Brown et al., 1990; Davis et al., 2001; Farrands et al., 1984; Price, 1993; Vernon, 1997; Wolf et al., 2001).

Physician failure to discuss and/or recommend appropriate CRC screening has been well documented (Holmes-Rovner et al., 2002; Levin et al., 2002; Ling et al., 2001, 2003; Malik & Sansone, 2002; Schroy, Barrison, Ling, Wilson, & Geller, 2002; Schroy et al., 2001; Taylor & Anderson, 2002; Wolf et al., 2006) This is particularly problematic because patients report that physicians are their main source of information about health and medicine (Hesse et al., 2005; Makoul, Arntson, & Schofield, 1995). Ling and colleagues reported that important CRC screening information was addressed in fewer than half of the physician–patient encounters during which the issue of CRC was raised: The pros and cons of screening were discussed in 40% of encounters, and available screening tests were discussed in only 36% (Ling et al., 2003). One of our recent studies indicated that while primary care physicians recognize and espouse the importance of recommending CRC screening to eligible patients, in practice these discussions tend to be truncated (Wolf, Baker, & Makoul, 2007). As noted by Helm and colleagues, "full disclosure of [CRC screening] benefits and risks is unlikely to occur, if only because of time limits on office visits" (Helm et al., 2003). The evidence on inconsistent physician recommendation of CRC screening, coupled with evidence that physicians are patients' main source of health information, suggests the need for interventions that can influence the physician–patient interaction.

Interventions designed to increase CRC screening have tended to focus on information targeted to either physicians or patients, in relative isolation from the interactive context of physician–patient encounters. We aim to provide patients with understandable information and motivational messages when waiting for their appointment, so that physicians can focus visit time and effort on answering questions, providing guidance, and tailoring recommendations. Our previous research indicates that well-designed multimedia patient education programs about CRC screening increase perceived risk, knowledge of relevant anatomy, knowledge of screening options, intention to discuss screening with the doctor, and willingness to consider screening tests (Cameron, Francis, Wolf, Baker, & Makoul, 2007; Makoul et al., 2009). Given high-quality messages, the primary aim of this study is to test a question with considerable theoretical and practical import: Do messages have a different impact on screening behavior when delivered by multimedia technology or print?

SPECIFIC AIMS

Based on our review of the literature, we believe this study is the first to explicitly compare the effects of message-equivalent print and multimedia materials that were developed with patient input and tested in community settings. A fundamental aim is to assess the effect of print and multimedia on knowledge relevant to CRC screening and impression of the patient education messages (e.g., clarity). In addition, we outlined a focused set of specific aims regarding screening completion:

Aim 1: Determine if multimedia and print interventions that provide patients with information and motivational messages about CRC screening increase screening rates above those for usual care.

Aim 2: Determine whether showing patients a multimedia program achieves higher CRC screening rates than does a print booklet with equivalent messages.

Aim 2a: Examine if the effects of these multimedia and print interventions on CRC screening rates differ with literacy level.

Aim 2b: Examine if the effects of these multimedia and print interventions on CRC screening rates differ with race/ethnicity.

METHODS

The Institutional Review Board (IRB)-approved study is designed and implemented as a randomized controlled trial in which patients between the ages of 50 and 80 years of age at the time of their clinic visit are assigned to one of three study arms: (1) usual care, which serves as the Control condition; (2) the Print intervention group; and (3) the Multimedia intervention group.

Usual Care

In terms of providing information about CRC and CRC screening (i.e., beyond physician–patient communication), usual care at our study clinics entails maintaining a supply of brochures produced by the ACS on *Cancer Facts for Women* and *Cancer Facts for Men* in the examination rooms of each clinic.Colon cancer is among the types of cancer addressed in these materials. All participants will receive usual care; the intervention groups also receive the print or multimedia materials described below.

The Interventions

The patient education materials in this study are based on the multimedia programs developed through grants from the ACS-Illinois Division and the National Cancer Institute (NCI) (Principal Investigator: Dr. Makoul). The multimedia program incorporates illustrations, animations, photographs, and voice-over; it was developed using Adobe Photoshop, AfterEffects, and Premiere. Using the multimedia program as our starting point, we reverse-engineered a print version by using the same script and graphics to yield message-equivalent materials. The print version was made with Adobe Photoshop, Illustrator, and InDesign. In addition, we made Spanish and English versions of both the print and multimedia tools. Our English script was translated into Spanish by four different Spanish-speakers from different countries and back-translated into English. The English and Spanish versions were then revised to ensure parallel content; we used an established protocol for the translation process (Cella et al., 1998; Eremenco, Cella, & Arnold, 2005; Lent, Hahn, Eremenco, Webster, & Cella, 1999). Lexile analysis indicates that the text is written at a fourth-grade reading level (Stenner, 1996; Stenner, Horablin, Smith, & Smith, 1988).

There are 584 words in the English version. The structure of the Spanish language requires more words (e.g., stool cards = *tarjetas de muestras fecales*); therefore the Spanish version runs to 651 words. Text in the English and Spanish print booklets uses the same font size and style. Voice-overs in the English and Spanish multimedia programs were done by the same bilingual woman. The print (27 pages, average of under 25 words per page, delivered in a spiral-bound 6.75 in. × 8.5 in. booklet) and multimedia (4 minutes, delivered as a Quicktime file) tools are available from Dr. Makoul (gmakoul@stfranciscare.org).

Graphics are an important component of both the print and multimedia tools. Particularly relevant to the print version is our use of *scaffolding* (i.e., providing cues) to enhance comprehension of material, helping less-able readers read more difficult text. One proven method of scaffolding is to include illustrations that support the text in telling the story. Since readers have two modes of receiving the information—text and illustration—they are more likely to remain engaged and to gain understanding (Lennon & Burdick, 2004). The logic of scaffolding also operates in the context of multimedia programs: Although voice-overs may obviate problems of reading, animation (e.g., showing the path of the colonoscopy tube) may help people grasp unfamiliar concepts.

Parameters of the Randomized Controlled Trial

Data are collected under the same conditions for all three arms of the randomized controlled trial: (1) physicians and staff know that we are doing a study; (2) physicians are reminded to talk with patients about CRC screening, and that diagnostic colonoscopies will be provided for patients who receive positive FOBT results during the study period; (3) research assistants

(RAs) ask patients a brief set of questions and conduct a literacy assessment in the waiting room before the doctor visit; (4) RAs conduct a brief post-visit interview with patients immediately after the doctor visit; (5) we conduct chart audits to determine the documentation of the screening discussion; (6) we use an electronic registry to collect test completion data at 3 months after the study visit; and (7) we conduct follow-up telephone interviews at 4 months after the study visit with patients who did not get screened, to assess their reasons.

Study Participants and Informed Consent

To ensure adequate statistical power for analyses, a target of 900 participants will be recruited into the study, and randomly assigned to one of the three arms. Participants will be randomized in a 1:1:1 ratio, yielding approximately 300 participants in each arm.

Inclusion and Exclusion Criteria

The inclusion criteria are that patients should be in the target age range (50–80 years), and registered for an appointment at the community health center. The exclusion criteria are that the patient reported CRC screening within the past year; is unable to speak English or Spanish; is blind, deaf, or otherwise unable to review study materials; or is too ill to participate (i.e., not well enough to approach the RA). Patients will be dropped from the analysis if the clinic system's database indicates that CRC screening was up to date at the time of their index visit. We anticipate that attrition due to past screening will be rare and randomly distributed across the sample. In addition, patients will be dropped from the study if their reading or viewing of intervention materials is interrupted by their clinic visit. Based on our prior multimedia study, we expect interruption to be an extremely rare event.

Recruitment and Pre-Screening Procedure

Upon registration at the community health center, patients in the target age group are handed a card inviting them to learn about the study or are approached by the RA after check-in. We used similar invitation cards written in plain language during a previous study. Personnel and patients responded positively to this approach, which encourages interested people to see the RA, but does not require much additional time or effort for busy clinic staff. The invitation cards are 8.5 in. × 5.5 in., with English text on one side and Spanish text on the other.

If a patient expresses interest, the RA thanks the patient and asks a brief set of questions to determine eligibility. The initial pre-screening question ("Have you participated in this study before?") is designed to help avoid recruiting people into the study more than once; the self-report will be verified. If a patient reports being new to the study, the RA then asks two questions, the first focusing on CRC screening within the past year, which is an appropriate timeframe because FOBT is the most practical and likely mode of screening at the study sites. The second question is intended to mask the purpose of the study and focuses on whether the patient's cholesterol has been checked within the past year. The intent of the pre-screen is to rapidly identify patients who report having been screened for CRC by any recommended method in the past year. If patients answer "Yes" to the question about CRC screening, they are not eligible for the study; the RA thanks them for their time and provides a plastic penlight as a token of appreciation.

Informed Consent Process

Patients who answer "No" or "Don't know," or otherwise express uncertainty in response to the question about CRC screening, have the opportunity to participate in the study. Even if they are mistaken (i.e., screening is up-to-date), participation can help patients better understand CRC screening, ascertain their screening status, and clarify the recommended frequency of screening. The RA engages in the informed consent and Health Insurance Portability and Accountability Act (HIPAA) in English or Spanish, whichever language the patient prefers. This process is intended to make clear that the RA will ask a brief set of questions before and after the visit, may ask the participant to view patient education materials, and will need access to the patient's medical record number, so that a member of the study team can access the record and review the status of preventive care as captured in the clinic system's database.

Patients are not told that we are explicitly looking at whether or not they complete CRC screening, as that information might function as an intervention in and of itself. The consent process notes that patients who complete the study will receive a $10 gift-card and a plastic penlight before leaving the clinic. We used this same incentive in a previous study; the level of compensation was seen as attractive, fair, and respectful (Cameron et al., 2007). In addition, the penlight generated interest amongst potential participants.

Pre-Visit Measures and Procedure

The RA collects data from participants before their scheduled doctor visit, via interaction in the waiting room. There are two parts to the initial data collection—(1) a brief structured interview to assess baseline knowledge and demographics, and (2) a literacy assessment—both of which can be done in either English or Spanish. Patients assigned to the intervention groups are asked to view the print or multimedia materials, and to answer brief sets of questions designed to measure response to the materials as well as to gauge change in knowledge.

Baseline Knowledge and Demographics

The structured interview protocol was derived from questions tested and used in our previous multimedia study (Makoul et al., 2009). The RA uses printed cards to display response options. The interview begins with two items that assess language preference (one for speaking, the other for reading), which serve to both describe our sample and direct the RA to proceed in the appropriate language. These are followed by an orienting statement ("Today, we are trying to learn what people know about a certain type of cancer") and a question asking if the participant has ever heard of colon cancer, rectal cancer, or CRC. The next eight items assess knowledge regarding CRC and CRC screening; items asking if a patient knows something (e.g., "Do you know what a polyp is?") are coupled with a follow-up for people who answer affirmatively (e.g., "Can you describe it to me?").

As the proposed study focuses on uptake of screening, we do not seek additional detail on CRC screening attitudes and intention to avoid a situation in which the data collection itself could conceivably prompt screening. The interview protocol includes a transitional statement, and proceeds to demographic items. The first asks patients to report in which country they grew up. Our previous study experience suggested that people were more comfortable answering this question than one about country of birth. Subsequent items assess self-reported race/ethnicity, age, education level, health rating, reliance on physicians, and insurance coverage. This interview can be completed in about 3 minutes.

Health Literacy

Reading fluency is measured with the short version of the Test of Functional Health Literacy in Adults (TOFHLA) (Baker, Williams, Parker, Gazmararian, & Nurss, 1999). The short version (S-TOFHLA) takes a maximum of 7 min to administer. It has been shown to have good internal consistency (Cronbach's alpha = .98 for all items combined) and validity compared to the long version of the TOFHLA (Spearman's rank correlation = .91) and the Rapid Estimate of Adult Literacy in Medicine (Spearman's rank correlation = .80) (Baker et al., 1999). For simplicity, we refer to the construct assessed by the TOFHLA as health literacy, while recognizing that this test does not measure all domains of health literacy (DeWalt & Pignone, 2005).

The S-TOFHLA uses actual materials that patients might encounter in the health care setting to test reading ability. The reading comprehension section is a 36-item test using the modified Cloze procedure (i.e., every fifth to seventh word in a passage is omitted and multiple choice options are provided). Participants read the passage and select the option that best completes the blank, given the context of the surrounding phrases. Correct responses receive 1 point per item; incorrect responses do not receive any points. Scores from 0 to 16 indicate *inadequate literacy*; these individuals will often misread relatively basic materials, including prescription bottles, appointment slips, and medical instructions. Inadequate literacy has been associated with lower knowledge of chronic disease, less use of preventive services and cancer screening, worse health status, higher hospitalization rates, and higher mortality rates (Baker et al., 2002, 2007; Scott, Gazmararian, Williams, & Baker, 2002; Williams, Baker, Honig, Lee, & Nowlan, 1998; Williams, Baker, Parker, & Nurss, 1998; Wolf, Gazmararian, & Baker, 2005).

One of the most interesting methodological findings of our work to date is that people who have low literacy tend to demonstrate very concrete thinking and often construe this assessment of literacy as something that applies directly to their own care. More specifically, they respond to the S-TOFHLA—which includes statements such as "Your blood test was _____" and "Your doctor has sent you to have a _____ X-ray"—as if the text referred to them (e.g., some patients will say "I didn't have a blood test" or "I didn't get an X-ray"). Although we quickly learned the importance of ensuring that the RAs state that the S-TOFHLA is not about the participant, some participants have refused to engage with that instrument.

Assignment to Study Group

After participants have answered the baseline knowledge and demographic questions, the study arm to which they have been randomly assigned appears on the tablet computer used for data collection.

Protocol for the Control Group

For patients assigned to the Control group (i.e., usual care), the RA administers the S-TOFHLA, records the score, gives participants a penlight as a token of appreciation, and then asks them to come back to the waiting room area immediately after their doctor visit, to answer a few more questions and receive payment for participation.

Protocol for the Intervention Groups

For patients assigned to the Print or Multimedia intervention groups, the RA asks them to view the intervention to which they have been randomly assigned. The RA notes both the format and language of the intervention used for each participant. The multimedia program is viewed on the tablet computer, and runs for 4 minutes. The length of time a participant will spend reading the print booklet—which contains exactly the same script—varies with reading ability. The RA records whether the patient asks for help or otherwise indicates trouble with the materials; interrupted reading or viewing will be noted as well. The RA also discreetly monitors and records time spent reading the booklet, using a clock on the tablet computer. The RA retrieves the print booklet from participants after they read it and before reinitiating data collection (i.e., the print and multimedia versions are for use in the waiting room only).

Immediately after participants finish viewing the intervention to which they have been assigned, the RA asks a series of nine items designed to gauge reaction to the intervention, asking the extent to which the multimedia program or print booklet was clear, informative, believable, interesting, relevant, and easy to understand; as well as if the words were easy to understand, if the pictures were easy to understand, and whether the material applied to them.These questions and 0–10 response scale are drawn from our earlier studies of a multimedia patient education program; they address perceptions related to targeted messages as well as cognitive load, while adding very little time to data collection (Cameron et al., 2007; Makoul et al., 2009).

The RA then conducts a posttest of knowledge relevant to CRC, using the same eight items used as a measure of baseline knowledge. This allows us to assess the extent to which viewing the intervention materials increases knowledge. After participants answer the posttest knowledge questions, the RA administers the S-TOFHLA and records the score. The RA then gives participants a penlight as a token of appreciation, and asks them to come back to the waiting room immediately after their doctor visit, to answer a few more questions and receive payment for participation. The interventions and the posttest increase the overall length of participant involvement: As noted above, viewing the multimedia tool takes approximately 4 minutes; we anticipate that most participants randomized to view the print booklet will require at least that amount of time (i.e., participants in low-literacy focus groups took less than 6 minutes to finish reading the booklet).The posttest questions take less than 2 minutes.

Immediate Post-Visit Measures

Immediately after their doctor visit, participants in all three study arms have a brief (5 minutes) follow-up encounter with the RA. The post-visit structured interview asks if the patient has seen this doctor before, saw the *Cancer Facts* brochure that the clinic puts in the examination room as part of usual care, read the *Cancer Facts* brochure, and/or talked with the doctor about CRC screening. Patients also gauge physician communication by responding to items in the Communication Assessment Tool, a practical instrument that yields reliable and valid results (Makoul, Krupat, & Chang, 2007). All participants receive a $10 gift-card upon completing this session with the RA.

Screening Measures

We focus on CRC screening recommendation as a process measure and CRC screening completion as an outcome.

CRC Screening Recommendation

Physicians complete encounter notes for their visits, which become part of each patient chart. These notes include screening recommendations as well as information regarding whether the patient declined screening. Charts are reviewed by qualified study staff on a periodic basis, to determine if CRC screening was recommended during the index interview.

CRC Screening Completion

Completion of CRC screening within 3 months of the index visit is determined using the clinic system's electronic registry. The registry documents whether a CRC screening test has been ordered, as well as if the test has been completed, and whether the results are negative or positive. While preliminary data suggest that nearly all screening will be done via FOBT, analyses will include other recommended screening options as well (e.g., colonoscopy); all are captured in CRC screening fields within the database. Patients enrolled in the study will be matched to registry data via their medical record number, and reports will focus on CRC screening.

Follow-up Telephone Interviews: An Opportunity for Evaluation

As the interventions provide what our preliminary studies indicate are optimal messages, it is important to learn the perspective of people who were exposed to the message but did *not* complete screening. If the records indicate that screening was not completed within 3 months of the index visit, the RAs make up to 7 attempts to call patients. This interview, which takes less than 5 minutes, focuses on barriers to completing CRC screening. We recognize that the RAs will be unable to contact every participant who does not complete CRC screening, but we expect to gain useful information in the event that our hypotheses are not supported by the data. Calls are initiated approximately 100 days after the index visit.

Data Capture

Research Assistants (RAs) use Toshiba Portege M200 tablet computers to collect data electronically. The RAs read each structured-interview question aloud and record patient responses directly onto the tablet computer. We use Snap Surveys software (Snap v8, Mercator Research Group Ltd., Boston) to facilitate data entry. This software allows for straightforward electronic entry of responses and can generate output data files compatible with statistical programs. In addition, we loaded a software program to ensure data security, and conducted specific training on proper encryption and transfer procedures.

Implementation Fidelity

There are two main components of overall program evaluation: outcome evaluation (e.g., whether the interventions increased screening rates above baseline) and implementation evaluation (e.g., whether the interventions were implemented as planned), which is also called process evaluation (Rossi & Freeman, 1989; Shadish, Cook, & Leviton, 1991). High-fidelity implementation is an often overlooked, yet essential, marker of research quality: Monitoring implementation fidelity allows researchers to reduce heterogeneity by calibrating processes if and when needed. Thorough training and frequent meetings of the research team ensure that the study protocol is clearly understood, all questions are answered, and the RAs are well calibrated in their approach to the study.

Statistical Analysis

This chapter provides a preliminary report of data collected to date. Full statistical analyses will be conducted once data collection has been completed. Before conducting formal analyses, we will perform descriptive studies to ensure an adequate balance of covariates and potential confounding factors among the Control, Print, and Multimedia groups. Variables found to have statistically significant differences ($p < .05$) across treatment groups will be controlled for in further analyses.

One strength of our design is that the same physicians will see patients in all groups, but will not be told which group the patient is in. However, since patients of the same physician may tend to make similar screening decisions, we will investigate the use of a random effect for physician in a generalized linear mixed model (GLMM) with physician as a random effect, nested within site. If the random effect for physician is significant, we will use GLMM in the analyses for each specific aim.

When planning the study, our estimated screening rates for the baseline and intervention groups were 10% for Control, 20% for Print, and 30% for Multimedia, based on current CRC screening rates documented by the clinic sites as well as published research. For the power calculations, a two-tailed test and a Type I error rate of 1.6% is assumed for each pairwise comparison. A sample size of 300 per arm provides 80% power to detect a the estimated differences (Hintze, 2005). Based on demographic information received from the clinic sites and publicly available programs (http://www.pfizerhealthliteracy.org/calculator.html) (Pfizer Clear Health Communication Initiative, 2003), we estimated that nearly 40% of the study sample will have inadequate literacy.

PRELIMINARY RESULTS

Data collection began in May 2009. Table 13.1 summarizes preliminary results representing index visits that occurred through the end of March 2010 as well as follow-up data. Discrete variable distributions were compared across intervention arms using chi-square tests. Means and standard deviations are reported for continuous variables and compared across intervention arms using ANOVA.

Across all arms of the study, 55% of the patients identified their race or ethni-city as Hispanic/Latino, and 50% of the surveys were conducted in Spanish. Most of the patients had eighth-grade education or less; just over one third of the patients had inadequate health literacy, as measured by the S-TOFHLA.

Knowledge

The data presented are preliminary and do not control for covariates. At baseline, approximately 40% of the patients in all three study arms reported knowing what a *polyp* is. As shown in Table 13.2, self-reported knowledge increased to 80% of the print group and 72% of the multimedia group at post test. A chi-square test indicates no significant difference in knowledge between these groups.

Similarly, less than half of the patients in all three study arms reported knowledge of FOBT at baseline. Table 13.3 illustrates that both print and multimedia produced significant knowledge gain (i.e., from not knowing to knowing). While the jump in knowledge for the video group was clearly larger than for patients in the booklet group (38% vs. 26%), there was virtually no difference in knowledge at post test (78% vs. 77%).

TABLE 13.1 The Demographics of the Sample

	All N = 547	All (%)	Control N = 178	Control %	Booklet N = 180	Booklet (%)	Video N = 189	Video %	p-Value
Sex									.519
Male	174	32	53	30	55	31	66	35	
Female	373	68	125	70	125	69	123	65	
Race/ethnicity									.131
White non-Hispanic	89	16	26	15	40	22	23	12	
Black non-Hispanic	112	20	34	19	37	21	41	22	
Hispanic/Latino	299	55	106	60	87	48	106	56	
Multi-/other	47	9	12	7	16	9	19	10	
Survey language									.133
English	273	50	83	47	101	56	89	47	
Spanish	273	50	95	53	79	44	99	53	
Education									.384
Eighth grade or less	237	43	80	45	66	37	91	48	
Some high school	76	14	25	14	24	13	27	14	
High school graduate	96	18	28	16	40	22	28	15	
Some college	77	14	27	15	29	16	21	11	
College degree	61	11	18	10	21	12	22	12	
Health rating									.026
Poor	108	20	30	17	31	18	47	25	
Fair	221	41	74	43	65	37	82	44	
Good	159	29	56	32	64	36	38	20	
Very good/excellent	49	9	13	8	16	9	20	11	
Health literacy[a]	448		150		155		143		.448
Inadequate	152	34	52	35	48	31	52	36	
Marginal	38	8	17	11	11	7	10	7	
Adequate	258	58	81	54	96	62	81	57	
Age	Mean	SD	Mean	SD	Mean	SD	Mean	SD	.713
	57.6	6.6	57.3	6.2	57.5	6.4	57.9	7.0	

[a] N for health literacy was lower because not all patients completed the S-TOFHLA.

TABLE 13.2   Self-Reported Knowledge of Polyps

	No Gain	Gain	Maintain
	Before = No After = No	Before = No After = Yes	Before = Yes After = Yes
Booklet	20%	37%	43%
Video	28%	32%	40%

The results for colonoscopy knowledge were similar. Participants who self-reported knowledge at pretest and/or posttest were asked to describe polyps, FOBT, and colonoscopy. We will code the responses to increase the validity of analyses regarding CRC-relevant knowledge.

TABLE 13.3   Self-Reported Knowledge of FOBT

	No Gain	Gain	Maintain
	Before = No After = No	Before = No After = Yes	Before = Yes After = Yes
Booklet	22%	26%	51%
Video	22%	38%	40%

Rating of the Print and Multimedia Interventions

Tables 13.4 and 13.5 display ratings of the interventions by subjects with adequate and inadequate health literacy as measured by the S-TOFHLA. There was very little difference in evaluations by the adequate literacy group. Subjects in the inadequate literacy group found the video more understandable.

TABLE 13.4   Rating of Interventions by Subjects With Adequate Health Literacy

	Booklet Mean	Booklet SD	Booklet N	Video Mean	Video SD	Video N	t-Test p-value
Clear	8.62	0.87	95	8.80	0.56	81	.10
Informative	8.71	0.70	95	8.68	0.80	81	.82
Believable	8.75	0.73	95	8.81	0.50	81	.47
Interesting	8.33	1.62	95	8.47	1.41	81	.53
Understand	8.85	0.46	95	8.83	0.47	81	.72
Understand words	8.83	0.65	95	8.83	0.47	81	.96
Understand pictures	8.87	0.42	95	8.85	0.45	81	.74

TABLE 13.5   Rating of Interventions by Subjects With Inadequate Health Literacy

	Booklet Mean	Booklet SD	Booklet N	Video Mean	Video SD	Video N	t-Test p-value
Clear	8.72	0.86	46	8.86	0.40	51	.30
Informative	8.63	0.95	46	8.92	0.27	51	.05
Believable	8.65	0.95	46	8.92	0.27	51	.07
Interesting	8.63	1.04	46	8.92	0.27	51	.07
Understand	8.40	1.18	46	8.88	0.33	51	.01
Understand words	8.36	1.37	46	8.55	1.53	51	.51
Understand pictures	8.50	1.36	46	8.71	1.14	51	.42

CRC Screening and Physician Discussion

We are in the process of validating data regarding actual screening, but we can report that screening rates appear to be low (i.e., in the 10%–20% range) across all three arms of the study. Our telephone follow-up with patients who did not get screened provides insight into this finding. More specifically, only 16% of the subjects we were able to reach for follow-up said that the physician talked with them about CRC screening and 17% reported that the doctor gave them a stool-card test to do at home. The final question of the telephone interview was: "People have their own reasons for not getting a screening test. Can you tell me why you did not do a test?" Of the subjects contacted at follow-up, 165 gave one reason for not getting screened; 18 gave two reasons, for a total of 201 responses. "The doctor did not recommend it" was the overwhelming reason for not getting screened, representing 109 (54%) of the responses. The next most frequent responses were "Never got around to it" (7%) and "I feel fine / I do not have symptoms" (7%).

SUMMARY

The interventions in this study draw on communication science to optimize message design, use communication technology to optimize message delivery, and include parallel content in both print and multimedia versions to allow comparison of format-related effects on both knowledge and screening rates. The interventions are brief and easy to use. Moreover, the multimedia and print tools are based on patient education programs that we developed with extensive attention to theory as well as community-member input. In research conducted at community health centers, our multimedia patient education program increased perceived risk, knowledge of relevant anatomy, knowledge of screening options, intention to discuss screening with the doctor, and willingness to consider each of the primary screening tests (Makoul et al., 2009). We are seeing similar results in this study and, thus far, it appears that the interventions are well accepted across literacy levels.

However, our preliminary data indicate that—despite the demonstrated quality of these interventions—physician recommendation is the most powerful vector for patient uptake of CRC screening. We delivered the patient education programs in the context of the clinic visit with the intention of giving patients sufficient knowledge to engage in discussions about CRC screening with their physicians. It appears that we are accomplishing that goal. But, at least in this sample of poor and underserved patients, it also appears highly unlikely that patients will initiate discussion of CRC screening. Although physicians at the study sites are periodically reminded to talk with patients about CRC screening, we expect that more robust physician-directed interventions need to be coupled with the patient education programs to achieve the ultimate goal of markedly increasing both communication about and completion of screening.

REFERENCES

American Cancer Society. (2006). *Cancer facts and figures 2006.* Atlanta, GA: Author.

American Cancer Society. (2009). *Cancer facts and figures 2009.* Atlanta, GA: Author.

American Cancer Society. (2010). American Cancer Society guidelines for the early detection of cancer. Retrieved April 24, 2011, from http://www.cancer.org/healthy/findcancerearly/cancerscreeningguidelines/american-cancer-society-guidelines-for-the-early-detection-of-cancer

American Cancer Society. (2011). *Can colorectal polyps and cancer be found early?* Retrieved April 24, 2011, from http://www.cancer.org/Cancer/Colonand RectumCancer/DetailedGuide/colorectal-cancer-detection

Anderson, L. M., & May, D. S. (1995). Has the use of cervical, breast, and colorectal cancer screening increased in the United States? *American Journal of Public Health, 85*(6), 840–842.

Baker, D. W., Gazmararian, J. A., Williams, M. V., Scott, T., Parker, R. M., Green, D., . . . Peel, J. (2002). Functional health literacy and the risk of hospital admission among Medicare managed care enrollees. *American Journal of Public Health, 92*(8), 1278–1283.

Baker, D. W., Williams, M. V., Parker, R. M., Gazmararian, J. A., & Nurss, J. (1999). Development of a brief test to measure functional health literacy. *Patient Education and Counseling, 38*(1), 33–42.

Baker, D. W., Wolf, M. S., Feinglass, J., Thompson, J. A., Gazmararian, J. A., & Huang, J. (2007). Health literacy and mortality among elderly persons. *Archives of Internal Medicibne, 167*(14), 1503–1509.

Behavioral Risk Factor Surveillance System Public Use Data Tape, 2004. (2005). National Center for Disease Prevention and Health Promotion, Centers for Disease Control and Prevention.

Blalock, S. J., DeVellis, B. M., Afifi, R. A., & Sandler, R. S. (1990). Risk perceptions and participation in colorectal cancer screening. *Health Psychology, 9*(6), 792–806.

Box, V., Nichols, S., Lallemand, R. C., Pearson, P., & Vakil, P. A. (1984). Haemoccult compliance rates and reasons for non-compliance. *Public Health, 98*(1), 16–25.

Brenes, G. A., & Paskett, E. D. (2000). Predictors of stage of adoption for colorectal cancer screening. *Preventive Medicine, 31*(4), 410–416.

Brown, M. L., Potosky, A. L., Thompson, G. B., & Kessler, L. G. (1990). The knowledge and use of screening tests for colorectal and prostate cancer: Data from the 1987 National Health Interview Survey. *Preventive Medicine, 19*(5), 562–574.

Bunn, J. Y., Bosompra, K., Ashikaga, T., Flynn, B. S., & Worden, J. K. (2002). Factors influencing intention to obtain a genetic test for colon cancer risk: A population-based study. *Preventive Medicine, 34*(6), 567–577.

Byers, T., Levin, B., Rothenberger, D., Dodd, G. D., & Smith, R. A. (1997). American Cancer Society guidelines for screening and surveillance for early detection of colorectal polyps and cancer: Update 1997. American Cancer Society Detection and Treatment Advisory Group on Colorectal Cancer. *CA: A Cancer Journal for Clinicians, 47*(3), 154–160.

Cameron, K. A., Francis, L., Wolf, M. S., Baker, D. W., & Makoul, G. (2007). Investigating Hispanic/Latino perceptions about colorectal cancer screening: A community-based approach to effective message design. *Patient Education and Counseling, 68*(2), 145–152.

Cella, D., Hernandez, L., Bonomi, A. E., Corona, M., Vaquero, M., Shiomoto, G., & Baez, L. (1998). Spanish language translation and initial validation of the functional assessment of cancer therapy quality-of-life instrument. *Medical Care, 36*(9), 1407–1418.

Centers for Disease Control and Prevention (CDC). (1999). Screening for colorectal cancer—United States. *Morbidity and Mortality Weekly Report, 48*, 116–121.

Coffield, A. B., Maciosek, M. V., McGinnis, J. M., Harris, J. R., Caldwell, M. B., Teutsch, S. M., . . . Haddix, A. (2001). Priorities among recommended clinical preventive services. *American Journal of Preventive Medicine, 21*(1), 1–9.

Davis, T. C., Dolan, N. C., Ferreira, M. R., Tomori, C., Green, K. W., Sipler, A. M., & Bennett, C. L. (2001). The role of inadequate health literacy skills in colorectal cancer screening. *Cancer Investigation, 19*(2), 193–200.

DeWalt, D. A., & Pignone, M. P. (2005). Reading is fundamental: The relationship between literacy and health. *Archives of Internal Medicine, 165*(17), 1943–1944.

Eremenco, S. L., Cella, D., & Arnold, B. J. (2005). A comprehensive method for the translation and cross-cultural validation of health status questionnaires. *Evaluation & the Health Professions, 28*(2), 212–232.

Farrands, P. A., Hardcastle, J. D., Chamberlain, J., & Moss, S. (1984). Factors affecting compliance with screening for colorectal cancer. *Community Medicine, 6*(1), 12–19.

Goldstein, M. M., & Messing, E. M. (1998). Prostate and bladder cancer screening. *Journal of the American College of Surgeons, 186*(1), 63–74.

Helm, J., Choi, J., Sutphen, R., Barthel, J. S., Albrecht, T. L., & Chirikos, T. N. (2003). Current and evolving strategies for colorectal cancer screening. *Cancer Control, 10*(3), 193–204.

Hesse, B. W., Nelson, D. E., Kreps, G. L., Croyle, R. T., Arora, N. K., Rimer, B. K., & Viswanath, K. (2005). Trust and sources of health information: The impact of the Internet and its implications for health care providers: Findings from the first Health Information National Trends Survey. *Archives of Internal Medicine, 165*(22), 2618–2624.

Hintze, J. (2005). *NCSS and PASS 2005.* Kaysville, UT: Number Cruncher Statistical Systems.

Holden, D. J., Harris, R., Porterfield, D.S., Jonas, D.E., Morgan, L.C., Reuland, D., . . . Lyda-McDonald, B. (2010). *Enhancing the use and quality of colorectal cancer screening. Evidence Report/Technology Assessment No.190. (Prepared by the RTI International–University of North Carolina Evidence-based Practice Center under Contract No. 290-2007-10056-I.) AHRQ Publication No. 10-E-002.* Rockville, MD: Agency for Healthcare Research and Quality.

Holmes-Rovner, M., Williams, G. A., Hoppough, S., Quillan, L., Butler, R., & Given, C. W. (2002). Colorectal cancer screening barriers in persons with low income. *Cancer Practice, 10*(5), 240–247.

Kelly, R. B., & Shank, J. C. (1992). Adherence to screening flexible sigmoidoscopy in asymptomatic patients. *Medical Care, 30*(11), 1029–1042.

Ko, C. W., Kreuter, W., & Baldwin, L. M. (2002). Effect of Medicare coverage on use of invasive colorectal cancer screening tests. *Archives of Internal Medicine, 162*(22), 2581–2586.

Leard, L. E., Savides, T. J., & Ganiats, T. G. (1997). Patient preferences for colorectal cancer screening. *Journal of Family Practice, 45*(3), 211–218.

Lennon, C., & Burdick, H. (2004). *The Lexile Framework as an approach for reading measurement and success.* Durham, NC: MetaMetrics, Inc.

Lent, L., Hahn, E., Eremenco, S., Webster, K., & Cella, D. (1999). Using cross-cultural input to adapt the Functional Assessment of Chronic Illness Therapy (FACIT) scales. *Acta Oncologica, 38*(6), 695–702.

Levin, B., & Murphy, G. P. (1992). Revision in American Cancer Society recommendations for the early detection of colorectal cancer. *CA: A Cancer Journal for Clinicians, 42*(5), 296–299.

Levin, B., Smith, R. A., Feldman, G. E., Colditz, G. A., Fletcher, R. H., Nadel, M., . . . National Colorectal Cancer Roundtable (2002). Promoting early detection tests for colorectal carcinoma and adenomatous polyps: A framework for action: The strategic plan of the National Colorectal Cancer Roundtable. *Cancer, 95*(8), 1618–1628.

Lieberman, D. A. (1995). Cost-effectiveness model for colon cancer screening. *Gastroenterology, 109*(6), 1781–1790.

Ling, B., Trauth, J. M., Jernigan, J., Whittle, J., Arndt, D., & Fine, M. J. (2003). Patient–provider communication for colorectal and prostate cancer screening. *Journal of General Internal Medicine, 18,* 268.

Ling, B. S., Moskowitz, M. A., Wachs, D., Pearson, B., & Schroy, P. C. (2001). Attitudes toward colorectal cancer screening tests. *Journal of General Internal Medicine, 16*(12), 822–830.

Makoul, G., Arntson, P., & Schofield, T. (1995). Health promotion in primary care: Physician–patient communication and decision making about prescription medications. *Social Science & Medicine, 41*(9), 1241–1254.

Makoul, G., Cameron, K. A., Baker, D. W., Francis, L., Scholtens, D., & Wolf, M. S. (2009). A multimedia patient education program on colorectal cancer screening increases knowledge and willingness to consider screening among Hispanic/ Latino patients. *Patient Education and Counseling, 76*(2), 220–226.

Makoul, G., Krupat, E., & Chang, C. H. (2007). Measuring patient views of physician communication skills: Development and testing of the Communication Assessment Tool. *Patient Education and Counseling, 67*(3), 333–342.

Malik, J., & Sansone, R. A. (2002). Physician compliance with colon cancer screening. *American Journal of Gastroenterology, 97*(4), 1078–1079.

Mandel, J. S., Bond, J. H., Church, T. R., Snover, D. C., Bradley, G. M., Schuman, L. M., & Ederer, F. (1993). Reducing mortality from colorectal cancer by screening for fecal occult blood. Minnesota Colon Cancer Control Study. *New England Journal of Medicine, 328*(19), 1365–1371.

McCaffery, K., Borril, J., Williamson, S., Taylor, T., Sutton, S., Atkin, W., & Wardle, J. (2001). Declining the offer of flexible sigmoidoscopy screening for bowel cancer: A qualitative investigation of the decision-making process. *Social Science & Medicine, 53*(5), 679–691.

Myers, R. E., Vernon, S. W., Tilley, B. C., Lu, M., & Watts, B. G. (1998). Intention to screen for colorectal cancer among white male employees. *Preventive Medicine, 27*(2), 279–287.

National Association of Community Health Centers. (2005). America's health centers: 40 years of commitment and success. Retrieved May 1, 2006, from http://www.nachc.com/research/Files/IntrotoHealthCenters8.05.pdf

Newcomb, P. A., Norfleet, R. G., Storer, B. E., Surawicz, T. S., & Marcus, P. M. (1992). Screening sigmoidoscopy and colorectal cancer mortality. *Journal of the National Cancer Institute, 84*(20), 1572–1575.

Parker, S. L., Davis, K. J., Wingo, P. A., Ries, L. A., & Heath, C. W., Jr. (1998). Cancer statistics by race and ethnicity. *CA: A Cancer Journal for Clinicians, 48*(1), 31–48.

Pfizer Clear Health Communication Initiative. (2003). *Prevalence calculator*. Retrieved May 15, 2006, from http://www.pfizerhealthliteracy.org/calculator.html

Pignone, M., Rich, M., Teutsch, S. M., Berg, A. O., & Lohr, K. N. (2002a). Screening for colorectal cancer in adults at average risk: A summary of the evidence for the U.S. Preventive Services Task Force. *Annals of Internal Medicine, 137*(2), 132–141.

Pignone, M., Rich, M., Teutsch, S. M., Berg, A. O., & Lohr, K. N. (2002b). Screening for colorectal cancer in adults. *Systematic Evidence Review No. 7* (No. 02-S003). Rockville, MD: Agency for Healthcare Research and Quality.

Price, J. H. (1993). Perceptions of colorectal cancer in a socioeconomically disadvantaged population. *Journal of Community Health, 18*(6), 347–362.

Rossi, P. H., & Freeman, H. E. (1989). *Evaluation: A systematic approach* (4th ed.). Newbury Park, CA: Sage Publications.

Schroy, P. C., III, Barrison, A. F., Ling, B. S., Wilson, S., & Geller, A. C. (2002). Family history and colorectal cancer screening: A survey of physician knowledge and practice patterns. *American Journal of Gastroenterology, 97*(4), 1031–1036.

Schroy, P. C., III, Geller, A. C., Crosier, W. M., Page, M., Sutherland, L., Holm, L. J., & Heeren, T. (2001). Utilization of colorectal cancer screening tests: A 1997 survey of Massachusetts internists. *Preventive Medicine, 33*(5), 381–391.

Scott, T. L., Gazmararian, J. A., Williams, M. V., & Baker, D. W. (2002). Health literacy and preventive health care use among Medicare enrollees in a managed care organization. *Medical Care, 40*(5), 395–404.

Selby, J. V., Friedman, G. D., Quesenberry, C. P., Jr., & Weiss, N. S. (1992). A case-control study of screening sigmoidoscopy and mortality from colorectal cancer. *New England Journal of Medicine, 326*(10), 653–657.

Shadish, W. R., Cook, T. D., & Leviton, L. C. (1991). *Foundations of program evaluation: Theories of practice.* Newbury Park, CA: Sage Publications.

Simon, J. B. (1998a). Fecal occult blood testing: Clinical value and limitations. *Gastroenterologist, 6*(1), 66–78.

Simon, J. B. (1998b). Should all people over the age of 50 have regular fecal occult-blood tests? Postpone population screening until problems are solved. *New England Journal of Medicine, 338*(16), 1151–1152.

Stenner, A. J. (1996). *Measuring reading comprehension with the Lexile Framework.* Durham, NC: MetaMetrics.

Stenner, A. J., Horablin, I., Smith, D. R., & Smith, M. (1988). *The Lexile Framework.* Durham, NC: MetaMetrics.

Taylor, M. L., & Anderson, R. (2002). Colorectal cancer screening: Physician attitudes and practices. *Wisconsin Medical Journal, 101*(5), 39–43.

U.S. Preventive Services Task Force. (2002). Screening for colorectal cancer: Recommendation and rationale. *Annals of Internal Medicine, 137*(2), 129–131.

U.S. Preventive Services Task Force. (2008). Screening for colorectal cancer: U.S. Preventive Services Task Force recommendation statement. *Annals of Internal Medicine, 149*(9), 627–637.

Vernon, S. W. (1997). Participation in colorectal cancer screening: A review. *Journal of the National Cancer Institute, 89*(19), 1406–1422.

Vernon, S. W., Myers, R. E., Tilley, B. C., & Li, S. (2001). Factors associated with perceived risk in automotive employees at increased risk of colorectal cancer. *Cancer Epidemiology, Biomarkers & Prevention, 10*(1), 35–43.

Weller, D. P., Owen, N., Hiller, J. E., Willson, K., & Wilson, D. (1995). Colorectal cancer and its prevention: Prevalence of beliefs, attitudes, intentions and behaviour. *Australian Journal of Public Health, 19*(1), 19–23.

Williams, M. V., Baker, D. W., Honig, E. G., Lee, T. M., & Nowlan, A. (1998). Inadequate literacy is a barrier to asthma knowledge and self-care. *Chest, 114*(4), 1008–1015.

Williams, M. V., Baker, D. W., Parker, R. M., & Nurss, J. R. (1998). Relationship of functional health literacy to patients' knowledge of their chronic disease. A study of patients with hypertension and diabetes. *Archives of Internal Medicine, 158*(2), 166–172.

Winawer, S., Fletcher, R., Rex, D., Bond, J., Burt, R., Ferrucci, J., . . . Gastrointestinal Consortium Panel. (2003). Colorectal cancer screening and surveillance: Clinical guidelines and rationale—Update based on new evidence. *Gastroenterology, 124*(2), 544–560.

Winawer, S. J., Flehinger, B. J., Schottenfeld, D., & Miller, D. G. (1993). Screening for colorectal cancer with fecal occult blood testing and sigmoidoscopy. *Journal of the National Cancer Institute, 85*(16), 1311–1318.

Winawer, S. J., Fletcher, R. H., Miller, L., Godlee, F., Stolar, M. H., Mulrow, C. D., . . . Meyer, R. J. (1997). Colorectal cancer screening: Clinical guidelines and rationale. *Gastroenterology, 112*(2), 594–642.

Winawer, S. J., & Shike, M. (1995). Prevention and control of colorectal cancer. In P. Greenwald, B. S. Kramer, & D. L. Weeds (Eds.), *Cancer prevention and control* (pp. 537–560). New York, NY: Marcel Dekker.

Winawer, S. J., Zauber, A. G., Ho, M. N., O'Brien, M. J., Gottlieb, L. S., Sternberg, S. S., Panish, J. F. (1993). Prevention of colorectal cancer by colonoscopic polypectomy. The National Polyp Study Workgroup. *New England Journal of Medicine, 329*(27), 1977–1981.

Wolf, M. S., Baker, D. W., & Makoul, G. (2007). Physician–patient communication about colorectal cancer screening. *Journal of General Internal Medicine, 22*(11), 1493–1499.

Wolf, M. S., Gazmararian, J. A., & Baker, D. W. (2005). Health literacy and functional health status among older adults. *Archives of Internal Medicine, 165*(17), 1946–1952.

Wolf, M. S., Satterlee, M., Calhoun, E. A., Skripkauskas, S., Fulwiler, D., Diamond-Shapiro, L., . . . Mukundan, P. (2006). Colorectal cancer screening among the medically underserved. *Journal of Health Care for the Poor and Underserved, 17*(1), 47–54.

Wolf, R. L., Zybert, P., Brouse, C. H., Neugut, A. I., Shea, S., Gibson, G., . . . Basch, C. E. (2001). Knowledge, beliefs, and barriers relevant to colorectal cancer screening in an urban population: A pilot study. *Family & Community Health, 24*(3), 34–47.

Wong, N. Y., Nenny, S., Guy, R. J., & Seow-Choen, F. (2002). Adults in a high-risk area are unaware of the importance of colorectal cancer: A telephone and mail survey. *Diseases of the Colon & Rectum, 45*(7), 946–950.

14

Partnering With Safety-Net Primary Care Clinics: A Model to Enhance Screening in Low-Income Populations—Principles, Challenges, and Key Lessons

Samantha Hendren, Sharon Humiston, and Kevin Fiscella

DISPARITIES IN CANCER SCREENING

Racial and ethnic minorities, particularly African Americans, have higher death rates from many types of cancer, including breast cancer (BC), cervical cancer (CC), and colorectal cancer (CRC) (American Cancer Society, 2009a, 2009b). Despite a higher risk of CC and CRC among poor and African American patients (American Cancer Society, 2009a; American Cancer Society, 2009b), these patients are paradoxically less likely to undergo cancer screening (American Cancer Society, 2009a, 2009b). Thus, poor, minority, and uninsured patients are more likely to be diagnosed at later stages (American Cancer Society, 2009a, 2009b). This is one important mechanism for observed disparities in cancer mortality.

Causes of Disparities in Screening

There is no single explanation for racial, ethnic, and socioeconomic disparities in cancer screening. Broadly speaking, screening disparities reflect the interaction of patient, clinician, practice systems, and societal factors. Patient-level barriers to cancer screening have been extensively studied. They include logistic barriers (distance, transportation, work, and child care constraints), financial barriers (out-of-pocket costs for visits and procedures, lost time from work), health literacy (knowledge, informed decision making), psychological barriers (self-efficacy, fear of discomfort and shame), and culture (language, beliefs, norms).

Physician-level barriers reflect a combination of competing demands and inadequate communication. Most physicians indicate that they recommend cancer screening, particularly breast, cervical, and colorectal screening (Klabunde et al., 2003; Yabroff et al., 2009). However, high rates of physician recommendations for screening are not supported by either chart documentation (DuBard, Schmid, Yow, Rogers, & Lawrence, 2008; Zack, DiBaise, Quigley, & Roy, 2001) or patient report (Seeff et al., 2004). Primary care is funneled through rushed visits, overcrowded with acute and preventive care needs (Fiscella & Epstein, 2008). Because the allowable visit time is brief, only approximately 5 minutes is devoted to the primary problem (Fiscella & Epstein, 2008). The remaining problems receive a minute or less of physician time. Rushed visits provide little time for informed patient decision making or discussion of new medications. Discussion of cancer screening is often deferred completely, due to competing demands from more pressing problems. When cancer screening is discussed, physicians frequently use medical jargon (Deuster, Christopher, Donovan, & Farrell, 2008) and there is often little time for informed decision making (Ling et al., 2008).

The structure of many medical practices also contributes to failures in cancer screening. In contrast, organized systems can improve cancer screening rates (Breen & Meissner, 2005; Thompson et al., 2000). Beneficial approaches include the use of flow sheets (Goodwin et al., 2001; Ruhe et al., 2005), prompts (Goodwin et al., 2001; Ruhe et al., 2005), and outreach (Dietrich et al., 2006), as well as physician delegation of roles (Thompson et al., 2000). Practices that adopt these typically have higher rates of cancer screening (Roetzheim et al., 2004). However, not all screening interventions are effective (Simon et al., 2010); context and details of design clearly make a difference, particularly for hard-to-reach patients.

Needs–Resources Mismatch

Cancer screening disparities reflect an imbalance between patient needs and the resources of the health care system to address those needs. Even in countries with National Health Insurance, such as the United Kingdom, care is often apportioned *inversely* according to need. This perverse phenomenon has been termed the "Inverse Care Law"(Hart, 1971). It holds with even greater force in the United States, due to much greater resource differentials among practices serving higher-need (low socioeconomic status) and lower-need (high socioeconomic status) patients (Zuckerman, Williams, & Stockley, 2009). Specifically, practices serving poor and minority patients are more likely to report that they lack critical resources (Bach, Pham, Schrag, Tate, & Hargraves, 2004), are less likely to have electronic medical records (EMRs) (Hing, Burt, & Woodwell, 2007), and tend to have more chaotic work environments (Varkey et al., 2009). There is a large evidence-base on interventions that promote cancer screening (Baron et al., 2008; Sabatino et al., 2008; Stone et al., 2002a). Disparities result, in part, from the lack of resources to implement these proven interventions within practices that serve poor and minority patients (Fiscella, 2007).

What resources are needed to decrease disparities in cancer screening? Simply stated, safety-net practices that care for poor and minority patients need the resources to:

1. Systematically identify patients who are past due for screening.
2. Reach out to these patients using modalities that are likely to reach diverse populations.
3. Utilize communication formats that are sensitive to differences in language and culture.
4. Promote clinician–patient discussions that facilitate informed decision making.

The Potential for Unintended Consequences

The notion of needs–resources mismatch suggests that the use of interventions that do not address structural inequities in the delivery of care will fail to alleviate cancer screening disparities. In fact, some interventions designed to promote overall cancer screening may, paradoxically, increase disparities in screening for some groups. For example, imagine an intervention designed to ensure that cancer screening would be discussed by clinicians at every annual health assessment. This would likely increase rates of informed decision making regarding cancer screening and probably boost rates for the practices that implemented this intervention. However, affluent patients are most likely to schedule annual health assessments and, thus, would be disproportionately advantaged by this intervention. Similarly, imagine that a private health plan elected to mail out reminders for cancer screening to its members. Such mailings would disproportionately benefit those who have private insurance, a current address recorded, written English proficiency, cultural beliefs that resonate with the content of the letter, and the ability to make the copayments needed for the screening. The notion of needs–resources mismatch suggests that addressing health care disparities requires that health care systems address many of these barriers to screening. Failure to do so will likely perpetuate, if not worsen, disparities.

The cancer screening intervention described in this chapter seeks to decrease cancer screening disparities by addressing the needs–resource mismatch described above, through progressively intensive outreach (also referred to as adaptive interventions) tailored to patients' needs within primary care practices that serve low-income patients. It is loosely modeled on a successful intervention to decreased immunization disparities in our community.

Addressing Needs–Resources Mismatch for Immunizations

A successful model for increasing immunization rates was based on the Task Force on Community Preventive Services recommendations. The Task Force disseminated broad categories of evidence-based strategies to improve immunization coverage in communities, including increasing community demand for vaccinations, enhancing access to vaccination services, and provider- or system-based interventions (Centers for Disease Control and Prevention, 2010). The Task Force recommended combination strategies including interventions from more than one of the above-mentioned categories. To that point, most studies of immunization strategies had used single interventions, and applied the interventions in single practices rather than across a community or network of practices. A tiered (adaptive) intervention integrating tracking for all patients, patient reminders and recall as needed, and outreach for hard-to-reach patients demonstrated improvement in immunization rates in children in the late 1990s (Rodewald et al., 1999) and has subsequently shown success in adult (Winston, Wortley, & Lees, 2006) and adolescent (Szilagyi et al., 2010) populations. We have adapted this approach to cancer screening.

There are several reasons why immunization is an appropriate model for cancer screening. First, the locus of the intervention for both activities is primary care practices' health promotion systems. Also, interventions used to promote immunizations seem to have generally similar effects for cancer screening (Stone et al., 2002). Finally, as with cancer screening, immunization rates are below the Healthy People 2010 goals (Department of Health and Human Services, 2010) and racial and ethnic disparities are notable (Centers for Disease Control and Prevention, 2009).

PRINCIPLES AND RATIONALE

Our American Cancer Society (ACS)–sponsored cancer screening project, "Get Screened," is modeled on a successful intervention for immunization promotion (Szilagyi et al., 2006, 2002). Specifically, it incorporates the following principles (see Table 14.1).

Principle 1: Focus on Primary Care

There are many different approaches to addressing cancer screening disparities. Our approach is to focus on primary care. The primary advantages to this approach include leveraging clinician–patient relationships, identification of patients using medical records, and focusing efforts on patients who have not been screened during the appropriate time interval. To conserve resources,

TABLE 14.1 Principles for Cancer Screening Promotion Intervention

OBJECTIVE: Decrease disparities in cancer screening

PRINCIPLES:
1. Focus on primary care
2. Focus on practices that care for underserved patients
3. Minimize disruption to practices while building partnerships
4. Employ multimodal, tailored approaches
5. Employ repeated, adaptive interventions
6. Simplify patient and clinician decision making in cancer screening
7. Establish community linkages
8. Use carefully selected, well-trained community health workers
9. Implement an organized tracking system
10. Adapt, learn, and adapt through PDSA cycles

PDSA = Plan-Do-Study-Act.

an outreach program needs to target active patients. However, determining whether a patient is still a member of the practice is often a confusing affair; the absence of a recent visit may not necessarily mean that the patient has left the practice. National data show that most of the adult population— particularly those aged 40 years and older—has visited a physician in the past year, but uninsured patients visit their physician much less often. Roughly 40% of all uninsured, nonelderly Whites and Blacks and 53% of Latinos without insurance report that they did not make such a visit in the past year, compared to 13%, 14%, and 21% of Whites, Blacks, and Latinos with insurance (Kaiser Family Foundation, 2010). These effects are minimized in communities with high rates of both health insurance and usual source of care, such as Monroe County, New York, the setting of our study. Here, 93% of residents over 50 years of age report having seen a physician in the past year (Monroe County Health Department, 2007). Community-based outreach (in contrast to primary care–based outreach) may be needed in communities where significant numbers of patients lack access to primary care.

Principle 2: Focus on Practices That Care for Underserved Patients

To increase community rates of cancer screening while decreasing screening disparities, it is best to intervene in a setting that cares for large numbers of poor and minority patients. Such patients tend to cluster within a relatively small number of primary care practices, particularly community health centers and hospital clinics (Forrest & Whelan, 2000). Nearly 80% of elderly Black patients with Medicare are cared for by 20% of physicians. This clustering likely reflects patterns of residential segregation, patterns of public insurance by race, ethnicity, and income, and physician attitudes. While racial, ethnic, and socioeconomic segregation in health care may have insidious effects, it also provides the opportunity to focus resources on practices with the greatest needs (Fiscella & Shin, 2005). Thus, improving cancer screening rates within practices that care for large numbers of poor and minority patients represents a key strategy for improving cancer screening rates at the population level. Because patients may be suspicious of interventions targeted only toward minorities or low-income patients, we believe that all eligible patients within these practices should be included.

Principle 3: Minimize Disruption to Practices While Building Partnerships

Primary care work has become increasingly stressful due to the pressing need to see a large number of patients, many with complex problems (Hoff, 2009). The work environment in safety-net practices is particularly stressful (Linzer et al., 2009). Because of this, systems designed to promote cancer screening must be minimally disruptive to the daily work of the practice (Fullerton, Aponte, Hopkins, Bragg, & Ballard, 2006; May et al., 2009). Successful implementation requires active engagement of clinicians and staff in the goal of promoting cancer screening, while at the same time working with them to implement systems and processes that require minimal effort and time.

Principle 4: Employ Multimodal, Tailored Approaches

Multimodal approaches generally improve cancer screening more than single interventions (Stone et al., 2002). This may be particularly true in inner-city practices (Crane, Leakey, Ehrsam, Rimer, & Warnecke, 2000; Sin & St. Leger, 1999). There are several reasons for this. Any one strategy may not reach all patients (Valanis et al., 2003). For example, telephone outreach will not be effective for patients without telephones or who have not provided current telephone numbers. The same applies to addresses or letters. Prompts at the point of care will miss those persons who do not present for a visit. Finally, some patients may respond more readily to one approach over the other. Physician recommendation is a particularly powerful intervention for promoting cancer screening (Han et al., 2009; Ling et al., 2009; Percac-Lima et al., 2009; Sohl & Moyer, 2007). Interventions that are tailored to the population and address financial and logistic barriers may be more effective, particularly in minority populations (Masi, Blackman, & Peek, 2007).

Principle 5: Employ Repeated, Adaptive Interventions

A single cancer screening message may not reach a patient when s/he is open to responding positively. Repeated outreach is based on sound behavior change theory, and empirically has been shown to be effective in promoting cancer screening in poor and minority populations (Crane et al., 2000; Dietrich et al., 2006). Repeated outreach increases participant response (Edwards et al., 2009), potentially by priming persons who do not respond to their first intervention. Optimally, more intensive, adaptive interventions are reserved for persons who fail to respond to previous low-intensity interventions (Gierisch et al., 2010).

Principle 6: Simplify Patient and Clinician Decision Making in Cancer Screening

The ACS currently recommends seven types of CRC screening modalities (McFarland et al., 2008). However, in practice, most primary care physicians recommend either some type of fecal occult blood testing (FOBT) or optical colonoscopy (Klabunde et al., 2009). Furthermore, providing clinicians and patients with a menu of seven options creates a burden of choice that may undermine informed decision making and patient autonomy (Ling et al., 2008; Schwartz, 2004), and may increase patient confusion (Jones, Vernon, & Woolf, 2010). Busy primary care clinicians do not have time to discuss the various merits and limitations of each of these approaches in the context of existing evidence. Simplification of patient and clinician decision making around CRC screening may help promote physicians' recommendations. Simplification can be accomplished by basing recommendations on options that are (1) widely available in the community, (2) covered by third-party payers, and (3) accurate. The use of FOBT screening during visits (i.e., following a rectal examination) and the use of low-sensitivity FOBT testing should be discouraged (Whitlock, Lin, Liles, Beil, & Fu, 2008). Because only average-risk patients are appropriately screened with FOBT testing, rapid risk stratification should be incorporated into screening tools for patients and clinicians.

Principle 7: Establish Community Linkages

Wagner's chronic care model is relevant to delivery of preventive services including cancer screening (Glasgow, Orleans, & Wagner, 2001). One of the core components of this model is community linkage. In the context of cancer screening, this means establishing partnerships with facilities that offer high-quality mammography and colonoscopy services. "High quality" refers not only to the technical quality of the service, but also to systems for efficiently communicating results to primary care clinicians and assistance in following up on abnormal results. Other key community partners are those that provide community outreach and payment for cancer screening to persons without health insurance. The most prominent examples are the National Breast and Cervical Cancer Early Detection Program (NBCCEDP) and the

Colorectal Cancer Control Program, which are explicitly designed to facilitate breast, cervical, and colorectal cancer screening among uninsured and underinsured women and men nationally (Khan et al., 2008). Unfortunately, these programs only serve a relatively small portion of eligible persons (Tangka et al., 2006). Strong bidirectional linkages between primary care practices and these programs—coupled with improved funding for these programs—could significantly improve cancer screening rates by addressing cost-related barriers.

Principle 8: Use Carefully Selected, Well-Trained Community Health Workers

Community health workers, sometimes referred to as patient navigators, have been shown to improve cancer screening (Christie et al., 2008; Jandorf, Gutierrez, Lopez, Christie, & Itzkowitz, 2005; Lewin et al., 2005; Percac-Lima et al., 2009). Training in cultural competence promotes worker self-efficacy (Yu et al., 2007). Proficiency in the language of the target population is also critical when face-to-face or telephone communication is needed (Wahab, Menon, & Szalacha, 2008). Use of motivational interviewing skills may facilitate adherence (Dietrich et al., 2006; Wahab et al., 2008), but requires training and supervision of the worker. Selection and training of the community health worker becomes paramount if the worker conducts in-reach (interventions delivered during patient visits) in addition to outreach (interventions delivered to patients in their homes through mail and telephone). In-reach requires collaboration with clinicians and office staff. It requires engagement of staff in the development of practical methods for implementing prompts at the point of care (Aspy, Enright, Halstead, Mold, & Oklahoma Physicians Resource/Research Network, 2008). Therefore, training community health workers to work effectively with practice staff (in-reach) and to communicate effectively with patients through outreach is critical (Nagykaldi, Mold, & Aspy, 2005).

Principle 9: Implement an Organized Tracking System

Identifying patients in need of screening, conducting outreach and in-reach, and implementing more intensive interventions for those who fail to respond each require strong skills in (1) organization, (2) use of appropriate health information technology, and (3) implementation of office systems. For example, organizational/tracking systems are needed at each step to:

- Identify patients who are overdue for screening and identify (in real time) patients who failed to respond to earlier outreach attempts.
- Conduct outreach by mail, telephone, or other means.

- Implement prompts to patients and clinicians at the point of care.
- Make screening appointments and track abnormal findings.

Optimally, these functions would be built-in functionality of practices' electronic medical records systems. Unfortunately, few current EMR systems possess all of these features (Shekelle, Morton, & Keeler, 2006).

Principle 10: Plan-Do-Study-Act (PDSA)

There is growing evidence that quality improvement in primary care is not a simple process (Carpiano, Flocke, Frank, & Stange, 2003; Crabtree, 2003; Solberg, 2007; Stroebel et al., 2005). Primary care practices can be understood as complex adaptive systems, each with its own unique culture, team functioning, and systems/tools for delivering preventive care (Carpiano et al., 2003). For this reason, interventions found to be effective in one practice often require considerable adaption to be effective in another (Cohen et al., 2008). One way to accomplish this adaptation is through a series of PDSA cycles (Speroff & O'Connor, 2004). Such cycles allow evidence-based interventions to be successfully adapted to local conditions. We piloted each intervention (e.g., point-of-care provider prompts) using PDSA cycles before starting the comprehensive program.

THE GET SCREENED PROGRAM

Overview

This ongoing project has three major aims:

1. To improve cancer screening for all patients within practices serving low-income and minority patients.
2. To eliminate racial and socioeconomic disparities in CRC and BC screening within the community.
3. To examine the impact of the intervention on practice- and community-wide disparities in cancer screening.

Consistent with principles 1 and 2, we focus on enrolling primary care safety-net practices within Rochester, New York. We use interventions that are minimally disruptive to the practice (principle 3) and are multimodal (principle 4). We repeat interventions among patients who remain unscreened after earlier interventions, using the tracking registry described below (principle 5). We incorporate a simplified CRC screening decision tool into our prompt for patients and clinicians (principle 6). We assist patients who are uninsured in completing the paperwork necessary to qualify for free screening (principle 7). We carefully select and train practice assistants in both the technical aspects of the work (running reports, using mail merges, and printing labels) in addition to motivational approaches to patients and staff (principle 8). We work collaboratively with the practices in real-time patient data tracking (principle 9). For example, we have arranged for persons within the practices who scan reports from colonoscopy, fecal immunochemical tests (FITs), and mammography into the EMR to also send us these results to inform our outreach efforts. We also use the practices' EMR-reporting functions to download data relevant to cancer screening and patient tracking for our program.

We will evaluate our intervention using a pragmatic, randomized trial design that seeks to identify the most effective interventions for improving cancer screening rates and reduces disparities in cancer screening (Zwarenstein et al., 2008). Pragmatic trials are designed primarily to inform clinical practice; these contrast with explanatory trials that are designed primarily to examine mechanisms and advance theory (Thorpe et al., 2009). Patients are the unit of randomization, based on the assumption that the interventions primarily target the patient and that sustained effects on clinician behavior will be small. Patients who serve as controls in the initial trial receive screening interventions in a subsequent time period. Sequential trials in different practice settings within the target community permit adaptation of trial design over time, to provide more informative findings (principle 10) (Brown et al., 2009).

Key Elements of the Intervention

Tracking Registry

A patient registry is a database tailored to capture, manage, and provide data on specific conditions necessary to provide organized chronic and preventive care using population health principles (Metzger, 2004). Registries facilitate identification of patients eligible for BC and CRC screening, generation of prompts at the point of care, and tracking of patients who remain unscreened. Registries also allow measurement of BC and CRC screening rates over time, for midpoint corrections and generation of feedback to providers. We reviewed commercially available tracking registries, but could not find one that met all our requirements, so we created a user-friendly electronic registry using Microsoft Access™. Research assistants enter data into the registry and generate reports by practice. Examples of our registry fields and other project materials described below are available by request from the authors.

Patient Recall

We have incorporated three types of recall messages to patients: automated telephone reminders (ATRs), personal letters, and personal telephone calls. ATRs show promise for improving cancer screening rates at low cost

(DeFrank et al., 2009; Feldstein et al., 2009). These are implemented either directly through programming of purchased software or through contract with commercial vendors, which our program used. ATRs require a list of patients' names and telephone numbers (exportable from a registry or directly through the practice management system) and a Health Insurance Portability and Accountability Act (HIPAA)-compliant script. The recorded message includes the patient's name in the message, and calls are repeated until the call is answered by a live person or an answering device.

Personal letters have a proven track record for improving rates of cancer screening (Stone et al., 2002), but are slightly more labor intensive and costly to implement. They can be implemented through mail merge using databases such as Microsoft Access or commercially available patient registries.

Personal telephone calls, particularly those that include elements of motivational interviewing and that are repeated over time, have been shown to increase rates of cancer screening among low-income patients (Dietrich et al., 2006). However, they are labor intensive to implement and language barriers should be anticipated. Often, many calls are required before the identified patient can be reached. In our program, a trained, nonmedical community health worker performs personal telephone calls to patients who request more information in response to ATRs or letters, and to patients who remain unscreened after lower-intensity interventions.

Point-of-Care Reminders

A systematic review of the literature shows that prompts at the point of care may improve cancer screening (Stone et al., 2002). However, contextual factors may also play a role. In a prior study, electronic prompts at the point of care failed to improve rates of CRC screening in a large group practice, possibly because clinicians began to doubt their reliability (Sequist, Zaslavsky, Marshall, Fletcher, & Ayanian, 2009). Similarly, we found that the clinicians in our participating practices felt that the electronic alerts in their EMRs were not user friendly. They seldom entered data necessary to trigger the prompts, or viewed the prompt when data had been entered for them. Consequently, we designed and implemented paper-based point-of-care prompts for both patients and clinicians. We adapted and piloted a low-literacy tool (previously used to prompt patients to request pneumococcal vaccination; Jacobson et al., 1999) for both mammography and CRC screening. The CRC prompt includes a brief summary of the advantages and limitations of colonoscopy and FOBT to facilitate patient decision making regarding screening modality (described below), and a brief screen for patient risk category. No more than three visit prompts are delivered for the same patient.

The outreach worker also delivers fecal immunochemical test kits to the practice and instructs medical assistants in how to counsel patients in their use and correct completion of the test requisition. These also are made available at the time of the patient visit.

Simplification of Clinician–Patient CRC Decision Making

As discussed above, we developed a tool designed to simplify CRC screening decision making. This tool lists advantages and limitations of optical colonoscopy compared with FOBT. Consistent with recent recommendations from the U.S. Preventive Services Task Force (USPSTF) (Whitlock et al., 2008), we encourage the practice to use high-sensitivity FOBT (either high-sensitivity, guaiac-based tests or FIT tests, rather than standard, lower-sensitivity FOBT tests). We worked with the locally prevalent health care systems and health plans to make these tests available and to approve reimbursement for them.

Engagement of Practices

It is axiomatic that any practice-based intervention requires engagement of clinicians and staff. Our approach is to meet first with practice leadership and next with all clinicians and staff. The purpose of these meetings is to solicit buy-in and prepare clinicians and staff for steps to follow: telephone calls and letters to patients (that will generate questions including requests for screening) and prompts at the point of care (that will generate the crucial provider recommendation). Clinician and staff buy-in are equally critical because each has necessary and unduplicated roles. For example, medical assistants are responsible for delivery of point-of-care prompts and for making sure that CRC screening kits are readily available to clinicians. Secretaries are responsible for generating referrals for mammography and colonoscopy.

Real-Time Feedback

Feedback loops are critical to quality improvement (Ozbolt et al., 2004). In this particular context, feedback loops are essential for triggering the next step (i.e., more intensive intervention). Feedback includes obtaining real-time data on recent screening to distinguish screened from unscreened patients. We do this via a system for accessing screening data as it comes into the practice, supplemented with chart audits.

The Role of Practice Assistants

Well-trained community health workers serve as "practice assistants" who conduct both outreach and in-reach. They create and mail recall letters, initiate and respond to patient calls, assist with screening referrals, work with staff to implement point-of-care prompts, and ensure that screening referral forms are available at the point of care. This work requires strong communication skills and the ability to engage patients and staff in screening-related activities.

Identification of Patients Who Are Past Due for Screening

We assist each participating practice, using their own billing data, to identify patients seen within the past 2 years who are the appropriate age (40–75 years for mammography and 50–75 years for CRC screening). Trained research assistants, working under business associate agreements with each practice, review charts for these patients and abstract relevant data using structured forms. The project coordinator ensures that inclusion criteria for participant eligibility are satisfied. Eligible participants within each practice are randomly assigned to an early intervention or delayed intervention group; the delayed intervention group serves as a control for the former, comparing cancer screening rates at the end of 1 year between patients who randomly were assigned to the intervention to the "delayed" group, which received usual care for the same time period.

Outcome Measures

We assess rates of cancer screening based on chart abstractions conducted by trained research assistants who use a structured abstraction instrument. Research assistants are blinded to the group to which participants are assigned. We assess the number of interventions that are delivered prior to screening and also the time and resources required to implement each component of the intervention, to assess the cost-effectiveness.

CHALLENGES AND LESSONS LEARNED

The Get Screened program has been implemented in several primary care practices in our community, and is ongoing. During early implementation, we have encountered challenges and learned valuable lessons.

Working Within Safety-Net Primary Care Practices

The basic structure of primary care, the 15-minute visit, does not lend itself well to preventive care due to competition from more acute and pressing needs. Therefore, any innovation that is introduced into primary care must take into account this context. We encountered clinicians who were motivated to increase cancer screening, but who also felt pressured to see more patients per day. This is not unlike the experience of primary care physicians in general (Hoff, 2009).

Team-based care, as envisioned within what is called the Patient Centered Medical Home (Bodenheimer, Grumbach, & Berenson, 2009), could help to offload some of the routine tasks from clinicians onto staff (Grumbach & Bodenheimer, 2002). This would free up the clinician to engage in more complex tasks such as informed decision making. Unfortunately, team-based care currently confronts several barriers to implementation in primary care. These include a paucity of open staff time, a lack of adequate health information technology (Bodenheimer & Grumbach, 2003), a lack of any mechanism for reimbursement for care provided outside of 15-min visits or by staff other than clinicians (Goroll, Berenson, Schoenbaum, & Gardner, 2007), and the need for a fundamental change in practice, from "clinicians doing it all" to "care that is shared between team members based on training" (Hoff, 2009; Schuetz, Mann, & Everett, 2010). Working for practical change in the current system, we found that we could not greatly increase the workload for either physicians or medical assistants and still enjoy their cooperation.

We also found that each practice is unique, with its own culture, procedures, and processes, and Health Information Technology with different functionalities (Grumbach & Mold, 2009). We are adapting the intervention to each practice.

The pressures above are encountered in all primary practices, but are exacerbated in safety-net practices. The combination of chronic understaffing and large numbers of patients with complex biomedical and psychosocial needs results in a particularly pressured work environment. Our experience is mirrored by a formal study of practice work environments (Varkey et al., 2009). Often, space is limited. A high turnover of ancillary staff requires frequent project orientations for new staff. While both clinicians and staff are motivated to promote cancer screening, tasks related to doing so compete with many other priorities for time and attention. Since current office personnel are simply not able to take on additional tasks, of necessity, our program relies on direct prompts to patients and on a project-dedicated practice assistant who promotes cancer screening.

Reaching and Engaging Practitioners

While practice leaders were genuinely enthusiastic about trying to improve cancer screening rates, it is difficult to get our message to all of the practitioners in large practices. We were warned that emails and written notices would be ineffective, and that a face-to-face presentation was required to obtain buy-in. We found that our presentations to the practice groups at their monthly meetings were attended by a minority of staff, and many practitioners continued to be unclear about the purpose of the alerts that they received. Resident and part-time clinicians tended to be absent from meetings. We, therefore, adopted a multimodal approach to communication, with emails, written notes, and periodic personal visits between study staff and practitioners to maintain interest and get feedback.

One of our most important lessons was that staff within practices may simply not attend to new tasks when already very busy. When our program was implemented, practice medical assistants were relied upon to flag charts with alerts. However, the consistency of this activity was affected by staff turnover, forgetfulness, or the feeling that they were too busy to add another task to their routine. Because point-of-care alerts were not being posted consistently and recent, published evidence shows the limited effectiveness of physician alerts for CRC screening (Sequist et al., 2009), the study was modified to emphasize direct-to-patient telephone and mailed alerts.

Health Information Technology

Less than half of the office-based physicians in the United States have any type of EMR (Hsiao et al., 2009). Furthermore, few EMRs offer adequate functionalities related to cancer screening (Taplin, Rollason, Camp, diDonato, & Maggenheimer, 2010). Even when these functionalities exist, they may not be used. For example, in one practice, most physicians reported that it simply took too much time to enter dates of screening into electronic alerts and to utilize electronic prevention reminders. Furthermore, even when electronic alerts are activated centrally, clinicians may ignore them (Sequist et al., 2009). For this reason, we piloted and implemented a combination of paper-based prompts for clinicians and patients.

The inefficiency of the EMR for finding screening information made it challenging for our study staff to "close the loop," that is, to determine whether a patient had completed screening. This was because the screening information was often scanned into the EMR in a variety of sections (e.g., with all test results, which then required manual searching), rather than into a single, clearly identified section for cancer screening results. Although study staff became facile at searching EMR records, it would not be feasible to replicate their effort in an underfunded primary care practice, raising questions of the program's sustainability. Nonetheless, we are optimistic that improved connectivity and functionalities in future Health Information Technology systems will automate many of these labor-intensive processes.

Access to Newer Screening Technology

Despite incentives to promote cancer screening, health plans may not always cover—and hospital laboratories may not always offer—newer, evidence-based testing. For example, the literature and the USPSTF promote the use of high-sensitivity (HS) FOBT including FIT (which has higher rates of adherence), compared to traditional FOBT testing (Whitlock et al., 2008). However, FIT was not covered by the area's major health plan at the time the project started and the hospital laboratory did not offer it. We addressed these challenges by: (1) persuading local health care insurers to cover FIT based on evidence of effectiveness and costs; (2) persuading local primary care practices, university colorectal surgeons and gastroenterologists, and, most importantly, the hospital clinical laboratory to emphasize HS-FOBT (both guiaic and FIT); and (3) promoting the use of FIT kits that patients mail to an outside laboratory as an option, given hospital bureaucratic delays in change over to HS-FOBT. We also use these same kits in mailings to selected patients, because this outside laboratory provides the kits free of charge. Billing is done when samples are received.

Barriers to Connecting Patients With Screening Programs

Working with patients in safety-net practices, we learned that a generous state program designed to pay for cancer screening for the uninsured was underutilized. The reason appeared to be that paperwork to connect patients with the program required a significant expenditure of time for both the referring medical provider and the patient. Practitioners' time constraints, as well as patient barriers (e.g., low literacy) helped to explain why the program had few people enrolled, despite the fact that patients reported cost as a barrier to cancer screening. We partnered with the state program to streamline their process for enrolling patients.

Contacting Patients

Reaching patients by telephone proved challenging. The telephone numbers recorded in the medical record often were incorrect, which may reflect lapses in updating procedures at registration and/or the secular trend toward dropping "land line" use. In many cases, our calls were answered by machine. We could not determine whether the message eventually reached the target patient. The challenges are summarized in Table 14.2.

CONCLUSIONS

In summary, the Get Screened program has been designed to address the challenging problem of cancer screening disparities identified in poor and minority patients. The program utilizes principles from a successful

TABLE 14.2 Challenges During Implementation of the Get Screened Program

- Primary care practitioners and staff are busy with competing demands.
- A multimodal approach to communication is required to educate and engage practitioners and staff across large practices that include part-time personnel and trainees, and frequent updates are needed, especially if staff turnover is high.
- The existence of an EMR does not ensure either delivery or response to cancer screening reminders.
- Health plans may not cover, and hospital laboratories may not perform, evidence-based cancer screening tests (e.g., FIT).
- Paperwork may prevent patients from using public health programs intended to ease financial barriers to cancer screening.
- It is difficult to contact patients and to be certain that you have succeeded in contacting them, given widespread call screening and the use of answering machines.

EMR = electronic medical record; FIT = fecal immunochemical testing.

immunization promotion program, including a partnership with primary care practices serving disadvantaged patients. The program has been tailored to each participating practice, and employs multimodal, repeated interventions. To address the mismatch between resources in the practices and high patient needs, carefully selected, well-trained, and supervised practice assistants perform much of the leg work. They provide increasingly intensive interventions to promote cancer screening amongst hard-to-reach patients. To address the lack of Health Information Technology support in these practices, a tracking registry has been designed and implemented. Simplified cancer screening decision-making tools have been designed, with input from the target community, to decrease practitioner and patient barriers to decision making. Finally, a PDSA approach has allowed the program to respond to challenges and improve over time. The long-term sustainability of this approach is unclear, and lower-intensity interventions are being piloted as well. The next step is for Get Screened to measure screening rates at the end of the early intervention period, to see whether this approach has improved screening rates in our community, and whether disparities by race and socioeconomic status have decreased.

Many of the challenges that we encountered reflect a broken system of primary care coupled with a lack of resources within safety-net practices. Potentially, the passage of the Patient Protection and Affordability Act in 2010 could begin to alleviate some of these challenges (Fiscella et al., 2011), through support for the Patient-Centered Medical Home, the promotion of meaningful Health Information Technology, the piloting of new payment models, increased funding for community health centers, and support for the establishment of community-based partnerships for underserved patients.

REFERENCES

American Cancer Society (2009a). *Cancer facts & figures for African Americans 2009–2010*. Atlanta, GA: Author.

American Cancer Society (2009b). *Cancer facts & figures for Hispanics/Latinos 2009–2011*. Atlanta, GA: Author.

Aspy, C. B., Enright, M., Halstead, L., Mold, J. W., & Oklahoma Physicians Resource/ Research Network. (2008). Improving mammography screening using best practices and practice enhancement assistants: An Oklahoma Physicians Resource/Research Network (OKPRN) study. *Journal of the American Board of Family Medicine, 21,* 326–333.

Bach, P. B., Pham, H. H., Schrag, D., Tate, R. C., & Hargraves, J. L. (2004). Primary care physicians who treat blacks and whites. *New England Journal of Medicine, 351,* 575–584.

Baron, R. C., Rimer, B. K., Breslow, R. A., Coates, R. J., Kerner, J., Melillo, S. . . . Task Force on Community Preventive Services. (2008). Client-directed interventions to increase community demand for breast, cervical, and colorectal cancer screening a systematic review. *American Journal of Preventive Medicine, 35* (1 Suppl.), S34–S55.

Bodenheimer, T., & Grumbach, K. (2003). Electronic technology: Aspark to revitalize primary care? *Journal of the American Medical Association, 290,* 259–264.

Bodenheimer, T., Grumbach, K., & Berenson, R. A. (2009). A lifeline for primary care. *New England Journal of Medicine, 360,* 2693–2696.

Breen, N., & Meissner, H. I. (2005). Toward a system of cancer screening in the United States: Trends and opportunities. *Annual Review of Public Health, 26,* 561–582.

Brown, C. H., Ten Have, T. R., Jo, B., Dagne, G., Wyman, P. A., Muthen, B., & Gibbons, R. D. (2009). Adaptive designs for randomized trials in public health. *Annual Review of Public Health, 30,* 1–25.

Carpiano, R. M., Flocke, S. A., Frank, S. H., & Stange, K. C. (2003). Tools, teamwork, and tenacity: An examination of family practice office system influences on preventive service delivery. *Preventive Medicine, 36,* 131–140.

Centers for Disease Control and Prevention. (2009). Influenza vaccination coverage among children and adults—United States, 2008–09 influenza season. *Morbidity & Mortality Weekly Report, 58,* 1091–1095.

Centers for Disease Control and Prevention. (2010). Vaccine—Preventable diseases: Improving coverage in children, adolescents, and adults. In *Guide to community preventive services*. Atlanta, GA: Author. Retrieved July 1, 2011, from http://www.thecommunityguide.org

Christie, J., Itzkowitz, S., Lihau-Nkanza, I., Castillo, A., Redd, W., & Jandorf, L. (2008). A randomized controlled trial using patient navigation to increase colonoscopy screening among low-income minorities. *Journal of the National Medical Association, 100,* 278–284.

Cohen, D. J., Crabtree, B. F., Etz, R. S., Balasubramanian, B. A., Donahue, K. E., Leviton, L. C., . . . Green. L. W. (2008). Fidelity versus flexibility: Translating evidence-based research into practice. *American Journal of Preventive Medicine, 35*(5 Suppl.), S381–S389.

Crabtree, B. F. (2003). Primary care practices are full of surprises! *Health Care Management Review, 28,* 279–283.

Crane, L. A., Leakey, T. A., Ehrsam, G., Rimer, B. K., & Warnecke, R. B. (2000). Effectiveness and cost-effectiveness of multiple outcalls to promote mammography among low-income women. *Cancer Epidemiology, Biomarkers & Prevention, 9,* 923–931.

DeFrank, J. T., Rimer, B. K., Gierisch, J. M., Bowling, J. M., Farrell, D., & Skinner, C. S. (2009). Impact of mailed and automated telephone reminders on receipt of repeat mammograms: Arandomized controlled trial. *American Journal of Preventive Medicine, 36,* 459–467.

Department of Health and Human Services. (2011). *Healthy People 2010.* Objective IID-12. Increase the percentage of children and adults who are vaccinated annually against seasonal influenza. Retrieved July 1, 2010, from http://www.healthypeople.gov/2020/topicsobjectives2020/objectiveslist.aspx?topicid=23

Deuster, L., Christopher, S., Donovan, J., & Farrell, M. (2008). A method to quantify residents' jargon use during counseling of standardized patients about cancer screening. *Journal of General Internal Medicine, 23,* 1947–1952.

Dietrich, A. J., Tobin, J. N., Cassells, A., Robinson, C. M., Greene, M. A., Sox, C. H., . . . Younge, R. G. (2006). Telephone care management to improve cancer screening among low-income women: A randomized, controlled trial. *Annals of Internal Medicine, 144,* 563–571.

DuBard, C. A., Schmid, D., Yow, A., Rogers, A. B., & Lawrence, W. W. (2008). Recommendation for and receipt of cancer screenings among medicaid recipients 50 years and older. *Archives of Internal Medicine, 168,* 2014–2021.

Edwards, P. J., Roberts, I., Clarke, M. J., Diguiseppi, C., Wentz, R., Kwan, I., . . . Pratap, S. (2009). Methods to increase response to postal and electronic questionnaires. *Cochrane Database of Systematic Reviews, (3),* MR000008.

Feldstein, A. C., Perrin, N., Rosales, A. G., Schneider, J., Rix, M. M., Keels, K., . . . Glasgow, R. E. (2009). Effect of a multimodal reminder program on repeat mammogram screening. *American Journal of Preventive Medicine, 37,* 94–101.

Fiscella, K. (2007). Eliminating disparities in health care through quality improvement. In R. Williams (Ed.), *Eliminating healthcare disparities in America: Beyond the IOM report.* Totowa, NJ: Humana Press.

Fiscella, K., & Epstein, R. M. (2008). So much to do, so little time: Care for the socially disadvantaged and 15-minute visits. *Archives of Internal Medicine, 168,* 1843–1852.

Fiscella, K., Humiston, S., Hendren, S., Winters, P., Jean-Pierre, P., Idris, A., & Ford, P. (2011). Eliminating disparities in cancer screening and follow-up of abnormal results: What will it take? *Journal of Health Care for the Poor and Underserved, 22(1),* 83–100.

Fiscella, K., & Shin, P. (2005). The inverse care law: Implications for healthcare of vulnerable populations. *Journal of Ambulatory Care Management, 28,* 304–312.

Forrest, C. B., & Whelan, E. M. (2000). Primary care safety-net delivery sites in the United States: A comparison of community health centers, hospital outpatient departments, and physicians' offices. *Journal of the American Medical Association, 284,* 2077–2083.

Fullerton, C., Aponte, P., Hopkins, R., Bragg, D., & Ballard, D. J. (2006). Lessons learned from pilot site implementation of an ambulatory electronic health record. *Baylor University Medical Center Proceedings, 19,* 303–310.

Gierisch, J. M., DeFrank, J. T., Bowling, J. M., Rimer, B. K., Matuszewski, J. M., Farrell, D., & Skinner, C. S. (2010). Finding the minimal intervention needed for sustained mammography adherence. *American Journal of Preventive Medicine, 39,* 334–344.

Glasgow, R. E., Orleans, C. T., & Wagner, E. H. (2001). Does the chronic care model serve also as a template for improving prevention? *Milbank Quarterly, 79,* 579–612.

Goodwin, M. A., Zyzanski, S. J., Zronek, S., Ruhe, M., Weyer, S. M., Konrad, N., . . . Stange, K. C. (2001). A clinical trial of tailored office systems for preventive service delivery. The Study to Enhance Prevention by Understanding Practice (STEP-UP). *American Journal of Preventive Medicine, 21,* 20–28.

Goroll, A. H., Berenson, R. A., Schoenbaum, S. C., & Gardner, L. B. (2007). Fundamental reform of payment for adult primary care: Comprehensive payment for comprehensive care. *Journal of General Internal Medicine, 22,* 410–415.

Grumbach, K., & Bodenheimer, T. (2002). A primary care home for Americans: Putting the house in order. *Journal of the American Medical Association, 288,* 889–893.

Grumbach, K., & Mold, J. W. (2009). A health care cooperative extension service: Transforming primary care and community health. *Journal of the American Medical Association, 301,* 2589–2591.

Han, H. R., Lee, J. E., Kim, J., Hedlin, H. K., Song, H., & Kim, M. T. (2009). A meta-analysis of interventions to promote mammography among ethnic minority women. *Nursing Research, 58,* 246–254.

Hart, J. T. (1971). The inverse care law. *Lancet, 1,* 405–412.

Hing, E. S., Burt, C. W., & Woodwell, D. A. (2007). Electronic medical record use by office-based physicians and their practices: United States, 2006. *Advance Data,*(393), 1–7.

Hoff, T. (2009). *Practice under pressure: Primary care physicians and their medicine in the twenty-first century.* Piscataway, NJ: Rutgers University Press.

Hsiao, C.-J., Beatty, P. C., Hing, E. S., Woodwell, D. A., Rechtsteiner, E. A., & Sisk, J. E. (2009). *Electronic medical record/electronic health record use by office-based physicians: United States, 2008 and preliminary 2009.* Hyattsville, MD: National Center for Health Statistics, Centers for Disease Control and Prevention.

Jacobson, T. A., Thomas, D. M., Morton, F. J., Offutt, G., Shevlin, J., & Ray, S. (1999). Use of a low-literacy patient education tool to enhance pneumococcal vaccination rates. A randomized controlled trial. *Journal of the American Medical Association, 282,* 646–650.

Jandorf, L., Gutierrez, Y., Lopez, J., Christie, J., & Itzkowitz, S. H. (2005). Use of a patient navigator to increase colorectal cancer screening in an urban neighborhood health clinic. *Journal of Urban Health, 82,* 216–224.

Jones, R. M., Vernon, S. W., & Woolf, S. (2010). Is discussion of colorectal cancer screening options associated with heightened patient confusion? *Cancer Epidemiology, Biomarkers & Prevention, 19*(11), 2821–2825.

Kaiser Family Foundation. (2010). *No doctor visit in past year for nonelderly adults by race/ethnicity and insurance status, 2005–2006.* Retrieved July 1, 2011, from http://facts.kff.org/chart.aspx?ch=369

Khan, K., Curtis, C. R., Ekwueme, D. U., Stokley, S., Walker, C., Roland, K., . . . Saraiya, M. (2008). Preventing cervical cancer: Overviews of the National Breast and Cervical Cancer Early Detection Program and 2 US immunization programs. *Cancer, 113*(10 Suppl.), 3004–3012.

Klabunde, C. N., Frame, P. S., Meadow, A., Jones, E., Nadel, M., & Vernon, S. W. (2003). A national survey of primary care physicians' colorectal cancer screening recommendations and practices. *Preventive Medicine, 36,* 352–362.

Klabunde, C. N., Lanier, D., Nadel, M. R., McLeod, C., Yuan, G., & Vernon, S. W. (2009). Colorectal cancer screening by primary care physicians: Recommendations and practices, 2006–2007. *American Journal of Preventive Medicine, 37,* 8–16.

Lewin, S. A., Dick, J., Pond, P., Zwarenstein, M., Aja, G., van, Wyk, B., . . . Patrick, M. (2005). Lay health workers in primary and community health care. *Cochrane Database of Systematic Reviews,* (1), CD004015.

Ling, B. S., Schoen, R. E., Trauth, J. M., Wahed, A. S., Eury, T., Simak, D. M., . . . Weissfeld, J. L. (2009). Physicians encouraging colorectal screening: A randomized controlled trial of enhanced office and patient management on compliance with colorectal cancer screening. *Archives of Internal Medicine, 169,* 47–55.

Ling, B. S., Trauth, J. M., Fine, M. J., Mor, M. K., Resnick, A., Braddock, C. H., . . . Whittle, J. (2008). Informed decision-making and colorectal cancer screening: Is it occurring in primary care? *Medical Care, 46* (9 Suppl. 1), S23–S29.

Linzer, M., Manwell, L. B., Williams, E. S., Bobula, J. A., Brown, R. L., Varkey, A. B., . . . MEMO (Minimizing Error, Maximizing Outcome) Investigators. (2009). Working conditions in primary care: Physician reactions and care quality. *Annals of Internal Medicine, 151,* 28–36.

Masi, C. M., Blackman, D. J., & Peek, M. E. (2007). Interventions to enhance breast cancer screening, diagnosis, and treatment among racial and ethnic minority women. *Medical Care Research & Review, 64*(5 Suppl.), 195S–242S.

May, C. R., Mair, F., Finch, T., Macfarlane, A., Dowrick, C., Treweek, S., . . . Montoir, V. M. (2009). Development of a theory of implementation and integration: Normalization Process Theory. *Implementation Science, 4,* 29.

McFarland, E. G., Levin, B., Lieberman, D. A., Pickhardt, P. J., Johnson, C. D., Glick, S. N., . . . American College of Radiology (2008). Revised colorectal screening guidelines: Joint effort of the American Cancer Society, U.S. Multisociety Task Force on Colorectal Cancer, and American College of Radiology. *Radiology, 248,* 717–720.

Metzger, J. (2004). *Using computerized registries in chronic disease care.* Oakland, CA: California HealthCare Foundation.

Monroe County Health Department. (2007). *Monroe County Adult Survey Health Report 2006.* Rochester, NY: Monroe County Health Department.

Nagykaldi, Z., Mold, J. W., & Aspy, C. B. (2005). Practice facilitators: A review of the literature. *Family Medicine, 37,* 581–588.

Ozbolt, J., Ozdas, A., Waitman, L. R., Smith, J. B., Brennan, G. V., & Miller, R. A. (2004). Decision support for patient care: Implementing cybernetics. *Studies in Health Technology & Informatics, 107,* 1–3.

Percac-Lima, S., Grant, R. W., Green, A. R., Ashburner, J. M., Gamba, G., Oo, S., . . . Atlas, S. J. (2009a). A culturally tailored navigator program for colorectal cancer screening in a community health center: A randomized, controlled trial. *Journal of General Internal Medicine, 24,* 211–217.

Rodewald, L. E., Szilagyi, P. G., Humiston, S. G., Barth, R., Kraus, R., & Raubertas, R. F. (1999). A randomized study of tracking with outreach and provider prompting to improve immunization coverage and primary care. *Pediatrics, 103,* 31–38.

Roetzheim, R. G., Christman, L. K., Jacobsen, P. B., Cantor, A. B., Schroeder, J., Abdulla, R., . . . Krischer, J. P. (2004). A randomized controlled trial to increase cancer screening among attendees of community health centers. *Annals of Family Medicine, 2,* 294–300.

Ruhe, M. C., Weyer, S. M., Zronek, S., Wilkinson, A., Wilkinson, P. S., & Stange, K. C. (2005). Facilitating practice change: Lessons from the STEP-UP clinical trial. *Preventive Medicine, 40,* 729–734.

Sabatino, S. A., Habarta, N., Baron, R. C., Coates, R. J., Rimer, B. K., Kerner, J., . . . Task Force on Community Preventive Services. (2008). Interventions to increase recommendation and delivery of screening for breast, cervical, and colorectal cancers by healthcare providers systematic reviews of provider assessment and feedback and provider incentives. *American Journal of Preventive Medicine, 35*(1 Suppl.), S67–S74.

Schuetz, B., Mann, E., & Everett, W. (2010). Educating health professionals collaboratively for team-based primary care. *Health Affairs, 29,* 1476–1480.

Schwartz, B. (2004). *The paradox of choice: Why more is less.* New York, NY: HarperCollins.

Seeff, L. C., Nadel, M. R., Klabunde, C. N., Thompson, T., Shapiro, J. A., Vernon, S. W., & Coates, R. J. (2004). Patterns and predictors of colorectal cancer test use in the adult U.S. population. *Cancer, 100,* 2093–2103.

Sequist, T. D., Zaslavsky, A. M., Marshall, R., Fletcher, R. H., & Ayanian, J. Z. (2009). Patient and physician reminders to promote colorectal cancer screening: A randomized controlled trial. *Archives of Internal Medicine, 169,* 364–371.

Shekelle, P. G., Morton, S. C., & Keeler, E. B. (2006). Costs and benefits of health information technology. *Evidence Report/Technology Assessment,* (132), 1–71.

Simon, S. R., Zhang, F., Soumerai, S. B., Ensroth, A., Bernstein, L., Fletcher, R. H., & Ross-Degnan, D. (2010). Failure of automated telephone outreach with speech recognition to improve colorectal cancer screening: A randomized controlled trial. *Archives of Internal Medicine, 170,* 264–270.

Sin, J. P., & St. Leger, A. S. (1999). Interventions to increase breast screening uptake: Do they make any difference? *Journal of Medical Screening, 6,* 170–181.

Sohl, S. J., & Moyer, A. (2007). Tailored interventions to promote mammography screening: A meta-analytic review. *Preventive Medicine, 45,* 252–261.

Solberg, L. I. (2007). Improving medical practice: A conceptual framework. *Annals of Family Medicine, 5,* 251–256.

Speroff, T., & O'Connor, G. T. (2004). Study designs for PDSA quality improvement research. *Quality Management in Health Care, 13,* 17–32.

Stone, E. G., Morton, S. C., Hulscher, M. E., Maglione, M. A., Roth, E. A., Grimshaw, J. M., . . . Shekelle, P. G. (2002a). Interventions that increase use of adult immunization and cancer screening services: Ameta-analysis. *Annals of Internal Medicine, 136,* 641–651.

Stroebel, C. K., McDaniel, R. R., Jr., Crabtree, B. F., Miller, W. L., Nutting, P. A., & Stange, K. C. (2005). How complexity science can inform a reflective process for improvement in primary care practices. *Joint Commission Journal on Quality & Patient Safety, 31,* 438–446.

Szilagyi, P. G., Humiston, S. G., Sandler, M., Gallivan, S., Albertin, C., & Blumkin, A. (2010). *Reminder/recall outreach for adolescent immunization: A RCT.* Pediatric Academic Society platform presentation, Vancouver, BC.

Szilagyi, P. G., Schaffer, S., Barth, R., Shone, L. P., Humiston, S. G., Ambrose, S., & Averhoff, F. (2006). Effect of telephone reminder/recall on adolescent immunization and preventive visits: Results from a randomized clinical trial. *Archives of Pediatrics & Adolescent Medicine, 160,* 157–163.

Szilagyi, P. G., Schaffer, S., Shone, L., Barth, R., Humiston, S. G., Sandler, M., & Rodewald, L. E. (2002). Reducing geographic, racial, and ethnic disparities in childhood immunization rates by using reminder/recall interventions in urban primary care practices. *Pediatrics, 110,* e58.

Tangka, F. K., Dalaker, J., Chattopadhyay, S. K., Gardner, J. G., Royalty, J., Hall, I. J., . . . Coates, R. J. (2006). Meeting the mammography screening needs of underserved women: The performance of the National Breast and Cervical Cancer Early Detection Program in 2002–2003 (United States). *Cancer Causes & Control, 17,* 1145–1154.

Taplin, S. H., Rollason, D., Camp, A., diDonato, K., & Maggenheimer, E. (2010). Imagining an electronic medical record for turning cancer screening knowledge into practice. *American Journal of Preventive Medicine, 38,* 89–97.

Thompson, N. J., Boyko, E. J., Dominitz, J. A., Belcher, D. W., Chesebro, B. B., Stephens, L. M., & Chapko, M. K. (2000). A randomized controlled trial of a clinic-based support staff intervention to increase the rate of fecal occult blood test ordering. *Preventive Medicine, 30,* 244–251.

Thorpe, K. E., Zwarenstein, M., Oxman, A. D., Treweek, S., Furberg, C. D., Altman, D. G., . . . Chalkidou, K. (2009). A pragmatic–explanatory continuum indicator summary (PRECIS): A tool to help trial designers. *Journal of Clinical Epidemiology, 62,* 464–475.

Valanis, B., Whitlock, E. E., Mullooly, J., Vogt, T., Smith, S., Chen, C., & Glasgow, R. E. (2003). Screening rarely screened women: Time-to-service and 24-month outcomes of tailored interventions. *Preventive Medicine, 37,* 442–450.

Varkey, A. B., Manwell, L. B., Williams, E. S., Ibrahim, S. A., Brown, R. L., Bobula, J. A., . . . MEMO Investigators. (2009). Separate and unequal: Clinics where minority and nonminority patients receive primary care. *Archives of Internal Medicine, 169,* 243–250.

Wahab, S., Menon, U., & Szalacha, L. (2008). Motivational interviewing and colorectal cancer screening: A peek from the inside out. *Patient Education & Counseling, 72,* 210–217.

Whitlock, E. P., Lin, J. S., Liles, E., Beil, T. L., & Fu, R. (2008). Screening for colorectal cancer: A targeted, updated systematic review for the U.S. Preventive Services Task Force. *Annals of Internal Medicine, 149,* 638–658.

Winston, C. A., Wortley, P. M., & Lees, K. A. (2006). Factors associated with vaccination of Medicare beneficiaries in five U.S. communities: Results from the racial and ethnic adult disparities in immunization initiative survey, 2003. *Journal of the American Geriatrics Society, 54,* 303–310.

Yabroff, K. R., Saraiya, M., Meissner, H. I., Haggstrom, D. A., Wideroff, L., Yuan, G., . . . Coughlin, S. S. (2009). Specialty differences in primary care physician reports of Papanicolaoutest screening practices: A national survey, 2006 to 2007. *Annals of Internal Medicine, 151,* 602–611.

Yu, M. Y., Song, L., Seetoo, A., Cai, C., Smith, G., & Oakley, D. (2007). Culturally competent training program: Akey to training lay health advisors for promoting breast cancer screening. *Health Education & Behavior, 34,* 928–941.

Zack, D. L., DiBaise, J. K., Quigley, E. M., & Roy, H. K. (2001). Colorectal cancer screening compliance by medicine residents: Perceived and actual. *American Journal of Gastroenterology, 96,* 3004–3008.

Zuckerman, S., Williams, A. F., & Stockley, K. E. (2009). Trends in Medicaid physician fees, 2003–2008. *Health Affairs, 28,* w510–w519.

Zwarenstein, M., Treweek, S., Gagnier, J. J., Altman, D. G., Tunis, S., Haynes, B., . . . Moher, D. (2008). Improving the reporting of pragmatic trials: An extension of the CONSORT statement. *British Medical Journals, 337,* a2390.

15

Hope and Life: Healthy Families Begin With Healthy Women

Deborah O. Erwin, Lina Jandorf, Linda D. Thélémaque,
Michelle Treviño, Frances G. Saad-Harfouche, Anabella G. Castillo,
Zoran Bursac, Jomary Colón, LeaVonne Pulley, Elvira Aguirre
Wendrell, María Hannigan, Elsa Iris Mendez, and Carol Horowitz

During the 1990s, the United States experienced a dramatic increase in immigration of Hispanic peoples, accounting for a significant proportion (40%) of the current Hispanic population. Hispanics are now considered to be the largest minority group in the United States, comprising over 42.7 million of the population (American Cancer Society, 2009). The diverse groups of women commonly aggregated into this single category, labeled "Latinas or Hispanic" in the United States, continue to be less likely to have undergone mammography, with 59.6% of Latina women aged 40 and older completing the examination within the past 2 years, compared to 68.1% of non-Latina Whites (American Cancer Society, 2009). Mexican (56.2%) and Puerto Rican women (57.8%), specifically, have lower rates (American Cancer Society, 2009). In the U.S., breast cancer is the most frequently diagnosed cancer in Latinas, although the incidence rate of breast cancer is 27% lower for Latinas (90.2 per 100,000) than for White non-Latina women (126.9 per 100,000) (American Cancer Society, 2009). This may be due to protective reproductive patterns (lower age at first birth and more children) or the possibility that many Latinas are not diagnosed at all due to low mammography utilization (American Cancer Society, 2009). Latinas are reported to have more advanced cancer with larger tumors and/or metastatic disease at the time of diagnosis, correlated with a poorer prognosis and a lower chance of successful treatment (Joslyn, Foote, Nasseri, Coughlin, & Howe, 2005; Li, Malone, & Daling, 2003). Low levels of mammography utilization and delayed follow-up of abnormal results might explain why Latina women are nearly 20% more likely to die of breast cancer than non-Latina White women diagnosed at a similar age and stage (American Cancer Society, 2009).

With regard to cervical cancer, incident rates for Latinas are more than 50% higher than those for White women (8.2 per 100,000 women for Caucasians vs. 13.2 per 100,000 for Hispanics), despite the decrease in rates of new cases of invasive cervical cancer over the past 30 years of about 50% (American Cancer Society, 2009). Only 74.6% of Latinas (aged 18 and older) have had a Pap test within the past 3 years, compared with 81.4% of non-Latina White women. Central and South American women are the least likely to have had a recent Pap test (71.3%). These higher incidences of cervical cancer and lower screening rates for both breast and cervical cancer indicate the need to develop and disseminate culturally and linguistically appropriate programs to promote cancer screening and ultimately help reduce survival disparities in this growing immigrant population.

Undoubtedly, these disparities are complicated by aggregating very different ethnic subgroups into a monolithic group reported as "Latina." For example, Vargas Bustamante, Chen, Rodriguez, Rizzo, and Ortega (2010) demonstrate that Latinos of Mexican and Central/South American origin are much less likely to receive guideline-recommended preventive care services than non-Latino Whites and other Latino subgroups. Puerto Ricans, Cubans, Dominicans, and other Latinos have less pronounced disparities for most preventive services, which are largely explained by socioeconomic, health system, and policy factors (Vargas Bustamante et al., 2010). Cross-sectional analysis of the 2000 National Health Interview Survey data shows that Latinas are less likely to be screened by mammography, but adjusting for health insurance attenuates these data (Echeverria & Carrasquillo, 2006). Latinas most likely to respond to outreach efforts in a Washington, DC study were those who had had a previous mammogram or other screening (e.g., Pap) (Warren, Londoño, Wessel, & Warren, 2006). Moreover, these participants were primarily from Central and South America, 43% had university-level educations, and 56% had been in the United States for over 10 years. Reaching recent, unscreened immigrants and those with fewer resources continues to be challenging. Suggested solutions for improving screening rates include removing economic concerns, and providing care and education through bilingual staff in culturally appropriate environments (Mayo, Erwin, & Spitler, 2003; Warren et al., 2006).

A comparison between African American and Latina women regarding knowledge and participation in mammography screening demonstrated how little we understand the cultural and ethnic variations that impact disparities (Darnell, Chang, & Calhoun, 2006). These results showed that knowledge and awareness about breast cancer and mammography correlated with screening for African American women, but not for Latinas. These findings suggest that acculturation and citizenship status, language, or various cultural factors may further complicate access to services and trump the potential impact of knowledge to positively increase screening. Mexican immigrant women are often reported to still hold what has been described as "fatalistic" views of breast cancer, where fatalism is defined as "the belief that death is inevitable when cancer is present" (Powe, 1995, p. 385). These views may be influenced by negative experiences in their home country, and cancer awareness may be much lower for this subgroup as compared to other women (Schettino, Hernández-Valero, Moguel, Hajek, & Jones, 2006). Moreover, many outreach efforts and educational campaigns are not reaching those whose primary language is Spanish, and language barriers continue to be a major factor impeding adequate health communication, contributing to health disparities for many immigrants (Jacobs, Karavolos, Rathouz, Ferris, & Powell, 2005). Demographic changes, cancer screening, and incidence and mortality rates, together with current research findings, clearly demonstrate that improved culturally appropriate interventions are needed to reduce the disparities in breast and cervical cancer for the diverse groups of women categorized as Latina.

THE DEVELOPMENT OF ESPERANZA Y VIDA

The intervention framework for the *Esperanza y Vida* (Hope and Life) model was adopted from the Witness Project, an evidence-based, culturally competent, faith- and community-based breast and cervical cancer education program designed to meet the specific cultural, educational, knowledge, and learning-style levels of underserved African American women (http://rtips.cancer.gov/rtips/index.do) (Erwin, 2009). Survivors and lay health advisors operate as teams to provide educational, inspirational, and empowerment messages to African American church and community groups, to increase breast self-examination (BSE), mammography, clinical breast exams (CBE), and Pap tests (Erwin, Spatz, & Stotts, 1999). The importance and credibility of survivors as messengers (Kreuter et al., 2007) and peer-to-peer communication of health messages, as in the case of community health workers or lay health advisors, is well documented for African American and minority communities (Carlson et al., 2006; Fowler, Rodney, Roberts, & Broadus, 2005; Lisovicz et al., 2006) and is an essential component of The Witness Project. However, we recognized that The Witness Project could only be a framework, and that we would need to culturally customize the intervention for diverse Latina subgroups to be an appropriate educational intervention for diverse Latinas. Full presentations of the qualitative findings of this process are available in Erwin et al. (2010).

Our goal was to incorporate crucial variables, issues, and program components most applicable to this heterogeneous population of Latinas, as well as recognize the cultural, social, and economic diversity within the population across the United States. We therefore used formative research in New York City (NYC) and Arkansas (AR) to understand the needs and cultural issues of diverse Latino immigrants, so that we could create a program that was potentially adaptable for multiple regions across the United States. Table 15.1 displays the various formative research that has been more fully described in other publications (Erwin et al., 2007, 2010; Erwin, Johnson, Feliciano-Libid, Zamora, & Jandorf, 2005). Community advisory boards (CABs) were created at each site, including breast cancer survivors, community gatekeepers (e.g., community center staff), and local clergy. Through our relationships with these community members, we were able to conduct our initial focus groups and in-depth interviews, test our study materials, recruit volunteers, and identify community- and faith-based organizations that serve and work with immigrant Latinas (Erwin et al., 2007; Jandorf et al., 2008). This formative research used the PEN-3 model (Airhihenbuwa, 1992; Airhihenbuwa & Webster, 2004) for analyzing the qualitative (focus groups and key informant interviews) findings, with three primary domains: cultural identity, relationships and expectations, and cultural empowerment (Erwin et al., 2005). PEN-3 was developed such that qualitative information from multiple sources (e.g., numerous focus group participants) can be categorized into domains that can then be openly discussed with CAB members for validation. Table 15.2 demonstrates how we interpreted, analyzed, and applied the qualitative data to the intervention program using the PEN-3 model (for more complete descriptions of the qualitative data analysis and interpretations into programmatic content, see Erwin et al., 2007, 2010). We used the PEN-3 model to categorize the themes and text into domains that can then be applied to educational messages, program format, and content. As described in Table 15.2, the analysis determined: (1) where the emphasis of the program would focus (e.g., the *Person, Extended Family*, or *Neighborhood*); (2) whether the responses and themes in the text reflected *Perceptions, Enablers* or *Nurturer* influences; (3) whether the belief, experience, or attitude exerted a *Positive, Existential,* or *Negative* value on the specific screening; (4) if there were variations in responses by women according to their country of origin or acculturation experiences, and if these were rooted within systemic domains such as culture (from their country of origin, or the U.S. immigration experience) or personal experience within individual behavioral control; and (5) how we needed to create the intervention to reinforce the Positive factors, revise or educate to minimize Negative factors, and account for the factors beyond the control of the intervention. Table 15.2 shows this stepwise process and the subsequent impact and program design application to the intervention, which we titled *Esperanza y Vida* (Hope and Life).

TABLE 15.1 Formative Research to Develop the Intervention

Method or Instrument	Sample Size	Participants/Focus for Methodology	Types of Measures	Method of Analysis
Focus groups	$N = 112$ individuals from 13 groups (9 groups New York City; 4 groups Arkansas)	Puerto Rican, Dominican, and Mexican women living in New York City; as well as recent Mexican immigrant women living in Arkansas	Questions about: (1) issues about cancer; (2) experiences with the medical system, folk medicine, and beliefs about illness; (3) the role of spirituality in their lives; (4) relations with local churches, community organizations, and family; and (5) ethnic variation and similarity among the diverse Latina groups in their communities	PEN-3 model
In-depth interviews	$N = 23$ key informant interviews in New York City ($N = 12$) and Arkansas ($N = 11$); 6 men and 17 women total	Participants selected to represent a large range of community organizations (e.g., church; outreach workers; professionals, community-based organizations, breast cancer survivors)	Semi-structured question guide	PEN-3 model
Survey questionnaires	Total $N = 119$ $n = 96$ focus group participants $n = 23$ key informant interviewees	Focus group and key informant participants recruited through churches, social and community organizations, and existing health programs; and local "gatekeepers," who were recent immigrants, or residents of rural and urban communities	49-item demographic questionnaire to assess acculturation issues and obtain demographic descriptors (e.g., years in U.S., preferred language, age, marital status, education, and religious orientation)	Descriptive statistics
9-item pre- and post-knowledge for pilot program assessments	$N = 242$ pre- and post-knowledge surveys	Items included screening guidelines for breast and cervical cancer, identification of a Pap test and mammogram, location of female anatomy, and what factors increase risk for these cancers	Three-choice answer set of questions in Spanish and English to assess baseline and post-intervention knowledge	Pre- and post-data individually matched by respondent for comparison and analysis
10-item satisfaction surveys for pilot program assessments	$N = 242$ participants at pilot educational programs	These surveys were anonymous, and additional comments were solicited for improving the program (e.g., suggested materials revisions, health issues that needed more or less discussion, and the length of the program)	Five-item Likert Scale to assess the participants' perceptions of the educational presentations (e.g., usefulness, new information, how well information was conveyed, whether they would recommend the program for others, and the convenience of the location)	Average Likert Scores across 10 items

TABLE 15.2   Application of Formative Findings to Intervention Using PEN-3 Analysis

	Purpose	Application to Findings	Program Impact
A	Determine the emphasis of the program to be on the person (P), the extended family (E), or the neighborhood (N)	The emphasis was consistently determined to be on the extended family, based on the comments that Latinas do not feel that is important to prioritize themselves, and that the family—both nuclear and extended—takes precedence	1. Intervention was customized to accommodate, focus, and include the extended Latino family, so men were trained as lay health advisors and partners were invited to attend programs 2. Tagline: *Familias saludables empiezan con mujeres saludables* (Healthy families begin with healthy women)
B	Categorize participant responses into the three components of the PEN-3 dimensions of Relationship and Expectations (see Figure 15.1) with the components being (1) Perceptions, (2) Enablers, or (3) Nurturers	Identified and categorized "individually held knowledge, beliefs, etc." (perceptions) vs. comments that reflect "societal, systematic, or structural influences" (enablers) vs. "influences that a person may receive from significant others" (nurturers) within the textual data	1. Created lists of experiences, beliefs, and perceptions that will need to be categorized as Positive, Existential, and/or Negative in a later step to determine potential program content
C	Determine the behavioral value of text categorized as Perceptions, Enablers, or Nurturer according to the cultural empowerment domain (e.g., Positive, Existential, or Negative) for the desired screening behavior	Created a 3 × 3 table to demonstrate the value for each theme category in light of breast and cervical cancer screening behaviors; compared how specific themes within the Relationship and Expectation domain crossed with the Cultural empowerment domain by Latino subgroup	1. Demonstrated specific experiences that positively impacted screening behaviors (e.g., spirituality/church, *machismo*) 2. Demonstrated specific themes and experiences that may not be either positive or negative 3. Demonstrated specific themes that negatively impacted screening behaviors (e.g., lack of knowledge; social/political status of women, *machismo*)

	Purpose	Application to Findings	Program Impact
D	Analyze the nature of sociocultural influences and the impact of these differences in customization process as to whether they are considered "historically rooted" within the Latino culture and lifestyle	Historically rooted: • Gender relations and roles of men • Myths/misinformation • *Machismo* • Monolingual Spanish language • Family values • Country of origin and immigration status	Determined which issues and concerns may be beyond the scope of any intervention to address (e.g., issues related to immigration), and issues that are historically rooted but may be positively impacted by educational messages or program components (e.g., *machismo*/encouraging men to be educated and protect wives' health; language challenges/provide navigation in Spanish)
E	Analyze the findings to determine what could and should be "reinforced" through the intervention vs. issues that need to be "revised"	Shaped and clarified messages and program content, and structured the intervention	Reinforced: • Acknowledge importance/roles of prayer and religious practice via narrative by survivor • Offer prayer to begin program • Inclusion of men (allow men to teach men) • Latinas to talk to other Latinas • Men should know about "their women . . ." • Encourage men to protect and nurture women by directing women to be screened Revised: • If church is not perceived as supportive, finding other community locations for programs • Survivors and narrative experiential demonstration that cancer ≠ death • Offer and navigate women through challenges of medical system (access) • Educate about system/availability/screening • Provide longer educational programs, with basic information such as anatomy

Once all data were collected and analyzed into tables and categories, we discussed the findings, and the interpretation of the meanings of these findings, with our CAB members. Some of the key findings that were determined to be essential in the development of the intervention program components were the patriarchal family structure, the lack of knowledge and understanding about cancer and screening practices, and the variations in attitudes about religion and the role of the church by geographic region and ethnicity (Erwin et al., 2010). CAB members suggested that men be included in the educational format—as educators for men, as well as participants with their partners—so that men would be able to understand their roles and responsibilities in a venue that traditionally has been considered only relevant to women's health. For example, men are taught about their potential role in the transmission of cervical cancer (i.e., Human Papillomavirus [HPV]); the importance of screening and early detection for both breast and cervical cancer; and to recognize their cultural influence (i.e., *machismo*, personal leadership for their families), to encourage the women in their lives to obtain screening examinations.

The medical cultures of all countries of origin of our participants are so different from those of the United States with regard to screening practices, educational outreach, and relationships for women with their doctors (e.g., not disrobing for examinations, not asking questions or questioning the doctor), that recently immigrated women demonstrated much lower knowledge levels about anatomy and cancer than the majority of African American women reached for The Witness Project (Erwin et al., 2007). Therefore, the CAB members and pilot participants suggested that the Esperanza y Vida educational programs spend more time explaining basic anatomy and health education concepts about cancer and screening for participants than had been included in The Witness Project. This enhanced information is presented in the form of anatomical graphics and expanded discussion of the relationship between HPV and the risk of cervical cancer. The goal is to increase the understanding of participants about the nuances of breast and cervical cancer, causation, and the relationship between early detection and increased survival. Furthermore, the program encouraged the participants to become more proactive with regard to their health and the decision making process.

The distinct geographic variations of our study sites (NYC and AR) provided an important qualitative insight for developing an intervention that would appeal to diverse Latino subgroups. For example, the nature of the spiritual and religious beliefs revealed in the focus groups was subtle, and the relationship with organized churches varied between the NYC and AR sites. Mexican American women in AR trusted and relied upon their local churches. This was not always the case for women in NYC. This resulted in allowing more variation in program placement than just faith-based site planning, as was the focus for The Witness Project programs (Erwin et al., 2007) and, further, program leaders and survivors were encouraged to incorporate spiritual issues as appropriate to their needs and audiences. Together, these cultural adaptations provided unique programming that distinguishes the Esperanza y Vida educational program from The Witness Project and other health promotion programs for Latino populations. In addition to these essential program development contributions, the CABs were instrumental in the recruitment of our initial volunteers. Our CABs continue to be active in our work, helping to recruit new sites and volunteers as well as running a forum for us to share our findings as they did for our pilot study (Jandorf et al., 2008).

RESEARCH DESIGN AND METHODS

Once the intervention was developed and piloted, the goal of the American Cancer Society–funded study was to investigate the effectiveness of Esperanza y Vida for reaching diverse members of the Latino population, to increase breast and cervical cancer knowledge and screening behaviors. Outcome efficacy was evaluated by a randomized controlled study measuring knowledge and screening outcomes, with a minimum of 672 Latino participants in 24 control and 24 intervention groups in rural and urban AR and 900 Latino participants in 30 control and 30 intervention groups in NYC. Leveraged funding from another foundation allowed us to add a third site in Buffalo, NY with an additional 300 Puerto Rican men and women. Second, this study evaluated specific factors within the intervention to understand how the intervention addressed cognitive, social, and access factors that may serve as deterrents or motivators for screening behaviors. The *specific aims* of the study were as follows:

1. To evaluate the effectiveness of the Esperanza y Vida intervention in increasing breast and cervical cancer knowledge and screening behaviors in Latina participants compared to Latinas in a control health education program on diabetes.
2. To determine the demographic, cognitive, access, and social factors of Latina participants in New York and Arkansas associated with and/or predictive of screening, intent to obtain screening, and acceptance of navigation, to describe how the intervention impacts deterrents and facilitators for screening in diverse Latino populations.

The primary hypothesis (H1) was that Esperanza y Vida intervention group participants would demonstrate greater knowledge and be more likely to increase cervical and breast screening behaviors than participants attending the control programs. Diabetes prevention and control was selected for the control programs because this disease is a significant health risk for Latino populations and, for a community-based study, it is important to provide participants in the control groups with important health information (Israel et al., 2003). Additional secondary hypotheses were as follows: (H2) Increases in breast and cervical cancer screening knowledge would be associated with increased screening behaviors; (H3) increases in breast and cervical cancer knowledge would be associated with increased acceptance of navigational services; (H4) intervention group participants would demonstrate a greater decrease in barriers to cancer screening related to access, social, and cognitive deterrents compared to participants in the control programs; and (H5) a decrease in reported barriers would correspond to an increase in screening behaviors.

The CONSORT guidelines (Moher, Schulz, & Altman, 2001) were followed from the onset of the study randomization, for each site's programs (control vs. intervention). We used cluster randomization within each site by randomizing program units (e.g., community centers or church groups) rather than individuals. Random assignment lists were generated for each site separately and programs were assigned as explained below. All sites hired bilingual/bicultural program coordinators. They, as well as the site host, were blinded to condition, until a site agreed to host an educational program. This process prevented selection bias by program staff or self-selection bias by the community groups and their members. Each group was then assigned to focus on breast and cervical cancer (intervention) or diabetes education (control), based on the predetermined randomization sequence (see Figure 15.1).

Attendance at the educational programs was voluntary. Oral consents were obtained at the end of each program and Institutional Review Boards at all institutional sites granted permission for a waiver of signed consent, allowing us to verbally explain the elements of the research and to have participants provide signatures for further contact (navigation and the 2- and 8-month follow-up telephone calls). The waiver was justified, as the immigration status of participants was unknown and signing consent forms could have the appearance of increased risk for undocumented immigrants.

All participants completed sociodemographic questions (age, country of birth, marital status, years in the United States, language preference), answered pre- and post-program knowledge questions, and reported their current participation in screening exams (BSE, CBE, mammogram, and Pap) and barriers (Sudarson, Jandorf, & Erwin, in press). This information was collected through an audience response system (ARS) in Spanish or English, depending upon participants' preferences. This system has been found to

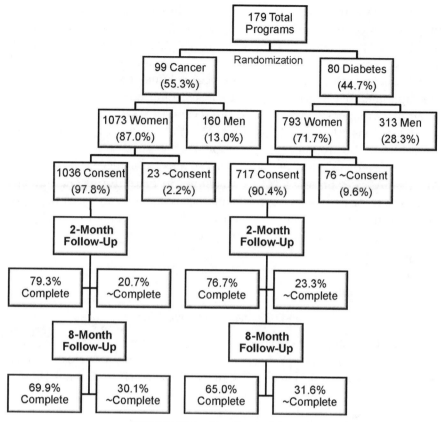

FIGURE 15.1   The Study Schema

be a useful tool when dealing with English as a second language (ESL), or with rural and/or low-literacy populations (Gamito, Burhansstipanov, Krebs, Bemis, & Bradley, 2005). Participants were able to confidentially and anonymously enter their answers by pressing the numbers matching their answer options on their individual wireless keypads. Questions and answer options were presented on PowerPoint™ slides and read by program leaders. The PowerPoint slides presented identical information and questions at all sites; program staff customized resources for diverse Latino subgroups and for geographic region to be offered to participants at the end of each program.

At each program, staff recorded program-specific factors, including the site (AR, NYC, or Western New York [WNY]), the setting (urban or rural/suburban), the type of site (community-based, faith-based, or private home), the length of the educational program, and the language in which the program was conducted (Spanish or English). Within each location, program staff actively recruited community sites at which to conduct group programs, including community-based and faith-based organizations, as well as private homes. At each program, bilingual, culturally matched program staff and peer volunteers (including breast and cervical cancer survivors) assisted with the programs. The peer volunteers specifically testify to the importance of early detection, regular screening, and the strength one has to survive a diagnosis of breast or cervical cancer.

Questions related to the participants' cancer screening practices were embedded in the program's presentation. For the purpose of analysis, these responses were recoded to assess participants' adherence, based on the American Cancer Society's (ACS) guidelines in place during the outreach time period for each respective screening examination. Analyses were performed using SPSS (version 16.0) software. Both chi-square and analysis of variance (ANOVA) statistical tests were used to compare the sites, with significance reported at $p = .05$.

PROGRAM COMPONENTS

To conduct the study, we needed to recruit and train volunteers, plan outreach strategies, recruit appropriate sites for programs, and create navigational and follow-up strategies to secure outcome data from the intervention.

Recruitment/Training of Volunteers

We recruited Latino men and women to serve as volunteer *Consejeros de Salud* (lay health advisors) or *Sobrevivientes* (breast or cervical cancer survivors). Intervention programs were conducted by the Esperanza y Vida research staff with assistance from the Consejeras/Consejeros de Salud and a testimony from a local Sobreviviente, seen as a blessing and proof that a cancer diagnosis is not a death sentence. The Consejeros de Salud, although not cancer survivors, volunteered their time by helping to organize and publicize programs, distribute appropriate program materials to study participants, supply facts about cancer during the educational program presentations, and answer questions about available services. All volunteers were required to attend an 8-hour training session designed and conducted by the staff and were given materials to guide their outreach efforts. During training, volunteers were informed on current breast and cervical cancer facts, early detection and screening methods, and how to organize and conduct educational programs. The Sobrevivientes were further trained on how to present their story of survival in a compelling, effective manner, mindful of the time constraints oftentimes posed by the site location or program participants (Saad-Harfouche et al., 2010).

Outreach Plan/Recruitment of Sites

Esperanza y Vida involves more than a translation of materials and messages; it is culturally tailored for appropriateness and competency and (1) is a distinct spiritual program, (2) provides direct access to survivors, and (3) provides a way to inform males in the Hispanic/Latino community about breast and cervical health. Presented to small groups in churches, community centers, and participants' homes, the program provides a method for building on the social capital of family and community relationships to affect the larger cultural context and promote behavior change. Program site selection was based on their relevance and accessibility by the local Latino community and recruited through the efforts of the local site Program Coordinators, with contacts in local religious, community, and health-related organizations.

Navigation/Follow-Up

Following the educational presentation, female participants were asked permission to be contacted in 2 months and again in 8 months to assess the program's impact on screening behaviors, and they granted consent by providing their signature and contact information on their individual IRB-approved Registration Cards. The 2-month call assessed current breast and cervical cancer screening adherence and reasons for being screened, or unscreened. Following the 2-month assessment, we offered navigation assistance to all nonadherent participants. Navigation assistance was provided in the form of appointment scheduling, enrollment in federally and/or state-funded programs, interpreting during cancer screening exams when language was a barrier, or transportation. For women who were screened and received a positive cancer diagnosis, we provided navigation assistance throughout the treatment and recovery process, and oftentimes assistance extended to include the needs of the entire family (e.g., billing assistance, food pantry referral). Six months after completing the 2-month assessment (8 months following the educational intervention) female participants were contacted again to reassess their exam adherence and determine whether additional navigation assistance was needed or desired. In addition, 12 months post-intervention, an annual appointment reminder letter was generated and sent to all females who had provided consent and an address, along with an up-to-date Community Resource Guide with information on free or low-cost clinics and resources in their area.

PRELIMINARY RESULTS

Randomization of programs began in August 2007 and ended in December 2009, resulting in 1,233 women and men participating in 99 cancer programs and 1,106 women and men participating in 80 diabetes programs. Figure 15.1 diagrams the randomization process and response rates. We focus on presenting only the results from the cancer programs in this chapter (diabetes program results and program outcomes will be published elsewhere). Of the women attending the cancer programs, 88% were immigrants, coming from four primary regions ($N = 939$), with Mexico having the largest group (436 women; 52.0%), followed by Puerto Rico (235; 28.0%), Central and South America (147; 17.5%), and the Dominican Republic (121; 14.4%).

Program Variations

Cancer program differences by geographic region were striking, as 14 different variables, from the site and the day of the week programs were conducted, to the length of programs, were found to be significant (see Table 15.3). Likewise, the sociodemographics of participants (see Table 15.4) and interpersonal and cultural variables (see Table 15.5) by site were also significantly different. These variations are repeated when we examine

TABLE 15.3   Program Differences[a]

Variables	Arkansas	New York City	Western New York	p-Value
Total number of programs	34	40	25	
# of Male participants Mean (SD)	3.15 (4.75)	0.90 (1.57)	3.28 (4.11)	.010
Location type				.000
Community	11.8	82.5	32.0	
Faith-based	55.9	7.5	28.0	
Private home	32.4	10.0	40.0	
Language				.030
Spanish	100.0	90.0	80.0	
English	0.0	10.0	20.0	
Opening prayer				.000
Yes	82.4	60.0	28.0	
Survivor				.002
Yes	70.6	95.0	96.0	

(continued)

Variables	Arkansas	New York City	Western New York	p-Value
Male advisor				.332
Yes	11.8	5.0	16.0	
Closing prayer				.000
Yes	82.4	57.5	24.0	
System used				.000
Paper	41.2	5.0	0.0	
ARS	44.1	80.0	68.0	
Both	14.7	15.0	32.0	
Day of the week				.004
Monday	2.9	0.0	4.0	
Tuesday	2.9	30.0	12.0	
Wednesday	11.8	15.0	12.0	
Thursday	11.8	32.5	12.0	
Friday	14.7	10.0	16.0	
Saturday	20.6	7.5	28.0	
Sunday	35.3	5.0	16.0	
Day of the week— Recoded				.010
Weekday	50.0	22.5	56.0	
Weekend	50.0	77.5	44.0	
Program time				.000
Morning	5.9	62.5	28.0	
Afternoon	50.0	32.5	32.0	
Evening	44.1	5.0	40.0	
Number of volunteers				.004
Zero	11.8	20.0	20.0	
One	76.5	72.5	40.0	
Two	11.8	7.5	24.0	
Three	0.0	0.0	16.0	
Length of program	192.79 (44.9)	98.63 (17.8)	158.46 (41.0)	.000
Mean volunteers	1.00 (0.5)	0.88 (0.5)	1.36 (1.0)	.018
Country of origin				.000
Mexico	69.3	29.9	0.3	
Dominican Republic	0.2	16.9	3.3	
Puerto Rico	0.0	18.8	67.6	
United States	3.3	14.2	18.5	
Central America	22.5	3.6	1.5	
South America	3.1	8.2	1.8	
Other	1.7	8.4	7.0	

[a]Cancer intervention program participants only.

TABLE 15.4   Sociodemographic Variable by Geographic Location[a]

Sociodemographic Variables	AR N	AR %	NYC N	NYC %	WNY N	WNY %	Total N	Total %	p-Value
Language preference									.000
Spanish	737	83.8	461	63.5	286	50.4	1484	68.3	
English	74	8.4	115	15.8	127	22.4	316	14.5	
No preference	69	7.8	150	20.7	154	27.2	373	17.2	
Years living in the U.S. (non-U.S.-born)									.000
Less than 4 years	187	21.1	49	8.7	30	14.5	266	16.1	
5–14 years	353	39.9	225	39.8	28	13.5	606	36.6	
15 or more years	345	39.0	291	51.5	149	72.0	785	47.4	
Marital status									.000
Married/Partnered	699	78.7	374	50.3	278	49.1	1351	61.5	
Not married	189	21.3	369	49.7	288	50.9	846	38.5	
Health insurance									.000
None	593	69.8	210	28.5	53	9.5	856	39.9	
Public (Medicaid/Medicare)	30	3.5	321	43.6	331	59.4	682	31.8	
Work/Self-paid/DK/Other	227	26.7	206	28.0	173	31.1	606	28.3	
Screening adherence (age-corrected)[b] Mammography									.000
Adherent	38	23.6	141	55.7	84	57.9	263	47.0	
Partially adherent	46	28.6	47	18.6	29	20.0	122	21.8	
Nonadherent	77	47.8	65	25.7	32	22.1	174	31.1	
Clinical breast exam									.000
Adherent	119	32.1	191	49.0	124	51.2	434	43.3	
Nonadherent	252	67.9	199	51.0	118	48.8	569	56.7	

[a]Cancer intervention program participants only.
[b]Female participants only.

sociodemographics by country of origin (see Table 15.6), demonstrating the enormous amount of variability that we have within and across sites. Table 15.7 demonstrates some of the qualitative differences noted by program site.

Screening Variations

Table 15.6 displays the baseline screening adherence data by country of origin, which is significantly different among groups for CBE and mammography, ranging from a high of 62.0% for women from the Dominican Republic for mammograms, to a low of 33.3% for women from Mexico. Mammography adherence for women over age 40 also varied by geographic site (23.6% in

TABLE 15.5   Interpersonal and Cultural Variables by Geographic Location[a]

Interpersonal and Cultural Variables	AR		NYC		WNY		Total		
	N	**%**	**N**	**%**	**N**	**%**	**N**	**%**	**p-Value**
How often is language a problem in getting the health care you want/need?									.000
Very/Somewhat	296	60.5	137	26.9	125	23.7	558	36.5	
Seldom/Never	193	39.5	373	73.1	403	76.3	969	63.5	
How well do you understand what your doctor or health care provider tells you?									.000
Very/Somewhat	127	26.6	231	45.7	253	50.5	611	41.2	
A little/Not at all	350	73.4	274	54.3	248	49.5	872	58.8	
Compared with people of other ethnic groups or races, how do you feel you have been treated when seeking health care in the past 12 months?									.000
Worse than other groups	142	30.5	31	7.1	24	5.7	197	14.9	
The same as other groups	189	40.6	230	52.4	240	57.3	659	49.8	
Better than other groups	19	4.1	40	9.1	41	9.8	100	7.6	
Have not sought health care in past 12 months	66	14.2	60	13.7	37	8.8	163	12.3	
Don't know	49	10.5	78	17.8	77	18.4	204	15.4	

[a]Cancer intervention program participants only.

AR, 55.7 in NYC, and 57.9% in WNY; see Table 15.4). CBE adherence rates (age-adjusted) also varied by geographic region (see Table 15.4), with an overall adherence rate of only 43.3% (32.1% in AR, 49.0% in NYC, and 51.2% in WNY). Interestingly, Pap adherence and breast self-examination (BSE) were not significantly different by country of origin or region; Pap was near the national rate for all Latinas at 74.4%, and BSE was practiced by only 21.4% of participants.

TABLE 15.6 Demographics and Baseline Screening by Country of Origin[a]

	Mexico		Puerto Rico		Central/South America		Dominican Republic/Other		Total		p-Value
	N	%	N	%	N	%	N	%	N	%	
Age											.000
18–29	124	30.0	40	13.5	23	13.8	20	13.8	207	20.3	
30–39	149	36.0	52	17.6	52	31.1	34	23.4	287	28.1	
40–49	93	22.5	52	17.6	39	23.4	30	20.7	214	20.9	
50–59	34	8.2	48	16.2	20	12.0	26	17.9	128	12.5	
60–64	6	1.4	29	9.8	13	7.8	6	4.1	54	5.3	
65 or older	8	1.9	75	25.3	20	12.0	29	20.0	132	12.9	
Age recoded											.000
18–40	273	65.3	92	30.6	75	44.6	54	36.7	494	47.8	
41 or older	145	34.7	209	69.4	93	55.4	93	63.3	540	52.2	
Marital status											.000
Married/partnered	333	80.6	121	40.5	115	70.1	77	55.0	646	63.6	
Not married	80	19.4	178	59.5	49	29.9	63	45.0	370	36.4	
Insurance											.000
No	303	78.1	20	7.2	91	61.1	29	23.2	443	47.2	
Yes	85	21.9	256	92.8	58	38.9	96	76.8	495	52.8	
Less than 5 years	68	16.6	59	19.9	25	15.0	22	15.5	174	17.1	
5–14 years	237	57.8	56	18.9	62	37.1	41	28.9	396	39.0	
15 or more years	105	25.6	182	61.3	80	47.9	79	55.6	446	43.9	
Language preference											.000
Spanish	358	89.7	181	61.4	136	81.9	81	75.7	756	75.7	
English	14	3.5	23	7.8	5	3.0	33	7.5	75	7.5	
No preference	27	6.8	91	30.8	25	15.1	25	18.0	168	16.8	
Barriers to screening											
Lack of insurance	86	20.6	29	9.6	33	19.6	15	10.2	163	15.8	.000
Lack of money	48	11.5	16	5.3	9	5.4	14	9.5	87	8.4	.011
Lack of transportation	5	1.2	43	14.3	2	1.2	3	2.0	53	5.1	.000

	Mexico		Puerto Rico		Central/South America		Dominican Republic/Other		Total		
	N	%	N	%	N	%	N	%	N	%	p-Value
All of the above	59	14.1	20	6.6	19	11.3	16	10.9	114	11.0	.019
None of the above	24	5.7	98	32.6	14	8.3	26	17.7	162	15.7	.000
BSE—Doctor or nurse recommendation?											.004
Yes	248	68.7	200	81.6	105	70.9	91	73.4	644	73.3	
No	96	26.6	35	14.3	38	25.7	23	18.5	192	21.9	
Don't know	17	4.7	10	4.1	5	3.4	10	8.1	42	4.8	
CBE adherence[b]											.000
Adherent	128	38.1	128	54.5	50	34.2	61	50.8	367	43.8	
Nonadherent	208	61.9	107	45.5	96	65.8	59	49.2	470	56.2	
I or my spouse know where to get a CBE											.000
Yes	141	70.1	196	91.2	49	67.1	66	82.5	452	79.4	
Mam—adherence[b]											.000
Adherent	39	33.3	97	59.5	31	36.5	49	62.0	216	48.6	
Partially adherent	33	28.2	36	22.1	19	22.4	12	15.2	100	22.5	
Nonadherent	45	38.5	30	18.4	35	41.2	18	22.8	128	18.8	
Mam—Doctor or Nurse recommendation?											.000
Yes	161	45.6	183	74.4	84	60.9	88	74.6	516	60.4	
No	178	50.4	52	21.1	53	38.4	26	22.0	309	36.1	
Don't know	14	4.0	11	4.5	1	0.7	4	3.4	30	3.5	
I or my spouse know where to get a mammogram											.000
Yes	129	58.6	187	87.8	56	64.4	64	79.0	436	72.5	

[a] Cancer intervention program participants only.
[b] Female participants only.

TABLE 15.7 Programmatic Differences by Site

Variables	Arkansas	WNY	NYC
Program implementation and site recruitment	Prior approval from Catholic diocese essential; programs primarily conducted in churches and participant homes	No prior approval needed (except for IRB); once we contacted an organization, we sent them the portfolio and set up a date; primarily programs conducted in community-based organizations, schools, as well as participants' homes	No prior approval needed (except for IRB); once we contacted an organization, we sent them the portfolio and set up a date; primarily programs conducted in community-based organizations, schools, as well as participants' homes
Site characteristics	Mostly urban/suburban; access to health care services and public transportation limited in rural areas	Urban	Urban
Program length	3.0 hours	2.1 hours	1.5 hours
Male attendees	Majority attend without partners; pose a barrier with navigation	Evenly distributed	Very few men attending program
Access to screenings and navigation	Limited access for underinsured and non-English-speakers; majority require appointment scheduling, interpretation, transportation	Good access to clinics with bilingual doctors; however, due to long waiting period women were referred to other non-Spanish-speaking clinics, which required appointment scheduling, interpretation, and need for transportation	Age requirement for places where screening would be provided free or at low cost—otherwise, women were referred to health clinics that bill using a sliding scale fee; lack of time is an issue for many of the women

Potential Barriers

Potential barriers to screening—such as insurance, language, and perceived discrimination—that were all significantly different by country of origin, are included in Table 15.6. While fear of going to the doctor/nurse/clinic and of hearing the results from a medical examination did not vary across sites, the degree to which language was a barrier in getting the health care they needed/wanted varied, particularly between AR and NYC/WNY women, similar to the preferred language, as noted in Table 15.4. Sixty percent of AR women reported that language was very often/sometimes a problem, compared to 27% of NYC and 24% of WNY women (see Table 15.5). These variations may be a function of length of time in the U.S., local availability of bilingual health care providers, or different geographic patterns of immigration. A related question—"How well do you understand what your doctor or health care provider tells you?"—also varied among the sites; this was not surprising, considering the problem of language variance. Again, the women in AR (Table 15.5) and/or of Mexican origin (Table 15.8) reported the lowest level of understanding of the doctor/health care provider. Participants were also asked about how they viewed their health care treatment compared to that received by other races/ethnicities. A greater proportion of women in AR (Table 15.5) and from Mexico (Table 15.8) believed that they had been treated worse than other ethnic groups or races (30.5% and 28%, respectively) versus women at the new NYC and WNY sites (7.1%, and 5.7%, respectively) or other countries of origin.

Participant Health Care Knowledge by Country of Origin

There were significant differences in people's knowledge of where to get cancer screening across sites and by country of origin (see Table 15.6). Latinas from Mexico were the least likely to know where to obtain breast screening (58.6%) and Puerto Rican women (87.8%) were most likely to know where to obtain screening. In WNY, 84% of women knew where to go to get a mammogram, compared to 60% in AR; 92% of WNY women knew where to get a CBE, compared to 70% of AR women. However, there was no significant difference among sites in terms of the percentages of women who knew where to obtain cervical screening, reflected in the similar adherence to Pap screening.

DISCUSSION AND LESSONS LEARNED

In an effort to meet the unique needs of the diverse Latino population, Esperanza y Vida, developed from the successful intervention framework of The Witness Project, has evolved into a culturally tailored and competent

TABLE 15.8 Potential Barriers to Screening[a]

	Mexico		Puerto Rico		Central/South America		Dominican Republic/ Other		Total		p-Value
	N	%	N	%	N	%	N	%	N	%	
Insurance											.000
None	303	75.9	20	6.9	91	57.2	29	21.6	443	45.1	
Public (Medicare/Medicaid)	25	6.3	213	73.2	21	13.2	66	49.3	325	33.1	
Private (Self-pay/Employer/Other)	71	17.8	58	19.9	47	29.6	39	29.1	215	21.9	
How often is language a problem in getting the health care you want/need?											.000
Very/Somewhat	141	55.7	71	29.3	43	46.7	18	18.9	273	40.0	
Seldom/Never	112	44.3	171	70.7	49	53.3	77	81.1	409	60.0	
How well do you understand what your doctor or health care provider tells you?											.000
Very/Somewhat	49	20.5	125	51.7	29	31.5	35	37.6	238	35.7	
Seldom/Never	190	79.5	117	48.3	63	68.5	58	62.4	428	64.3	
Compared with people of other ethnic groups or races, how do you feel you have been treated when seeking health care in the past 12 months?											.000
Worse than other groups	57	24.1	4	2.2	15	17.4	3	4.0	79	13.7	
The same as other groups	94	39.7	104	58.1	39	45.3	45	60.0	282	48.9	
Better than other groups	13	5.5	27	15.1	6	7.0	7	9.3	53	9.2	
Have not sought health care in the past 12 months	43	18.1	21	11.7	14	15.3	8	10.7	86	14.9	
Don't know	30	12.7	23	12.8	12	14.0	12	16.0	77	13.3	

[a]Cancer intervention program participants only.

health education program for Latino-based cultural groups from a variety of backgrounds and countries of origin. Along with updated cancer information relevant to Latino groups living in the United States, a special emphasis on the patriarchal structure of the Latino family, and a modern and sophisticated electronic data collection system, Esperanza y Vida offers an educational and research experience for less acculturated, new immigrant Latino groups. Significant efforts spent on formative data and appropriate intervention development have provided a strong foundation for a rigorous, randomized control study that has resulted in high program attendance, rapid accrual, robust sample sizes (exceeding program estimates), and high follow-up rates. As demonstrated in Figure 15.1, obtaining multiple contact telephone numbers, telling women who the person calling them will be, and promoting the gift card incentive for completing the brief telephone calls have positively impacted the response rates at 2 months (79.3%) and again at 8 months (69.9%) for a population that is often characterized as transient between countries, mobile within locations, and otherwise challenging to follow.

The ARS methodology, which captures participant data via small electronic keypads, was incorporated to alleviate common barriers faced by the use of traditional pen-and-paper methods, such as missing data due to participant error, lengthy data entry, and data entry errors. The ARS allowed the users to answer personal, health-related questions in group settings in a confidential and anonymous manner, in Spanish or English. Even participants with low literacy skills could easily participate in the surveys, as the staff member read each question and answer and the participants gave their responses via keypads that resemble a small television remote control and are easy to use. Research questions were embedded within the educational PowerPoint slides and allowed for engaged participation from the audience throughout the presentation. This method made it easier to collect demographics, knowledge, attitude, beliefs, and barrier data related to cancer screening, and it allowed us to overcome literacy barriers and collect information from a high proportion of participants (over 90% completion of questions). An important component of this multisite study was the centralization of the data. Using an Access database, each site uploaded local program data which was then merged, providing overall information for program reports and future data analysis. The data manager was able to troubleshoot any problems that each site encountered in its electronic data collection.

Use of the PowerPoint program delivery also allowed us to use illustrations to address topics such as female reproductive anatomy and HPV, which were topics of high interest and low knowledge. The nature of community-based research, with participants arriving late, leaving early, and programs conducted in sites not conducive to electronic hardware and projectors, sometimes forced staff to rely upon pen-and-paper surveys for data collection, so flexibility in response to participants' and community needs was important.

Preliminary outcomes of intervention effectiveness, at 2-months post-intervention, are demonstrating that the participants from the cancer programs were more likely to be screened for CBE, mammogram, and Pap tests than participants from the diabetes program (manuscript in process). Approximately 40% of women who reported being nonadherent to current screening guidelines at the time of a program (baseline) reported receipt of the Pap, CBE, and/or mammography by the initial follow-up period at 2 months. These are exciting results and, at the time of this writing, analyses were expected to be completed and published in 2011. In addition, demographic characteristics demonstrate significant geographic variability as well as differences in program implementation. These ethnic and geographic variations demonstrate the heterogeneity of the Latino subgroups, the importance of assessing country of origin, and the potential impact of these variations on cancer control outcomes, all of which is worthy of further scientific explorations and analyses (Jandorf et al., in press; Sudarson et al., 2010).

Regardless of the final outcomes, the baseline results and rigorous methods give us confidence in the validity of our data and the representativeness of the participants. Although complete outcome analyses are not yet available, these preliminary results suggest that the theoretical domains of social capital, transculturation/transmigration, and relational culture may offer important theoretical explanations to predict breast and cervical cancer screening among these immigrant Latina groups (Pasick, Burke, et al., 2009). Our outcomes suggest that personalized outreach within groups that build on women's cultural identities, negotiating skills, and community support (social capital), as well as the caring and trust demonstrated by outreach staff (relational culture), may be equally important factors influencing subsequent screening behaviors for participants as cognitive constructs such as cancer knowledge, self-efficacy, or perceptions of risk (Erwin et al., 2010; Pasick, Barker, et al., 2009). Likewise, themes related to experiences of immigration, discrimination, and therapeutic engagement (transculturation/transmigration) are especially important considerations for recent immigrant groups (Pasick, Burke, et al., 2009).

We have crafted and conducted what we believe to be an innovative and effective study and educational program, thereby honoring key principles of community-based participatory research (CBPR) principles—appropriate attention to services, driven by community perspectives, resulting in rigorous and valid research outcomes. We included and invited spouses, partners, and even single men in the community to participate and learn about these cancers that impact the women in their lives. We recruited and trained cancer survivors to discuss their experiences and the importance of early detection, offering a relatively rare window on an often frightening and stigmatized disease experience among Latino groups. The testimony of the survivor deeply resonated with many participants. In many Latino communities, cancer is not openly discussed, so to see that a woman has survived, and is speaking out to encourage others to get screened, impacts their lives. Many times, it is not until after the end of a program, when the most of the participants have left and only a few linger on to speak to the staff or survivors, that the extent of the impact becomes clear.

As this is a multisite program, and the pace of life in different locations and among different cultural groups varied, so did the program scheduling and the length of time taken to conduct the educational program. It was somewhat surprising that the same PowerPoint program would result in average time variations from 1.5 (NYC) hours to over 3.0 (AR) hours with different groups, based on questions and audience discussion and participation. The program length may vary from site to site, regardless of the use of the ARS, oftentimes depending on the audience, location, or individuals who require detailed assistance. These differences also correspond to variations in weekly program scheduling requested by community members, as a higher proportion of AR and WNY programs were conducted on weekends (53% and 49%, respectively), when families can gather together without strict time schedules. In contrast, community members in NYC preferred weekdays (84%) and these programs were primarily scheduled on Tuesdays and Thursdays, during lunchtimes or late afternoons when participants were in the city, but tended to be more time-limited. Future data analysis will examine the influence of these factors in screening outcomes for a "dose–response" effect.

This educational program covered in-depth information about breast and cervical cancer (or diabetes) risk, screening and/or prevention, attempting to maximize the benefit for the time invested by participants. Interestingly, Pap test rates at baseline were relatively high among all groups, while mammography and CBE varied by site and country of origin. Related to breast cancer, there were integral topics that were omitted in our programs, although we believe that participants may have benefitted from their inclusion, such as how to perform a breast self-examination (BSE). BSE is not considered a screening tool and has been dropped from most recommended screening or awareness guidelines. It is, however, arguably a behavior change modifier in moving women toward being more likely to obtain CBE and mammography (Bloom, Grazier, Hodge, & Hayes, 1991). For those subgroups in our sample with low baseline mammogram and CBE screening rates, such as Mexican and Dominican women and newer immigrant women, BSE may need to be considered as an educational process for improving awareness and potential behavior change to screening adherence.

The numbers of Mexican and South and Central American immigrants are increasing steadily throughout many areas of the United States, and there are few evidence-based outreach and screening interventions for this diverse group (e.g., the Research Tested Intervention Programs [RTIPS] on the Cancer Control P.L.A.N.E.T. do not include any breast or cervical interventions specifically for Latino populations). One of the positive aspects of *Esperanza y Vida* for potential replication to other sites is that it can be customized to appropriately meet the needs of diverse communities in vastly different geographic regions. The program goes beyond some of the more traditional programs, explores new methodologies and approaches, and embraces the family, partners, and spouses of women within its programming to reach the community. Our staff have great passion for their work and report weekly about how excited women are to learn about their bodies and these health topics; what a sense of relief participants experience when they learn that they can receive free or low-cost screenings regardless of documentation status; and how these new immigrants are so impressed when doors are opened for them in this country, which can sometimes feel so intimidating. Most importantly, we have been successful in this research not only because we serve our communities' specific needs, but because we are also part of the communities that we serve.

ACKNOWLEDGMENTS

In addition to the generous support of our research by the American Cancer Society Research Scholars Grant, we would like to acknowledge the formative research support from the Susan G. Komen for the Cure (POP0201290 and POP0503950), and the additional funding from the John R. Oishei Foundation of Western New York to include the study site in Buffalo. We also gratefully acknowledge the thousands of Latino participants and the community members and organizations without whose passionate, honest, and selfless contribution of time and energy, none of this would have been possible. Supported by American Cancer Society grant: RSGT-07-021-01-CPPB.

REFERENCES

Airhihenbuwa, C. O. (1992). Health promotion and disease prevention strategies for African Americans: A conceptual model. In R. L. Braithwaite & S. E. Taylor (Eds.), *Health issues in the Black community* (pp. 267–280). San Francisco, CA: Jossey-Bass.

Airhihenbuwa, C. O., & Webster, J. D. (2004). Culture and African contexts of HIV/AIDS prevention, care and support. *Journal of Social Aspects of HIV/AIDS Research Alliance, 1*(1), 4–13.

American Cancer Society. (2009). *Cancer facts and figures for Hispanics/Latinos 2009–2011*. Atlanta, GA: American Cancer Society.

Bloom, J. R., Grazier, K., Hodge, F., & Hayes, W. A. (1991). Factors affecting the use of screening mammography among African American women. *Cancer Epidemiology Biomarkers & Prevention, 1*(1), 75–82.

Carlson, B. A., Neal, D., Magwood, G., Jenkins, C., King, M. G., & Hossler, C. L. (2006). A community-based participatory health information needs assessment to help eliminate diabetes information disparities. *Health Promotion Practice, 7*(3 Suppl.), 213S–222S.

Darnell, J. S., Chang, C., & Calhoun, E. A. (2006). Knowledge about breast cancer and participation in a faith-based breast cancer program and other predictors of mammography screening among African American women and Latinas. *Health Promotion Practice, 7*(3 Suppl.), 201S–212S.

Echeverria, S. E., & Carrasquillo, O. (2006). The roles of citizenship status, acculturation, and health insurance in breast and cervical cancer screening among immigrant women. *Medical Care, 44*(8), 788–792.

Erwin, D. O. (2009). The Witness Project: Narratives that shape the cancer experience for African American women. In J. McMullin & D. Weiner (Eds.), *Confronting cancer: Metaphors, advocacy, and anthropology* (pp. 125–146). Santa Fe, NM: School for Advanced Research Seminar Series.

Erwin, D. O., Johnson, V. A., Feliciano-Libid, L., Zamora, D., & Jandorf, L. (2005). Incorporating cultural constructs and demographic diversity in the research and development of a Latina breast and cervical cancer education program. *Journal of Cancer Education, 20*(1), 39–44.

Erwin, D. O., Johnson, V. A., Trevino, M., Duke, K., Feliciano, L., & Jandorf, L. (2007). A comparison of African American and Latina social networks as indicators for culturally tailoring a breast and cervical cancer education prevention. *Cancer, 109*(2), 368–377.

Erwin, D. O., Spatz, T. S., & Stotts, R. C. (1999). Increasing mammography practice by African American women. *Cancer Practice, 7*, 78–85.

Erwin, D. O., Trevino, M., Saad-Harfouche, F. G., Rodriguez, E. M., Gage, E., & Jandorf, L. (2010). Contextualizing diversity and culture within cancer control interventions for Latinas: Changing interventions, not cultures. *Social Science and Medicine, 71*, 693–701.

Fowler, B. A., Rodney, M., Roberts, S., & Broadus, L. (2005). Collaborative breast health intervention for African American women of lower socioeconomic status. *Oncology Nursing Forum. Online, 32*(6), 1207–1216.

Gamito, E. J., Burhansstipanov, L., Krebs, L. U., Bemis, L., & Bradley, A. (2005). The use of an electronic audience response system for data collection. *Journal of Cancer Education, 20*(3), 80–86.

Israel, B. A., Schulz, A. J., Parker, E. A., Becker, A. B., Allen, A., & Guzman, J. R. (2003). Critical issues in developing and following community based participatory research principles. In M. Minkler & N. Wallerstein (Eds.), *Community-based participatory research for health* (pp. 53–76). San Francisco, CA: Jossey-Bass.

Jacobs, E. A., Karavolos, K., Rathouz, P. J., Ferris, T. G., & Powell, L. H. (2005). Limited English proficiency and breast and cervical cancer screening in a multiethnic population. *American Journal of Public Health, 95*(8), 1410–1416.

Jandorf, L., Bursac, Z., Pulley, L., Trevino, M., Castillo, A., & Erwin, D. O. (2008). Breast and cervical cancer screening among Latinas attending culturally specific educational programs. *Progress in Community Health Partnerships: Research, Education and Action, 2*(3), 195–204.

Jandorf, L., Ellison, J. L., Shelton, R. C., Thelemaque, L. D., Castillo, A. G., Mendez, E. I., . . . Erwin, D. (in press). *Esperanza y Vida*: A culturally and linguistically customized breast and cervical education program for diverse Latinas: At three different U.S. sites. *Journal of Health Communication.*

Joslyn, S. A., Foote, M. L., Nasseri, K., Coughlin, S. S., & Howe, H. L. (2005). Racial and ethnic disparities in breast cancer rates by age: NAACCR breast cancer project. *Breast Cancer Research and Treatment, 92*(2), 97–105.

Kreuter, M. W., Green, M. C., Cappella, J. N., Slater, M. D., Wise, M. E., Storey, D., . . . Woolley, S. (2007). Narrative communication in cancer prevention and control: A framework to guide research and application. *Annals of Behavioral Medicine, 33*(3), 221–235.

Li, C. I., Malone, K. E., & Daling, J. R. (2003). Differences in breast cancer stage, treatment, and survival by race and ethnicity. *Archives of Internal Medicine, 163*, 49–56.

Lisovicz, N., Johnson, R. E., Higginbotham, J., Downey, J. A., Hardy, C. M., Fouad, M. N., . . . Partridge, E. E. (2006). The Deep South network for cancer control. Building a community infrastructure to reduce cancer health disparities. *Cancer, 107*(8 Suppl.), 1971–1979.

Mayo, R. M., Erwin, D. O., & Spitler, H. D. (2003). Implications for breast and cervical cancer control for Latinas in the rural south: A review of the literature. *Cancer Control, 10*(5 Suppl.), 60–68.

Moher, D., Schulz, K. F., & Altman, D. (2001). The CONSORT statement: Revised recommendations for improving the quality of reports of parallel-group randomized trials. *Journal of the American Medical Association, 285*, 1987–1991.

Pasick, R. J., Barker, J. C., Otero-Sabogal, R., Burke, N. J., Joseph, G., & Guerra, C. (2009). Intention, subjective norms, and cancer screening in the context of relational culture. *Health Education & Behavior, 36*(5 Suppl.), 91S–110S.

Pasick, R. J., Burke, N. J., Barker, J. C., Joseph, G., Bird, J. A., Otero-Sabogal, R., . . . Guerra, C. (2009). Behavioral theory in a diverse society: Like a compass on Mars. *Health Education & Behavior, 36*(5 Suppl.), 11S–35S.

Powe, B. D. (1995). Fatalism among elderly African Americans: Effects on colorectal cancer screening. *Cancer Nursing, 18*(5), 385–392.

Saad-Harfouche, F. G., Jandorf, L., Gage, E., Thélémaque, L., Colón, J., Castillo, A. G., . . . Erwin, D. O. (2010). *Esperanza y Vida*: Training lay health advisors and cancer survivors to promote breast and cervical cancer screening in Latinas. *Journal of Community Health, 36*(2), 219–227. (DOI: 10.1007/s10900-010-9300-3).

Schettino, M. R., Hernández-Valero, M. A., Moguel, R., Hajek, R. A., & Jones, L. A. (2006). Assessing breast cancer knowledge, beliefs, and misconceptions among Latinas in Houston, Texas. *Journal of Cancer Education: The Official Journal of the American Association for Cancer Education, 21*(1 Suppl.), S42–S46.

Sudarson, N. R., Jandorf, L., & Erwin, D. O. (2010). Multi-site implementation of health education programs for Latinas. *Journal of Community Health, 36*(2), 193–203. (DOI: 10.1007/s10900-010-9297-7).

Vargas Bustamante, A., Chen, J., Rodriguez, H. P., Rizzo, J. A., & Ortega, A. N. (2010). Use of preventive care services among Latino subgroups. *American Journal of Preventive Medicine, 38*(6), 610–619.

Warren, A. G., Londoño, G. E., Wessel, L. A., & Warren, R. D. (2006). Breaking down barriers to breast and cervical cancer screening: A university-based prevention program for Latinas. *Journal of Health Care for the Poor and Underserved, 17*(3), 512–521.

16

A Decision-Support Intervention for Black Women Eligible for Adjuvant Systemic Therapy: Sisters Informing Sisters[SM] About Breast Cancer Treatment—An Intervention to Reduce Treatment Disparities

Vanessa B. Sheppard, Sherrie Flynt Wallington,
Karen Patricia Williams, and Wanda Lucas

Breast cancer is the leading cancer diagnosed in women and the second cause of cancer death (American Cancer Society, 2010). Over the next 5 years, approximately 100,000 African American women will be diagnosed with breast cancer. Unfortunately, a disproportionate number of these women will have less than optimal outcomes. Compared to White women, African American (hereinafter referred to as Black) women have higher breast cancer mortality rates, despite lower age-adjusted incidence rates (Menashe, Anderson, Jatoi, & Rosenberg, 2009). Recent data suggest that this disparity is widening (Klassen et al., 2002; O'Malley, Forrest, & Mandelblatt, 2002). Adjuvant systemic therapies, such as chemotherapy and endocrine therapy, are beneficial for survival of both node-positive and node-negative disease (Goldhirsch et al., 2003). However, disparities persist in referral and uptake of adjuvant treatment for Black women (Ashing-Giwa et al., 2004; Chu, Lamar, & Freeman, 2003; Joslyn & West, 2000). For example, compared with Whites, Black women have fewer oncology consults, receive less aggressive chemotherapy regimens, are more likely to discontinue chemo-therapy, and are less likely to have endocrine therapy prescribed for ER/PR-positive tumors (Ashton et al., 2003; Bickell et al., 2006; Gordon, 2003; Guidry, Matthews-Juarez, & Copeland, 2003; Schleinitz, DePalo, Blume, & Stein, 2006). When Black women do receive systemic treatment, their survival outcomes are similar to those for Whites (Dignam, 2000, 2001). Thus, survival disparities may be partly explained by the lower use of adjuvant therapies (Bickell et al., 2006). A prescription of adjuvant therapy generally occurs within the context of the patient–provider relationship; therefore, communication between these parties may influence its use (Coulter, Entwistle, & Gilbert, 1999; Gafni, Charles, & Whelan, 1998; Halkett, Arbon, Scutter, & Borg, 2005; Janz et al., 2004).

Previous studies have found that Black patients report fewer participatory medical encounters, ask fewer questions, receive less medical information in consultations for cancer treatment, and have more problems communicating with physicians than Whites (Gordon, Street, Sharf, & Souchek, 2006; Hack, Degner, & Parker, 2005; Halbert, Armstrong, Gandy, & Shaker, 2006; Hall, Roter, & Katz, 1988; Kreling, Figueiredo, Sheppard, & Mandelblatt, 2006). In one study, Blacks' lower receipt of information from physicians than Whites was explained by Blacks' lower engagement in active communication behaviors (e.g., asking questions, voicing concerns, etc.) that typically elicit information from physicians (Gordon et al., 2006). Other research has documented that women who ask more questions report better patient–provider communication, are more informed, and tend to follow treatment recommendations more than women who ask fewer questions (Schleinitz et al., 2006). Thus, less participatory patient–provider encounters could result in inadequate knowledge about and use of adjuvant therapy among Black women (Hack et al., 2005; Kreling et al., 2006). In non-Black populations, communication skill practice and peer role model interventions have been effective in improving communication skills and promoting patients' involvement in care (Cegala, McClure, Marinelli, & Post, 2000; Krupat et al., 1999; Towle, Godolphin, Manklow, & Wiesinger, 2003). Researchers have found that Black women were more likely to have full staging of their tumors ordered if they were more assertive with their physicians (Krupat et al., 1999). These studies and others suggest that improving patient communication skills may positively influence provider communication (Epstein & Street, 2007; Janz et al., 2004; Krupat et al., 1999; Sayer, 2000).

There are limited interventions and patient decision aids to address patient–provider interactions or support Black women's decision-making processes afterwards. To address the limitations, we developed an intervention to improve patient-centered cancer care for Black breast cancer patients (Sheppard et al., 2010). This chapter begins with a historical overview of the evolution of patient-centered approaches to clinical decision making, followed by descriptions of some well-discussed physician–patient decision-making models, starting with the paternalistic model and moving forward. Next, we specifically discuss skill interventions and patient decision aids and their benefits, and the lack of similar tools for Black women making decisions regarding adjuvant therapy treatment. This will be followed by a discussion of an American Cancer Society–funded skill intervention and patient decision aid example, and lastly insights and lessons learned for skill intervention and patient decision aid development targeting Black women for adjuvant therapy decision making.

HISTORICAL UNDERPINNINGS OF PATIENT-CENTERED APPROACHES TO CLINICAL DECISION MAKING

Cancer treatments have become increasingly more sophisticated as a result of research and technological advances (Stacey, Samant, & Bennett, 2008). Thus, for cancer patients, some clinical decisions about treatment are straightforward, with clear supporting evidence, whereas others are more difficult. Consequently, there has been a major shift in the approaches to clinical decision making within the most recent generation of practicing physicians. For much of the 20th century, physicians took a very paternalistic approach (Charles, Gafni, & Whelan, 1997). Physicians were considered the keeper of all medical lore and the sole decision makers. However, since the 1970s, there has been an increasing recognition that cancer patients need to be better informed and take more of an active role in decisions concerning their medical care (Stacey et al., 2008).

First, more emphasis, as well as legislation, has focused on the importance of informed consent (Mazur, 1986; Schultz, 1998; Wills & Holmes-Rovner, 2003). Guidelines on informed consent intend to protect patients and promote ethical research conduct through the full explanation of a proposed treatment, including any possible harm, and through the requirement that people freely consent (Jefford & Moore, 2008). In the research setting, the idea of written informed consent dates back to the 1900s and has shifted the emphasis from medical paternalism to that of a duty to respect patient autonomy (Dowd & Wilson, 1995; Schultz, 1998; Wills & Holmes-Rovner, 2003). Several states have laws aimed at improving informed consent by requiring the disclosure of options for the treatment of breast cancer, particularly for breast-conserving surgery (Nattinger, Hoffman, Shapiro, Gottlieb, & Goodwin, 1996). However, although informed consent generally implies that patients are informed of a particular treatment, consent forms typically focus on the side effects of the chosen treatment rather than strategies to engage patients in making cancer decisions (Stacey et al., 2008). We are now in an era in which patients want to be more involved in their health and medical care. A growing number of patients have shifted from being passive bystanders to active participants in the clinical decision-making process (O'Connor et al., 2003). Patient surveys across several health domains have given evidence to patient empowerment and report that patients want and expect to be involved in the making of health decisions (Davison et al., 2002; Degner et al., 1997; O'Connor et al., 2003; Goold & Fessler, 2002). Moreover, with the recent breast cancer advances and technologies, unlike previous generations, women diagnosed with breast cancer have several choices to make, including the type of surgery, whether to have radiation, the type of adjuvant therapy (chemotherapy or hormonal therapy), and the type of reconstruction, if any (Zuckerman, 2000). Also important is that there is emerging evidence that indicates that women with breast cancer who have been actively involved in making decisions about their treatment tend to be more satisfied with their overall quality of life, have higher physical and social functioning, and experience fewer side effects (Hack, Degner, Watson, & Sinha, 2006; Street & Voigt, 1997). However, many women will not have access to all the available and balanced information that they need to make the most informed choices appropriate for them. Thus, informed consent and shared decision making with their physician or health provider becomes increasingly important (Zuckerman, 2000).

PATIENT INVOLVEMENT APPROACHES: MODELS OF PHYSICIAN–PATIENT DECISION MAKING

This patient empowerment in health decisions has been due in part to a rapid expansion in and access to medical information, particularly with the Internet, improved access to health information for patients, and an evolution of the patient's role in decision making (Stacey et al., 2008). Likewise, health professional organizations are also emphasizing the need for client-centered care and the expectation that patients will be involved in making their health decisions (Institute of Medicine, 2001). This is considered to now be an important aspect of patient-centered care. As such, these evolutionary changes have yielded several models of patient involvement in the decision-making process. Benefits to patient involvement in the decision-making process can help improve satisfaction, understanding, and confidence in the decisions that are made (Institute of Medicine, 2001). It is now recognized that there are several distinct approaches to treatment decision making that physicians can use with their patients—the paternalistic approach, the informed or consumerist approach, and the shared approach (Charles, Gafni, & Whelan, 1999). Table 16.1 provides a brief summary of key distinctions between paternalistic interactions and those that are regarded as shared or collaborative interactions.

First, as mentioned earlier, physicians who adopt a paternalistic approach take on the burden of making the primary health decisions. The paternalistic model has been well articulated in the literature (Deber, 1994; Emanuel & Emanuel, 1992; Levine et al., 1992), and research suggests that physicians adopting this approach are unlikely to have much interest in

TABLE 16.1   A Summary of Key Aspects of Paternalistic and Shared Decision Making

Characteristic	Paternalistic Decision Making	Shared Decision Making
Partial disclosure of facts, benefits, and options to patient	X	
Full disclosure of facts, benefits, and options to patient		X
Considers patient's values		X
Includes or relies on physician opinions	X	
Promotes patient autonomy		X
Provides physician with authority	X	
Balanced patient–physician relationship		X
Patient is able to make informed decision		X
Potential to cause anxiety to patient		X

discussing patient concerns; they are more likely to want short descriptions of physical symptoms that they can transform into diagnostic categories, thus allowing them to then make a treatment decision that they think is in their patient's best interest without having to explore each patient's values and concerns (Gafni et al., 1998). The next two models, the informed or consumer model and the shared decision-making (SDM) model, were developed largely in part to the flaws of the paternalistic model (Charles et al., 1999).

In the informed or consumer model, one of the more often mentioned and promoted models among patient advocacy groups, patients are accorded a more active role in both defining the problem for which they want help and determining appropriate treatment (Gafni et al., 1998). Key characteristics involve the physician or health care team diagnosing the problem, providing options and information, and subsequently allowing the patient to make an informed decision in a fairly autonomous manner (Charles et al., 1997). The information exchange is one-way, from physician to patient (Charles et al., 1999).

Research suggests that some patients prefer either a passive or completely active decision-making role (Brown et al., 2002; Bruera, Sweeney, Calder, Palmer, & Benisch-Tolley, 2001; Bruera, Willey, Palmer, & Rosales, 2002; Mazur & Hickam, 1997). However, within the past decade, a prevailing approach is shared decision making, whereby patients together with their clinician discuss the current evidence on options and arrive at a mutually agreed-upon choice (Charles et al., 1997; Elwyn et al., 2001; Towle et al., 2003). The information exchange between the physician and patient is two-way; at minimum, the physician must inform the patient of all information that is relevant to making the decision, information about available treatment options, the benefits and risks of each option, and potential effects on the patient's psychological and social well-being. Likewise, the patient needs to provide information to the physician on issues just mentioned, along with his or her values, preferences, lifestyle, beliefs, and knowledge about his or her illness and its treatment (Charles et al., 1999). Only in this model do physicians commit themselves to an interactive relationship with patients in developing treatment recommendations that are consistent with the patient's values and preferences (Gafni et al., 1998). There is limited information about decision preferences of minority breast cancer patients, but some data suggest that Latinas and Blacks are more likely to involve their family members than Whites (Maly, Umezawa, Ratliff, & Leake, 2006). Additionally, data from general health studies suggest that Blacks are less likely than Whites to be actively involved in their treatment decisions (Cooper-Patrick et al., 1997).

Strategies and Tools for Increasing Skill Development and Patient Involvement

The decisions that breast cancer patients have to make are difficult, and women often must navigate through massive amounts of information, some of which is explained to them adequately and some of which is not. As a result, breast cancer patients require targeted approaches to prepare them for the physician–patient encounter and to promote their ability to make the most informed and appropriate decision for them (Stacey et al., 2008). Patient decision aids can help patients recognize that a decision needs to be made, understand the current scientific evidence, clarify their values associated with outcomes of options, and achieve a quality decision (Elwyn et al., 2006). Patient decision aids are tools that translate evidence into a patient-friendly form by providing, at a minimum, information on the options, benefits and risks, and methods to clarify personal values (O'Connor et al., 1999). Most patient decision aids are self-administered and available in many formats—paper-based, such as question prompt sheets (Gaston & Mitchell, 2005), videos and DVDs, and on the Internet (Stacey et al., 2008)—and some are practitioner-based, involving more complex approaches, as is the case with many breast cancer decision aids (Green, Biesecker, McInerney, Mauger, & Fost, 2001; Green et al., 2004; Whelan et al., 2004). Based on a systematic review of randomized trials of cancer patient decision aids, patients exposed to decision aids are more likely to participate in decision making and achieve higher-quality decisions (Stacey et al., 2008). Other reviews have also examined breast cancer and other cancer patient decision aids in detail (Gaston & Mitchell, 2005; Gravel, Legare, & Graham, 2006; Kinnersley et al., 2007; Matsuyama, Reddy, & Smith, 2006; O'Connor et al., 2001; Waljee, Hawley, Alderman, Morrow, & Katz, 2007). Unfortunately, there is a paucity of skill interventions and patient decision aids for Black women considering adjuvant therapy. However, shared decision making (SDM) appears to be acceptable in Black men regarding prostate cancer screening. Williams et al. (2008) found that 57% of African American men preferred SDM compared to 36% who preferred to make their own decision; only 7% wanted their doctor to decide. A higher level of education and older age were associated with preferring SDM, whereas men with greater prostate cancer screening knowledge were more likely to prefer to make the decision independently (Williams et al., 2008).

BLACK WOMEN AND ADJUVANT THERAPY: SKILLS INTERVENTIONS AND PATIENT DECISION AIDS

In general, some studies show that many patients are not necessarily given quantitative information about prognosis with and without adjuvant therapy and often make inaccurate estimates (Ravdin et al., 2001; Whalan & Loprinzi, 2005). These potential estimates then affect the decisions that patients make (Kassirer, 1994; Llewellyn-Thomas, 1995). Without accurate and balanced information about treatment outcomes as a point of reference, patients cannot play a role as adequately informed partners in deciding whether to take adjuvant therapy and what specific treatment might be most appropriate.

For instance, one study was designed to examine the impact of a novel computer program decision aid, *Adjuvant!*, on treatment decisions made during consultations between oncologists and patients with breast cancer, and its implications for practice (Siminoff, Gordon, Silverman, Budd, & Ravdin, 2006). The program estimates outcomes with or without adjuvant therapy. This study showed that a decision aid made a difference in the choice of whether or not to take adjuvant therapy. The decision aid allowed patients and physicians to consider the benefits of adjuvant therapy in an easy-to-understand format. Treatment decisions were more individualized for patients in the intervention than in the control group. The use of the decision aid was acceptable to both patients and physicians (Siminoff et al., 2006). This study did not report data specifically for Blacks or other racial and ethnic groups; women were categorized as either White or non-White (20%). Further, the extent to which Black women were involved in the development of existing decision aids is unclear from current reports.

Due to the scarcity of skill interventions for Black women considering adjuvant therapy, as well as evidence showing that skill interventions and decision aids play an important role in decision making, more research is needed that focuses on women. Moreover, researchers have suggested that building upon important cultural values may strengthen interventions with Black women (Airhihenbuwa, 1995). In doing so, both the physician and the patient need to be aware of the cultural assumptions underlying the development and use of decision aids, and must access their cultural sensitivity to the needs and preferences of patients in diverse cultural groups (Charles, Gafni, Whelan, & O'Brien, 2006). The following sections present an example of the formative and pilot data of a decision-support intervention for newly diagnosed Black breast cancer patients.

INTERVENTION EXAMPLE: SISTERS INFORMING SISTERS[SM] ABOUT BREAST CANCER TREATMENT—AN INTERVENTION TO REDUCE TREATMENT DISPARITIES

In an effort to reduce treatment disparities, we developed an intervention targeting Black women. In the following sections, we describe the formative process we used to develop a decision-support intervention for Black women eligible for adjuvant therapy. We sought to first qualitatively describe the factors that influence Black women's adjuvant therapy decisions, use these formative data to develop messages for a treatment decision-support intervention, and pilot test the acceptability and utility of the intervention with community members and newly diagnosed women. The overall goal of the intervention was to empower Black women to engage in their interactions with providers when making decisions about adjuvant systemic therapy. To do this, we focused on increasing women's skills in communicating with their provider.

Intervention Development: Formative Phase

Overview

As described earlier, there is limited information about decision-support interventions for Black women with breast cancer or the involvement of Black women in the development of existing decision aids. Therefore, we collected formative data to inform the intervention. Formative research is conducted at the beginning of an intervention or program, to help researchers or program managers decide on appropriate strategies for the intervention, and to better understand the factors that influence the behavior of their target audience and determine the best ways to reach them. The purpose of the formative phase of this work was to build upon existing knowledge about treatment decisions and use a cultural health behavior model to develop a culturally appropriate intervention for newly diagnosed Black women. In this section, we describe: (1) our approach to collecting and analyzing formative data to inform our intervention messages and approach: (2) key perceptions, enablers, and nurturers that are important to women when making adjuvant therapy decisions; and (3) how we used these data to develop an intervention strategy to promote better patient–provider communication. The Institutional Review Board (IRB) approved the data collection activities of the study, which were conducted in the Washington, DC metro area. First, qualitative data were collected and analyzed. Next, these formative findings, analyzed according to the PEN-3 Health Behavior Cultural Model (PEN-3), were translated into specific intervention activities and messages using domains of a cultural behavioral model. Lastly, community members, researchers/clinicians, and newly diagnosed patients (who were all Black) reviewed the intervention materials and provided feedback for revisions, and then the resulting intervention workbook was pilot tested.

Theoretical Framework

The PEN-3 Health Behavior Cultural Model provided the primary framework for formative data collection and analysis and the development of intervention messages (see Figure 16.1). We selected this framework because it has been successfully used to analyze qualitative data and inform the development of other culturally appropriate interventions (Airhihenbuwa, 1993, 1995). PEN-3 has three interrelated domains: (1) cultural identity, (2) relationships and expectations, and (3) cultural empowerment as applied to cancer chemotherapy communication (Airhihenbuwa, 1993, 1995). The cultural identity domain determines the intervention focus (i.e., person, extended family, and/or neighborhood). The relationships and expectations domain

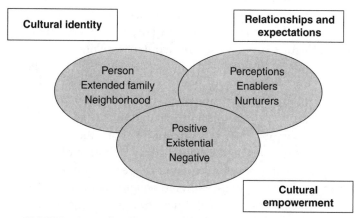

FIGURE 16.1 The PEN-3 Health Behavior Cultural Model

Source: From *Health and Culture: Beyond the Western Paradigm*, by C. O. Airhihenbuwa, 1995, Thousand Oaks, CA: Sage. Adapted with Permission.

is used to determine the perceptions, enablers, and nurturers that impact health behaviors, such as uptake of adjuvant therapy. Perceptions include the knowledge, attitudes, values, and beliefs that either facilitate or hinder a woman's motivation to use adjuvant therapy. Enablers are community and/or structural factors (e.g., resources, accessibility, etc.) that facilitate behavior. Nurturers are reinforcing factors, such as those from one's social network. The third domain, cultural empowerment, assesses the cultural appropriateness of health beliefs from the second domain and categorizes these as "positive" (practices that improve use of adjuvant therapy), "existential" (practices that neither positively nor negatively influence health treatment), or "negative" (practices that decrease the likelihood of using adjuvant therapy) (Airhihenbuwa, 1995).

The Results of the Formative Phase

We conducted in-depth interviews with Black women newly diagnosed in active treatment ($n = 14$), Black survivor mentors ($n = 10$), and cancer providers that treated large numbers of Black breast cancer patients (see Table 16.2). All interviews were audio-recorded and transcribed verbatim into transcripts. The transcripts were analyzed by members of the research team and followed the process of the PEN-3 domains described. In Table 16.3, the key themes from the formative data are described according to each PEN-3 domain. They are summarized and organized according to cultural empowerment categories of *perceptions, nurturers,* and *enablers. Positive perceptions* included hope, determination, faith in God, and acceptance of breast cancer. *Negative perceptions* were fear of adjuvant treatment side effects (nausea and hair loss), beliefs that systemic adjuvant therapies were experimental, concerns about being unable to care for family members, and feelings of mistreatment by the medical community. Several women expressed negative perceptions about breast cancer treatment, which were largely derived from observations of others' treatment experiences. One woman explained why she decided against chemotherapy: *"I know what* [chemotherapy] *did to my husband. It made all his hair fall out."* Myths about breast cancer treatment included the belief that chemotherapy and/or hormonal therapies were experimental, and that an injury led to breast cancer. In some instances, these myths influenced women to decide against chemotherapy or hormone therapy.

Existential perceptions that did not directly influence treatment decisions included fatalism, fear for the future, and preference for mastectomy to avoid chemotherapy and additional treatment. Several women held fatalistic beliefs about breast cancer prior to, but not after, their diagnosis. All respondent groups commented that Black women held strong spiritual beliefs that aided their ability to cope with the disease and treatment, but these were not a primary decision-making resource. *Enablers* of adjuvant therapy decisions

TABLE 16.2 Characteristics of Patients and Survivor Participants ($N = 32$)

Characteristic	Total N (%)	Women in Active Treatment[a] $N = 14$	Survivor Advocates[a] $N = 10$	Newly Diagnosed Women[b] $N = 8$
Education				
<12 years	1 (3)	1	–	–
>12 years	26 (81)	13	5	8
Unknown	5 (16)	–	5	–
Marital/Partner Status				
Unmarried/Unpartnered	16 (50)	6	4	6
Married/Partnered	9 (31)	6	1	2
Unknown	7 (22)	2	5	–
Stage				
0	1 (3)	1	–	–
I	8 (25)	7	–	1
II	11 (34)	6	1	4
III	3 (9)	–	1	2
IV	1 (3)	–	–	1
Unknown	8 (25)	–	8	–
Type of Surgery				
Mastectomy	18 (56)	8	6	4
Lumpectomy	7 (22)	–	3	4
Unknown	7 (22)	6	1	–
Chemotherapy				
Yes	19 (59)	6	7	6
No	12 (38)	8	2	2
Unknown	1 (3)	–	1	–
Radiation				
Yes	12 (38)	5	5	2
No	18 (56)	9	3	6
Unknown	1 (6)	–	1	–

[a]Women who completed in-depth interviews for formative data collection.
[b]Newly diagnosed women who provided feedback on intervention.

were patient–provider communication, access factors, and the availability of anti-nausea medications. Women who reported good communication were more satisfied with their treatment decisions, were more knowledgeable about their treatment, and proceeded with recommended adjuvant therapies. Women who reported adhering to physician recommendations for adjuvant therapies described providers' explanations as responsive and thorough. As one woman shared, "*I have excellent communication with* [providers]. *They explain things. They take time with me. They always call me back. They've been very open about the prognosis.*"

Women who reported poor patient–provider communication, or who were uncomfortable asking questions, reported feeling less confident about their adjuvant treatment decisions. Other women felt that they did not

TABLE 16.3   A Summary of Treatment Perceptions, Enablers, and Nurturers That Influence Adjuvant Treatment Decisions

Domain Description	Positive	Existential	Negative
Perceptions knowledge, attitudes, values, and beliefs that may facilitate or hinder personal motivation to maintain or change health beliefs and/or practices	Faith in God Hope, determination Acceptance Need to be strong for family Sharing stories of survival	Cancer myths Spiritual beliefs Fear/fatalism Finality/mastectomy Concerns about recurrence	Fear of treatment side effects/tolerating treatment Experience of others; cancer myths Ability to take care of family/children Belief that chemotherapy is experimental Concerns about hormonal therapy side effects, long-term Doctors do not have time to address questions Treatment impacts daily life and activities Silence and privacy (re: sharing the diagnosis) Mistreatment from the medical system
Enablers community and structural factors that may affect treatment decisions	Access issues Strong relationships with providers Social support Spiritual beliefs Women should speak up for themselves Good patient–provider communication Writing down questions	Decision-making preferences Prefers professional to make decisions Does not know as much about cancer as cancer providers	Poor patient–provider communication Limited knowledge about treatment options Uncomfortable asking questions of providers Base decision on—future concerns (fertility, etc.) Neglected by providers
Nurturers reinforcing factors from a person's social network that may influence a person	Supportive spouse and family Survivors, faith community Close relationship with providers Empathetic providers Family Faith in God	Religious beliefs No help with emotional aspects of the disease	Family members' negative reactions and concerns Lack of empathetic providers Family members who lack knowledge Provider bias Uninformed family and community members

receive all necessary information and attributed this to the fact that they were passive in their interactions with providers: *"You know, they always ask* [if] *I have anything to say, and I never have anything to say so it's mostly my fault."* This lack of participation in decision making and limited questioning affected treatment decisions, as several women rejected chemotherapy because they perceived few benefits relative to the risks. Others opted to receive mastectomies to avoid additional treatment and reduce the chance of recurrence. As one survivor summarized, *"The problem is that you just don't get the right information at the right time."* A few women felt that some doctors talked down to them or assumed that they did not understand the medical terms because of their race or economic status.

Taken together, these findings were used to inform the intervention components (see Table 16.4). For example, given the importance of sharing and hearing the stories of others, we confirmed that our strategy would

TABLE 16.4 Examples of Integration of Formative Findings for the T.A.L.K. Back!® Intervention Strategy

Formative Findings	Exemplar Messages/Strategies for Survivor Coach	Examples From Patient Guidebook
Perceptions Sharing/hearing stories of survival Strong faith Concern about negative side effects	• Encourage reliance on faith. • Address key fears about treatment. • Help is available for potential side effects. • Survival rates are higher with appropriate treatment.	**Message 1: You Are Not Alone** Presentation of facts, list of support resources, and glossary of oncologic terms. Worksheet of values, preferences, related to key decision, and stories from other survivors.
Enablers Patient-provider relationship Need/desire for better communication	• Identify values, preferences for decision making. • Help patient handle negative physician responses.	**Message 2: Sharing in Treatment Decisions** Definition and diagram of informed decision making, information to consider when weighing treatment options, sample and blank worksheets to weigh pros and cons of treatment options, and issues to discuss with physicians.
Nurturers Other survivors Family Faith in God Interaction w/providers	• Use of a Black breast cancer survivor. • Review strategies to share information with family members. • Role-play patient–physician interactions.	**Message 3: T.A.L.K. Back!®** Focus on: Telling Story, Asking Questions, Listening Actively, and Knowing treatment options; provides sample conversations on how to use the communication-decision model, sample questions to ask physicians, blank sheets for patient's use.

involve survivors as interventionists. Similarly, the importance of faith in God during one's diagnosis was integrated within our first message. The intervention approach, messages, and strategies were reviewed by eight newly diagnosed Black breast cancer patients and revisions were made as necessary. The following section provides an overview of the intervention approach and materials.

Intervention Overview

Figure 16.2 provides an overview of the Sisters Informing Sisters[SM] (SIS) intervention. The intervention included an in-person coaching session, a patient guidebook, and detailed training and implementation materials for the interventionist. The interventionist (survivor coach) is integral to the success of the intervention. While it was decided to use peers, it was necessary to identify key criteria for the selection of appropriate peers and also develop training materials. A detailed facilitator's manual was developed for use with clients. Additionally, a coaches' training institute was employed to train more coaches. Three survivor coaches who self-identified as Black/African American were hired: one full-time coach/program manager and two part-time coaches. Survivors selected to become coaches had completed their primary treatment and had experience as advocates or in the fields of

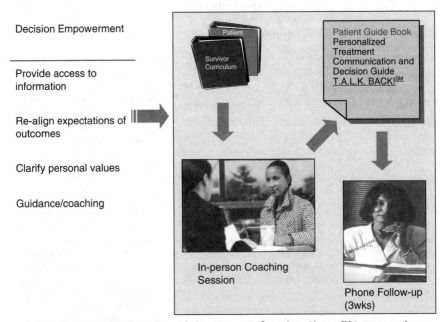

FIGURE 16.2   An Overview of the Sisters Informing Sisters[SM] Intervention

counseling and/or wellness coaching. In addition, they were trained to understand basic terminology, breast cancer etiology, and treatments for breast cancer. Although the intention was not to create breast cancer experts, they were prepared to counter misconceptions and myths about the disease found in formative work and published studies. Special care was made to ensure that they were aware of the boundaries of their work, that is, they were not to provide medical advice to their patients, despite the fact that they were survivors. Furthermore, they were trained to use active and reflective listening techniques, motivational interviewing, and appreciative inquiry (Chen et al., 2009; Shiboski, Schmidt, & Jordan, 2007). Finally, coaches were encouraged to demonstrate empathy without becoming a crutch to patients, as the goal was to coach patients into becoming their own best advocate.

Training Modules for Interventionists/Survivor Coaches

To maximize instruction and information acquisition among coaches, the institute utilized the 4MAT model of learning as a way to capitalize on the various learning styles of students. The model maintains that learners possess four unique learning styles (innovative, analytic, dynamic, and common sense) that are influenced by whether individuals are right-brained or left-brained. This approach was proven successful in both the initial acquisition and retention of health-related information, and was utilized as the foundation for training breast cancer survivors to provide cancer support through the Witness Program® developed at the University of Arkansas (Spatz, 1991).

The SIS Training of Coaches (TOC) curriculum and training program created for this study utilized various techniques to make information accessible to its learners. For example, lecture-style instruction was used to impart information on breast cancer terminology, treatment options, types of physicians/providers involved in breast cancer care, and implications of breast cancer staging. Experiential learning took place through role-play activities, in which coaches and patients were paired to simulate a coaching activity.

Coaches were trained by integrating a variety of techniques to prepare them for working with newly diagnosed cancer patients. These techniques, made popular in the field of counseling and wellness coaching, were modified to support women through their cancer treatment journey and help them become more informed, mindful, and active members of their treatment team. What follows is a brief description of some of the techniques that were used to prepare SIS survivor coaches to effectively work with newly diagnosed women. Survivor coaches received training in the etiology, diagnosis, and treatment of breast cancer. The training was offered in two parts: Breast Cancer 101 and Breast Cancer 201. Although not intended to create breast cancer experts, it prepared them to counter misconceptions and myths about the disease. Special care was made to ensure that survivor coaches did not provide medical advice to their patients, but instead used their personal stories as a way of connecting and building relationships and trust. They presented a face of survivorship that clients could identify with (i.e., if I survived it, you can too) and provided real-life experiences and information (not myths and misconceptions) about breast cancer treatment and survivorship.

In addition to preparing survivor coaches for their work with program participants, program staff monitored and tracked coaching activities through progress notes and monthly program meetings. Additionally, survivor coaches were provided with ongoing emotional support for any issues that arose for them on their own survivorship journeys. Coaches had the opportunity to work together to support each other, discuss challenges encountered, and brainstorm solutions. It was hoped that this type of ongoing support would prevent survivor coach burnout and ensure the longevity and viability of the program.

Intervention Implementation: Process Data

To assess the feasibility of the intervention, we conducted a pilot study using a pretest/posttest design. After receiving Institutional Review Board approval, breast cancer patients were recruited from surgical and oncology practices, cancer navigators, and breast cancer support groups. Colorful tri-folded brochures that described the study and included a study voicemail line, e-mail, and telephone numbers were mailed to local support groups, cancer providers, and mammography clinics.

Eligible women were those who self-identified as being Black and had histologically confirmed breast cancer. All patient interviews were conducted by telephone by a research assistant, who read all materials, including the consent and survey, to the patient over the telephone using a computer-assisted telephone interview (CATI) format. Patients returned consent forms by mail and received a $25 American Express gift check for their time after their coaching session. After the coaching session, women were recontacted within 3 months by the survivor coach to complete a telephone follow-up survey to assess intervention outcomes. Participants received $15 after the follow-up survey. *Programmatic data* from survivor coaches' tracking sheets were also reviewed to assess the location of the coaching sessions, the lengths of the sessions, key observations (e.g., patients' mood, etc.), and referrals.

Preliminary Results and Lessons Learned

This section summarizes preliminary information regarding women seen through the SIS intervention. Forty-seven Black women were seen by a survivor coach; their ages ranged from 32–54 years, and 38% were married or living as married. Women were referred to the program from a variety of sources, including surgeons ($n = 41$), medical oncologists ($n = 6$), and community sources ($n = 22$), or from friends/self-referral ($n = 73$). On average, the time from the initial contact to the first appointment was 27 days. The most common reason for this delay was because of scheduling issues, generally because of a patient's ill health (due to recovery from surgery). In two instances, coaches assisted women prior to the in-person session by helping to recognize that the patient was likely having unusual problems with recovery, and assisted women in contacting their providers. Even after agreeing to see the coach, there were some women who were unreachable; a few of these women were faced with additional social challenges of homelessness and substance recovery issues. Overall, coaches made up to five calls to contact women and a letter was also mailed to the address on record. Sixty-four percent of the participants were recruited to the program prior to their surgery, while the remaining women were in various stages of their treatment. Most participants agreed that it would be best to see a coach either before surgery or right after surgery, to prepare themselves for talking with their doctor about treatment. Most (95%) women seen by coaches were insured and most had completed high school. In the District of Columbia, regardless of income, most residents have some form of health insurance.

Patient coaching sessions were held in coffee shops (40%), patients' homes (30%), and hospitals or other medical facilities (12%). Seventy-four percent of the patients attended the sessions alone, without family members and/or friends. Coaches observed that more than half of the patients appeared to be optimistic (55%) in the face of their diagnosis. Other patients were observed by coaches as being anxious (20%), afraid (15%), or sad (10%). Coaches used the patient guidebook and T.A.L.K. Back!© model to facilitate sessions with patients. Steps within T.A.L.K. Back!© were tailored to each woman's case (e.g., emphasis on treatment options vs. emphasis on getting certain questions answered by providers). Common patient concerns noted by coaches were: The ability to conceive later on in life, the effects of chemotherapy, decisions about whether to have a double mastectomy, recurrence, and financial matters. In most instances, these issues were related to women's weighing of their treatment options or their concerns about recommended treatment options.

Additional assistance that was offered to patients included: General survivor-to-survivor support (82%), sharing of personal story (66%), development of questions for providers (50%), dissemination of resources (46%), help with medical terminology (34%), assistance with decision making (26%), assistance with communication skills (24%), and explanation of treatment (20%). Survivor coaches made referrals to nutritionists and patient navigators at various cancer centers, for assistance with transportation- or insurance-related issues. Typical post-session activities were as follows: Referral to support groups, distribution of recipes (for use during treatment), appointment setting for follow-up telephone calls, homework to request and obtain pathology from providers, and delivery of information about clinical trials.

Shared Decision-Making Model

Most (86%) patients reported that the steps in the T.A.L.K. Back!© model helped them communicate better with their provider; 10% responded that they did not and 5% were uncertain. After using the guidebook, 98% of participants were informed and 98% reported increased knowledge about their treatment options. Two focus groups were held (one with participants and one with coaches) to gain each group's experience with and perspectives on the intervention (see the summary in Table 16.5). Overall, both groups were very satisfied with their experiences with the program. Women in both

TABLE 16.5   A Summary of the Evaluation Focus Groups

Perspectives from Survivor Coaches

Overall, coaches felt that the training prepared them for the role of being an "empowerer."

Participants reported that being an example of survivorship was the most powerful of the interactions with newly diagnosed women.

Coaches rated the patient guidebook and the facilitator guide as extremely easy to use.

For most coaches, it took two to three telephone calls to reach the patient.

All coaches strongly believed that the SIS program is valuable and would like it to be extended to more women.

Coaches also felt that the relationship with a survivor coach would be beneficial to women who are finished with treatment and are entering survivorship.

The importance of reaching women prior to surgery was stressed as important to influencing patient outcomes.

All would be interested in participating in a support group, if initiated by the SIS program.

Patient Perspectives

Overall, participants were satisfied with the intervention.

Women expressed the desire to speak to the survivor coach more frequently and earlier in the treatment journey.

Upon diagnosis, women stated that they needed more information on the side effects of treatment, especially from chemotherapy.

Suggestions for recruitment included community outreach about SIS using brochures posted in various places, etc.

Some participants had referred other patients to the SIS program.

Several women expressed interest in being trained as a survivor coach.

Women expressed a strong desire to have a SIS support group. They stated that a support group or more information on "what to expect when you're a cancer survivor" would be helpful.

groups stated the importance of reaching women earlier in the treatment process, to facilitate the best assistance and support with decision making. Interestingly, coaches felt that the T.A.L.K. method of communicating with providers and decision support would be useful to women during the survivorship phase of treatment. Several patients were interested in serving as coaches, and women in both groups wanted to continue the process by having a support group. An evaluation of the effects of the intervention on intermediate intervention outcomes is underway. Lessons learned from this phase will be used to refine recruitment efforts and to streamline coordination of intervention components.

Lessons Learned and Next Steps

Although most women initiate and complete adjuvant systemic therapies such as chemotherapy and hormonal therapy, a substantial number of Black women do not. Clinical trials demonstrate that benefits and outcomes of these therapies in Black women are comparable to outcomes in Whites. Thus, the lower use of adjuvant systemic therapy in African American breast cancer patients may contribute to poorer outcomes in this group. Unfortunately, interventions to eliminate disparities after a woman is diagnosed with breast cancer are limited. Our formative work from providers, patients, and survivor coaches supported the need of interventions in this area for newly diagnosed women. The SIS intervention was developed to begin to fill this gap and assist African American women who are newly diagnosed with breast cancer. We focused on increasing the patient's involvement in her treatment decisions, given that patient-centered care—which includes shared decision making—has been suggested as an ideal framework to guide interactions with providers. To identify culturally relevant approaches and messages for our empowerment model, we used the PEN-3 health education model and collected rich in-depth qualitative data. This approach identified the type of messages, the delivery mechanism (e.g., survivors) and education/skills (e.g., treatment knowledge, communicating with providers), and cultural targets for the intervention. The resulting intervention builds upon successful models of peer education that have been used to educate women about breast cancer screening and early detection methodologies.

Overall, we learned that women found the approach of using trained peers acceptable and that it is feasible to recruit newly diagnosed women into a decision-support intervention. We also found good support for the print materials that were developed for this project. The T.A.L.K. Back!© shared decision-making approach is in concordance with key elements of the National Cancer Institute (NCI) model for patient-centered cancer care and was grounded in information gleaned from in-depth interviews with providers, newly diagnosed women, and peer advocates. The PEN-3 health education model provided us with the framework to identify intervention targets and to build upon cultural assets within the Black American community.

Preliminary data suggest high satisfaction for the intervention. Both formative data and those from intervention participants support the employment of peers. It was necessary to have intense training and also retraining to ensure that all coaches followed protocols. Additionally, given that a few women died, it was necessary to have supports in place for the coaches themselves. We worked with a clinically trained psychologist to both refer patients and coaches when necessary. Partnerships within the health care system will be key to identifying and holding the in-person session as early as possible after diagnosis. It will be important to balance recruitment into the intervention with the need for a woman to adjust to the diagnosis before meeting with a coach. One challenge to seeing women early in the process was that women were seen by coaches from various health care systems across the Washington, DC metro area. Thus, the coaches were not integrated within just one health care system, and women often needed to make time for a separate appointment. While the in-person session is important for building trust, and facilitating development of communication and decision-making skills, we are considering the possibility of conducting the initial session by telephone. The training was well received by survivors. Several of the SIS coaches were experienced peer volunteers with other breast cancer advocacy groups, but expressed that they had not received training specific to helping newly diagnosed women make treatment decisions or a detailed communication guide, particularly for African American women. To our knowledge, this is the first treatment-focused intervention aimed to promote shared decision making in newly diagnosed African American women that included Black women in its development. To reduce disparities, more focus on this phase of the cancer control continuum is necessary. Given these promising preliminary results, steps are under way to complete analysis of shared decision making and communication outcomes, and eventually to evaluate long-term outcomes using a rigorous research design.

ACKNOWLEDGMENTS

This chapter draws in part from a prior paper: Sheppard, V.B., Williams, K.P., Harrison, T. M., Jennings, Y., Lucas, W., Stephen, J., . . . Taylor, K.L. (2010). Development of a decision-support intervention for Black women with breast cancer. *Psychooncology, 19,* 62–70. This research has been supported by funding from the American Cancer Society (MRSGT-06-132-01CPPB) and the Susan G. Komen Foundation (POP0503398) to Dr. Vanessa B. Sheppard.

REFERENCES

Airhihenbuwa, C. (1993). Health promotion for child survival in Africa: Implications for cultural appropriateness. *Hygie, 12,* 10–15.

Airhihenbuwa, C. O. (1995). *Health and culture: Beyond the western paradigm.* Thousand Oaks, CA: Sage.

American Cancer Society (2010). *Breast cancer facts and figures 2009–2010.* Atlanta, GA: Author.

Ashing-Giwa, K. T., Padilla, G., Tejero, J., Kraemer, J., Wright, K., & Coscarelli, A. (2004). Understanding the breast cancer experience of women: A qualitative study of African American, Asian American, Latina and Caucasian cancer survivors. *Psychooncology, 13,* 408–428.

Ashton, C. M., Haidet, P., Paterniti, D. A., Collins, T. C., Gordon, H. S., O'Malley, K., . . . Street, R. L., Jr. (2003). Racial and ethnic disparities in the use of health services: Bias, preferences, or poor communication? *Journal of General Internal Medicine, 18,* 146–152.

Bickell, N. A., Wang, J. J., Oluwole, S., Schrag, D., Godfrey, H., Hiotis, K., . . . Guth, A. A. (2006). Missed opportunities: Racial disparities in adjuvant breast treatment. *Journal of Clinical Oncology, 24,* 1357–1362.

Brown, R. F., Butow, P. N., Henman, M., Dunn, S. M., Boyle, F., & Tatters all, M. H. (2002). Responding to the active and passive patient: Flexibility is the key. *Health Expectations, 5,* 236–245.

Bruera, E., Sweeney, C., Calder, K., Palmer, L., & Benisch-Tolley, S. (2001). Patient preferences versus physician perceptions of treatment decisions in cancer care. *Journal of Clinical Oncology, 19,* 2883–2885.

Bruera, E., Willey, J. S., Palmer, J. L., & Rosales, M. (2002). Treatment decisions for breast carcinoma: Patient preferences and physician perceptions. *Cancer, 94,* 2076–2080.

Cegala, D. J., McClure, L., Marinelli, T. M., & Post, D. M. (2000). The effects of communication skills training on patients' participation during medical interviews. *Patient Education and Counseling, 41,* 209–222.

Charles, C., Gafni, A., & Whelan, T. (1997). Shared decision-making in the medical encounter: What does it mean? (Or it takes at least two to tango). *Social Science & Medicine, 44,* 681–692.

Charles, C., Gafni, A., & Whelan, T. (1999). Decision-making in the physician–patient encounter: Revisiting the shared treatment decision-making model. *Social Science & Medicine, 49,* 651–661.

Charles, C., Gafni, A., Whelan, T., & O'Brien, M. A. (2006). Cultural influences on the physician-patient encounter: The case of shared treatment decision-making. *Patient Education and Counseling, 63,* 262–267.

Chen, L. M., Li, G., Reitzel, L. R., Pytynia, K. B., Zafereo, M. E., Wei, Q., & Sturgis, E. M. (2009). Matched-pair analysis of race or ethnicity in outcomes of head and neck cancer patients receiving similar multidisciplinary care. *Cancer Prevention Research (Philadelphia, PA), 2,* 782–791.

Chu, K. C., Lamar, C. A., & Freeman, H. P. (2003). Racial disparities in breast carcinoma survival rates: Separating factors that affect diagnosis from factors that affect treatment. *Cancer, 97,* 2853–2860.

Cooper-Patrick, L., Powe, N. R., Jenckes, M. W., Gonzales, J. J., Levine, D. M., & Ford, D. E. (1997). Identification of patient attitudes and preferences regarding treatment of depression. *Journal of General Internal Medicine, 12,* 431–438.

Coulter, A., Entwistle, V., & Gilbert, D. (1999). Sharing decisions with patients: Is the information good enough? *BMJ, 318,* 318–322.

Davison, B. J., Gleave, M. E., Goldenberg, S. L., Degner, L. F., Hoffart, D., & Berkowitz, J. (2002). Assessing information and decision preferences of men with prostate cancer and their partners. *Cancer Nursing, 25,* 42–49.

Deber, R. B. (1994). Physicians in health care management: 8. The patient-physician partnership: decision making, problem solving and the desire to participate. *Canadian Medical Association Journal, 151,* 423–427.

Degner, L. F., Kristjanson, L. J., Bowman, D., Sloan, J. A., Carriere, K. C., O'Neil, J., . . . Mueller, B. (1997). Information needs and decisional preferences in women with breast cancer. *Journal of the American Medical Association, 277,* 1485–1492.

Dignam, J. J. (2000). Differences in breast cancer prognosis among African-American and Caucasian women. *CA: A Cancer Journal for Clinicians, 50,* 50–64.

Dignam, J. J. (2001). Efficacy of systemic adjuvant therapy for breast cancer in African-American and Caucasian women. *Journal of the National Cancer Institute Monograph,* 36–43.

Dowd, S. B., & Wilson, B. (1995). Informed patient consent: A historical perspective. *Radiologic Technology, 67,* 119–124.

Elwyn, G., Edwards, A., Mowle, S., Wensing, M., Wilkinson, C., Kinnersley, P., & Grol, R. (2001). Measuring the involvement of patients in shared decision-making: A systematic review of instruments. *Patient Education and Counseling, 43,* 5–22.

Elwyn, G., O'Connor, A., Stacey, D., Volk, R., Edwards, A., Coulter, A., . . . International Patient Decision Aids Standards (IPDAS) Collaboration. (2006). Developing a quality criteria framework for patient decision aids: Online international Delphi consensus process. *BMJ, 333,* 417.

Emanuel, E. J., & Emanuel, L. L. (1992). Four models of the physician-patient relationship. *Journal of the American Medical Association, 267,* 2221–2226.

Epstein, R. M., & Street, R. L. (2007). *Patient-centered communication in cancer care: Promoting healing and reducing suffering.* National Cancer Institute. NIH Publication No. 07-6225. Bethesda, MD: National Cancer Institute.

Gafni, A., Charles, C., & Whelan, T. (1998). The physician-patient encounter: The physician as a perfect agent for the patient versus the informed treatment decision-making model. *Social Science & Medicine, 47,* 347–354.

Gaston, C. M., & Mitchell, G. (2005). Information giving and decision-making in patients with advanced cancer: A systematic review. *Social Science & Medicine, 61,* 2252–2264.

Goldhirsch, A., Wood, W. C., Gelber, R. D., Coates, A. S., Thurlimann, B., & Senn, H. J. (2003). Meeting highlights: Updated international expert consensus on the primary therapy of early breast cancer. *Journal of Clinical Oncology, 21,* 3357–3365.

Goold, S. D., & Fessler, D. (2002). Development of an instrument to measure trust in health insurers. *Journal of General Internal Medicine, 15* (Suppl.1), S118–S119.

Gordon, H. S., Street, R. L., Jr., Sharf, B. F., & Souchek, J. (2006). Racial differences in doctors' information-giving and patients' participation. *Cancer, 107,* 1313–1320.

Gordon, N. H. (2003). Socioeconomic factors and breast cancer in black and white Americans. *Cancer and Metastasis Reviews, 22,* 55–65.

Gravel, K., Legare, F., & Graham, I. D. (2006). Barriers and facilitators to implementing shared decision-making in clinical practice: A systematic review of health professionals' perceptions. *Implementation Science, 1,* 16.

Green, M. J., Biesecker, B. B., McInerney, A. M., Mauger, D., & Fost, N. (2001). An interactive computer program can effectively educate patients about genetic testing for breast cancer susceptibility. *American Journal of Medical Genetics, 103,* 16–23.

Green, M. J., Peterson, S. K., Baker, M. W., Harper, G. R., Friedman, L. C., Rubinstein, W. S., & Mauger, D. T. (2004). Effect of a computer-based decision aid on knowledge, perceptions, and intentions about genetic testing for breast cancer susceptibility: A randomized controlled trial. *Journal of the American Medical Association, 292,* 442–452.

Guidry, J. J., Matthews-Juarez, P., & Copeland, V. A. (2003). Barriers to breast cancer control for African-American women: The interdependence of culture and psychosocial issues. *Cancer, 97,* 318–323.

Hack, T. F., Degner, L. F., & Parker, P. A. (2005). The communication goals and needs of cancer patients: A review. *Psychooncology, 14,* 831–845.

Hack, T. F., Degner, L. F., Watson, P., & Sinha, L. (2006). Do patients benefit from participating in medical decision making? Longitudinal follow-up of women with breast cancer. *Psychooncology, 15,* 9–19.

Halbert, C. H., Armstrong, K., Gandy, O. H., & Shaker, L. (2006). Racial differences in trust in health care providers. *Archives of Internal Medicine, 166,* 896–901.

Halkett, G. K., Arbon, P., Scutter, S. D., & Borg, M. (2005). The experience of making treatment decisions for women with early stage breast cancer: A diagrammatic representation. *European Journal of Cancer Care (England), 14,* 249–255.

Hall, J. A., Roter, D. L., & Katz, N. R. (1988). Meta-analysis of correlates of provider behavior in medical encounters. *Medical Care, 26,* 657–675.

Institute of Medicine (2001). *Crossing the quality chasm: A new health system for the 21st century* (Rep. No. 2). Washington, DC: National Academies Press.

Janz, N. K., Wren, P. A., Copeland, L. A., Lowery, J. C., Goldfarb, S. L., & Wilkins, E. G. (2004). Patient-physician concordance: Preference, perceptions, and factors influencing the breast cancer surgical decision. *Journal of Clinical Oncology, 22,* 3091–3098.

Jefford, M., & Moore, R. (2008). Improvement of informed consent and the quality of consent documents. *Lancet Oncology, 9,* 485–493.

Joslyn, S. A., & West, M. M. (2000). Racial differences in breast carcinoma survival. *Cancer, 88,* 114–123.

Kassirer, J. P. (1994). Incorporating patients' preferences into medical decisions. *New England Journal of Medicine, 330,* 1895–1896.

Kinnersley, P., Edwards, A., Hood, K., Cadbury, N., Ryan, R., Prout, H., . . . Butler, C. (2007). Interventions before consultations for helping patients address their information needs. *Cochrane Database of Systematic Reviews,* CD004565.

Klassen, A. C., Smith, A. L., Meissner, H. I., Zabora, J., Curbow, B., & Mandelblatt, J. (2002). If we gave away mammograms, who would get them? A neighborhood evaluation of a no-cost breast cancer screening program. *Preventive Medicine, 34,* 13–21.

Kreling, B., Figueiredo, M., Sheppard, V., & Mandelblatt, J. (2006). A qualitative study of factors affecting chemotherapy use in older women with breast cancer: Barriers, promoters, and implications for intervention. *Psychooncology, 15(12),* 1065–1076.

Krupat, E., Irish, J. T., Kasten, L. E., Freund, K. M., Burns, R. B., Moskowitz, M. A., & McKinlay, J. B. (1999). Patient assertiveness and physician decision-making among older breast cancer patients. *Social Science &Medicine, 49,* 449–457.

Levine, D. M., Becker, D. M., Bone, L. R., Stillman, F. A., Tuggle, M. B., Prentice, M., . . . Filippeli, J. (1992). A partnership with minority populations: A community model of effectiveness research. *Ethnicity & Disease, 2,* 296–305.

Llewellyn-Thomas, H. A. (1995). Patients' health-care decision making: A framework for descriptive and experimental investigations. *Medical Decision Making, 15,* 101–106.

Maly, R.C., Umezawa, Y., Ratliff, C.T., & Leake, B. (2006). Racial/ethnic group differences in treatment decision-making and treatment received among older breast carcinoma patients. *Cancer, 106*(4), 957–965.

Matsuyama, R., Reddy, S., & Smith, T. J. (2006). Why do patients choose chemotherapy near the end of life? A review of the perspective of those facing death from cancer. *Journal of Clinical Oncology, 24,* 3490–3496.

Mazur, D. J. (1986). What should patients be told prior to a medical procedure? Ethical and legal perspectives on medical informed consent. *American Journal of Medicine, 81,* 1051–1054.

Mazur, D. J., & Hickam, D. H. (1997). Patients' preferences for risk disclosure and role in decision making for invasive medical procedures. *Journal of General Internal Medicine, 12,* 114–117.

Menashe, I., Anderson, W. F., Jatoi, I., & Rosenberg, P. S. (2009). Underlying causes of the black-white racial disparity in breast cancer mortality: A population-based analysis. *Journal of the National Cancer Institute, 101,* 993–1000.

Nattinger, A. B., Hoffman, R. G., Shapiro, R., Gottlieb, M. S., & Goodwin, J. S. (1996). The effect of legislation requirements on the use of breast-conserving surgery. *New England Journal of Medicine, 335,* 1035–1040.

O'Connor, A. M., Drake, E. R., Wells, G. A., Tugwell, P., Laupacis, A., & Elmslie, T. (2003). A survey of the decision-making needs of Canadians faced with complex health decisions. *Health Expectations, 6,* 97–109.

O'Connor, A. M., Rostom, A., Fiset, V., Tetroe, J., Entwistle, V., Llewellyn-Thomas, H., . . . Jones, J. (1999). Decision aids for patients facing health treatment or screening decisions: Systematic review. *BMJ, 319,* 731–734.

O'Connor, A. M., Stacey, D., Rovner, D., Holmes-Rovner, M., Tetroe, J., Llewellyn-Thomas, H., . . . Jones, J. (2001). Decision aids for people facing health treatment or screening decisions. *Cochrane Database of Systematic Reviews,* CD001431.

O'Malley, A. S., Forrest, C. B., & Mandelblatt, J. (2002). Adherence of low-income women to cancer screening recommendations. *Journal of General Internal Medicine, 17,* 144–154.

Ravdin, P. M., Siminoff, L. A., Davis, G. J., Mercer, M. B., Hewlett, J., Gerson, N., & Parker, H. L. (2001). Computer program to assist in making decisions about adjuvant therapy for women with early breast cancer. *Journal of Clinical Oncology, 19,* 980–991.

Sayer, H. (2000). Meeting the information needs of cancer patients. *Professional Nurse, 4,* 244–247.

Schleinitz, M. D., DePalo, D., Blume, J., & Stein, M. (2006). Can differences in breast cancer utilities explain disparities in breast cancer care? *Journal of General Internal Medicine, 21,* 1253–1260.

Schultz, E. A. (1998). Informed consent: An overview. *CRNA, 9,* 2–9.

Sheppard, V. B., Williams, K. P., Harrison, T. M., Jennings, Y., Lucas, W., Stephen, J., . . . Taylor, K. L. (2010). Development of decision-support intervention for Black women with breast cancer. *Psychooncology, 19,* 62–70.

Shiboski, C. H., Schmidt, B. L., & Jordan, R. C. (2007). Racial disparity in stage at diagnosis and survival among adults with oral cancer in the US. *Community Dentistry and Oral Epidemiology, 35,* 233–240.

Siminoff, L. A., Gordon, N. H., Silverman, P., Budd, T., & Ravdin, P. M. (2006). A decision aid to assist in adjuvant therapy choices for breast cancer. *Psychooncology, 15*(11), 1001–1013.

Spatz, T. S. (1991). Improving breast self-examination training by using the 4MAT instructional model. *Journal of Cancer Education, 6,* 179–183.

Stacey, D., Samant, R., & Bennett, C. (2008). Decision making in oncology: A review of patient decision aids to support patient participation. *CA: A Cancer Journal for Clinicians, 58,* 293–304.

Street, R. L., Jr. & Voigt, B. (1997). Patient participation in deciding breast cancer treatment and subsequent quality of life. *Medical Decision Making, 17,* 298–306.

Towle, A., Godolphin, W., Manklow, J., & Wiesinger, H. (2003). Patient perceptions that limit a community-based intervention to promote participation. *Patient Education and Counseling, 50,* 231–233.

Waljee, J. F., Hawley, S., Alderman, A. K., Morrow, M., & Katz, S. J. (2007). Patient satisfaction with treatment of breast cancer: Does surgeon specialization matter? *Journal of Clinical Oncology, 25,* 3694–3698.

Whelan, T., Levine, M., Willan, A., Gafni, A., Saunders, K., Mirsky, D., . . . Dubois, S. (2004). Effect of a decision aid on knowledge and treatment decision making for breast cancer surgery. *Journal of the American Medical Association, 292,* 435–441.

Whalan, T., & Loprinzi, C. (2005). Physician/patient decision aids for adjuvant therapy. *Journal of Clinical Oncology, 23,* 1627–1630.

Williams, R. M., Zincke, N. L., Turner, R. O., Davis, J. L., Davis, K. M., Schwartz, M. D., . . . Taylor, K. L. (2008). Prostate cancer screening and shared decision-making preferences among African-American members of the Prince Hall Masons. *Psychooncology, 17,* 1006–1013.

Wills, C. E., & Holmes-Rovner, M. (2003). Patient comprehension of information for shared treatment decision making: State of the art and future directions. *Patient Education and Counseling, 50,* 285–290.

Zuckerman, D. M. (2000). The need to improve informed consent for breast cancer patients. *Journal of the American Medical Women's Association, 55,* 285–289.

17

Prostate Cancer Patient Education Project (PC^{PEP}): Prostate Cancer Symptom Management in Low-Literacy Men

David M. Latini, Stacey L. Hart, Heather Honoré Goltz, Stephen J. Lepore, and Leslie R. Schover

Few psychosocial interventions exist for men living with prostate cancer (PCa), and none of these interventions has been developed to address survivorship concerns for men with low health literacy. In this chapter, we describe the development and evaluation of Prostate Cancer Patient Education Project (PC^{PEP}), a PCa patient-education program for men with low health literacy, treated for localized disease that is tailored to the participant's particular symptom profile. The program was developed using input from PCa survivors to determine the most effective symptom-management practices (Latini et al., 2008).

In 2005, PCa surpassed lung cancer as the most common cancer diagnosis in American men (American Cancer Society, 2005). There will be an estimated 217,730 new PCa cases in 2010, up from 192,280 cases in 2009 (American Cancer Society, 2009, 2010). PCa represents 28% of all new male cancer diagnoses expected in 2010, the same proportion represented by breast cancer in women (American Cancer Society, 2010). It continues to disproportionately affect minority men (American Cancer Society, 2007).

TREATMENT OF LOCALIZED PCA

Patients with early, localized PCa have several treatment options and alternatives for active treatment. Surgery involves complete removal of the prostate. Radiotherapy can be accomplished using the external-beam method or implantation of radioactive "seeds" (brachytherapy). Based on their clinical condition, some men may opt for hormonal therapy (HT), freezing the prostate (cryoablation), or "active surveillance" (i.e., observation of disease progression, sometimes in conjunction with later HT) (Talcott, 1996).

Most PCa develops in older men and grows very slowly (American Cancer Society, 2001). However, because of the use of the prostate-specific antigen (PSA) screening test to identify PCa in its very early stages, the average age at diagnosis has fallen rapidly; and the number of patients diagnosed has increased. Thus, patients are receiving a PCa diagnosis earlier, allowing more patients to receive possibly curative therapy. However, these early diagnoses are forcing more men to choose a cancer therapy several years earlier than if PSA tests were unavailable, and if PCa diagnoses were simply based on the appearance of symptoms or on an abnormal digital rectal exam (Talcott, 1996). There also continues to be controversy about whether earlier diagnosis translates to better survival or simply subjects more men to morbidity associated with unnecessary treatment (Wilt et al., 2008).

TREATMENT-RELATED SYMPTOMS

Currently available treatments for localized PCa carry the risk of a number of possible iatrogenic symptoms, primarily urinary and bowel incontinence and erectile dysfunction (ED). These symptoms have important implications for health-related quality of life (HRQOL) (Litwin et al., 1995). Because the prognosis for men diagnosed with localized PCa is quite good, men who develop iatrogenic symptoms will likely experience them for years (Talcott, 1996).

Side effects vary by treatment. Men who receive a radical prostatectomy are more likely to have problems with urinary and sexual functioning. Radiotherapy patients are more likely to experience bowel problems (Litwin et al., 1995; Talcott, 1996). However, this symptom picture may change over time. Surgery patients frequently report substantial improvements in urinary and sexual functioning 12 months after treatment (Lubeck et al., 1999), but radiotherapy patients have a different prognosis. Although their urinary functioning remains fairly stable over time, their sexual functioning declines steadily over time (Lubeck et al., 1999; Talcott et al., 1998); and they also report substantial declines in bowel function (Potosky et al., 2000). HT patients report both localized problems (e.g., ED) and systemic concerns, such as fatigue, depression, and hot flashes (Holzbeierlein, McLaughlin, & Thrasher, 2004).

One important consideration for urinary, sexual, bowel, and hormonal symptoms is the amount of bother they cause a patient. The level of perceived bother may vary by patient characteristics. For example, older men tend to have poorer sexual function and slower recovery after treatment for PCa, but younger men tend to be more distressed by poorer sexual function than older men (Roberts, Lepore, Hanlon, & Helgeson, 2010). HRQOL also may vary on the basis of other characteristics (e.g., men with lower socioeconomic status having worse HRQOL; Penson et al., 2001). Thus, while the need for symptom management may vary by treatment type because of different symptoms for different treatments, perceived symptom-management needs also may vary, based on the characteristics of the patient.

Patients receive a great deal of information immediately after treatment. However, one relevant study by Steginga et al. has shown that men do not process much of this information because of the emotional burden of receiving a cancer diagnosis (Moore & Estey, 1999). Steginga and her colleagues suggested that patients receive telephone follow-up and ongoing support to manage their symptoms. In another descriptive study, one third of the men interviewed reported moderate-to-high unmet needs that were related to sexuality, psychological concerns, and use of the health care system (Steginga et al., 2001). Respondents reported a need for information about specific symptoms, such as urinary and bowel function and sexual dysfunction, with younger men being more interested in information about sexual functioning than older men.

The need for symptom-management education is greater for men with low health literacy. Health literacy—"the ability to which individuals have the capacity to obtain, process, and understand health-information services needed to make appropriate health decisions" (Ratzan & Parker, 2000)—has been shown to be strongly related to health status and health outcomes (Baker et al., 2002; Bennett et al., 1998; Kalichman & Rompa, 2000). Persons with low health-literacy skills are significantly less likely to take preventive actions to improve their health (Gazmararian, Parker, & Baker, 1999; Scott, Gazmararian, Williams, & Baker, 2002). Health literacy is a particular concern because African American men, a group with a significantly higher prevalence of PCa, are overrepresented among low-literacy men with PCa (Bennett et al., 1998).

TAILORED INTERVENTIONS AND STEPPED CARE

One approach to psychosocial interventions is to "tailor" the intervention to the individual, usually based on some previously defined characteristic. A related concept is "stepped care," usually motivated by cost concerns. Patients are provided with lower-cost treatment initially and "stepped up" to more costly interventions as needed (Newman, 2000; Otto, Pollack, & Maki, 2000; Wilson, Vitousek, & Loeb, 2000).

One tailored self-care intervention has particular relevance to the intervention described here. It was developed and delivered to patients with multiple sclerosis (MS) (Likosky, Starr-Schneidkraut, & Wilson, 1994; Likosky, Starr-Schneidkraut, Wilson, & Javerbaum, 1995; Starr et al., 1996). The intervention components were developed based on the results of a qualitative examination of the self-care strategies of current MS patients, using the Critical Incident Technique, a semi-structured technique used to elicit effective and ineffective symptom-management strategies (Flanagan, 1954). The intervention was also delivered, at least in part, over the telephone. Efforts were made to tailor it by providing modules to participants with impairment in a specific area, as indicated by their responses to a disease-specific HRQOL instrument. Although this study enrolled a small number of patients, the authors were able to show significant improvement in some disease-specific HRQOL measures.

As mentioned previously, PCa survivors experience different symptoms, depending on their treatment; and the perceived importance of these symptoms varies, based on an individual's characteristics (e.g., age, relationship status). A tailored intervention is particularly appropriate for these men.

INTERVENTIONS FOR PCa

Although most research on psychosocial aspects of PCa has focused on describing impairments in HRQOL and psychological functioning of men with PCa (Bokhour, Clark, Inui, Silliman, & Talcott, 2001; Eton & Lepore, 2002; Helgeson & Lepore, 1997; Litwin et al., 1995; Lubeck et al., 1999, 2001; Meade, Calvo, Rivera, & Baer, 2003), the number of interventions developed specifically for PCa survivors has been limited (Visser & van Andel, 2003). Two main support-group networks—the American Cancer Society's "Man to Man" and "US Too"—exist around the nation to provide ongoing support. A small number of behavioral medicine researchers have tried to move beyond this model, with didactic and more intensive supportive interventions. These fall into three categories—diet/lifestyle interventions, interventions to improve psychological functioning, and disease-specific interventions—although some interventions span these categories.

Of the few interventions that exist, two have come from nurse researchers. One intervention by Maliski et al. (2004) used a nurse case-manager approach to improve quality of life in low-income men with PCa. The intervention by Maliski et al. used retrospective record review to describe interventions offered to patients, making it difficult to replicate in later research. The nurse case managers provided each patient with an intervention tailored to his particular needs, rather than developing standard materials and targeting patients with intervention components based on patient characteristics.

Another nurse-led intervention based on Mishel's Uncertainty in Illness Theory focused on psychological outcomes, such as problem-solving, cognitive reframing, cancer knowledge, and patient–provider communications, as well as disease-specific outcomes, including symptom distress, number of symptoms, urinary and sexual functioning, and satisfaction with sexual functioning (Mishel et al., 2002). Some participants received the intervention alone, whereas others received the intervention and a family member received a modified form of the intervention. Both groups were compared to a usual-care control group. In addition to providing techniques to reduce uncertainty, the patient educator provided didactic information about symptom management. The investigators reported significant improvement in cognitive-reframing and problem-solving scales at 4 months, but this effect did not hold up at the 7-month assessment. For some men, PCa symptoms tend to resolve over time anyway; and men in all three groups reported fewer symptoms over time, with significant improvements in urinary incontinence and satisfaction for treatment-group men (Mishel et al., 2002).

Another intervention used a group approach to provide didactic information about PCa to treatment-group men. Some treatment-group men were randomized to also participate in a discussion group held after each didactic session. Men in both treatment conditions also received printed materials summarizing the lectures. Men in the education plus discussion condition had the best outcomes. Men in the education conditions reported significantly better outcomes for PCa knowledge, physical functioning, positive health behaviors, and sexual bother. No significant differences were found in sexual or urinary functioning. Importantly, the investigators found a differential effect by educational level, with less-educated men benefiting more from the intervention. Whereas college-educated men evidenced improvements in knowledge about PCa and positive health behaviors from pre- to post-intervention in both the control and intervention conditions, men with less than a college-level education improved more if they received the intervention than if they were in the control condition. These findings suggest that men with less formal education do not have easy access to information about PCa, do not know how to access such information, or need more help in understanding the information than men with relatively more formal education (Lepore, Helgeson, Eton, & Schulz, 2003).

NEEDS FOR PCa EDUCATION FOCUSING ON SYMPTOM MANAGEMENT

Boberg et al. (2003) found that the greatest unmet need for improvement in PCa education programs related to treatment-related symptoms and cancer recurrence. Among men on HT, treatment symptoms and ways to manage them were the two most commonly reported areas of unmet informational needs (Templeton & Coates, 2003). Although the interventions described above meet some needs of men with PCa, most do not address this need for specific information about managing treatment-related side effects. For programs that provide an information component about symptom management, the interventions' effect on symptom management has been mixed. Mishel et al. (2002) reported that their intervention reduced sexual bother and improved urinary functioning, but they did not find significant differences in sexual functioning. Lepore et al. (2003) also reported significant decreases in sexual bother, but no effect of their intervention on urinary or sexual functioning. PC^{PEP} was developed to improve symptom management in men with PCa, with an emphasis on tailoring the intervention to men's needs and making the intervention accessible to men with low health literacy.

THEORETICAL FRAMEWORKS

The intervention described here is based on two broad theoretical and conceptual frameworks: the Symptom Management Model (SMM) (Dodd et al., 2001; UCSF Faculty Group in Symptom Management, 1994), developed by faculty members in the University of California at San Francisco (UCSF) School of Nursing Center for Symptom Management; and Self-Efficacy Theory (Bandura, 1986, 1997). Since it was published in 1994 and revised in 2001, the SMM has been used in numerous studies of symptoms in cancer and chronic disease (Dodd et al., 2001; UCSF Faculty Group in Symptom Management, 1994). The SMM characteristics and their conceptualized relationships to one another are depicted in Figure 17.1. To further define important aspects of the symptom-management experience, we used Self-Efficacy Theory to refine the SMM. Self-Efficacy Theory has been used in numerous studies of chronic disease management (Lorig et al., 1999, 2001; S. R. Wilson et al., 1996). In particular, two points where we will try to intervene to improve symptom management are outcome efficacy (confidence that an outcome can be affected) and self-efficacy (confidence that one can personally accomplish an outcome) (Bandura, 1986). In the SMM, self-efficacy is part of the symptom experience.

Figure 17.2 shows the resulting biopsychosocial model derived from combining the UCSF SMM and Self-Efficacy Theory. According to the model, men who improve their functional status will have reduced symptom distress, the primary outcome in our intervention. Further, men who attend the intervention session and consistently do their assigned homework are more likely to reduce their symptom distress. Adherence also is likely to increase the number of mastery experiences that a participant has and his sense of outcome and self-efficacy. Figure 17.2 includes the basic variables describing PCa symptom management.

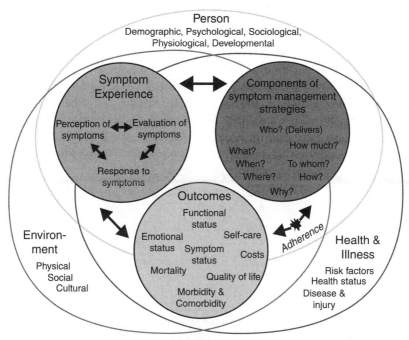

FIGURE 17.1   The University of California at San Francisco Symptom Management Model

Source: "Advancing the Science of Symptom Management" by M. Dodd, S. Janson, N. Facione, J. Faucett, E. S. Froelicher, J. Humphreys, et al. (2001), *Journal of Advanced Nursing* 33, pp. 668–676. Used with permission.

FORMAT AND CONTENT

PC^PEP intervenes on the symptom experience by providing symptom-management strategies to facilitate better symptom outcomes. In particular, it is designed to reduce symptom distress by increasing participants' symptom-management knowledge and providing them with more effective symptom-management strategies, based on their current symptom presentation.

Several general principles guided this program's development. Participants receive information and resources that will help them see their symptoms as ultimately manageable problems (i.e., Bandura's Concept of Outcome Efficacy). A set of validated measures of PCa symptom distress and functional status is used to determine areas that are most problematic and important to the participant. Based on the participant's needs, the patient educator and the participant establish symptom-management goals. The intervention provides resources and opportunities for mastery over reported symptoms. An important distinction between PC^PEP and others is that PC^PEP includes a 6-month follow-up that allows reassessment and repetition of

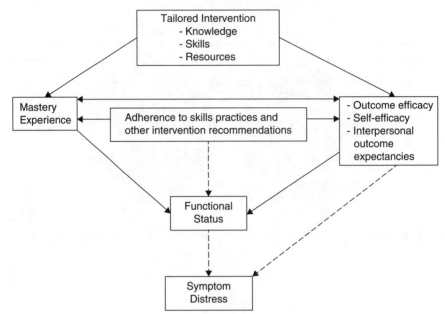

FIGURE 17.2   The Biopsychosocial Model of Prostate Cancer Symptom
Management

Source: "Sexual Rehabilitation After Localized Prostate Cancer: Current Interventions and Future
Directions" by D. M. Latini, S. L. Hart, D. W. Coon, and S. J. Knight, 2009, *Cancer Journal*,
15, p. 34–40. Used with permission.

parts of the intervention related to areas where the participant continues to
report problems. The 6-month follow-up period also offers further opportunities at each follow-up to address the changing symptom profile typical in
PCa survivors.

The resources provided include factual information about symptom
management, lists of community and Internet-based resources, and referrals to outside resources for specific problems (e.g., a referral to a support
group or counselor to deal with emotional concerns related to having cancer
or changes in sexual performance). Each intervention module includes skill-
building exercises that provide mastery experiences, leading to greater feelings of control over symptoms. For example, one component in the Mishel
et al. (2002) intervention that was particularly useful in controlling urinary
incontinence was teaching participants Kegel exercises to strengthen pelvic-
floor muscles. Given their results, the present intervention has included
Kegel exercises as one skill component of the urinary-functioning module(s).

The PC^{PEP} intervention format builds on previous symptom-
management education programs in other disease areas (Likosky et al., 1994,
1995; McNabb, Wilson-Pessano, Hughes, & Scamagas, 1985; Wilson et al.,
1983), other self-management programs based on Self-Efficacy Theory, and

earlier PCa interventions by Lepore et al. (2003) and Mishel et al. (2002)—although some information provided in the PC^PEP intervention may duplicate information that participants received at their initial cancer diagnosis. However, many patients feel overwhelmed with information at the time of diagnosis; and the emotional burden of learning that they have a potentially life-threatening disease may interfere with information processing (Moore & Estey, 1999). Thus, repetition can be beneficial. The PC^PEP intervention is conducted as one-on-one telephone sessions, when the educator addresses the specific needs of each patient, as indicated by (1) changes in functional status or symptom-distress scores or (2) requests for information or referrals from the participant. The telephone approach is convenient to intervention staff and patients alike, and does not require special computer equipment or knowledge for participants.

To provide a better understanding of how the PC^PEP intervention works, it is useful to consider a specific example. ED is a symptom frequently reported by men treated with surgery, radiotherapy, and HT. Participants who report erectile difficulties receive a module including information about noninsertive sexual practices that they might incorporate into their relationship to provide pleasure to them and their partner. This information might help change a participant's attitude about what constitutes a fulfilling sexual experience. The skills component might include practice in communication skills for talking with a partner about ED and ways of incorporating other sexual techniques into a relationship. Patients also are referred to resources such as a urologist who can provide pharmacological treatment for their ED, or a mental health professional who can provide more in-depth counseling about adapting to the patient's ED.

THE BASIS OF PC^PEP

PC^PEP resembles most closely the interventions developed by Lepore et al. (2003), Mishel et al. (2002), and Maliski et al. (2004). It includes a tailored telephone intervention with a defined symptom-management component similar to the intervention by Mishel et al. and the MS symptom-management program described above. Like the intervention by Maliski et al., it is based on a conceptualization of change in the symptom experience as a product of changing patients' feelings of outcome efficacy and self-efficacy. Change in self-efficacy is a potential mediator of the intervention effects on primary outcomes (see Figure 17.2).

PC^PEP also builds on these previous intervention studies to extend our understanding of psychosocial programs for PCa survivors. Although previous interventions used sexual and urinary functioning as primary outcomes, the focus of both programs was primarily on other outcomes, such as cognitive reframing (Mishel), PCa knowledge (both Mishel and Lepore), and positive health behaviors (Lepore). The PC^{PEP} intervention focuses primarily on symptom management. In addition, while some information about managing feelings is included in PC^{PEP}, the main focus is on managing *physical symptoms*. We took this approach because Ullrich et al. showed that men with PCa reporting emotional distress tended to do so because of poorly managed physical symptoms (Ullrich, Carson, Lutgendorf, & Williams, 2003).

The study by Mishel et al. (2002) included information about managing symptoms such as sexual functioning. However, their data were collected before the introduction of sildenafil and other oral ED medications, and focused on facilitating insertive sexual practices, mainly through the use of mechanical devices that helped participants to develop erections. One reason participants who received the intervention did not significantly improve sexual functioning is that they also reported being troubled by the intrusiveness of the erectile aids. Currently, three oral medications are available to improve erectile functioning; and it is possible that other medications will be approved before much longer. In addition, because many men with PCa do not benefit from oral erectile aids (Penson et al., 2005; Schover et al., 2002), PC^{PEP} includes other means for improving erectile functioning. It also provides information about noninsertive practices men can use if they are unable to restore their potency.

Another important lesson from the study by Mishel et al. (2002) is that symptom-management education may be more effective if it is available over a longer time period. Mishel et al. offered participants telephone sessions for eight consecutive weeks. PC^{PEP} offers education at six time points—baseline, 2 weeks, and 1, 2, 4, and 6 months. The follow-up points offer participants a chance to request more information about their current symptoms or learn about newly emerging symptoms. This is an important distinction, as symptoms vary over time based on the treatment selected (Lubeck et al., 1999). Adding assessment and intervention points allows a better understanding of changes in symptom profiles over time, intervention closer in time to when symptoms occur, and tracking of adherence more closely.

DEVELOPMENT OF THE PC^{PEP} MODULES

In creating new materials for low-literacy patients, several principles were kept in mind (Doak, Doak, & Root, 1996; National Cancer Institute, 2003). Materials were written in active voice, using common words and short sentences, and using examples to illustrate difficult words. Materials also included an interactive component so that the learner could demonstrate mastery of the material and where he might need further instruction (Doak et al., 1996). As the modules were developed, the investigators used the readability statistics provided in Microsoft Word as one indication of readability, with a target of sixth grade reading level. The investigators used the Suitability Assessment of Materials (SAM) method (Doak et al., 1996), which provided a systematic method for evaluating written patient-education materials. The method incorporates a number of criteria already discussed (e.g., layout, writing style, and level of interactivity). After the modules were developed, they were reviewed in a series of three group cognitive interviews, with three to four patients per group. The groups were composed of both high- and low-literacy PCa survivors. Group members were asked about meaning, readability, the types of graphics used, and the amount of white space. Suggestions from group members were reviewed by the investigators as a whole and incorporated into the final version of the PC^PEP materials.

DESIGN OF THE PC^PEP RANDOMIZED CLINICAL TRIAL

The PC^PEP study was a randomized controlled trial (RCT) with 200 participants randomized one-to-one to either a wait-list control group or the new intervention. We used the random permuted blocks within strata method to randomize participants to study groups (Pocock, 1983). The groups were stratified on health-literacy level and PCa treatment type to ensure that there were (1) equivalent numbers of low-literacy men in each group, and (2) equivalent numbers of patients with different treatment histories in each group. To participate in the RCT, a potential participant had to: (1) be male; (2) be 18 years or older, with biopsy-proven PCa; (3) be diagnosed with localized disease; (4) have a telephone at the time of enrollment; (5) have an address where he could receive intervention materials by mail (a street address or post office box); and (6) be able to speak and understand English. Potential participants were excluded if they: (1) had another form of active cancer; (2) had metastasis; (3) had a recurrence of disease (PCa); (4) had co-occurring serious medical illnesses that would affect erectile functioning and urinary incontinence (e.g., diabetes) in the problem list, or ability to respond to the questions and take an active part in the intervention (e.g., dementia, cognitive dysfunction) in the problem list; (5) received non-VA surgery follow-up care (i.e., the patient had been seeing physicians for cancer follow-up outside of the VA); (6) were unable to provide informed consent; or (7) had not been treated for PCa (i.e., had not completed surgery, radiation, or cryotherapy) and were not on HT.

STUDY OUTCOMES

The primary outcomes for PC^PEP were the urinary and sexual symptom-distress measures from the Expanded Prostate Cancer Index (EPIC) (Wei, Dunn, Litwin, Sandler, & Sanda, 2000). The measure has subscales that assess urinary, bowel, sexual, and hormonal symptom frequency and perceived bother. We hypothesized that men who received the tailored symptom-management intervention would report significantly less symptom distress than they would if they received only the usual psychosocial care available to Veterans in a large VA medical center. Measures to be included in the assessments are shown in Table 17.1 and described more fully below.

MODERATING VARIABLES

Health Literacy

In Lepore's previous psychosocial intervention, men with less education benefited more than men with more education (Lepore et al., 2003). In particular, less-educated men showed significantly greater improvements in physical functioning, positive health behaviors, and sexual bother. On the basis of his earlier results, we hypothesized that health literacy would moderate the effect of PC^{PEP}, with lower-literacy men reporting greater improvements in sexual and urinary bother than higher-literacy men. Although health literacy was not measured in the Lepore study, it is likely that men with less formal education had lower health literacy. However, more formal schooling is no guarantee of literacy within the health system. Therefore, we chose to focus on health literacy as a moderating variable. Health literacy was measured with the Rapid Assessment of Adult Literacy in Medicine—Short Form (REALM-SF) at baseline. Using the REALM-SF scoring rules, men in our intervention were considered lower literacy if they correctly pronounced three or fewer of the seven words (i.e., sixth-grade level or below).

PCa Treatment

A man's symptom profile is heavily influenced by the type of PCa treatment that he received. Because symptom profiles differ by treatment type over time and data were collected for 6 months post-enrollment, we included treatment type as a possible mediator to account for the differential effect of the intervention.

POTENTIAL MEDIATING VARIABLES

Self-Efficacy

Self-efficacy was measured using an 11-item instrument developed by Lepore for use in his previous psychosocial intervention for men with PCa (Lepore & Helgeson, 1999). Its internal consistency was .93.

TABLE 17.1   Measures Mapped Onto the PC^PEP Model Components

SMM Component	Construct	No. of Items	Coefficient Alpha	Measure
Primary outcomes				
Symptom evaluation	Sexual bother	4	.78	EPIC (Wei et al., 2000)
Symptom evaluation	Urinary bother	7	.87	EPIC (Wei et al., 2000)
Potential moderators				
Person	Health literacy	7	na	REALM-SF (Wolf et al., 2004)
Health and illness	Prostate cancer treatment	1	na	CaPSURE (CaPSURE Investigators, 1995)
Potential mediators				
Symptom experience	Self-efficacy for managing treatment-related symptoms	6	.82	Lepore (Lepore & Helgeson, 1999)
Functional status	Sexual functioning	9	.90	EPIC (Wei et al., 2000)
Functional status	Urinary functioning	5	.83	EPIC (Wei et al., 2000)
Adherence	Homework compliance	1	na	
Other variables				
Outcome	Cancer knowledge	13	na	Lepore (Lepore et al., 2003)
Environment	Relationship status	1	na	CaPSURE (CaPSURE Investigators, 1995)
Symptom status	General HRQOL	12	na	SF-12 (Ware, Kosinski, Turner-Bowker, & Gandek, 2002)
Health and illness	Health care utilization		na	CaPSURE (CaPSURE Investigators, 1995)
Health and illness	Disease severity	3	na	Gleason, PSA, Stage
Health and illness	Comorbid conditions	14	na	CaPSURE (CaPSURE Investigators, 1995)

Functional Status

Functional status was assessed using the EPIC urinary functioning and sexual functioning subscales (Wei et al., 2000). The psychometric properties of the EPIC have already been described in the primary outcomes section. While functional status is an outcome in the SMM, in the PC^{PEP} conceptual model, functional status was hypothesized to mediate the intervention effect.

Adherence

Adherence was a critical component of the underlying model. Research on psychosocial interventions has shown that homework adherence is an important predictor of positive outcomes (Coon & Thompson, 2003). Homework is an important part of each module in the PC^{PEP} intervention. For example, if a participant reports urinary incontinence at the 1-month follow-up, the patient educator provides the urinary-incontinence module, which includes Kegel exercises as homework. At the 6-month follow-up, the educator discusses the Kegel-exercise homework and determines the participant's level of adherence on a scale from 0 to 100.

OTHER VARIABLES

Cancer Knowledge

Knowledge about PCa symptom management was assessed using a brief true–false knowledge test modeled on the 13-item measure used by Lepore in his previous study (Lepore et al., 2003). Cancer knowledge was a secondary outcome.

General Quality of Life

General HRQOL was assessed with the Short Form Health Survey 36, version 1.0. The scales measuring mental health, vitality, and bodily pain were used to determine whether participants needed assistance in managing these more systemic problems. If so, they were offered a module addressing their particular concern. All three scales show good reliability (range .76–.87) in validation studies with adults aged 65 years and above (Ware et al., 2002).

Disease Severity

Information was obtained from the patient's medical record regarding disease stage (T stage), Gleason grade (primary and secondary), serum PSA level, and the medical treatment plan (surgery, external-beam radiotherapy, brachytherapy, cryotherapy, HT).

Comorbid Conditions

At baseline and 6 months, participants were asked about comorbid conditions. Questions captured both the total number of comorbidities as well as the presence or absence of specific comorbid conditions that could affect a participant's symptom profile.

STUDY PROCEDURES

Recruitment was accomplished through an opt-out letter to Veterans identified in the local VA Cancer Registry. The letter provided an overview of the study; patients could indicate that they declined to participate in further study activities by initialing a section of the letter and returning it. Those who did not opt-out within 10 business days were contacted by phone to determine if they were interested in enrolling in the study. In this phone call, patients were informed of the study's purpose, procedures, risk and benefits of participation, and reimbursement. Patients who expressed an interest in the study were sent written consent forms. All recruitment and consent procedures were carried out by mail and telephone, because many Veterans live far from the local VA hospital. Once informed consent was obtained, participants completed the baseline assessment. Figure 17.3 shows the flow of participants through the study.

Participants were asked to complete assessments at baseline, and at 2 weeks and 1, 2, 4, and 6 months post-enrollment. The health-literacy assessment was included in the baseline assessment, and participants were randomized as soon as the baseline assessment was completed. Participants were asked about their demographic background (age, ethnicity, educational level, income level, relationship status), utilization of the health care system since they received their PCa diagnosis, symptom distress, functional status, general HRQOL, and self-efficacy for cancer-related symptom management. Portions of the baseline assessment were re-administered at the follow-up interviews. All assessments were carried out by an Outcomes Assessment Research Coordinator, who was blinded to the participant's study condition.

Because discussing their cancer might be distressing, all participants were provided with a letter that provided lists of counseling resources, with contact information. At the end of the baseline assessment, each participant in both groups received a copy of the National Cancer Institute's booklet, *Taking Time: Support for People with Cancer*. Participants randomized to the intervention condition also received the tailored symptom-management intervention. The package was accompanied by a cover letter that encouraged the subject to read and listen to the materials, so as to obtain the most benefit from the program. On the basis of an intervention-group participant's

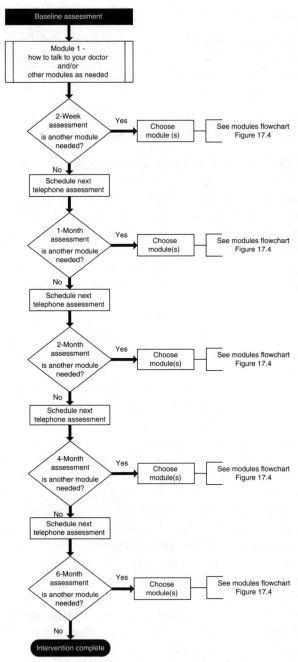

FIGURE 17.3   Intervention Flowchart

responses to the EPIC and SF-36 at each time point, a participant was provided with the symptom-management-intervention modules appropriate to his current concerns. To determine whether a patient receives a particular module, his score on each EPIC or SF-36 subscale is compared to his score on the same subscale at the previous assessment. If the difference is 10 points or more in the direction of poorer functioning or more bother, then he is provided with the relevant intervention module. The 10-point cutoff was chosen because it is one half a standard deviation for each subscale, reported to be a clinically meaningful difference on the EPIC. Participants who reported a concern in a specific area also were provided with the relevant module, even if their EPIC or SF-36 score did not indicate a statistically significant change from their previous assessment. The same procedure was followed for intervention-group participants at each follow-up.

The modules include patient–provider communication, memory problems, fatigue, emotional health, urinary frequency, exercise, ED treatments, bowel problems, hot flashes, and breast-area changes. Figure 17.4 shows the list of modules. In addition to the specially developed easy-readability patient-education materials, each participant received an audio recording that was the verbatim contents of the written materials. Each recording was made using a trained voice actor. This approach was intended to broaden the impact of the intervention by providing audio materials that can be listened to in a car or on a portable stereo, and are accessible—even to someone who cannot read.

Besides the written and audio versions of each module, each participant received a follow-up phone call from the patient educator about a week after each assessment point (Figure 17.3), to ensure that he had received and understood the materials and to help him incorporate the information into his life. For example, if a participant had received the module on Kegel exercises to strengthen his pelvic-floor muscles, the patient educator helped him to incorporate Kegel exercises into his daily routine by suggesting that he use mealtimes as a trigger to remember to do his exercises. The phone calls were intended to answer questions about materials, problem-solve implementing new behaviors and skills, and increasing adherence to the intervention.

At 6 months, intervention participants completed the 6-month assessment and received the module(s) appropriate to their symptom-management needs, but were not assessed again. The investigators felt that conducting the 6-month assessment and then not offering needed intervention modules to participants would be unethical. At the end of the RCT (after the 6-month follow-up assessment), control-group participants were offered the opportunity to receive the intervention to address any current symptom concerns they had.

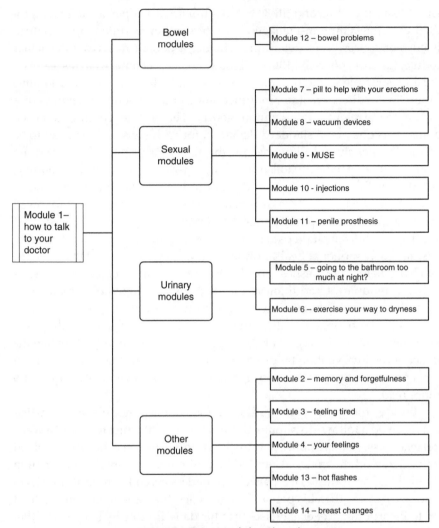

FIGURE 17.4   Modules Flowchart

PLANS FOR FURTHER RESEARCH

Preliminary analyses suggest that PC^{PEP} is more efficacious in improving symptoms and reducing symptom distress than earlier psychosocial interventions. Given the limited resources of most cancer centers and other service organizations, the tailored-intervention approach increases the likelihood that such a program will be sustainable. Effectiveness studies are needed to understand whether or not the intervention can achieve similar results in non-Veteran populations. Additional tailoring could be done to include themes, images, and other culturally specific information to make the program more appropriate for specific groups (Kreuter et al., 2004). Our results suggest that using the Critical Incident Technique approach to identify effective symptom-management practices and then incorporating them into tailored symptom-management education programs is a successful approach that should be considered as a way of improving symptom management among cancer survivors, particularly when programs are developed using literacy-appropriate methods.

REFERENCES

American Cancer Society. (2001). *The National Comprehensive Cancer Network prostate cancer treatment guidelines for patients.* Atlanta, GA: Author.

American Cancer Society. (2005). *Cancer facts and figures 2005.* Atlanta, GA: Author.

American Cancer Society. (2007). *Cancer facts and figures for African-Americans 2007–2008.* Atlanta, GA: Author.

American Cancer Society. (2009). *Cancer facts & figures.* Atlanta, GA: Author.

American Cancer Society. (2010). *Cancer facts and figures 2010.* Atlanta, GA: Author.

Baker, D. W., Gazmararian, J. A., Williams, M. V., Scott, T., Parker, R. M., Green, D., . . . Peel, J. (2002). Functional health literacy and the risk of hospital admission among Medicare managed care enrollees. *American Journal of Public Health, 92*(8), 1278–1283.

Bandura, A. (1986). *Social foundations of thought and action: A social cognitive theory.* Englewood Cliffs, NJ: Prentice-Hall.

Bandura, A. (1997). *Self-efficacy: The exercise of control.* New York, NY: W. H. Freeman.

Bennett, C. L., Ferreira, M. R., Davis, T. C., Kaplan, J., Weinberger, M., Kuzel, T., . . . Sartor, O. (1998). Relation between literacy, race, and stage of presentation among low-income patients with prostate cancer. *Journal of Clinical Oncology, 16*(9), 3101–3104.

Boberg, E. W., Gustafson, D. H., Hawkins, R. P., Offord, K. P., Koch, C., Wen, K. Y., . . . Salner, A. (2003). Assessing the unmet information, support and care delivery needs of men with prostate cancer. *Patient Education and Counseling, 49*(3), 233–242.

Bokhour, B. G., Clark, J. A., Inui, T. S., Silliman, R. A., & Talcott, J. A. (2001). Sexuality after treatment for early prostate cancer: Exploring the meanings of "erectile dysfunction." *Journal of General Internal Medicine, 16*(10), 649–655.

CaPSURE Investigators. (1995). *Cancer of the Prostate Strategic Research Endeavor (CaPSURE) baseline questionnaire.* Lake Forest, IL: TAP Pharmaceutical Products.

Coon, D. W., & Thompson, L. W. (2003). The relationship between homework compliance and treatment outcomes among older adult outpatients with mild-to-moderate depression. *American Journal of Geriatric Psychiatry, 11*(1), 53–61.

Doak, C. C., Doak, L. G., & Root, J. H. (1996). *Teaching patients with low literacy skills* (2nd ed.). Philadelphia, PA: J. B. Lippincott.

Dodd, M., Janson, S., Facione, N., Faucett, J., Froelicher, E. S., Humphreys, J., . . . Taylor, D. (2001). Advancing the science of symptom management. *Journal of Advanced Nursing, 33*(5), 668–676.

Eton, D. T., & Lepore, S. J. (2002). Prostate cancer and health-related quality of life: A review of the literature. *Psychooncology, 11*(4), 307–326.

Flanagan, J. C. (1954). The critical incident technique. *Psychological Bulletin, 51,* 327–358.

Gazmararian, J. A., Parker, R. M., & Baker, D. W. (1999). Reading skills and family planning knowledge and practices in a low-income managed-care population. *Obstetrics & Gynecology, 93*(2), 239–244.

Helgeson, V. S., & Lepore, S. J. (1997). Men's adjustment to prostate cancer: The role of agency and unmitigated agency. *Sex Roles, 37*(3–4), 251–267.

Holzbeierlein, J. M., McLaughlin, M. D., & Thrasher, J. B. (2004). Complications of androgen deprivation therapy for prostate cancer. *Current Opinion in Urology, 14*(3), 177–183.

Kalichman, S. C., & Rompa, D. (2000). Functional health literacy is associated with health status and health-related knowledge in people living with HIV-AIDS. *Journal of Acquired Immune Deficiency Syndromes, 25*(4), 337–344.

Kreuter, M. W., Skinner, C. S., Steger-May, K., Holt, C. L., Bucholtz, D. C., Clark, E. M., Haire-Joshu, D. (2004). Responses to behaviorally vs culturally tailored cancer communication among African American women. *American Journal of Health Behavior, 28*(3), 195–207.

Latini, D. M., Hoffmann, D. J., Flores, D. V., McNeese, T. D., Hart, S. L., & Knight, S. J. (2008, February 14–16). *Symptom management strategies of men treated for localized prostate cancer.* Paper presented at the Genitourinary Cancer Symposium, San Francisco, CA.

Lepore, S. J., & Helgeson, V. S. (1999). Psychoeducational support group enhances quality of life after prostate cancer. *Cancer Research, Therapy and Control, 8,* 81–91.

Lepore, S. J., Helgeson, V. S., Eton, D. T., & Schulz, R. (2003). Improving quality of life in men with prostate cancer: A randomized controlled trial of group education interventions. *Health Psychology, 22*(5), 443–452.

Likosky, W. H., Starr-Schneidkraut, N. J., & Wilson, S. R. (1994). "Coping with MS Effectively": A proactive psychosocial intervention for patients with multiple sclerosis. *Neurology, 44,* A393.

Likosky, W. H., Starr-Schneidkraut, N. J., Wilson, S. R., & Javerbaum, J. R. (1995). Impact of the "Coping with MS Effectively" program on adaptive coping in MS patients. *Neurology, 45,* A334.

Litwin, M. S., Hays, R. D., Fink, A., Ganz, P. A., Leake, B., Leach, G. E., & Brook, R. H. (1995). Quality-of-life outcomes in men treated for localized prostate cancer. *Journal of the American Medical Association, 273*(2), 129–135.

Lorig, K. R., Ritter, P., Stewart, A. L., Sobel, D. S., Brown, B. W., Jr., Bandura, A., . . . Holman, H. R. (2001). Chronic disease self-management program: 2-year health status and health care utilization outcomes. *Medical Care, 39*(11), 1217–1223.

Lorig, K. R., Sobel, D. S., Stewart, A. L., Brown, B. W., Jr., Bandura, A., Ritter, P., . . . Holman, H. R. (1999). Evidence suggesting that a chronic disease self-management program can improve health status while reducing hospitalization: A randomized trial. *Medical Care, 37*(1), 5–14.

Lubeck, D. P., Kim, H., Grossfeld, G., Ray, P., Penson, D. F., Flanders, S. C., & Carroll, P. R. (2001). Health related quality of life differences between black and white men with prostate cancer: Data from the cancer of the prostate strategic urologic research endeavor. *Journal of Urology, 166*(6), 2281–2285.

Lubeck, D. P., Litwin, M. S., Henning, J. M., Stoddard, M. L., Flanders, S. C., & Carroll, P. R. (1999). Changes in health-related quality of life in the first year after treatment for prostate cancer: Results from CaPSURE. *Urology, 53*(1), 180–186.

Maliski, S. L., Kwan, L., Krupski, T., Fink, A., Orecklin, J. R., & Litwin, M. S. (2004). Confidence in the ability to communicate with physicians among low-income patients with prostate cancer. *Urology, 64*(2), 329–334.

McNabb, W. L., Wilson-Pessano, S. R., Hughes, G. W., & Scamagas, P. (1985). Self-management education of children with asthma: AIR WISE. *American Journal of Public Health, 75*(10), 1219–1220.

Meade, C. D., Calvo, A., Rivera, M. A., & Baer, R. D. (2003). Focus groups in the design of prostate cancer screening information for Hispanic farmworkers and African American men. *Oncology Nursing Forum, 30*(6), 967–975.

Mishel, M. H., Belyea, M., Germino, B. B., Stewart, J. L., Bailey, D. E., Jr., Robertson, C., Mohler, J. (2002). Helping patients with localized prostate carcinoma manage uncertainty and treatment side effects: Nurse-delivered psychoeducational intervention over the telephone. *Cancer, 94*(6), 1854–1866.

Moore, K. N., & Estey, A. (1999). The early post-operative concerns of men after radical prostatectomy. *Journal of Advanced Nursing, 29*(5), 1121–1129.

National Cancer Institute. (2003). *Making Health Communication Programs Work*. Retrieved 24, August 2004, from http://www.cancer.gov/pinkbook

Newman, M. G. (2000). Recommendations for a cost-offset model of psychotherapy allocation using generalized anxiety disorder as an example. *Journal of Consulting and Clinical Psychology, 68*, 549–555.

Otto, M. W., Pollack, M. H., & Maki, K. M. (2000). Empirically supported treatments for panic disorder: Costs, benefits, and stepped care. *Journal of Consulting and Clinical Psychology, 68*, 556–563.

Penson, D. F., McLerran, D., Feng, Z., Li, L., Albertsen, P. C., Gilliland, F. D., . . . Stanford, J. L. (2005). 5-year urinary and sexual outcomes after radical prostatectomy: Results from the Prostate Cancer Outcomes Study. *Journal of Urology, 173*(5), 1701–1705.

Penson, D. F., Stoddard, M. L., Pasta, D. J., Lubeck, D. P., Flanders, S. C., & Litwin, M. S. (2001). The association between socioeconomic status, health insurance coverage, and quality of life in men with prostate cancer. *Journal of Clinical Epidemiology, 54*(4), 350–358.

Pocock, S. J. (1983). *Clinical trials: A practical approach*. New York, NY: Wiley.

Potosky, A. L., Legler, J., Albertsen, P. C., Stanford, J. L., Gilliland, F. D., Hamilton, A. S., . . . Harlan, L. C. (2000). Health outcomes after prostatectomy or radiotherapy for prostate cancer: Results from the Prostate Cancer Outcomes Study. *Journal of the National Cancer Institute, 92*(19), 1582–1592.

Ratzan, S. C., & Parker, R. M. (2000). Introduction. In C. R. Selden, M. Zorn, S. C. Ratzan, & R. M. Parker (Eds.), *National Library of Medicine current bibliographies in medicine: Health literacy* (Vol. NLM Pub. No. CBM 2000-1). Bethesda, MD: National Institutes of Health, U.S. Department of Health and Human Services.

Roberts, K. J., Lepore, S. J., Hanlon, A. L., & Helgeson, V. (2010). Genitourinary functioning and depressive symptoms over time in younger versus older men treated for prostate cancer. *Annals of Behavioral Medicine, 40*(3), 275–283.

Schover, L. R., Fouladi, R. T., Warneke, C. L., Neese, L., Klein, E. A., Zippe, C., Kupelian, P. A. (2002). The use of treatments for erectile dysfunction among survivors of prostate carcinoma. *Cancer, 95*(11), 2397–2407.

Scott, T. L., Gazmararian, J. A., Williams, M. V., & Baker, D. W. (2002). Health literacy and preventive health care use among Medicare enrollees in a managed care organization. *Medical Care, 40*(5), 395–404.

Starr, N. J., Likosky, W. H., Hayes, B. W., Casey, D., Wilson, S. R., & Javerbaum, J. (1996). Improved quality of life (QOL) outcomes in MS patients after participation in the "Coping with MS Effectively" program. *Neurology, 46,* S63.004.

Steginga, S. K., Occhipinti, S., Dunn, J., Gardiner, R. A., Heathcote, P., & Yaxley, J. (2001). The supportive care needs of men with prostate cancer. *Psychooncology, 10*(1), 66–75.

Talcott, J. A. (1996). Quality of life in early prostate cancer: Do we know enough to treat? *Hematology/Oncology Clinics of North America, 10,* 691–701.

Talcott, J. A., Rieker, P., Clark, J. A., Propert, K. J., Weeks, J. C., Beard, C. J., . . . Kantoff, P. W. (1998). Patient-reported symptoms after primary therapy for early prostate cancer: Results of a prospective cohort study. *Journal of Clinical Oncology, 16,* 275–283.

Templeton, H., & Coates, V. (2003). Informational needs of men with prostate cancer on hormonal manipulation therapy. *Patient Education and Counseling, 49*(3), 243–256.

UCSF Faculty Group in Symptom Management. (1994). A model for symptom management. *Image: Journal of Nursing Scholarship, 26*(4), 272–276.

Ullrich, P. M., Carson, M. R., Lutgendorf, S. K., & Williams, R. D. (2003). Cancer fear and mood disturbance after radical prostatectomy: Consequences of biochemical evidence of recurrence. *Journal of Urology, 169*(4), 1449–1452.

Visser, A., & van Andel, G. (2003). Psychosocial and educational aspects in prostate cancer patients. *Patient Education and Counseling, 49*(3), 203–206.

Ware, J. E., Jr., Kosinski, M., Turner-Bowker, D. M., & Gandek, B. (2002). *How to score Version 2 of the SF-12 Health Survey (with a supplement documenting Version 1).* Lincoln, RI: QualityMetric.

Wei, J. T., Dunn, R. L., Litwin, M. S., Sandler, H. M., & Sanda, M. G. (2000). Development and validation of the Expanded Prostate Cancer Index composite (EPIC) for comprehensive assessment of health-related quality of life in men with prostate cancer. *Urology, 56*(6), 899–905.

Wilson, G. T., Vitousek, K. M., & Loeb, K. L. (2000). Stepped care treatment for eating disorders. *Journal of Consulting and Clinical Psychology, 68,* 564–572.

Wilson, S. R., Latini, D., Starr, N. J., Fish, L., Loes, L. M., Page, A., & Kubic, P. (1996). Education of parents of infants and very young children with asthma: A developmental evaluation of the Wee Wheezers program. *Journal of Asthma, 33*(4), 239–254.

Wilson, S. R., Scamagas, P., German, D. F., Hughes, G. W., Lulla, S., Coss, S., . . . Stancavage, F. B. (1993). A controlled trial of two forms of self-management education for adults with asthma. *American Journal of Medicine, 94*(6), 564–576.

Wilt, T. J., MacDonald, R., Rutks, I., Shamliyan, T. A., Taylor, B. C., & Kane, R. L. (2008). Systematic review: Comparative effectiveness and harms of treatments for clinically localized prostate cancer. *Annals of Internal Medicine, 148*(6), 435–448.

Wolf, M. S., Heckinger, E. A., Arozullah, A. M., Costello, S. R., Yarnold, P. R., Soltysik, R. C., Bennette, C. L. (2004, May). *Identifying persons with poor health literacy in 7-seconds: An important adjunct to improving cancer screening and treatment.* Paper presented at the American Society for Clinical Oncology, New Orleans, LA.

18

Automated Pain Intervention for Underserved African American and Latina Women With Breast Cancer

Karen O. Anderson, Guadalupe R. Palos, Araceli Garcia-Gonzalez, Tito R. Mendoza, Eric Kai-Ping Liao, Karin M. Hahn, Arlene Nazario, Vicente Valero, Michael Fisch, and Richard Payne

During the past three decades, effective clinical practice guidelines for cancer pain management have been developed and evaluated (Benedetti et al., 2000; Jacox, Carr, & Payne, 1994; World Health Organization, 1996, 1998). When the guidelines are implemented, the vast majority of patients with cancer-related pain experience good control of their pain (Zech, Grond, Lynch, Hertel, & Lehmann, 1995). Unfortunately, the guidelines are not always followed, and many patients continue to receive inadequate management of pain (Cleeland et al., 1994). Racial- and ethnic-minority patients are particularly at risk for undertreatment of cancer-related pain (Anderson, Green, & Payne, 2009; Cleeland, Gonin, Baez, Loehrer, & Pandya, 1997). When minority patients are underserved due to socioeconomic and health care system factors, they may be even more vulnerable to inadequate pain management. A multifaceted approach that targets patients, physicians, and health care system barriers is needed to optimize pain treatment for underserved minority patients. Multicomponent interventions, however, are difficult to implement in large understaffed public hospitals that typically serve socioeconomically disadvantaged minority patients. In the present chapter, we describe an interactive voice response (IVR) system that measures patients' pain levels and alerts providers when pain is moderate to severe in intensity. The IVR system also assesses patient and health care system-related obstacles to pain control. Thus, the intervention targets patients, providers, and health care system barriers to optimal pain treatment.

Individuals from racial and ethnic minorities, as well as low-income families of any race or ethnicity, often are in poorer health than other Americans (Agency for Healthcare Research and Quality, 2008). Minority patients also are at risk for disparities in the quality of health care delivery. Health care disparities have been defined as racial and ethnic differences in the quality of care that are not due to access-related factors, clinical needs, preferences, or appropriateness of intervention (Smedley, Stith, Nelson, Institute of Medicine, & Committee on Understanding and Eliminating Racial and Ethnic Disparities in Health Care, 2003). Eliminating disparities in health care delivery is a major strategy for reducing disparities in health. Minority patients with cancer are at risk for disparities in the quality of care, including pain management.

Inadequate treatment of cancer-related pain among minority patients has been documented in multiple studies (Anderson et al., 2000, 2009; Green et al., 2003). The results of our descriptive studies suggested that underserved minority patients might benefit from education about pain management that empowered them to expect good pain management from their providers. We completed a randomized clinical trial that evaluated pain management education for underserved African American and Hispanic patients with cancer-related pain (Anderson et al., 2004). The patients randomly assigned to the education group received a culture-specific video and booklet on pain management. The educational materials presented actual minority patients who received good pain control and modeled how to assertively discuss pain with health care providers. Each patient also met with a bilingual research nurse who reviewed the materials. The results of our clinical trial indicated that education alone was not sufficient to improve pain management for underserved minority patients. We concluded that a multicomponent intervention that targets patient, health care provider, and health care system barriers is needed to optimize pain management for underserved minority patients.

BARRIERS TO OPTIMAL PAIN TREATMENT FOR UNDERSERVED MINORITY PATIENTS WITH CANCER

The barriers to optimal pain treatment for underserved minority patients with cancer-related pain include barriers related to health care providers, patients, and the health care system. *Provider-related barriers* include lack of knowledge and training related to pain treatment, concerns about prescribing opioid medications, inappropriate concerns about patient addiction to opioids, and inadequate assessment of patients' pain (Von Roenn, Cleeland, Gonin, Hatfield, & Pandya, 1993). In our survey study of underserved minority patients with cancer-related pain, the physicians and nurses treating the patients were asked to rank a list of potential barriers to optimal cancer pain management in their setting (Anderson et al., 2000). Inadequate pain assessment, patient reluctance to report pain, and inadequate staff knowledge regarding pain management were reported as the top barriers by more than half of the health care professionals.

A number of *patient-related barriers* to the assessment of cancer pain have been identified (Cleeland et al., 1997; Thomason et al., 1998; Ward et al., 1993; Ward & Hernandez, 1994). Patients with a serious medical illness such as cancer may underreport pain and pain severity. For example, patients with cancer often do not want to be labeled as complainers, do not want to distract their physicians from treating the cancer, or are afraid that pain means that their cancer is progressing. Although minority patients share many of the concerns that limit pain control in non-Hispanic White patients, data from several studies suggest that specific concerns may be reported more frequently among minority patients (Anderson et al., 2002; Ward & Hernandez, 1994). For example, many Hispanic and African American patients describe stoicism and the belief that pain is an inevitable part of having cancer and must be accepted (Juarez, Ferrell, & Borneman, 1998; Juarez, Ferrell, & Borneman, 1999; Thomason et al., 1998). African American and Hispanic patients are often concerned about taking potent opioids because they fear that they will become addicts, will develop tolerance, or will experience intolerable side effects from the analgesics (Anderson et al., 2000; Cleeland et al., 1997). Studies of Hispanic and African American cancer patients also have found that many patients rely on alternative and complementary pain treatments, and prefer to take analgesics only when pain is very severe (Juarez et al., 1998, 1999).

In addition to patient and provider barriers, underserved minority patients face *barriers in the health care system* that can adversely impact optimal pain treatment. For example, minority patients who receive analgesic prescriptions may face the additional barrier of limited availability of opioids in their hospital or neighborhood pharmacy (Green, Ndao-Brumblay, West, & Washington, 2005; Morrison, Wallenstein, Natale, Senzel, & Huang, 2000). In our survey of providers treating underserved minority patients, higher percentages of the health professionals in minority as compared to nonminority settings ranked lack of access to a wide range of analgesics as an important barrier (Anderson et al., 2000).

In sum, inadequate assessment and treatment by health care providers and patient beliefs are major factors contributing to undertreatment of pain for minority cancer patients. Underserved patients also face barriers related to the health care system, such as lack of insurance and difficulty obtaining opioid medications. Given the multiple barriers, a multifaceted intervention that involves health care providers and patients probably is needed to improve cancer pain treatment for underserved minority patients. With regard to patients, previous research suggested that patients could benefit from education in pain management that addresses patient-related barriers. Several randomized clinical trials with largely nonminority samples of cancer patients found that education on pain management produced significant reductions in pain intensity ratings (de Wit et al., 1997; Miaskowski et al., 2004; Oliver, Kravitz, Kaplan, & Meyers, 2001; Syrjala et al., 2008; Wells, Hepworth, Murphy, Wujcik, & Johnson, 2003). Our recent trial of underserved African American and Hispanic cancer patients, however, found that education alone did not improve the pain experience of the minority patients (Anderson et al., 2004). The results suggested that patients might benefit more from individualized education that targets specific patient-related barriers.

With regard to health care provider barriers, recent clinical trials with samples of mainly nonminority patients have demonstrated that documenting pain assessment information in patients' charts and implementing standardized pain treatment are effective strategies for improving pain management outcomes (Cleeland et al., 2005; Du Pen et al., 1999; Trowbridge et al., 1997). In the Trowbridge et al. (1997) study, the largely nonminority patients were asked to rate their average and worst pain during the previous week, as well as satisfaction with their pain management and the degree of pain relief received. The oncologists treating the patients in the intervention group were asked to review a summary of the patients' pain scale scores prior to seeing the patients. The results revealed a decrease in the incidence of pain in the intervention group. In addition, the oncologists treating the intervention group were more likely to make changes in the patients' analgesic prescriptions, as compared to the oncologists treating the control group patients. Additional research is needed to determine if these physician interventions are effective for improving pain treatment of underserved minority cancer patients.

In our project, we are evaluating the feasibility of a novel IVR intervention that targets patient, provider, and health care system barriers. This multicomponent intervention addresses multiple barriers that underserved minority patients face.

AUTOMATED PAIN ASSESSMENT WITH THE IVR SYSTEM

One patient-related barrier to optimal pain treatment is patients' reticence in reporting symptoms. Patient reluctance to report pain is identified by both oncologists and oncology nurses as one of the major barriers to adequate control of cancer pain (Larson, Viele, Coleman, Dibble, & Cebulski, 1993; Von Roenn et al., 1993). Patients report a variety of reasons for not reporting pain, including not wanting to distract the doctor from attending to their cancer, wanting to be a "good" patient, and fatalism about the possibility of achieving pain control (Anderson et al., 2002; Ward et al., 1993). Patients' reluctance to report symptoms is often compounded by the difficulty of finding time for adequate symptom assessment in a busy clinic. Patients with breast cancer often have multiple symptoms that need monitoring in addition to pain, including fatigue, nausea, diarrhea, psychological distress, sleep disturbance, and changes in appetite.

Telephone systems have been widely used in outpatient health care settings for communicating with patients, identifying symptoms that need medical attention, and following patients after treatment (Korcz & Moreland, 1998). However, traditional telephone communication requires considerable staff time and is not feasible for assessing symptoms on a regular basis. Combining the use of touch-tone telephones with computers and the Internet may be an effective way to follow patients who have symptoms, such as pain, that need to be monitored closely while away from the hospital. At the most sophisticated level, these systems can decode the actual spoken response of patients. More typically, however, a patient can respond to spoken instructions by using the keypad of a touch-tone telephone. For example, a patient might be asked to rate his or her pain at its worst in the last day from 0 (no pain) to 10 (pain as bad as you can imagine). Information obtained in this way can be used to update a patient file on an Internet or intranet site and can be configured to alert providers.

Computer-generated IVR systems provide information similar to that obtained from paper-and-pencil questionnaires or in clinical interviews (Agel, Rockwood, Mundt, Greist, & Swiontkowski, 2001; Mundt et al., 1998). One study examined the relationship of IVR-administered depression rating scales and scales administered by human raters (Mundt et al., 1998). The short IVR-based rating of depression correlated well with interviewer-obtained ratings and produced equivalent scores. Similar concordance between clinician-obtained and IVR-obtained symptom reporting was found in a study by Kobak et al. (1997). Prevalence rates for psychiatric disorders were similar between diagnoses made by the computer and those made by a mental health professional. However, patients were twice as likely to report such issues as alcohol and drug abuse or suicidal ideation in response to the IVR system's questions. Similarly, interviewer and IVR administration of the SF-12 Health Survey found that patients acknowledge greater emotional problems when using the IVR format (Millard & Carver, 1999).

Novel IVR systems have been tested in several studies as a method of providing adjunctive therapy for psychiatric conditions as well as for persons under stress. For example, patients with depression made telephone calls to an IVR system that made self-help recommendations to patients based on information that the patient entered (Osgood-Hynes et al., 1998).

More than half of the IVR users demonstrated at least a 50% reduction in scores on standard depression rating scales. IVR-based behavioral interventions have also been used with patients with obsessive-compulsive disorder (Baer & Greist, 1997). IVR systems have been designed to monitor the stress of caregivers of people with Alzheimer's disease, and to provide stress reduction recommendations and, when necessary, referrals to providers (Mahoney, Tarlow, & Jones, 2003).

In a study of patients with chronic noncancer pain, an IVR system was used to enhance the efficacy of group cognitive-behavioral therapy (Naylor, Helzer, Naud, & Keefe, 2002; Naylor, Keefe, Brigidi, Naud, & Helzer, 2008). The IVR system asked patients to rate their pain and related symptoms. In addition, the patients could access information on pain coping skills, they could rehearse skills, and they received personalized feedback messages from their therapist. The results of the study indicated that the use of the IVR system was associated with significant pain reduction and improvements in quality of life and coping. A variety of IVR systems have been used to facilitate substance abuse programs and to prevent relapse (Curry, McBride, Grothaus, Louie, & Wagner, 1995; Gustafson, Bosworth, Chewning, & Hawkins, 1987; Shiffman, Paty, Gnys, Kassel, & Hickcox, 1996).

An IVR system specifically designed to assess the special needs of cancer patients receiving chemotherapy was reported by Siegel et al. (1988). The questions focused on such issues as transportation, help with self-care, and managing bills. When patients reported a specific need, a social work consult was initiated. The authors reported that patients readily accepted the system and were able to use the IVR accurately and reliably. The results of other recent studies found that patients with cancer used an IVR system successfully and described it as very helpful for symptom assessment and management. In a pilot study of patients with advanced lung cancer, an IVR system was used to assess multiple symptoms during a 12-week study (Davis et al., 2007). Compliance with the weekly symptom ratings was excellent, and the majority of the patients reported that the symptom survey helped them to discuss symptom issues with their oncologist. A randomized clinical trial comparing the efficacy of automated telephone symptom management and nurse-assisted symptom management for patients with solid tumors or non-Hodgkin's lymphoma found that both interventions produced a clinically significant reduction in symptom severity during the 10-week study (Sikorskii et al., 2007). The patients contacted by the automated voice response system reported higher severity of symptoms, as compared to the patients contacted by a nurse. The investigators speculated that patients might have been more willing to report symptoms to the automated system. These results indicate that cancer patients can benefit from an automated assessment and triage system. An IVR system should be especially helpful for assessing a symptom such as pain that patients may be reluctant to report to their physicians. Accurate and regular pain assessment, when provided to the physicians, should facilitate pain management.

DEVELOPMENT OF THE UNIVERSITY OF TEXAS M. D. ANDERSON CANCER CENTER IVR SYMPTOM ASSESSMENT SYSTEM

In a pilot study at the M. D. Anderson Cancer Center, an IVR system was used to assess pain intensity in a sample of cancer outpatients receiving treatment in a pain and symptom management clinic (Chandler & Payne, 2005). The patients used an 800 number to call the IVR computer-telephone system one time per day. The system asked patients to rate their present pain intensity and their worst, least, and average pain during the past 24 hours, using 0–10 scales. The IVR system paged a provider (a clinical pharmacist or nurse) when patients reported that the severity of their worst pain in the past 24 hours was 7 or greater. In consultation with the patient's physician, the provider made appropriate adjustments in analgesic medications. The results of this pilot study indicated that patients used the IVR system successfully and described it as very helpful in improving their pain management.

The success of this pilot study encouraged the Department of Symptom Research to pursue the development of an IVR system for the assessment of multiple symptoms. The IVR system is based on the M. D. Anderson Symptom Inventory (MDASI), a brief, easily understood, and validated symptom assessment tool that measures the severity of cancer-related symptoms and their impact on daily functioning (Cleeland et al., 2000). The core symptoms include: Pain, fatigue, nausea, vomiting, disturbed sleep, diarrhea, shortness of breath, lack of appetite, numbness or tingling, dry mouth, difficulty remembering things, sadness, and feeling distressed. Six interference items assessing symptom-related interference in general activity, walking, mood, work, relations with other people, and enjoyment of life also are included in the IVR system.

The IVR system automatically contacts patients using telephone information from study databases. The system is programmed to contact patients at their preferred times on specified dates. If a patient does not answer the IVR call, then the system continues to call the patient at specified intervals, up to a maximum of four calls. Once a contact is made, the symptom assessment script runs. Patient responses to the symptom and interference questions are deposited into a web-based database, with real-time updates.

The IVR technology incorporates the use of telephones with computers to follow patients who have symptoms that require close monitoring outside of a clinical setting. We conducted a study to show how data obtained using an IVR system compared with data collected using a traditional paper-and-pencil method (Mendoza et al., 2001). Equivalency testing was used to examine similarity of (a) severity ratings, (b) correlations of the two methods across time, and (c) measures of internal consistency. Data from 33 cancer patients who underwent blood and marrow transplantation showed that the severity of symptom ratings is equivalent for the two methods. Both methods are similarly reliable and sensitive to change over time. Overall, we concluded that the two methods are similar enough to be used interchangeably when assessing cancer-related symptoms. However, the IVR approach offers several advantages: First, missing data are minimized, especially in longitudinal studies. Second, the IVR system may be more cost-effective over time. Finally, the availability of immediate feedback through the IVR system may be critical in managing symptoms more effectively.

In our project, we are evaluating the feasibility of the IVR system, which is designed to overcome common patient, health care provider, and health system barriers to pain management. Our specific aims are: (1) to evaluate the feasibility of an IVR intervention for pain management that targets both underserved minority patients with breast cancer and their health care providers; (2) to pilot test the efficacy of the IVR intervention for improving pain management of underserved minority patients with breast cancer, as compared to the current standard of care; and (3) to pilot test the efficacy of the IVR intervention for improving pain-related symptoms (fatigue, sleep disturbance, sadness) of underserved minority patients with breast cancer, as compared to the current standard of care.

In the present chapter, we describe the development and implementation of the IVR intervention. In addition, we present evidence of the feasibility of the intervention. After we complete our data collection and analyses, we will report the potential efficacy of the IVR intervention in future publications. We hypothesized that the feasibility of the IVR intervention for underserved African American and Latina women with breast cancer would be demonstrated by good rates of patient recruitment and retention and patient evaluation of the IVR intervention. The feasibility also will be evaluated by health care provider responses to the IVR alerts.

METHODS

Setting and Patients

The study sample consisted of underserved African American and Latina patients with a primary diagnosis of breast cancer, who were receiving treatment at a public hospital in Houston, Texas. Eligible patients were at least 18 years of age, English- or Spanish-speaking, currently living in the United

States, and socioeconomically disadvantaged. Eligible patients also reported a "pain worst" score on the Brief Pain Inventory of 4 or greater. Patients treated at the public hospital are required to meet strict income-based economic eligibility criteria before being treated in the oncology clinics. These criteria are based on federal poverty-level guidelines used for means-tested programs such as Medicaid. Exclusion criteria included patients who were unable to use the IVR system or had a current diagnosis of psychosis or dementia. Permission to conduct the study was obtained from the Institutional Review Boards of the University of Texas M. D. Anderson Cancer Center, the University of Texas Health Science Center, and the Harris County Hospital District.

Table 18.1 presents the demographic and disease-related clinical variables for the study sample. The mean age of the patients was 50 years, and most of the women had less than a high school education. Almost half of the women were married, and most were not currently working outside the home. Among the Latina women, 74% were born in another country,

TABLE 18.1   Baseline Demographic and Clinical Variables of African American and Latina Women With Breast Cancer

Characteristic	IVR Group (*n* = 31)	Control Group (*n* = 29)
Mean age SD	**50 years (9.9)**	**50 years (11.0)**
Ethnic group (*n*)		
African American	13 (42%)	12 (41%)
Hispanic	18 (58%)	17 (59%)
Mean years of education SD	11 (4.1)	10 (2.9)
Marital status (*n*)		
Married	15 (48%)	13 (45%)
Single	16 (52%)	16 (55%)
Employment status (*n*)		
Unemployed	18 (39%)	24 (52%)
Employed	5 (11%)	5 (11%)
Homemaker	10 (22%)	8 (17%)
Retired	8 (17%)	6 (13%)
Other	5 (11%)	3 (7%)
Disease stage (*n*)		
IIA/B	7 (22%)	7 (24%)
IIIA/B	12 (39%)	12 (41%)
IV	12 (39%)	10 (35%)
Good performance status (*n*)[a]	14 (45%)	15 (52%)

[a]Good performance status is defined as a score of 0–1 on the 5-point ECOG scale, in which 0 is fully active and 4 is completely disabled.

with Mexico the most common (58%) country of origin. The mean number of years living in the United States for the Latina women was 22 years ($SD = 16$). One of the African American women was born in another country.

Procedures

IVR Intervention

The IVR system was demonstrated at baseline to patients who were randomly assigned to the IVR intervention group. The research staff explained that the system would call the patient two times per week. Patients were asked to designate their preferred language for the IVR calls (English or Spanish) and convenient times for the system to call them. If a patient did not answer or an answering machine was activated, the IVR system repeated the call three times. If not answered after these repeats, the system notified the research staff, who contacted the patient or the patient's family. The system asked patients to identify themselves using a study number. After patients identified themselves, the IVR symptom assessment script began. Patients were asked to report their responses using the touch-tone keypad. They also had the option of changing an answer, if they inadvertently entered a wrong number.

IVR Treatment Components for Patients

The IVR intervention targeted both patients and physicians. The IVR intervention components for patients addressed both patient and health care system barriers to optimal pain treatment. The IVR intervention included (1) assessment of patients' pain and related symptoms by the IVR, (2) assessment of possible barriers to optimal pain management, (3) educational information for patients that promotes optimal pain treatment, and (4) notification to the patient treatment team of reported barriers. The barriers assessed by the IVR system included: (1) nonadherence to analgesic medication regimens ("Are you taking your pain medicine the way the doctor told you to?"); (2) difficulty obtaining analgesic medications ("Are you having any problems getting your pain medicine?"); (3) side effects from analgesic medications ("Are you having any problems with side effects from your pain medicine?"); (4) concerns about opioids, such as fear of addiction ("Are you worried about becoming addicted to your pain medicine?"); (5) reliance on alternative strategies (e.g., herbs, prayer) for pain management ("Are you using other ways to control your pain, such as herbs or teas?"); and (6) lack of family support for pain management ("Does your family help you to manage your pain?"). The patient provided a simple "Yes" or "No" answer to each question, using the telephone keypad (1 = "Yes" and 2 = "No"). When a patient reported a possible barrier, the research staff contacted the patient to obtain additional information about the barrier and to provide appropriate patient education, if indicated.

IVR Treatment Components for the Health Care Provider

The IVR intervention for the oncology providers included: (1) determination of pain and other symptoms that exceeded the symptom severity threshold; and (2) feedback of information about supra-threshold symptoms to the oncology provider. Thus, the IVR assessment/feedback intervention for providers combined timely assessment with immediate feedback that could trigger a symptom management action plan. The oncology providers also were notified of any patient-reported barriers to optimal pain management.

The National Comprehensive Cancer Network (NCCN) clinical practice guidelines for treatment of cancer-related pain indicate that a pain level of 5 or greater on a 0–10 scale is moderate pain that should be treated promptly (Benedetti et al., 2000). When the patient's reported pain level was 5 or greater, then this information was immediately forwarded by e-mail to the oncology fellow who was following the patient. The fellows were encouraged to follow the NCCN-based pain treatment guidelines. When the patient's pain level was 5 or greater, the physician also received, via e-mail alert, the information on the patient's reported barriers to pain treatment. Thus, the physician was able to address the patient's individual barriers (e.g., fear of opioids, side effects from analgesics) when he or she talked with the patient by return telephone call or during a clinic visit.

When the patient's pain level was less than 5, then the physician did not receive an immediate e-mail alert regarding pain intensity and related barriers. The patient's pain and symptom ratings and barrier information were summarized in a report that was provided to the physician prior to the patient's next clinic visit. The project research staff monitored the IVR alerts in the web-based intranet site for the IVR system. Following an alert, the staff sent an e-mail to the physician who received the alert. The e-mail contained a simple form for documentation of the action taken. The options for "actions taken" included: A recommendation for new analgesic medication or new dose of existing medication, a recommendation for other pain management intervention, and recommendations for a clinic or emergency room visit.

Other Symptoms

Although the project focused on pain management, the IVR system assessed 12 additional symptoms. One aim of the project is to determine if an IVR intervention that focuses on pain management will also produce a positive impact on pain-related symptoms, such as fatigue, sleep disturbance, and emotional distress. The treatment team received an e-mail alert when a symptom reached a predetermined threshold. For example, if the patient reported a distress or sadness level of 5 or greater, then the treatment team received an e-mail alert. The symptoms nausea, vomiting, and drowsiness also triggered an e-mail alert to the treatment team when the level was 5 or greater. For the symptom shortness-of-breath, the alert threshold was 3 or greater. The symptom alert levels were developed in consultation with oncologists and oncology nurses at the M. D. Anderson Cancer Center.

Control Group

Patients in the control group received the usual standard of care for pain and symptom management that is followed at the public hospital. The hospital has pain treatment guidelines that are based on the NCCN clinical practice guidelines (Benedetti et al., 2000). The patients completed the paper-and-pencil assessments at baseline and at the two follow-up clinic visits.

Baseline Assessment

Eligible patients for the study were recruited in the outpatient oncology clinics. Once a patient agreed to participate and signed a written informed consent, baseline assessment was conducted. Research staff also followed a standard script to demonstrate the IVR and teach patients how to use the system. The assessment instruments included the Brief Pain Inventory (Cleeland & Ryan, 1994), the MDASI paper form (Cleeland et al., 2000), the SF-12 Health Survey (Ware, Kosinski, & Keller, 1996), the Profile of Mood States (McNair, Lorr, & Droppleman, 1992), the Barriers Questionnaire (Ward et al., 1993), and demographic variables. The patients were given the choice of completing the English- or Spanish-language versions of the assessment instruments. The Latina patients completed a brief acculturation scale consisting of two items: Length of time in the United States and place of birth. Although there are many validated tools to measure acculturation, we were concerned about respondent burden and we selected two strong indicators of acculturation. Acculturation is defined as a process in which members of one cultural group, generally a minority or immigrant group, learn the beliefs and behaviors of another group, typically the dominant group in a society (Palos, 1994).

Outcomes Assessment

Symptom assessment using the IVR system was conducted twice weekly during the study. The study questionnaires were readministered at clinic visits at Timepoint 1 at 4–6 weeks and Timepoint 2 at 8–10 weeks following enrollment in the study. Research staff obtained clinical information from

TABLE 18.2 Patient Survey on the Interactive Voice Response (IVR) System

Survey item (0–10 scale)	Mean	SD
How comfortable are you now using the telephone system to rate your symptoms?	8.5	2.0
How easy is it to use the telephone system to rate your symptoms?	9.1	1.4
Do you think the telephone system should be part of routine patient care?	8.8	1.7
What would be the ideal number of calls per week?	1.8	0.4

patient records (i.e., medical chart and the institutional patient database), such as laboratory values, cancer treatment information, pain and symptom management, and emergency room visits and/or hospitalizations. Fifty of the 60 (83%) enrolled patients completed the Timepoint 1 assessment, and 46 (77%) completed the Timepoint 2 assessment. Seven patients were lost to follow-up, three expired, and four left the study due to personal reasons (e.g., feeling overwhelmed or too ill).

Patient Evaluation of the IVR System

At the end of the study, each patient in the intervention group completed an IVR evaluation form that assessed their reactions to the intervention and suggestions for improvements in the IVR program. The areas assessed in the evaluation included patient satisfaction with the number of IVR calls, any difficulty using the IVR system, and patient satisfaction with pain treatment. Table 18.2 presents the patient responses to the survey administered at the completion of the study. Most of the patients reported feeling very comfortable using the IVR system and rated the telephone system as easy to use. The majority of the women felt that the telephone system should be a part of routine patient care. Among the Latina women, degree of acculturation did not appear to influence their evaluation of the IVR system. In addition, there were no significant differences between the survey responses of the Latina and African American women.

INITIAL CONCLUSIONS

Our initial results support the feasibility of the IVR system for the longitudinal assessment of pain and other cancer-related symptoms of underserved minority women with breast cancer. We reached our enrollment goal of 60 patients, and more than 76% of the patients completed all three assessments. The patients in the IVR intervention group were willing to report their pain and other symptoms on a regular basis, using the automated telephone method, and reported good satisfaction with the IVR system. The English- and Spanish-language versions of the IVR system were both rated very positively. Moreover, the African American and Latina women reported the belief that the IVR system would be a helpful addition to routine patient care.

The IVR system has the capacity to monitor pain and related symptoms while patients are away from the clinic or hospital. The system also can assess symptoms such as drowsiness that may be side effects from medications or other treatments. The telephone-based IVR system is readily accessible to underserved patients who often lack access to Internet-connected computers. Additional data analyses are planned to analyze the efficacy of the IVR intervention for reducing pain and related symptoms of underserved minority women with breast cancer.

ACKNOWLEDGMENT

This work was supported by American Cancer Society Grant # RSGT-05-219-01-CPPB.

REFERENCES

Agel, J., Rockwood, T., Mundt, J. C., Greist, J. H., & Swiontkowski, M. (2001). Comparison of interactive voice response and written self-administered patient surveys for clinical research. *Orthopedics, 24*, 1155–1157.

Agency for Healthcare Research and Quality. (2008). *Disparities in health care quality among racial and ethnic minority groups: Findings from the National Healthcare Quality and Disparities Reports*. Retrieved April 1, 2010, from http://www.ahrq .gov/qual/nhqrdr08/nhqrdrminority08.htm

Anderson, K. O., Green, C. R., & Payne, R. (2009). Racial and ethnic disparities in pain: Causes and consequences of unequal care. *Journal of Pain, 10*, 1187–1204.

Anderson, K. O., Mendoza, T. R., Payne, R., Valero, V., Palos, G. R., Nazario, A., . . . Cleeland, C. S. (2004). Pain education for underserved minority cancer patients: A randomized controlled trial. *Journal of Clinical Oncology, 22*, 4918–4925.

Anderson, K. O., Mendoza, T. R., Valero, V., Richman, S. P., Russell, C., Hurley, J., . . . Cleeland, C. S. (2000). Minority cancer patients and their providers: Pain management attitudes and practice. *Cancer, 88*, 1929–1938.

Anderson, K. O., Richman, S. P., Hurley, J., Palos, G., Valero, V., Mendoza, T. R., . . . Cleeland, C. S. (2002). Cancer pain management among underserved minority outpatients: Perceived needs and barriers to optimal control. *Cancer, 94*, 2295–2304.

Baer, L., & Greist, J. H. (1997). An interactive computer-administered self-assessment and self-help program for behavior therapy. *Journal of Clinical Psychiatry, 58*(Suppl. 12), 23–28.

Benedetti, C., Brock, C., Cleeland, C., Coyle, N., Dube, J. E., Ferrell, B., . . . National Comprehensive Cancer Network. (2000). NCCN Practice Guidelines for Cancer Pain. *Oncology (Williston Park), 14,* 135–150.

Chandler, S. W., & Payne, R. (2005). Computerized tools to assess and manage cancer pain. *Highlights in Oncology Practice, 14,* 114–117.

Cleeland, C. S., Gonin, R., Baez, L., Loehrer, P., & Pandya, K. J. (1997). Pain and treatment of pain in minority patients with cancer. The Eastern Cooperative Oncology Group Minority Outpatient Pain Study. *Annals of Internal Medicine, 127,* 813–816.

Cleeland, C. S., Gonin, R., Hatfield, A. K., Edmonson, J. H., Blum, R. H., Stewart, J. A., & Pandya, K. J. (1994). Pain and its treatment in outpatients with metastatic cancer. *New England Journal of Medicine, 330,* 592–596.

Cleeland, C. S., Mendoza, T. R., Wang, X. S., Chou, C., Harle, M. T., Morrissey, M., & Engstrom, M. C. (2000). Assessing symptom distress in cancer patients: The M. D. Anderson Symptom Inventory. *Cancer, 89,* 1634–1646.

Cleeland, C. S., Portenoy, R. K., Rue, M., Mendoza, T. R., Weller, E., Payne, R., . . . Marcus, A. (2005). Does an oral analgesic protocol improve pain control for patients with cancer? An intergroup study coordinated by the Eastern Cooperative Oncology Group. *Annals of Oncology, 16,* 972–980.

Cleeland, C. S., & Ryan, K. M. (1994). Pain assessment: Global use of the Brief Pain Inventory. *Annals Academy of Medicine Singapore, 23,* 129–138.

Curry, S. J., McBride, C., Grothaus, L. C., Louie, D., & Wagner, E. H. (1995). A randomized trial of self-help materials, personalized feedback, and telephone counseling with nonvolunteer smokers. *Journal of Consulting and Clinical Psychology, 63,* 1005–1014.

Davis, K., Yount, S., Del Ciello, K., Whalen, M., Khan, S., Bass, M., . . . Cella, D.(2007). An innovative symptom monitoring tool for people with advanced lung cancer: A pilot demonstration. *Journal of Supportive Oncology, 5,* 381–387.

de Wit, R., van Dam, F., Zandbelt, L., van Buuren, A., van der Heijden, K., Leenhouts, G., & Loonstra, S. (1997). A pain education program for chronic cancer pain patients: Follow-up results from a randomized controlled trial. *Pain, 73,* 55–69.

Du Pen, S. L., Du Pen, A. R., Polissar, N., Hansberry, J., Kraybill, B. M., Stillman, M., . . . Syriala, K. (1999). Implementing guidelines for cancer pain management: Results of a randomized controlled clinical trial. *Journal of Clinical Oncology, 17,* 361–370.

Green, C. R., Anderson, K. O., Baker, T. A., Campbell, L. C., Decker, S., Fillingim, R. B., . . . Vallerand, A. H. (2003). The unequal burden of pain: Confronting racial and ethnic disparities in pain. *Pain Medicine, 4,* 277–294.

Green, C. R., Ndao-Brumblay, S. K., West, B., & Washington, T. (2005). Differences in prescription opioid analgesic availability: Comparing minority and white pharmacies across Michigan. *Journal of Pain, 6,* 689–699.

Gustafson, D. H., Bosworth, K., Chewning, B., & Hawkins, R. P. (1987). Computer-based health promotion: Combining technological advances with problem-solving techniques to effect successful health behavior changes. *Annual Review of Public Health, 8,* 387–415.

Jacox, A., Carr, D. B., & Payne, R. (1994). New clinical-practice guidelines for the management of pain in patients with cancer. *New England Journal of Medicine, 330,* 651–655.

Juarez, G., Ferrell, B., & Borneman, T. (1998). Influence of culture on cancer pain management in Hispanic patients. *Cancer Practice, 6,* 262–269.

Juarez, G., Ferrell, B., & Borneman, T. (1999). Cultural considerations in education for cancer pain management. *Journal of Cancer Education, 14,* 168–173.

Kobak, K. A., Taylor, L. H., Dottl, S. L., Greist, J. H., Jefferson, J. W., Burroughs, D., . . . Serlin, R. C. (1997). A computer-administered telephone interview to identify mental disorders. *Journal of the American Medical Association, 278,* 905–910.

Korcz, I. R., & Moreland, S. (1998). Telephone prescreening enhancing a model for proactive healthcare practice. *Cancer Practice, 6,* 270–275.

Larson, P. J., Viele, C. S., Coleman, S., Dibble, S. L., & Cebulski, C. (1993). Comparison of perceived symptoms of patients undergoing bone marrow transplant and the nurses caring for them. *Oncology Nursing Forum, 20,* 81–87.

Mahoney, D. F., Tarlow, B. J., & Jones, R. N. (2003). Effects of an automated telephone support system on caregiver burden and anxiety: Findings from the REACH for TLC intervention study. *Gerontologist, 43,* 556–567.

McNair, D. M., Lorr, M., & Droppleman, L. F. (1992). *EdITS manual for the profile of mood states.* San Diego, CA: Educational and Industrial Testing Service.

Mendoza, T. R., Anderson, K. O., Wang, X. S., Easley, M., Mobley, G., & Cleeland, C. S. (2001). Phone it in or fill it in? Comparing symptom assessment using the interactive voice response system with the traditional paper and pencil method [abstract]. International Society for Quality of Life Research.

Miaskowski, C., Dodd, M., West, C., Schumacher, K., Paul, S. M., Tripathy, D., & Koo, P. (2004). Randomized clinical trial of the effectiveness of a self-care intervention to improve cancer pain management. *Journal of Clinical Oncology, 22,* 1713–1720.

Millard, R. W., & Carver, J. R. (1999). Cross-sectional comparison of live and interactive voice recognition administration of the SF-12 health status survey. *American Journal of Managed Care, 5,* 153–159.

Morrison, R. S., Wallenstein, S., Natale, D. K., Senzel, R. S., & Huang, L. L. (2000). "We don't carry that"—Failure of pharmacies in predominantly nonwhite neighborhoods to stock opioid analgesics. *New England Journal of Medicine, 342,* 1023–1026.

Mundt, J. C., Kobak, K. A., Taylor, L. V., Mantle, J. M., Jefferson, J. W., Katzelnick, D. J., & Greist, J. H. (1998). Administration of the Hamilton Depression Rating Scale using interactive voice response technology. *M.D. Computing, 15,* 31–39.

Naylor, M. R., Helzer, J. E., Naud, S., & Keefe, F. J. (2002). Automated telephone as an adjunct for the treatment of chronic pain: a pilot study. *Journal of Pain, 3,* 429–438.

Naylor, M. R., Keefe, F. J., Brigidi, B., Naud, S., & Helzer, J. E. (2008). Therapeutic Interactive Voice Response for chronic pain reduction and relapse prevention. *Pain, 134,* 335–345.

Oliver, J. W., Kravitz, R. L., Kaplan, S. H., & Meyers, F. J. (2001). Individualized patient education and coaching to improve pain control among cancer outpatients. *Journal of Clinical Oncology, 19,* 2206–2212.

Osgood-Hynes, D. J., Greist, J. H., Marks, I. M., Baer, L., Heneman, S. W., Wenzel, K. W., ... Vitse, H. M. (1998). Self-administered psychotherapy for depression using a telephone-accessed computer system plus booklets: An open U.S.–U.K. study. *Journal of Clinical Psychiatry, 59,* 358–365.

Palos, G. (1994). Cultural heritage: Cancer screening and early detection. *Seminars in Oncology Nursing, 10,* 104–113.

Shiffman, S., Paty, J. A., Gnys, M., Kassel, J. A., & Hickcox, M. (1996). First lapses to smoking: Within-subjects analysis of real-time reports. *Journal of Consulting and Clinical Psychology, 64,* 366–379.

Siegel, K., Mesagno, F. P., Chen, J. Y., Klein, L., Bowles, M. E., McKenna, M., . . . Christ, G. (1988). Computerized telephone assessment of the "concrete" needs of chemotherapy outpatients: A feasibility study. *Journal of Clinical Oncology, 6,* 1760–1767.

Sikorskii, A., Given, C. W., Given, B., Jeon, S., Decker, V., Decker, D., . . . McCorkle, R. (2007). Symptom management for cancer patients: A trial comparing two multimodal interventions. *Journal of Pain and Symptom Management, 34,* 253–264.

Smedley, B. D., Stith, A. Y., Nelson, A. R., Institute of Medicine, & Committee on Understanding and Eliminating Racial and Ethnic Disparities in Health Care (2003). *Unequal treatment—Confronting racial and ethnic disparities in health care.* Washington, DC: National Academies Press.

Syrjala, K. L., Abrams, J. R., Polissar, N. L., Hansberry, J., Robison, J., DuPen, S., . . . DuPen, A. (2008). Patient training in cancer pain management using integrated print and video materials: A multisite randomized controlled trial. *Pain, 135,* 175–186.

Thomason, T. E., McCune, J. S., Bernard, S. A., Winer, E. P., Tremont, S., & Lindley, C. M. (1998). Cancer pain survey: Patient-centered issues in control. *Journal of Pain and Symptom Management, 15,* 275–284.

Trowbridge, R., Dugan, W., Jay, S. J., Littrell, D., Casebeer, L. L., Edgerton, S., . . . O'Toole, J. B. (1997). Determining the effectiveness of a clinical-practice intervention in improving the control of pain in outpatients with cancer. *Academic Medicine, 72,* 798–800.

Von Roenn, J. H., Cleeland, C. S., Gonin, R., Hatfield, A. K., & Pandya, K. J. (1993). Physician attitudes and practice in cancer pain management. A survey from the Eastern Cooperative Oncology Group. *Annals of Internal Medicine, 119,* 121–126.

Ward, S. E., Goldberg, N., Miller-McCauley, V., Mueller, C., Nolan, A., Pawlik-Plank, D., . . . Weissman, D. E. (1993). Patient-related barriers to management of cancer pain. *Pain, 52,* 319–324.

Ward, S. E. & Hernandez, L. (1994). Patient-related barriers to management of cancer pain in Puerto Rico. *Pain, 58,* 233–238.

Ware, J., Jr., Kosinski, M., & Keller, S. D. (1996). A 12-Item Short-Form Health Survey: construction of scales and preliminary tests of reliability and validity. *Medical Care, 34,* 220–233.

Wells, N., Hepworth, J. T., Murphy, B. A., Wujcik, D., & Johnson, R. (2003). Improving cancer pain management through patient and family education. *Journal of Pain and Symptom Management, 25,* 344–356.

World Health Organization (1996). *Cancer pain relief and palliative care.* Geneva: Author.

World Health Organization (1998). *Cancer pain relief and palliative care in children.* Geneva: Author.

Zech, D. F., Grond, S., Lynch, J., Hertel, D., & Lehmann, K. A. (1995). Validation of World Health Organization Guidelines for cancer pain relief: A 10-year prospective study. *Pain, 63,* 65–76.

19

Psycho-Educational and Psycho-Spiritual Interventions for Low-Income Cancer Patients: Results of Randomized and Patient Preference Trials on Adherence and Quality-of-Life Outcomes

*Alyson B. Moadel, Melanie Harris, Evelyn Kolidas,
Ruth Santizo, Kimala Harris, and Doru Paul*

There has been substantial research documenting ethnic disparities in cancer outcomes with regard to disease stage, treatment, and survival. Comparatively little attention, however, has been directed toward identifying and addressing ethnic disparities with regard to another important and related area of cancer outcome: namely psychosocial well-being and quality of life (QOL) (Aziz & Rowland, 2002; Meyerowitz, Richardson, Hudson, & Leedham, 1998). In general, research in this area suggests that ethnic/cultural differences in the QOL concerns of cancer patients exist with Hispanic and African American patients who are vulnerable to certain aspects of psychosocial impairment (Ashing-Giwa, 1999; Bourjolly, Kerson, & Nuamah, 1999; Moadel, Perez, Gharraee, Jones, & Sparano, 2002; Rodrigue, 1997; Spencer, Lehman, Wynings, et al., 1999).

A number of studies highlight the central role that spiritual beliefs play in coping with cancer for disadvantaged populations (Ashing-Giwa & Ganz, 1997; Ashing-Giwa, Padilla, Tejero, Kraemer, et al., 2004; Dapueto, Servente, Francolino, & Hahn, 2005; Hoffman-Goetz, 1999; Musick, Koenig, Larson, & Matthews, 1998; Potts, 1996; Taylor, 1997; Wan et al., 1999). One finding that emerges consistently is that both Hispanic and African American cancer patients report a greater level of spirituality/religiosity (Bourjolly, 1998; Mickley & Soeken, 1993) and use of spiritual coping (Culver, Arena, Antoni, & Carver, 2002; Culver, Arena, Wimberly, Antoni, & Carver, 2004) than their White counterparts. These cultural variations are mirrored in surveys of complementary medicine use and practices where "spiritual healing" was one of the most common modalities used among Blacks (36–57%) and Hispanics (26%) (Alferi, Carver, Antoni, Weiss, & Duran, 2001; Lee, Lin, Wrensch, Adler, & Eisenberg, 2000).

Behavioral interventions have shown some success in mitigating distress and QOL impairment among cancer patients, as well as potentially longer survival rates (Devine, 2003; Meyer & Mark, 1995; Rehse & Pukrop, 2003). These interventions are mainly based in psychosocial and educational (hereinafter called "psycho-educational") approaches, which comprise any of the following components: (a) cognitive–behavioral (coping skills, progressive muscle relaxation, hypnotherapy, behavior modification); (b) educational (providing medical or procedural information); (c) counseling/ psychotherapy; and (d) nonprofessional support (support groups run by fellow patients) (Meyer & Mark, 1995). Insufficient social support has been found to be associated with higher distress levels among patients from across ethnic groups (Alferi et al., 2001; Beder, 1995; Meyerowitz, Formenti, Ell, & Leedham, 2000; Michael, Berkman, Colditz, Holmes, & Kawachi, 2002; Northouse et al., 1999). As such, the psycho-educational *group* model, which relies on patient support and connection, has shown great efficacy in reducing distress and improving coping, and may even be associated with enhanced survival (Blake-Mortimer, Gore-Felton, Kimerling, Turner-Cobb, & Spiegel, 1999; Fawzy & Fawzy, 1998).

Although the "state of the art" in QOL intervention for non-Hispanic White populations is well established, its applicability and relevance to the ethnic-minority cancer patient is unknown. There are several arrows pointing to areas of need among these vulnerable groups, but a clear road map for intervention has yet to be developed. The rationale to direct attention to the spiritual/existential needs of cancer patients is strong on several fronts. First, our own findings of a psychosocial needs assessment shows that spiritual needs are important to ethnic-minority cancer patients (Moadel et al., 1999; Moadel, Morgan, & Dutcher, 2007). Although not all patients are religious, patients may still seek solace in spiritual coping (Stolley & Koenig, 1997). Second, the need for meaning is universal; it provides a sense of purpose and connection in people's lives. The most common sources of meaning stem from connections with something greater than one's self, that is, family, career, or a religious or philosophical system of belief. When terminally ill patients lose their ability to work, they often turn to community or the transcendent realm for a renewed sense of meaning and connection (Baumesiter, 1991). Finally, there is some evidence that spiritual and religious beliefs/practices may be positively associated with health outcomes (Koenig & Cohen, 2002).

Despite evidence that mind–body interventions offer benefits to QOL after cancer, effects are modest, and at times, inconsistent (Fawzy, 1999; Meyer & Mark, 1995; Ross, Boesen, Dalton, & Johansen, 2002). The reasons for this may be small sample sizes, low enrollment rates, and poor intervention adherence plaguing the field of mind–body research (Bottomley, 1997; Irwin & Ainsworth, 2004; Richardson, Post-White, Singletary, & Justice, 1998). The vast majority of published studies on psychosocial/mind–body interventions in cancer survivors include sample sizes of less than 100 participants (Ross et al., 2002), and enrollment rates of 30–50% (Richardson et al., 1998). Enrollment and adherence are lowest among underserved populations and ethnic-minority cancer survivors, who may face socioeconomic barriers to participation including travel costs, and child care and work-related responsibilities (Ashing-Giwa, Padilla, Tejero, & Kim, 2004; Richardson et al., 1998). Moreover, research on preferences, needs, and practices regarding mind–body and psychosocial interventions among cancer patients clearly indicates that it is not "one-size-fits-all" (Powell, Shahabi, & Thoresen, 2003; Sanson-Fisher et al., 2000; Steele & Fitch, 2008).

In 1991, Thomas Burish put forth a report discussing the past, present, and recommendations for the future of behavioral cancer research as discussed at the American Cancer Society's second workshop on Methodology in Behavioral and Psychosocial Cancer Research (Burish, 1991). Two major conclusions were the need for greater application of research findings to the clinical setting, and greater representation of minority groups. Although progress has been made over the past 15–20 years, these needs are still salient (Helgeson, 2005). Rapkin and Trickett, in a discussion about behavioral prevention interventions, raise concerns about the randomized controlled trial pertaining to ecological validity and the clinical relevance of an intervention outside of the research context (Rapkin & Trickett, 2005). They assert that given that people often have preferences for interventions, the lack of choice in regard to what intervention they are given may result in poor adherence and drop-out at best, and mistrust of the researcher/health care community at worst. In direct response to the question of what directions are most useful for mind–body research in psycho-oncology, more than 10 years ago, Alastair Cunningham suggested that alternative designs to the randomized controlled trial are needed and should include a "smorgasbord" of interventions in which patients can choose (Cunningham, 1999).

Using our needs assessment as a base, The *Mind–Body Cancer Research Program* was developed to meet the psychosocial needs of the ethnic-minority cancer patient with advanced disease and those on active treatment by comparing two different interventions. In an effort to help contribute to the road map for addressing cancer disparities in QOL, this chapter will describe the development and piloting of these interventions, a spiritual support group, and the standard-of-care psycho-educational group, to address salient areas of psychosocial need among underserved cancer patients. It will also describe two phases used in the study design: (1) randomized comparison trial, and (2) patient preference trial, whereby patients can choose their group of choice. The study aims addressed are as follows:

1. To describe the characteristics of cancer patients who enroll in a Mind–Body Support Group Program, with and without group preferences considered.
2. To describe the characteristics of patients who choose a "Stress Management Support Group" and those who choose a "Spiritual Support Group," within the patient preference phase.
3. To examine intervention adherence and satisfaction among randomized and patient preference arms.
4. To explore within-group changes in quality of life and psychosocial outcomes by intervention group and study design (randomized vs. preference).

METHODS

Study Design

In Figure 19.1, an overview of the two-phase study design for this Mind–Body Support Group Program is provided. Below is a description of this American Cancer Society–funded randomized intervention trial designed to develop and compare a *Psycho-Spiritual Intervention* to a *Psycho-Educational Intervention* for English- and Spanish-speaking, underserved patients with advanced cancer.

The Mind–Body Cancer Research Program was implemented between 2004 and 2010 within a major cancer center in the Bronx, New York. The Bronx community is made up of nearly 1.4 million residents, many of whom are indigent and ethnic minorities. According to the 2000 U.S. Census data, the Bronx is the poorest borough in New York City, with 31% of the population living below the poverty line (U.S. Census Bureau, 2000). The major racial/ethnic groups represented are Hispanics (48%), Blacks (36%), and non-Hispanic Whites (15%). The subpopulations include African American, Puerto Rican, West Indian, Dominican, and Eastern European. As with most disadvantaged, minority populations in the United States, the Bronx suffers from high cancer morbidity and mortality rates (New York Department of Health, 2006).

This psychosocial intervention study proposed to directly address two major areas of need, supportive and spiritual, while incorporating attention to informational and practical needs. Eligibility includes English- or Spanish-speaking patients with stage III or IV cancer, and sufficient functional performance (ECOG < 3). Eligible patients were identified through self-referral (via flyers) or medical staff referral and informed by research

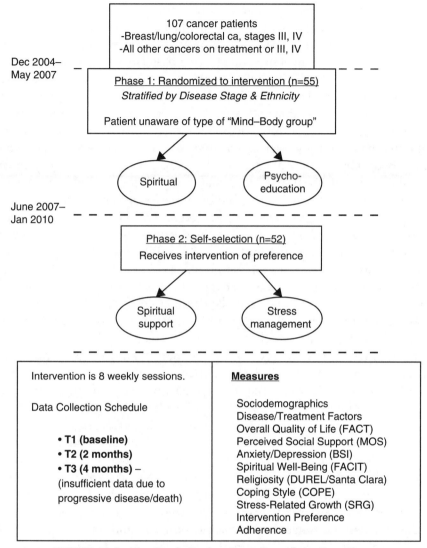

FIGURE 19.1 The Study Design Overview of the Two-Phase
Mind–Body Support Group Program

assistants that the goal of the study was (a)—randomized phase—"to examine the helpfulness of two different types of mind–body groups in helping patients to cope with the emotional and physical stresses related to living with cancer and its treatment"; or (b)—patient preference phase—"We have a Mind–Body Support Group Program where we are offering two different types of groups for patients to choose from, a Spiritual Support Group or a Stress Management Support Group." Assessments via interview were planned at three time points: T1 = baseline, T2 = 2 months, and

T3 = 4 months, utilizing standardized measures assessing various aspects of QOL, distress, religiosity, spiritual well-being, perceived social support, coping styles, and stress-related growth. An additional endpoint that will be explored in the future is survival at 1 year based on medical chart review.

Following acquisition of patients' written informed consent to participate and completion of the baseline assessment, patients were either randomized to intervention in Phase I (however, they remained unaware of the specific nature of the differences in interventions), or chose their intervention (Phase II). They then began attendance at an eight-session, weekly Mind–Body Group held at the hospital/clinic. In an effort to minimize sociocultural and medical factors that could influence the outcome in Phase I, randomization was stratified by disease stage and ethnicity.

Six major objectives were considered when designing the interventions for this study: (1) to respond to the documented psychosocial needs of the target underserved population; (2) to design a culturally relevant and accessible intervention for the underserved ethnic-minority population; (3) to focus on late-stage disease, which is overrepresented among minority populations (Jemal et al., 2004; Li, Malone, & Daling, 2003) and associated with great psychosocial morbidity (Walsh, Donnelly, & Rybicki, 2000); (4) to identify and include relevant quality of life endpoints to measure intervention efficacy; (5) to incorporate knowledge of previous behavioral research and clinical experience, indicating *what works and doesn't work* in psychosocial intervention (Fawzy, 1999); and (6) to produce measurable, replicable, and clinically applicable interventions.

The development of both interventions took several stages: (1) the selection of an overall name, Mind–Body Cancer Program (and in Spanish, *El Programa de Cancer para La Mente y El Cuerpo*), that would accurately reflect the nature of both interventions (NCCAM, 2002) as well as being accessible and meaningful to the population—the opinions of clinicians, researchers, and cancer patients were garnered in the name selection process; (2) the identification of basic principles, themes, and techniques utilized in published psychosocial/spiritual interventions with cancer patients; (3) the development and adaptation of specific topics, themes, exercises, and patient materials, with a focus on literacy and cultural relevance—evaluation of the topics and materials was included in the measures of the study to ensure acceptability; (4) pilot-testing of the interventions with the underserved target population; and (5) the generation of additional topics/themes and materials in weekly group debriefing meetings that followed each session.

The logistic format for each intervention is identical. They are administered through 8 weekly 1.5-hour group sessions held at three medical sites within the cancer center; however, patients who wish to continue past the assigned intervention period are allowed to, with such activity being documented. The interventions are based on an open-enrollment format so that new patients can join the class upon recruitment, rather than having to wait for the "next available group to start" (a widely used format, which can result in loss of valuable time, impairment of health, and hence, less potential to participate). To maintain the progress and flow of the program, each session is self-contained, and the series is noncumulative. However, each session for both interventions contains a defined and replicable format as follows: (a) Introduction, (b) Review of Week, (c) Topic of the Day, (d) Education *or* Reflection, (e) Skill-Building *or* Existential Group Exercise, (f) Open Discussion, (g) Homework, and (h) Closing Relaxation/Imagery exercise. The theoretical and practical components of each intervention are described next.

INTERVENTIONS

Psycho-Educational Intervention

The psycho-educational intervention is based on the well-established "standard of care" psychosocial intervention group model (Fawzy & Fawzy, 1998). The intention is to provide individuals with information and coping skills that will assist them in achieving and maintaining an optimal state of physical, emotional, and social functioning. It does this by reducing the sense of helplessness and uncertainty regarding their disease through educational, problem-solving, and goal-setting approaches.

The psycho-educational intervention used in the Mind–Body Program was based on the following three intervention strategies that are described widely in the literature (Cunningham, Edmonds, & Williams, 1999; Fawzy & Fawzy, 1994; Spiegel & Diamond, 1998):

1. Educational (i.e., providing education and information to promote coping).
2. Cognitive–behavioral (i.e., coping skills training, progressive muscle relaxation, behavior modification, assertiveness/communication skills training).
3. Supportive (i.e., facilitator-guided feedback and peer support).

Following introductions and the review of the week, the intervention takes its unique shape through topical discussion and exercises as described below:

Topic of the day: Topics address salient themes that have emerged in the needs assessment study as well as those raised during the intervention sessions themselves. Examples include "Befriending Anxiety," "Coping with Stress," "Communicating Your Needs," "Angry—Who Me?" "You Are What You Think," "Caretaking vs. Caring For," "Living with Change," "Assertiveness Training," and "Intimacy & Sexuality."

Education: All topics are discussed within the framework of cognitive–behavioral theory through helping patients identify their emotions, explore the beliefs that may underlie them, and create behavioral change to get their needs met and improve quality of life.

Skill-building exercise: These exercises are directed toward enhancing coping skills in managing cancer and its consequences through hands-on learning. Examples include having members role-playing questions that they want to ask their physicians with another group member, writing a list of short-term goals, learning and practicing diaphragmatic breathing, and implementing thought-monitoring exercises.

Open discussion: This follows directly from the group exercise, in which themes and experiences are discussed and processed.

Homework: A homework activity is assigned that is geared toward promoting utilization and practice of skills learned/discussed in the session.

Closing exercise: A progressive muscle relaxation or visual imagery exercise is led by the facilitator.

Psycho-Spiritual Intervention

The psycho-spiritual intervention was conceived and developed to address an area that has received little empirical attention, namely the spiritual needs of cancer patients, while drawing on the coping style and interests of the ethnic-minority cancer patient. This approach to the psychosocial intervention model is, hence, centered around helping patients find meaning, hope, peace, and spiritual resources in the face of advanced cancer. Whereas "religion" generally refers to a way of relating to a higher power, "spirituality" suggests a process by which individuals examine and define broader concepts such as meaning, values, transcendence (appreciation of a dimension beyond the self), connection, and becoming (personal reflection of life's unfolding) (Martsolf, 1997). As such, this intervention is of a "spiritual" nature, with participants encouraged to use or apply the terminology that best fits with their understanding of the *spiritual* (i.e., God, higher power, higher self, nature, oneness, humanity), thus accommodating both religious and nonreligious persons.

Drawing from the established theory and practice of existential psychotherapy, the psycho-spiritual intervention addresses existential themes of death, freedom, isolation, and meaninglessness—considered to be, at once, the main catalysts and challenges to adaptation in life (Frankl, 1988;

Yalom, 1980). It is further informed by published work regarding existential/ spiritual interventions used with cancer patients (Breitbart, Gibson, Poppito, & Berg, 2004; Cole & Pargament, 1999; Fitchett & Handzo, 1998).

The existential topics (e.g., "meaning," "suffering") central to the intervention are better described as *themes* to be explored, addressed, and resolved as a process throughout the intervention in ongoing discussions, sharing, and experiential activities. In this vein, readings and materials from various religious and nonreligious traditions are used as a medium for exploring patients' search for meaning, control, connection, and hope in the face of life-threatening disease.

Following introductions and the review of the week, each session follows the outline described below:

Topic of the day: Topics address salient spiritual/existential themes that have emerged from the needs assessment as well as in the group itself. Examples include "Acceptance," "Meaning of Suffering," "Transcendence," "Transformation," "Finding Peace," "Loneliness & Connection," "Forgiveness," "Creativity & Self-Expression," and "Ritual & Meaning."

Reflection period: To stimulate reflection, quotes, inspirational readings, prayers, or stories pertaining to the theme of the week are read and discussed. Examples include poems/prayers written by African American motivational figures such as Maya Angelou, Iyanla Vanzant, and Martin Luther King. Themes of the week and inspirational messages are translated as needed into Spanish; quotes are also chosen from Spanish motivational figures as well.

Group exercise: These exercises are directed toward resolving existential conflicts and strengthening spiritual connection for each member. Examples include having members write answers to such questions as: "Why me? Why did I get cancer?"; "What have I learned about myself or life from having cancer?" Other exercise options include: storytelling, with the focus on discovering universal truths, courage, hope, or meaning; having members enter and select anonymous fears, regrets, and hopes from a basket, for discussion by the group; and guiding participants to write their own personal affirmations and/or prayers toward cultivating inner peace.

Open discussion: This follows directly from the group exercise, in which reactions are discussed and processed.

Homework: A homework activity is assigned that is geared toward promoting further reflection and processing of the theme of the session (e.g., reading a daily affirmation).

Closing meditation: A guided imagery exercise that directly addresses the theme/s of the session is led by the facilitator.

RESULTS

1. To describe the characteristics of cancer patients who enroll in a Mind–Body Support Group Program, with and without group preferences considered.

    Due to limited availability and funding for bilingual staff to translate materials and facilitate the groups, piloting of the Spanish-speaking intervention phase experienced many external challenges in recruitment and implementation, resulting in excessive incomplete data among the 19 Spanish-speaking patients accrued. As such, results will focus on findings relevant to the English-speaking sample only. There were 107 patients accrued to study that completed T1 and T2 assessments, 55 in the randomized phase and 52 in the patient preference phase. Table 19.1 describes and compares the socio-demographic and medical characteristics of both samples. On the whole, the sample was predominantly female, African American or Hispanic, made up of U.S. immigrants, and not college educated. The groups did not differ on demographics with the exception of religion, with much fewer Protestants and many more "Other religions" participating in the preference trial than the randomized trial, where the vast majority was Protestant or Catholic. Interestingly, only half of the patient preference arm endorsed being religious, compared to 75% of those randomized. The differences in disease site, stage, and treatment was likely related to an amendment made to the study toward the end of the randomized phase, to expand "advanced-stage" eligibility to "active treatment, any stage" (except breast, lung, and colorectal which still had to be later-stage), due to low enrollment. Among the psychosocial variables, two emerged as different between the two phases: those in the Preference trial reported lower social support but higher active coping than those in the randomized trial (Table 19.2).

2. To describe the characteristics of patients who choose a Stress Management Support Group and those who choose a Spiritual Support Group, within the patient preference phase.

    In Table 19.3, baseline sociodemographic and psychosocial differences between patients in each intervention group are shown for each study phase. As can be seen, the randomization for Phase I seemed to minimize "natural" differences between groups, with the exception of one: those in the psycho-educational group have higher scores on the "BSI—Somatization" subscale compared to the spiritual group. On the other hand, the patient preference trial revealed many differences between those choosing each group. Those choosing the Spiritual Support Group endorsed higher education, more private religious activity, better quality of life, lower anxiety, and greater use of humor as a coping strategy.

TABLE 19.1 Sociodemographic and Medical Characteristics of the Sample (*n* = 107)

Baseline	Randomized Phase (*n* = 55)	Patient Preference Phase (*n* = 52)
Age	55 ± 11 *M* years (range 32–74)	57 ± 10 *M* years (range 32–74)
Gender	80% Female	81% Female
Education	77% ≤ High school degree	74% ≤ High school degree
Marital status	27% Married	31% Married
Ethnicity	55% African American 27% Hispanic 15% Caucasian	44% African American 23% Hispanic 21% Caucasian
U.S. immigrant	78%	65%
Religion**	53% Protestant 35% Catholic 6% Other	27% Protestant 35% Catholic 25% Other
Religious/spiritual**	75% Religious 86% Spiritual	50% Religious 77% Spiritual
Cancer diagnoses*	24% Breast 18% Lung 15% Colorectal 12% Hematologic 11% Ovarian 22% Other	14% Breast 14% Lung 4% Colorectal 8% Hematologic 10% Ovarian 51% Other
Disease stage**	24% III 73% IV	26% I–II 24% III 50% IV
Time since diagnosis	2.8 ±3.2 *M* years (range 1 month to 14 years)	2.11 ±2.7 *M* years (range 1 month to 12 years)
Chemotherapy**	76% Currently on	43% Currently on

*$p < .05$; **$p < .01$.

TABLE 19.2 Psychosocial Differences Between Randomized and Patient Preference Samples (*n* = 107)

Baseline	Randomized Phase (*n* = 55)	Patient Preference Phase (*n* = 52)
MOS—Social support* • Emotional support* • Affection*	73 ± 24 *M* years (range 66–79)	63 ± 26 *M* years (range 56–70)
COPE—Active coping*	5.3 *M* ± 2.0 (range 4.8–5.9)	6.2 *M* ± 1.5 (range 5.8–6.6)

*$p > .05$; **$p > .01$.

TABLE 19.3 Baseline Sociodemographic and Psychosocial Differences Between Intervention Groups by Study Phase

Baseline	Randomized Phase (*n* = 55)	
	Psycho-educational group (46%)	**Spiritual group (54%)**
BSI—Somatization*	52.89	46.57
	Patient preference phase (*n* = 52)	
	Stress Management Support Group (69%)	Spiritual Support Group (31%)
Education*	100% < HS	0% < HS
	76% HS	24% HS
	43% > HS	57% > HS
Frequency of private religious activity (DUREL)**	3.8	5.2
FACT-G: Overall QOL*	59.81	72.36
• Physical well-being*	15.58	19.50
• Emotional well-being*	14.31	18.19
• Functional well-being*	12.50	16.14
BSI—Anxiety*	54.01	46.93
COPE—Humor*	3.92	5.31

*$p > .05$; **$p > .01$.

3. To examine intervention adherence and satisfaction among randomized and patient preference arms.

   Intervention adherence based on attendance sheets and self-reported satisfaction is described in Table 19.4. As can be seen, both study phases demonstrated equally high *non*adherence, with nearly 23% not attending a single session. On the other hand, there were more patients in the Preference arm represented among those who were most adherent. Expectations, comfort, satisfaction, and the helpfulness of the program were also rated more highly among the Preference arm. Major barriers to adherence included feeling ill and competing medical appointments.

4. To explore within-group changes in quality of life and psychosocial outcomes by intervention group and study design (randomized vs. preference).

   Due to high nonadherence rates and small sample sizes, limited power precludes conducting a between-group analysis to examine the impact of the intervention on QOL. Instead, within-group pre- and post-analyses were conducted among patients who attended more than two sessions, to explore changes in QOL. Although patients in

TABLE 19.4 Intervention Adherence and Evaluation

	Intervention Adherence Between T1 and T2 (8 Weeks)	
	Randomized phase	Patient preference phase
Mean number of sessions attended (0–8)	3.30 (±3)	3.10 (±3)
Attended 0 sessions	22%	23%
Attended > 2 sessions	48%	56%
Attended > 3 sessions	37%	52%
Evaluation		
Expectations fulfilled (quite a bit/ very much)	54%	57%
Comfort in program (quite a bit/ very much)	62%	83%
Satisfaction (quite a bit/very much)	62%	70%
Helpful (quite a bit/very much)	62%	65%
Reasons for missing sessions		
Not feeling well	54%	40%
Medical appointments	30%	36%
Transportation barriers	12%	13%
Weather	11%	15%

the randomized phase did not experience any significant changes at the .05 alpha level, changes that met the $p < .1$ level are depicted in Figure 19.2. Patients randomized to the *spiritual group* experienced (nonsignificant) reduced social well-being and intrinsic religiosity, and increased somatization, but also increased coping through active coping, religion, instrumental support, and distraction. On the other hand, patients randomized to the *psycho-educational group* experienced (nonsignificant) reduced levels of affectional support and coping through emotional support.

In Figure 19.3, depicting the patient preference arm, patients in the Spiritual Support Group reported significantly ($p < .05$) reduced chemotherapy side effects/neurologic symptoms, but also significantly reduced tangible support. Among those in the Stress Management Support Group, significantly reduced tangible support was also reported, along with reduced use of venting as a coping strategy ($p < .05$).

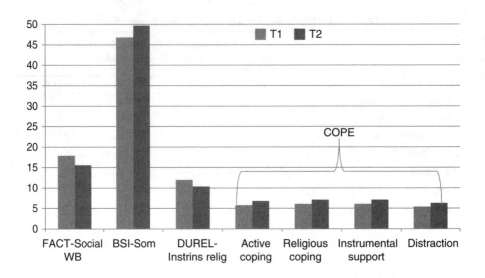

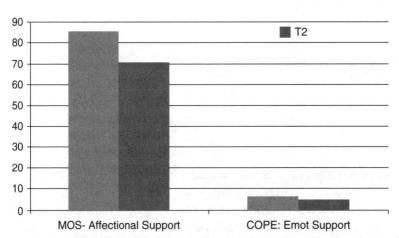

FIGURE 19.2 Noteworthy Pre- and Post-Intervention Changes in Psychosocial Variables Among Those Who Attended More Than Two Group Sessions; $p \leq .1$ (No Changes Reached a p-Value of .05 or Less)

DISCUSSION

This chapter presents a glimpse into the challenges and successes related to implementing a psychosocial intervention study to underserved, active treatment cancer patients, as well as the importance of enhancing enrollment, participation, and outcome in psychosocial research.

Hispanic and African American cancer patients reported greater *informational, practical, supportive,* and *spiritual* needs than non-Hispanic Whites. These "need disparities" are not surprising, given the factors that

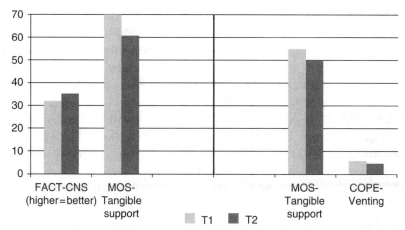

FIGURE 19.3 Significant Pre- and Post-Intervention Changes in Psychosocial Variables Among Those Who Attended More Than Two Group Sessions; $p < .05$

generally contribute to ethnic disparities, including deficient socioeconomic resources, education, and medical access (American Cancer Society, 2004). Further, among interventions that address the psychosocial care of the cancer patient, most have been developed with and for White, middle-class, and early-stage patients (Taylor et al., 2003). Few interventions have addressed the spiritual concerns of cancer patients, or sought to revise the psychosocial model for patients from ethnic-minority populations (Barg & Gullatte, 2001).

This intervention study presents the development of a psycho-educational to a psycho-spiritual group intervention for underserved and ethnic-minority cancer patients with advanced disease or on active treatment. It also describes the results of two methodological approaches used, randomized versus patient preference, to offer greater ecological validity to the population's needs. There were only 150 patients accrued to the study over a period of 5 years, and only 74% who completed the first 2 of 3 assessments. While the target sample focused on the most ill patients, often with poor and deteriorating performance status, this low accrual rate is a strong statement that support group interventions are limited in their reach. Clearly, medical concerns and appointments are major barriers to attending groups among those on active treatment and/or with advanced disease, and with limited resources. The low accrual rate rivals that of many other psychosocial intervention studies targeting less-advanced-stage patients (Richardson et al., 1998).

But, then, to whom does such an intervention appeal? It seems that middle-aged women, who are ethnic minorities and non-U.S. born, are interested in support groups. Other research has shown the saliency of formal and informal support groups in coping and information-gathering among minority cancer patients (Guidry, Aday, Zhang, & Winn, 1997). Men are generally less likely to participate in "support group" programs (Deans, Bennett-Emslie, Weir, Smith, & Kaye, 1988), which may reflect the fact that men tend to use more action-based, information-seeking coping strategies in comparison to women, who rely more on emotional expression and support (Volkers, 1999). While ethnic-minority men find comfort in spiritual modes of coping as well as faith-based groups, they may be more apt to participate in such groups with their partners than alone (Barg & Gullatte, 2001). Future research may benefit from designing and evaluating psychosocial interventions that include patients and family caregivers together.

Interestingly, patients who choose to participate in a general "mind–body" support group study differ from those who choose to participate in one that gives them a choice of a spiritual versus stress management support group. It appears that the latter group tended to endorse nondominant religious traditions or beliefs, including no religion, Eastern religions, and lower religiosity in general. Further, they are also those with the least social support, but with a more active coping style. The traditional medical model is built on an authoritative premise, where the doctor advises and the patient follows the advice. Although the concept of patient choice and autonomy in medical care is up and coming, it has yet to become fully integrated into the culture of medicine. As such, it may be no surprise that the less conventional patients, with limited social support yet proactive coping skills, are the most interested in participating in a study that offers them a choice.

Within the patient preference model, there is also a clear distinction between those who choose stress management and those who choose spiritual support. Contrary to expectations, more than two thirds of patients chose the former. This may reflect the fact that the group was less spiritually/ religiously oriented, or it may have more to do with specific needs at the time. Clearly, those who chose stress management support reported less religious activity, but they also had lower QOL and higher anxiety. For them, the need may have been focused on day-to-day living, and on managing the side effects of treatment and living with cancer. On the other hand, those who chose spiritual support were more highly educated and used humor as a form of coping. Perhaps their need was to find a place to get a "bigger perspective" on what they were going through.

Despite very formidable health and logistic barriers to participation, nearly three-fourths attended some level of the intervention among both trials, which suggests that the groups may, in fact, be addressing their needs. For who attended some sessions, attendance was highest among those in the preference trial. Program evaluation ratings suggest that the interventions are meeting patients' needs, particularly in the case of those who were able to choose their intervention. Notably, more of the preference patients felt very comfortable in their groups than the randomized patients.

The final question of import is whether or not mind–body groups improve QOL, and if choice of group affords an added benefit. Our within-group analyses can only offer some theories. First, it appears that patients who experience deteriorating support tend to be the ones who attend the groups. For those in the randomized phase, it also appears that the spiritual group may offer benefits to learning adaptive coping strategies which are not found in the psycho-educational group. In the preference phase, patients receiving spiritual support had improved medical side effects; but whether they attended more sessions due to better QOL or the sessions improved their QOL is not known. However, those in the stress management group experienced a reduction in venting. Perhaps, the opportunity to share their experiences with others who understood helped them to learn more adaptive ways of coping.

A question of interest for future studies is whether patients who participate in more of the psycho-educational group sessions have better treatment adherence, miss fewer medical visits, and engage in more assertive communication with their doctors about health-related needs.

LIMITATIONS

There are a number of limitations to be noted. First, this intervention study lacks a no-treatment (attention-only) control group, which is necessary to examine the absolute effects of the experimental interventions. However, ethical considerations prevailed in deciding not to withhold a treatment (i.e., psycho-education) that is known to offer a measurable and positive impact on quality of life. Second, given the small sample size, this chapter was meant to offer preliminary findings of such programs. This brings up the issue of the challenges in recruitment of underserved, ethnic-minority, late-stage cancer patients. Financial barriers, competing life/medical demands, and cultural beliefs can present formidable barriers to patient participation in a "nonessential" and/or "psychological" service. Further, patients diagnosed with later-stage cancers (i.e., stages III and IV) often experience challenges due to acute and lingering side effects from treatment that may affect their ability to enroll in and regularly attend programs. The demands of an eight-session support group, which requires patients to travel to attend, may be too great. These group interventions also attracted many more women than men, as is commonly found in support groups. Future research may consider spiritual and psycho-educational interventions that are home-based, via video- or telephone-counseling, or church- or community-center based, and may perhaps include family participation to enhance accessibility and acceptability. Lastly, the relevance of the interventions to the Spanish-speaking patient is pending future recruitment and development through qualitative interviews on psychosocial needs with patients who have completed their participation in the program, as well as with collaboration and focus groups with community members. In addition, ongoing needs assessments in English and Spanish are being implemented to help shed direct light on patient preferences for specific services.

CONCLUSIONS

It is believed that spirituality or religion promotes adjustment through its ability to give meaning and hope by providing an explanation for the experience of illness and suffering (Musick et al., 1998). African American and Hispanic cancer patients have a considerable need to find meaning and hope, and seem particularly receptive to coping with advanced disease within a supportive, structured group. Future research is needed to help identify the optimal healing environment for enhancing patient response to such psychosocial interventions, and taking the patient's preferences, cultural beliefs, and psychosocial needs into consideration is an important place to start. In addition to patient preference trials, community-based participatory methods can play an important role, so that we can not only identify if, how, and for whom such groups may reduce physical, emotional, social, and spiritual suffering, but refine and improve them along the way.

REFERENCES

American Cancer Society. (2004). Cancer: Basic facts. In *Cancer facts & figures 2004* (pp. 1–2). Atlanta, GA: Author.

Alferi, S. M., Carver, C. S., Antoni, M. H., Weiss, S., & Duran, R. E. (2001). An exploratory study of social support, distress, and life disruption among low-income Hispanic women under treatment for early stage breast cancer. *Health Psychology, 20*(1), 41–46.

Ashing-Giwa, K. (1999). Quality of life and psychosocial outcomes in long-term survivors of breast cancer: A focus on African-American women. *Journal of Psychosocial Oncology, 17*(3–4), 47–62.

Ashing-Giwa, K., & Ganz, P. A. (1997). Understanding the breast cancer experience of African-American women. *Journal of Psychosocial Oncology, 15*(2), 19–35.

Ashing-Giwa, K. T., Padilla, G., Tejero, J., Kraemer, J., Wright, K., Coscarelli, A., . . . Hills, D. (2004). Understanding the breast cancer experience of women: A qualitative study of African American, Asian American, Latina and Caucasian cancer survivors. *Psycho-Oncology, 13*, 408–428.

Ashing-Giwa, K. T., Padilla, G. V., Tejero, J. S., & Kim, J. (2004). Breast cancer survivorship in a multiethnic sample: Challenges in recruitment and measurement. *Cancer, 101*(3), 450–465.

Aziz, N. M., & Rowland, J. H. (2002). Cancer survivorship research among ethnic minority and medically underserved groups. *Oncology Nursing Forum, 29*(5), 789–801.

Barg, F. K., & Gullatte, M. M. (2001). Cancer support groups: Meeting the needs of African Americans with cancer. *Seminars in Oncology Nursing, 17*(3), 171–178.

Baumesiter, R. F. (1991). *Meanings of life*. New York, NY: Guilford Press.

Beder, J. (1995). Perceived social support and adjustment to mastectomy in socioeconomically disadvantaged Black women. *Social Work in Health Care, 22*(2), 55–71.

Blake-Mortimer, J., Gore-Felton, C., Kimerling, R., Turner-Cobb, J. M., & Spiegel, D. (1999). Improving the quality and quantity of life among patients with cancer: A review of effectiveness of group psychotherapy. *European Journal of Cancer, 35*(11), 1581–1586.

Bottomley, A. (1997). Where are we now? Evaluating two decades of group interventions with adult cancer patients. *Journal of Psychiatric and Mental Health Nursing, 4*(4), 251–265.

Bourjolly, J. N. (1998). Differences in religiousness among Black and White women with breast cancer. *Social Work in Health Care, 28*(1), 21–39.

Bourjolly, J. N., Kerson, T. S., & Nuamah, I. F. (1999). A comparison of social functioning among Black women with breast cancer. *Social Work in Health Care, 28*(3), 1–20.

Breitbart, W., Gibson, C., Poppito, S. R., & Berg, A. (2004). Psychotherapeutic interventions at the end of life: A focus on meaning and spirituality. *Canadian Journal of Psychiatry, 49*(6), 366–372.

Burish, T. G. (1991). Behavioral and psychosocial cancer research. Building on the past, preparing for the future. *Cancer, 67*(3 Suppl), 865–867.

Cole, B., & Pargament, K. (1999). Re-creating your life: A spiritual/psychotherapeutic intervention for people diagnosed with cancer. *Psycho-Oncology, 8*, 395–407.

Culver, J. L., Arena, P. L., Antoni, M. H., & Carver, C. S. (2002). Coping and distress among women under treatment for early stage breast cancer: Comparing African Americans, Hispanics and non-Hispanic Whites. *Psycho-Oncology, 11*, 495–504.

Culver, J., Arena, P. L., Wimberly, S. R., Antoni, M. H., & Carver, C. S. (2004). Coping among African-American, Hispanic, and non-Hispanic White women recently treated for early stage breast cancer. *Psychology & Health, 19*(2), 157–166.

Cunningham, A. J. (1999). Mind–body research in psychooncology: What directions will be most useful? *Advances in Mind–Body Medicine, 15*(4), 252–255.

Cunningham, A. J., Edmonds, C. V. I., & Williams, D. (1999). Delivering a very brief psychoeducational program to cancer patients and family members in a large group format. *Psycho-Oncology, 8*, 177–182.

Dapueto, J. J., Servente, L., Francolino, C., & Hahn, E. A. (2005). Determinants of quality of life in patients with cancer: A South American study. *Cancer, 103*(5), 1072–1081.

Deans, G., Bennett-Emslie, G. B., Weir, J., Smith, D. C., & Kaye, S. B. (1988). Cancer support groups—Who joins and why? *British Journal of Cancer, 58*, 670–674.

Devine, E. C. (2003). Meta-analysis of the effect of psychoeducational interventions on pain in adults with cancer. *Oncology Nursing Forum, 30*(1), 75–89.

Fawzy, F. I. (1999). Psychosocial interventions for patients with cancer: What works and what doesn't. *European Journal of Cancer, 35*(1), 1559–1564.

Fawzy, F. I., & Fawzy, N. W. (1994). A structured psychoeducational intervention for cancer patients. *General Hospital Psychiatry, 16*(3), 149–192.

Fawzy, F. I., & Fawzy, N. W. (1998). Group therapy in the cancer setting. *Journal of Psychosomatic Research, 45*(3), 191–200.

Fitchett, G., & Handzo, G. (1998). Spiritual assessment, screening, and intervention. In J. Holland (Ed.), *Psycho-oncology* (pp. 790–808). New York, NY: Oxford University Press.

Frankl, V. F. (1988). *The will to meaning: Foundations and applications of logotherapy, expanded edition.* New York, NY: Penguin.

Guidry, J. J., Aday, L. A., Zhang, D., & Winn, R. J. (1997). The role of informal and formal social support networks for patients with cancer. *Cancer Practice, 5*(4), 241–246.

Helgeson, V. S. (2005). Recent advances in psychosocial oncology. *Journal of Consulting & Clinical Psychology, 73*(2), 268–271.

Hoffman-Goetz, L. (1999). Cancer experiences of African American women as portrayed in popular mass magazines. *Psycho-Oncology, 8,* 36–45.

Irwin, M. L., & Ainsworth, B. E. (2004). Physical activity interventions following cancer diagnosis: Methodologic challenges to delivery and assessment. *Cancer Investigation, 22*(1), 30–50.

Jemal, A., Clegg, L. X., Ward, E., Wu, X., Jamison, P. M., Wingo, P. A., . . . Edwards, B. K. (2004). Annual report to the nation on the status of cancer, 1975–2001, with a special feature regarding survival. *Cancer, 101*(1), 3–27.

Koenig, H. G., & Cohen, H. J. (2002). *The link between religion and health: Psychoneuroimmunology and the faith factor.* Oxford, UK: Oxford University Press.

Lee, M. M., Lin, S. S., Wrensch, M. R., Adler, S. R., & Eisenberg, D. (2000). Alternative therapies used by women with breast cancer in four ethnic populations. *Journal of the National Cancer Institute, 92*(1), 42–47.

Li, C. I., Malone, K. E., & Daling, J. R. (2003). Differences in breast cancer stage, treatment, and survival by race and ethnicity. *Archives of Internal Medicine, 163,* 49–56.

Martsolf, D. S. (1997). Cultural aspects of spirituality in cancer care. *Seminars in Oncology Nursing, 13*(4), 231–236.

Meyer, T. J., & Mark, M. M. (1995). Effects of psychosocial interventions with adult cancer patients: A meta-analysis of randomized experiments. *Health Psychology, 14*(2), 101–108.

Meyerowitz, B. E., Formenti, S. C., Ell, K. O., & Leedham, B. (2000). Depression among Latina cervical cancer patients. *Journal of Social and Clinical Psychology, 19*(3), 352–371.

Meyerowitz, B. E., Richardson, J., Hudson, S., & Leedham, B. (1998). Ethnicity and cancer outcomes: Behavioral and psychosocial considerations. *Psychological Bulletin, 123*(1), 47–70.

Michael, Y. L., Berkman, L. F., Colditz, G. A., Holmes, M. D., & Kawachi, I. (2002). Social networks and health-related quality of life in breast cancer survivors. A prospective study. *Journal of Psychosomatic Research, 52,* 285–293.

Mickley, J., & Soeken, K. (1993). Religiousness and hope in Hispanic- and Anglo-American women with breast cancer. *Oncology Nursing Forum, 20*(8), 1171–1177.

Moadel, A., Morgan, C., Fatone, A., Grennan, J., Carter, J., Laruffa, G., . . . Dutcher, J. (1999). Seeking meaning and hope: Self-reported spiritual and existential needs among and ethnically-diverse cancer patient population. *Psycho-Oncology, 8,* 378–385.

Moadel, A., Perez, A., Gharraee, Z., Jones, C., & Sparano, J. (2002). Examining quality of life after breast cancer: Cultural, treatment, and menstrual factors. *Psychosomatic Medicine, 64*(1), 106.

Moadel, A. B., Morgan, C., & Dutcher, J. (2007). Psychosocial needs assessment among an underserved, ethnically diverse cancer patient population. *Cancer, 109*(S2), 446–454.

Musick, M., Koenig, H. G., Larson, D., & Matthews, D. (1998). Religion and spiritual beliefs. In J. Holland (Ed.), *Psycho-oncology* (pp. 780–789). New York, NY: Oxford University Press.

NCCAM. (2002). *What is Complementary and Alternative Medicine (CAM)?* Retrieved October 16, 2010, from http://nccam.nih.gov/health/whatiscam/

New York Department of Health. (2006, April 2006). *Cancer incidence and mortality by region, 1999–2003, New York State, County Bronx.* Retrieved January 29, 2007, from http://www.health.state.ny.us/nysdoh/cancer/nyscr/vol1/v1rnyc.htm

Northouse, L. L., Caffey, M., Deichelbohrer, L., Schmidt, L., Guziatek-Trojniak, L., West, S., . . . Mood, D. (1999). The quality of life of African American women with breast cancer. *Research in Nursing & Health, 22,* 449–460.

Potts, R. G. (1996). Spirituality and the experience of cancer in an African-American community: Implications for psychosocial oncology. *Journal of Psychosocial Oncology, 14*(1), 1–19.

Powell, L. H., Shahabi, L., & Thoresen, C. E. (2003). Religion and spirituality: Linkages to physical health. *American Psychologist, 58*(1), 36–52.

Rapkin, B. D., & Trickett, E. J. (2005). Comprehensive dynamic trial designs for behavioral prevention research with communities: Overcoming inadequacies of the randomized controlled trial paradigm. In E. J. Trickett & W. Pequegnat (Eds.), *Community Interventions and AIDS* (1st ed., p. 352). New York, NY: Oxford University Press.

Rehse, B., & Pukrop, R. (2003). Effects of psychosocial interventions on quality of life in adult cancer patients: Meta analysis of 37 published controlled outcome studies. *Patient Education & Counseling, 50*(2), 179–186.

Richardson, M. A., Post-White, J., Singletary, S. E., & Justice, B. (1998). Recruitment for complementary/alternative medicine trials: Who participates after breast cancer. *Annals of Behavioral Medicine, 20*(3), 190–198.

Rodrigue, J. R. (1997). An examination of race differences in patients' psychological adjustment to cancer. *Journal of Clinical Psychology in Medical Settings, 4*(3), 271–280.

Ross, L., Boesen, E. H., Dalton, S. O., & Johansen, C. (2002). Mind and cancer: Does psychosocial intervention improve survival and psychological well-being? *European Journal of Cancer, 38*(11), 1447–1457.

Sanson-Fisher, R., Girgis, A., Boyes, A., Bonevski, B., Burton, L., & Cook, P. (2000). The unmet supportive care needs of patients with cancer. *Cancer, 88*(1), 226–237.

Spencer, S. M., Lehman, J. M., Wynings, C., Arena, P., Carver, C. S., Antoni, M. H., . . . Love, N. (1999). Concerns about breast cancer and relations to psychosocial well-being in a multiethnic sample of early-stage patients. *Health Psychology, 18*(2), 159–168.

Spiegel, D., & Diamond, S. (1998). *Psychosocial interventions.* Paper presented at the Thirty-Fourth Annual Meeting of the American Society of Clinical Oncology, Atlanta, GA.

Steele, R., & Fitch, M. I. (2008). Supportive care needs of women with gynecologic cancer. *Cancer Nursing, 31*(4), 284–291.

Stolley, J. M., & Koenig, H. (1997). Religion/spirituality and health among elderly African Americans and Hispanics. *Journal of Psychosocial Nursing, 35*(11), 32–38.

Taylor, E. J. (1997). The story behind the story: The use of storytelling in spiritual caregiving. *Seminars in Oncology Nursing, 13*(4), 252–254.

Taylor, K. L., Lamdan, R. M., Siegel, J. E., Shelby, R., Moran-Klimi, K., & Hrywna, M. (2003). Psychological adjustment among African American breast cancer patients: One year follow-up results of a randomized psychoeducational group intervention. *Health Psychology, 22*(3), 316–323.

U.S. Census Bureau. (2000). State and County QuickFacts. Retrieved October 16, 2010, from http://quickfacts.census.gov/qfd/

Volkers, N. (1999). In coping with cancer, gender matters. *Journal of the National Cancer Institute, 91*(20), 1712–1714.

Walsh, D., Donnelly, S., & Rybicki, L. (2000). The symptoms of advanced cancer: Relationship to age, gender, and performance status in 1,000 patients. *Support Care Cancer, 8*, 175–179.

Wan, G. J., Counte, M. A., Cella, D. F., Hernandez, L., McGuire, D. B., Deasay, S., . . . Hahn, E. A. (1999). The impact of socio-cultural and clinical factors on health-related quality of life reports among Hispanic and African-American cancer patients. *Journal of Outcome Measurement, 3*(3), 200–215.

Yalom, I. D. (1980). *Existential psychotherapy*. New York, NY: Basic Books.

20

Psycho-Educational Intervention Among Underserved Cervical Cancer Survivors

*Kimlin T. Ashing-Giwa, Jung-won Lim,
and Mayra Serrano*

BACKGROUND AND SIGNIFICANCE

Cervical cancer remains a national and global health challenge. Cervical cancer is primarily caused by cellular changes due to the human papillomavirus (HPV) infection. The behavioral risk factors for cervical cancer include early sexual initiation, multiple sex partners, and smoking. However, the major risk factor of cervical cancer is limited access and utilization of the Pap test. The Pap test can detect abnormal cellular changes and precancerous legions in the cervix, and it is therefore a reliable and cost-effective diagnostic test that can prevent cervical cancer.

The incidence rates among African, Asian, and Latina American women are 11.4, 8.0, and 13.8, respectively, per 100,000, indicating that their incidence rate is significantly higher compared to European Americans (8.5 per 100,000) (SEER, 2004). Moreover, the mortality rate for all ethnic groups is 2.5 per 100,000 women per year, whereas those for African, Asian, and Latina American women are 4.9, 2.4, and 3.4, respectively. Additionally, the 5-year survival rate among African American (AA) women (61.4%) is lower than that of their European American counterpart (72%) (American Cancer Society, 2009a). In 2010, it was estimated that 12,200 women will be diagnosed with and 4,210 women will die of cancer of the cervix uteri (American Cancer Society, 2009b). Even though incidence and mortality rates have decreased over most of the past several decades, in 2010 there was a significant increase in the incidence and mortality figures, particularly among Latina Americans. Ethnic disparities in most illnesses and cancers exist, and disparities in cervical cancer persist despite this cancer being preventable. Given that ethnic-minority groups are the fastest-growing populations in the United States, and experience greater incidence, greater morbidity, and a lower survival rate, extra attention should be paid to cancer survivorship outcomes with ethnic-minority and underserved populations.

Cervical cancer is known to be most prevalent among the socio-economically disadvantaged and medically underserved who have limited access to health care, including the regular Pap test (Ashing-Giwa, 2008; Krieger et al., 1999). National data suggest a significant increase in the numbers of Americans who are underinsured, uninsured, and medically underserved; 20% of African Americans and 34% of Latina Americans in the United States are uninsured (State Health Access Data Assistance Center, 2009). A significant number of African Americans (25%) and Latinos (22%) live at or near the poverty level (U.S. Census Bureau, 2009). Thus, cervical cancer incidence and mortality rates seem to be a function of socioeconomic status, health insurance status, access to health care factors, as well as ethnic and cultural dimensions. Recent studies report that ethnic-minority and underserved populations suffer an increased cancer burden (Ashing-Giwa, 2000; Ashing-Giwa et al., 2010; Ashing-Giwa et al., 2004, 2009; Institute of Medicine, 1999). Many women may fall through the care net because we have not addressed the risk factors for poor utilization of care as well as health-related quality of life (HRQOL) among ethnic-minority and underserved women (Ashing-Giwa, 1999; Ashing-Giwa & Ganz, 1997). A recent study documented that African and Latina Americans reported greater diagnostic and therapeutic delay for breast and cervical cancer detection and treatment (Ashing-Giwa et al., 2010).

Several studies with multiethnic population of cervical cancer survivors note a negative impact of the illness on HRQOL (Ashing-Giwa et al., 2004; Ashing-Giwa, Kim, & Tejero, 2008; Ashing-Giwa et al., 2006; Basen-Engquist et al., 2003). Moreover, these medical, physical, psychological, social, functional, and sexual sequelae persist into long-term survivorship, and the burden is greatest among ethnic-minority and lower-income women (Ashing-Giwa et al., 2004; Ashing-Giwa et al., 2006, 2008; Basen-Engquist et al., 2003). The physical effects of the disease and its treatment can include fatigue, pain, bladder dysfunction, vaginal and bowel problems, and menopausal symptoms (Angen, MacRae, Simpson, & Hundleby, 2002; Lutgendorf et al., 2000; Steginga & Dunn, 1997; Whelan et al., 1997). In addition to the physical sequelae, psychological challenges can include depression, sleeping difficulties, difficulty concentrating, and anxiety (Anderson, Anderson, & deProsse, 1989; Auchincloss, 1995; Basen-Engquist et al., 2003; Corney, Everett, Howells, & Crowther, 1992; Eisemann & Lalos, 1999; Greimel, Thiel, Peintinger, Cegnar, & Pongratz, 2002; Lutgendorf et al., 2000; Whelan et al., 1997). Several risk factors for psychological problems among cervical cancer survivors have been identified, including a lack of social support, younger age, limited socioeconomic and comprehensive health care resources, and Latina ethnicity. In addition, changes in self-perception related to lost fertility, menopause and sexual function, and changes in the marital relationship are noted challenges experienced by cervical cancer survivors (Andersen, Woods, & Copeland, 1997; Andersen & van Der Does, 1994; Anderson, 1985, 1993, 1994; Cull et al., 1993; Greimel et al., 2002; Klee, Thranov, & Machin, 2000; Krumm & Lamberti, 1993; Lamb, 1995; Paavonen, 1999; Schover, Fife, & Gershenson, 1989; Zacharias, Gilg, & Foxall, 1994). Further, many cervical cancer survivors lack adequate information about the overall HRQOL impact of the illness, as well as knowledge of resources and relational communication strategies to help sustain their well-being after cancer diagnosis. As a result, a substantial number of cervical cancer patients may experience significant physical, psychological, and sexual dysfunction and overall HRQOL concerns, particularly those who are among the underserved and ethnic minorities (Ashing-Giwa et al., 2004, 2006; Aziz & Rowland, 2002; Meyerowitz, Formenti, Ell, & Leedham, 2000).

There is growing evidence that psychosocial intervention improves HRQOL of cancer patients (Allison et al., 2004; Heiney et al., 2003; Nelson et al., 2008; Rehse & Pukrop, 2003). Nevertheless, the effectiveness of psychosocial intervention on HRQOL and survival for cancer survivors still remains controversial (Falagas et al., 2007; Ross, Boesen, Dalton, & Johansen, 2002; Smedslund & Ringdal, 2004). For example, two meta-analyses confirmed a significant, small-to-moderate effect on HRQOL (Meyer & Mark, 1995; Sheard & Maguire, 1999), whereas several studies did not find differences in survival and well-being between before and after psychosocial intervention (Chow, Taso, & Harth, 2004; Goodwin, Leszcz, & Ennis, 2001; Spiegel, 2001). Unfortunately, such intervention studies mostly focused on breast cancer patients/survivors and did not include ethnic-minority and underserved populations. As a result, there is a challenge in applying the study results in a meaningful and relevant way to cervical cancer survivors, particularly ethnic-minority and underserved women.

Several studies found that cervical cancer survivors show significant HRQOL disruption compared to other cancer populations (Frumovitz et al., 2005; Wenzel, DeAlba, et al., 2005; Wenzel, Dogan-Ates, Habbal, et al., 2005), such that cervical cancer survivors may have more opportunities for significant improvement in HRQOL. A recent study demonstrated the efficacy of psychosocial telephone counseling on HRQOL for cervical cancer survivors (Nelson et al., 2008). Even though ethnic-minority and underserved women with cervical cancer were underrepresented in the intervention study due to socioeconomic barriers, resistance to psychosocial interventions, and prominent sexual and functional concerns (Frumovitz et al., 2005; Nelson et al., 2008; Wenzel, DeAlba, et al., 2005), an ethnically, and culturally tailored, telephonic psychosocial intervention may be beneficial in improving their psychological and social functioning.

This study is a behavioral trial that examines the utility of a culturally responsive telephone counseling intervention to improve psychosocial functioning and overall HRQOL. This study reports results from the preliminary findings of the intervention with a population-based sample of European and Latina American cervical cancer survivors. In this chapter, we describe (1) the methods and intervention protocol, (2) the demographic and medical characteristics of the sample, and (3) changes in HRQOL outcomes for intervention and control groups.

METHODOLOGY

Research Design

This study implemented a population-based, randomized controlled, culturally responsive telephone counseling intervention designed for cervical cancer survivors. The clinical research assistants (CRAs) were linguistically matched and received an intensive 1-week training program on cultural competence, health disparities, and the impact of cervical cancer. They received ongoing training and supervision during our biweekly staff meetings. The intervention condition received six individual psycho-educational telephone counseling sessions. All women in the intervention and control conditions were provided with the same "Survivorship Booklet" that contained written information on all the domains addressed in the telephone session (see Table 20.1), including cervical cancer treatment, emotional well-being, sexuality, stress management, communication with doctors, family communication, nutrition, and finances, as well as available psychological and medical resources.

Overall, this study is based on a behavioral change intervention model that integrates a problem solving-solution focused model with a *Contextual Model of HRQOL* to reduce the psychosocial burden of cervical cancer (Ashing-Giwa, 2005b) (Figure 20.1). The study utilizes the *Contextual Model of HRQOL* as a framework for integrating cultural and socio-ecological dimensions into the theoretical foundations of this intervention study. Therefore, the *Contextual Model* expands the traditional HRQOL and behavior change models by enhancing these frameworks' cultural and socio-ecological relevance. Cultural and socio-ecological relevance takes into consideration that contextual dimensions including cultural, ethnic, economic, political, social, neighborhood, and demographic factors influence HRQOL, including medical outcomes (Ashing-Giwa, 2005b). The *Model* presents constructs that can vary between and within ethnic groups; nonetheless, the domains presented below contain some generalizations about group membership. However, great caution must be taken to avoid stereotyping. The expansion of the traditional HRQOL framework to include these contextual domains may increase the validity and utility of the HRQOL framework to assess overall

TABLE 20.1   Domains for the Psycho-Educational Intervention

Session	Domain	Content
1	Managing Medical Issues, Health Education, and Cancer Resources	• Treatment side effects: Incontinence, bowel problems, lymphedema, sexual dysfunction, etc. • Relationship with health care professionals: Communication and trust
2	Coping Skills and Problem Solving Training	• Coping style • Self-care • Communication with loved ones
3	Balancing Emotions and Managing Stress	• Identify and validate emotions • Reactions to stress • Stress management techniques • Social support networks
4	Addressing Family and Social Concerns	• Family issues: Family confidant/advocate • Social issues: Social network • Communication
5	Addressing Relational and Sexual Concerns	• Relationship with partner/spouse: Communication and support • Sexual dysfunction: Loss of sexual desire/drive, vaginal dryness, narrowing/shortening of vagina, body image issues due to scarring
6	Finances and Employment	• Health insurance • Medical debt • Social services • Resources • Employment concerns: Disability and supplemental security income

functioning among ethnically and socioeconomically diverse populations of survivors (Ashing-Giwa, 2005b).

In this intervention program, targeted areas of concern are identified from the literature and the investigators' previous work. Additionally, survivors are asked to rank the order of distress for each areas of concern presented. Therefore, the intervention addresses concerns identified by the investigatory team and the literature, with a particular focus on the issues of greatest concern for each survivor. The six intervention domains are: (1) managing medical issues, health education, and cancer resources; (2) coping skills and problem solving training; (3) balancing emotions and managing stress; (4) addressing family and social concerns; (5) addressing relational and sexual concerns; and (6) finances and employment. For each domain, the goal, behavioral, and self-help strategies are discussed. The counselors guide each survivor in choosing realistic strategies and they rehearse the new skills or behaviors. In addition, problem-focused strategies, including effective communication and visualizations, are taught and practiced during the sessions. When the

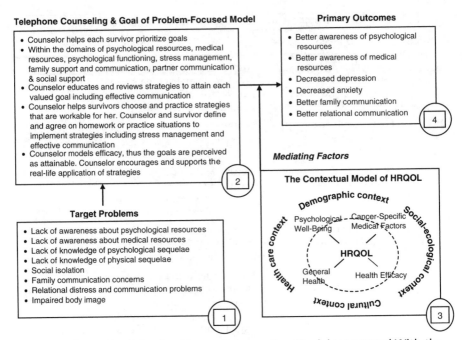

FIGURE 20.1 The Behavior Change Intervention Model Integrated With the Contextual Model of HRQOL

strategies are successfully taught, the amount of distress associated with each concern is reduced. During the counseling, psychological and physical experiences common to cervical cancer survivors are validated and normalized. The counseling incorporates active listening, active support, and active verbal reinforcement for adaptive coping practices. Further, the counseling is tailored to each woman and incorporates culturally sensitive practices. For example, when working with a Latina American survivor, the counselor will practice apt, respectful salutations because among most Latinos, appropriate salutations at the beginning and end of social interactions are critical to relationship building. Additionally, having a counselor who is ethnically matched can provide an empowering role model for effective communication and self-efficacy, as well as a source of support.

Participants and Sampling

The participants in this preliminary study were self-identified as European or Latina Americans. Eligible participants: (1) were within 6 months to 3 years of a cervical cancer diagnosis; (2) were diagnosed with stages I–III invasive cervical cancer; (3) had not been diagnosed with another type of cancer; (4) were between the ages of 18 and 65; and (5) did not have any other major disabling medical or psychiatric condition. Survivors within 6 months to 3 years post diagnosis were included because years since diagnosis did not influence overall HRQOL, psychological, or medical functioning in our previous study (Ashing-Giwa et al., 2009). Specifically, this preliminary study includes women who reported moderate to high burden (a baseline Functional Assessment of Cancer Therapy— General [FACT-G] score < 60) and below-median household income (< $60,000 per year). Women with metastatic disease were excluded because the medical characteristics are significantly different for these women. Women with a moderate-to-severe depression and anxiety were also excluded; however, women with a history of diagnosis of mild depression or anxiety were not excluded. The level of symptomatology for depression and anxiety was assessed using a self-report tool during the screening. The CRAs asked if the women had received any psychiatric diagnosis such as depression and anxiety that has interfered with their day-to-day activities, and if yes, the extent to which such psychiatric diagnosis conditions interfered with their day-to-day activities (a 5-point Likert scale from 0 = not at all to 4 = very much). If they responded 2 = fair amount, 3 = much, or 4 = very much, they were excluded.

Participants in Southern California were recruited from the California Cancer Surveillance Program—Los Angeles and Desert Sierra Regions. After identifying potential participants: (1) We mailed the study invitation package for recruiting samples. This study invitation letter detailed the study procedures; for example, a description of the study that involved the completion of two survey questionnaires, possible selection into the telephone psycho-educational sessions, and the duration of participation. (2) A bilingual, female CRA contacted potential participants by telephone, 2 weeks after the mailing of the study invitation package. During this telephone conversation, participants were informed that they would be contacted after the completed questionnaire was received, and at that time they would be assigned to either (a) the 6-week psycho-educational telephone intervention condition, or (b) the control condition. (3) Subjects desiring to participate in the study were screened for eligibility: Eligible participants were then mailed a baseline self-report assessment packet (see "Measurements" below) with the consent form. (4) After a participant had completed the baseline assessment, he or she received a $20 gift certificate. All study protocols, including the telephone sessions, were conducted in either English or Spanish. All study documents were translated and back-translated, and then verified by a certified translations company. This study was approved by the City of Hope (COH) and California State Institutional Review Board (IRB), and all participants were fully informed and their consent obtained.

Trial Procedures

Assignment and Randomization

After the baseline assessments had been collected, the demographic (e.g., ethnicity, language, income) and medical characteristics (e.g., stage at diagnosis, treatment) were entered into our database, and further inclusion was based on participant responses to the baseline questionnaire. Thus, participants were included if they indicated a moderate to high burden or a poorer HRQOL (score < 60) on the FACT-G and reported an income below the state median of $60,000 per year.

Protocol for Comparison Group

The comparison group was mailed a packet that included information about their participation and the "Survivorship Booklet," which is available in English and Spanish. Participants were recontacted in approximately 5–6 months to complete the first follow-up, and contacted again at 12 months after the initial screening, to complete a final follow-up questionnaire. This preliminary study reports findings from the baseline and 6-month follow-up only. After all participants had completed the baseline, 6-month, and 12-month follow-up questionnaires, they received a $20, $25, and $40 gift certificate, respectively.

Protocol for Intervention Group

Telephone session participants were notified by mail as well as receiving a reminder telephone call regarding the time and telephone number where they could be reached for a telephone session. The intervention consisted of six weekly, 40-minute sessions. The sessions addressed: (1) managing medical issues, health education, and cancer resources; (2) balancing emotions and managing stress; (3) coping skills and problem solving; (4) family and social concerns; (5) relational, intimacy, and sexual concerns; and (6) financial and employment concerns (see Table 20.1). These session domains were informed by the principal authors' research with multiethnic samples and the literature. In addition to the topics mentioned above, participants received a booster and debriefing session about 1 month after the end of the telephone sessions. The key to the first session was to establish rapport and orient the survivor to the counseling sessions. Beyond the first session, each session began with an inquiry into the survivor's status, a follow-up of issues from the previous session, and an introduction to the existing session's content and themes. All telephone sessions were tailored to the specific ethnic group, based on a culturally and linguistically responsive approach. A culturally and linguistically responsive approach includes the following: (1) language competency, (2) cultural competency (knowledge and sensitivity for the cultural origins and context of the survivor), (3) ethnical conduct, (4) empathy, (5) credibility, (6) purpose, and (7) graciousness (Ashing-Giwa, 2005a). A telephone conversation with a linguistic and culturally competent CRA who practices the above 7 principles enhances the likelihood that participants will develop an appropriate trust level and will be interested in sharing their experiences about cervical cancer and participating in the research study. Thus, well-trained CRAs who have at least 2 years of behavioral cancer research experience conducted the telephone sessions, and each participant was assigned a linguistically matched CRA. Approximately 5–6 months (after intervention) and 12 months after enrollment into the study, participants were mailed a packet containing the follow-up, posttest survey questionnaires. The detailed structure of the psycho-educational telephone intervention is shown in Figure 20.2.

Measurements

HRQOL was measured using the Functional Assessment of Cancer Therapy—Cervix (FACT-CX) to investigate the baseline and follow-up outcome differences after psycho-educational intervention. The FACT-CX is known to be an internally consistent and reliable self-report tool (Cella et al., 1993). The FACT-CX is comprised of the 27-item general cancer concerns (FACT-G), and an additional 10-item cervical cancer specific scale. The FACT-G generates

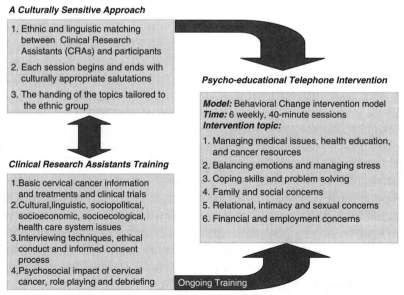

A Culturally Sensitive Approach

1. Ethnic and linguistic matching between Clinical Research Assistants (CRAs) and participants
2. Each session begins and ends with culturally appropriate salutations
3. The handing of the topics tailored to the ethnic group

Clinical Research Assistants Training

1. Basic cervical cancer information and treatments and clinical trials
2. Cultural, linguistic, sociopolitical, socioeconomic, socioecological, health care system issues
3. Interviewing techniques, ethical conduct and informed consent process
4. Psychosocial impact of cervical cancer, role playing and debriefing

Ongoing Training

Psycho-educational Telephone Intervention

Model: Behavioral Change intervention model
Time: 6 weekly, 40-minute sessions
Intervention topic:

1. Managing medical issues, health education, and cancer resources
2. Balancing emotions and managing stress
3. Coping skills and problem solving
4. Family and social concerns
5. Relational, intimacy and sexual concerns
6. Financial and employment concerns

FIGURE 20.2   The Structure of the Psycho-Educational Telephone Intervention

subscales on four domains, including physical, social/familial, emotional, and functional well-being. Items are rated from 0 (not at all) to 4 (very much), with a higher score indicating better HRQOL. Scale scores are computed by summing across items in the same scale and then transforming raw scale scores to range from 0 (worst outcome) to 100 (best outcome). Individual subscale scores are then summed and standardized to form a total FACT-G score. The total FACT-CX score is obtained by adding the FACT-CX additional items score to the FACT-G score. High reliability and good validity were reported in this study (Cronbach's coefficient $\alpha = .78-.91$).

Demographic (age, ethnicity, marital relationship, education, and income) and medical information (age at diagnosis, years since diagnosis, cancer stage, treatment type, and the number of comorbidities) were also obtained from the self-report and the cancer registries. The number of comorbidities was included by counting self-reported medical (i.e., asthma, diabetes, heart disease) and mental health (i.e., anxiety, depression) conditions from a list of 31 nonmajor disabling health conditions. These variables were collected at the baseline assessment.

Data Management and Analyses

The data for this preliminary analysis include the baseline and follow-up scores on the FACT measure. This study was analyzed by an intent-to-treat statistical methodological approach. An intent-to-treat analysis is an analysis based on the initial treatment intent, not on the treatment eventually administered, with the purpose of avoiding various misleading artifacts that can arise in intervention research, such as dropout (Hollis, 1999; Lachin, 2000). Because our preliminary study uses the pretest/posttest form and is in the ongoing recruitment stage, the sole requirement for evaluability was based on availability of baseline data on HRQOL. Thus, any evaluable subjects who were unavailable for the follow-up assessment were included in the analysis. In our preliminary study, 53.4% of the eligible sample was retained at follow-up assessment, indicating that there were 23 dropouts and all of them were assigned to the control group. To determine the imputation methods that fill data in missing values at 6-month follow-up, whether dropout at the follow-up was related to demographic and medical information and HRQOL outcomes was then examined, using t-test and chi-square statistics. Preliminary analyses found there were no significant differences in demographic and medical information between study completers at the follow-up and study dropouts at a $p < .05$ level. Additionally, no significant differences were found in the baseline HRQOL outcomes between study completers and dropouts. Therefore, data missing at the follow-up was replaced with the mean change of participants who completed the follow-up assessment considering the treatment condition (Chakraborty & Gu, 2009; Fisher & Dixon, 1990).

To examine the effectiveness of the intervention, first, *t*-test and chi-square statistics were used to investigate the differences in demographic and medical information between the intervention and control groups. Next, we employed matched-pair *t*-test and repeated measures analysis of variance (ANOVA) methods to examine differences between the intervention and control groups at two timepoints. To adjust for the possibility that an improvement in HRQOL might be related to HRQOL at baseline, we also investigated change over time in HRQOL outcomes, after controlling for the covariable HRQOL at the baseline and other covariates, using the repeated measure analysis of covariance (ANCOVA). Covariates were based on the significant differences by demographic and medical information between the intervention and control groups. The analyses were conducted using Statistical Package for the Social Sciences (SPSS) 18.0. All hypotheses were tested with a $p < .05$ criterion of significance for a two-sided test.

RESULTS

Recruitment

The recruitment results are described in Figure 20.3. As of December, 2009, 367 cervical cancer survivors were accessible and screened. Of these, 54 (14.7%) were ineligible, 74 (20.2%) refused, and 239 (65.1%) agreed to participate in this study. Of the women who agreed to participate, 125 cervical cancer survivors (52.3%) completed the baseline at the time of this preliminary study. In this analysis, no significant difference in demographic and medical information (ethnicity, age, cancer stage, chemotherapy, radiation therapy, surgery, and age at diagnosis) was found according to the study participation status (refusal vs. participation; intervention vs. control).

Considering the purpose of this study, first, ethnic groups other than European and Latina Americans ($n = 19$) were excluded for this preliminary analysis, since no African American survivor completed the follow-up measure at the time of this analysis. Survivors who reported a good HRQOL or a higher FACT-G score (≥ 60), or a high income level ($\leq \$60,000$ per year) at baseline ($n = 63$) were excluded. As a result, this preliminary study included a total of 43 cervical cancer survivors: 10 in the intervention condition and 33 in the control condition (Figure 20.4). The mean time between the baseline and follow-up assessments for the intervention group was 4.7 months (range 1–7 months). The mean follow-up time for the control group was 5.8 months

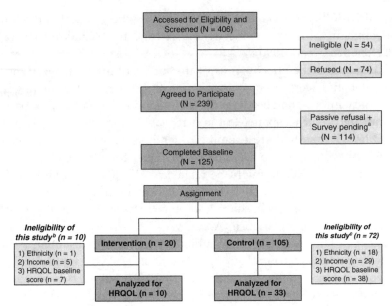

FIGURE 20.3   The Recruitment Diagram

[a]This study is based on the preliminary analysis for participants who completed the baseline as of December 2009; thus, "Survey pending" is considered as a passive refusal (no direct written or verbal refusal).

[b]This study focuses on the ethnic-minority and underserved population, considering ethnicity, income (< $60,000 per year), and HRQOL baseline scores < 60. In the intervention group, two survivors endorsed in both income and HRQOL baseline score eligibility.

[c]In the control group, 13 women endorsed in both income and HRQOL baseline score eligibility.

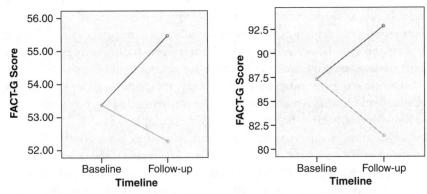

FIGURE 20.4   FACT-G and FACT-CX Scores for the Intervention and Control Groups

Note: The upward line refers to the intervention group and the downward line refers to the control group. FACT-G, $F = 4.256$, $p < .05$; FACT-CX, $F = 4.807$, $p < .05$. Analyses were controlled for comorbidities and each corresponding HRQOL baseline score.

(range 3–7 months). There was no significant difference in the follow-up time between the intervention and control groups at a $p < .05$ level.

Sample Characteristics

Table 20.2 indicates the study sample characteristics. The mean age of the participants was 47 years ($SD = 10.6$). About 86% of the participants were Latina Americans and 14% were European Americans. The majority of respondents endorsed having less than a high school degree (67%), earning less than $25,000 per year (60%), not working outside the home (62%), and holding public insurance coverage (72%). The mean time since cancer diagnosis was 2.8 years ($SD = 1.0$). About half of the participants were diagnosed with cervical cancer at stage I (56%), and received chemotherapy (44%) and radiation therapy (56%). Overall, a significant difference in the demographic and medical information between the intervention and control groups was not found. However, there was a significant difference in the number of comorbidities between the intervention and control groups, indicating that survivors in the intervention group were more likely to report medical and mental health conditions. Thus, the number of comorbidities was controlled for the main analyses.

Changes in HRQOL Outcomes

For these cervical cancer survivors, the overall HRQOL outcomes represent low-to-moderate mean scores, ranging from 52.6 to 64.0 at baseline. The physical well-being score was the highest in both the intervention and the control groups, while the social well-being score was the lowest.

Overall, we found a significant intervention benefit, from baseline to follow-up, for the intervention group on HRQOL outcomes. The intervention group showed a 2.1-point improvement in the FACT-G score, whereas the score of control group was decreased by 5.9 points ($F = 8.24$, $p < .01$). In the FACT-CX, a 5.1-point improvement in the intervention group was observed, whereas a 1.1-point decrease in the control group was observed ($F = 6.49$, $p < .05$). Then, we controlled for factors that may influence improvement in HRQOL outcomes; thus, we adjusted for the corresponding HRQOL outcome scores at baseline, as well as the number of comorbidities. Differences between the intervention and control groups persisted after adjusting for covariates (improvement in the FACT-G for intervention group = 2.1 vs. control group = −1.1; improvement in the FACT-CX for intervention group = 5.06 vs. control group = −5.76). Figure 20.4 illustrates the differences

TABLE 20.2 Demographic and Medical Information on the Participants

		Sample (%)			
		Total (N = 43)	Group		
			Intervention (n = 10)	Control (n = 33)	t or x^2
Demographic information					
Mean age (years)		47.1 (10.6)	47.9 (10.2)	46.9 (10.9)	0.26
Ethnicity	European American	6 (14)	3 (30)	3 (9)	2.79
	Latina American	37 (86)	7 (70)	30 (91)	
Relationship	Partnered	31 (72)	8 (80)	23 (70)	0.41
	Unpartnered	12 (28)	2 (20)	10 (30)	
Education	< High school	29 (67)	6 (60)	23 (70)	0.65
	High school	5 (12)	1 (10)	4 (12)	
	> High school	9 (21)	3 (30)	6 (18)	
Yearly household income	< $25,000	26 (60)	4 (40)	22 (67)	4.29
	$25,000–$45,000	14 (33)	4 (40)	10 (30)	
	> $45,000–$60,000	3 (7)	2 (20)	1 (3)	
Occupation	Homemaker	26 (62)	7 (70)	19 (59)	3.24
	Managerial/ professional	4 (10)	0	4 (13)	
	Technical	2 (5)	1 (10)	1 (3)	
	Service	4 (10)	1 (10)	3 (9)	
	Operator	3 (7)	1 (10)	2 (6)	
	Other	3 (7)	0	3 (9)	
Health Insurance	No insurance	4 (9)	1 (10)	3 (10)	3.43
	Public only	31 (72)	5 (50)	23 (82)	
	Private	8 (19)	4 (40)	4 (13)	
Medical information					
Mean age at diagnosis (years)		44 (11.0)	45 (10.1)	44 (11.4)	0.34
Years since diagnosis (years)		2.8 (1.0)	2.6 (1.0)	2.8 (1.0)	−0.54
Cancer stage	I	20 (56)	5 (50)	15 (58)	2.62
	II	12 (33)	3 (30)	9 (35)	
	II	4 (11)	2 (20)	2 (8)	
Surgery	Minor	10 (25)	2 (29)	6 (23)	2.25
	Simple hysterectomy	5 (13)	1 (14)	3 (12)	
	Total hysterectomy	8 (20)	2 (29)	4 (15)	
	Radical hysterectomy	8 (20)	0	6 (23)	
	No surgery	9 (23)	2 (29)	7 (27)	
Chemotherapy (yes)		19 (44)	5 (50)	14 (42)	0.18
Radiation (yes)		24 (56)	6 (60)	18 (55)	0.09
Number of comorbidities (before cancer) (M, SD)		3.0 (2.8)	4.3 (3.9)	2.7 (2.4)	1.64
Numberof comorbidities (now) (M, SD)		6.0 (4.9)	8.9 (4.3)	5.1 (4.8)	2.23*

*$p < 0.05$.

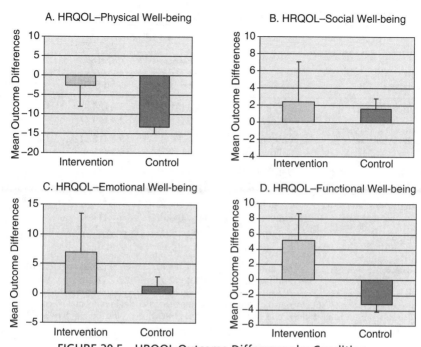

FIGURE 20.5   HRQOL Outcome Differences by Condition

Note: Each figure shows mean differences in each HRQOL sub-domain score between baseline and follow-up assessments by condition. Error bars represent standard errors. A. Physical well-being: $F = 10.14$, $p < .01$; B. Social well-being: $F = 2.90$, $p > .05$; C. Emotional well-being: $F = 1.70$, $p > .05$; D. Functional well-being: $F = 7.75$, $p < .01$.

in the baseline and follow-up mean scores by treatment condition, after controlling for covariates.

Table 20.3 and Figure 20.5 show the differences in the baseline and follow-up mean scores as measured by FACT-G sub-domain. The results indicate significant differences in physical ($F = 6.37$, $p < .05$) and functional ($F = 10.02$, $p < .01$) well-being by condition. After controlling for each corresponding FACT-G sub-domain score at baseline and for the number of comorbidities, the differences between the physical ($F = 10.14$, $p < .01$) and functional ($F = 7.75$, $p < .01$) well-being scores by condition were still significant. More specifically, unlike the expectations, physical well-being in both groups decreased after the 6-month follow-up; however, the decrease in the intervention group was much smaller than that in the control group ($F = 10.14$, $p < .01$). With regard to functional well-being, the score of the intervention group improved by 5.2 points, whereas that of the control group decreased by 3.3 points ($F = 7.75$, $p < .01$). The social and emotional well-being scores were somewhat—but not significantly—improved for the intervention group.

TABLE 20.3   Means and Standard Deviation of HRQOL Outcomes

Variables	Period	Intervention Mean (SD)	Control Mean (SD)	F^a
Physical well-being	Baseline	64.0 (21.0)	65.8 (24.3)	10.14**
	Follow-up	61.5 (11.5)	52.4 (19.4)	
Social well-being	Baseline	52.6 (7.4)	53.7 (16.0)	2.90
	Follow-up	55.0 (11.7)	55.3 (16.3)	
Emotional well-being	Baseline	57.6 (13.3)	58.1 (13.7)	1.70
	Follow-up	64.5 (11.3)	59.3 (12.8)	
Functional well-being	Baseline	51.6 (11.5)	55.6 (11.1)	7.75**
	Follow-up	56.8 (14.0)	52.3 (11.2)	
FACT-G	Baseline	52.7 (3.6)	53.6 (5.8)	4.26*
	Follow-up	54.8 (5.1)	52.5 (5.4)	
FACT-CX	Baseline	85.3 (13.8)	87.9 (22.2)	4.81*
	Follow-up	90.4 (17.7)	82.2 (20.4)	

[a]Repeated measure of ANCOVA were conducted to examine the changes in outcomes by condition, after controlling for comorbidities and each corresponding HRQOL outcome score at baseline.
*$p < .05$; **$p < .01$.

DISCUSSION

The medical community is charged with psychosocial care for the whole person according to the IOM report (Institute of Medicine, 2008). However, research and practice that addresses the psychosocial needs of ethnic and linguistic minorities, and of lower-income survivors, lags far behind. Indeed, cervical cancer survivors are probably among our most economically and psychologically vulnerable cancer survivors. However, few studies investigate strategies to improve survivorship outcomes.

Disparities in cancer outcomes exist for ethnic-minority survivors; in particular, women diagnosed with cervical cancer experience greater physical and psychosocial challenges and are often isolated (Ashing-Giwa et al., 2004, 2006). The need for increased intervention studies with cervical cancer survivors is compelling. This study assessed the effectiveness of a problem-solution focused, culturally and clinically responsive behavioral intervention with low-income cervical cancer survivors. Our findings suggest that the intervention is feasible, and associated with a change in the physical and functional well-being and overall HRQOL in moderate to highly distressed cervical cancer survivors. The culturally responsive approach necessitates that the CRAs are linguistically matched; and that they receive adequate training on the cultural (e.g., spirituality, beliefs, and practices relevant to illness and family contexts), socio-ecological (e.g., neighborhood resources), sociopolitical (e.g., immigration, social status), psychosocial (e.g., life burden, support), and health care system (e.g., access and utilization) aspects of our study population. In addition, the clinically or survivor-centered approach dictated that we should tailor the order and tone of the telephone session to the needs of each survivor. For example, if the survivor expresses a lot of sadness relating to an issue, the tone of the session—or the method for addressing that issue—will be more compassionate, while still implementing the psycho-educational or role-modeling content. Increasing the cultural and clinical responsiveness of the CRAs was the major focus of our biweekly staff supervision meetings. This clinically centered approach may have also contributed to the changes that were observed. The specific effects of such an approach on outcomes require further investigation; however, the present study did indicate that this type of intervention tailoring can be accomplished in a telephone-based intervention with cultural sensitivity.

Although culturally and socio-ecologically tailored interventions for this group of survivors have not been reported in the literature (Nelson et al., 2008), the present findings are consistent with other psychologically based interventions using these approaches to assist European American cancer survivors (Allison et al., 2004; Heiney et al., 2003; Meyerowitz, Richardson, Hudson, & Leedham, 1998; Rehse & Pukrop, 2003; Sheard & Maguire, 1999; Wenzel, Dogan-Ates, & Habbal, 2005; Wenzel, Robinson, & Blake, 1995). Recent research suggests that the concerns and challenges of nonminority survivors are also pertinent to ethnic-minority and underserved populations (American Cancer Society, 2007; Ashing-Giwa, 1999, 2005a; Meyerowitz et al., 2000; Office of Minority Health, 2001). The current study indicates that a psycho-educational intervention conducted over the telephone can improve physical and functional well-being and overall HRQOL. Additionally, trends were found, although not significant, for improvements in family/social and emotional measures in the intervention group. However, the emotional well-being scores were the most unfavorable HRQOL outcome at baseline, particularly among Latina Americans. This suggests that the level of burden in this domain may necessitate interventions to incorporate both professional and face-to-face components. Further, emotional aspects may not be readily responsive to the type of short-term intervention implemented in this study, because this dimension of HRQOL should be considered within the context of broader socio-ecological conditions (e.g., income, family stability, and distress) observed in subgroups of ethnic-minority cancer survivors and lower-income cancer survivors, in general. Therefore, more comprehensive (e.g., inclusion of family members) and longer-term interventions may be necessary to demonstrate improvements in emotional well-being among underserved cancer survivors. This requires further study.

Process Outcomes

We encountered many challenges in implementing this behavioral trial with underserved cancer survivors. The primary issue was their level of life burden. These survivors' lived experiences included high levels of financial, job, living situation, familial, and emotional distress. Many of these socio-ecological challenges are the realities of their premorbid contexts. These survivors are to be admired, as they are practicing adaptive coping and managing very difficult life circumstances. These competing life demands potentially influenced the study's enrollment, attrition, and adherence to protocol timeline.

From the principal investigator's perspective, psycho-educational interventions with underserved populations require clinical, cultural, and some protocol flexibility. The participants' level of life burden and competing life demands influenced the schedule, sequencing, and at times the content of the intervention sessions. Therefore in this intervention, we were responsive to the survivors' overall health status, life burdens, cultural practices, and linguistic capacities to improve the acceptability and the probable utility of the intervention. One specific example of how we implemented protocol flexibility was that we were willing to change the appointment times for the intervention sessions to accommodate survivors' schedules. Another example was that we allowed survivors to devote about half of one session to an urgent family, noncancer-related matter, and then provided them with appropriate referrals to better address this situation. Of course, this clinical and practical approach to behavioral–interventional trials needs further methodological and outcomes studies to establish scientifically acceptable guidelines.

Participants' Experiences

In addition, the qualitative process evaluation indicated that these survivors were very grateful for the intervention, and for the opportunity to discuss their disease-related and other life burdens with empathetic, culturally, and linguistically competent, and skilled, study staff. For example:

> **Emotional domain:** *"It was emotionally and intellectually stimulating, and surprised me by enriching my life . . . I feel lighter in spirit like I'm not dragging as many hang-ups around."* (European American)

> **Informational/medical issue domain:** *"I really appreciate the info provided with this study. It is so much more than anything my doctor or the research I have done has provided. Knowledge makes the stress of worry much less."* (Latina American)
>
> *"It helped me see/face how cancer was impacting my life. It also helped and encouraged me to make changes in the way I thought about my cancer."* (European American)

Cancer resources domain: *"The questions made me aware that there are resources I can utilize in the community for free. Thank you. I am feeling motivated to get well."* (European American)

Future Directions and Clinical Implications

Finally, given that Latina Americans are one of the fastest-growing populations in the United States and that they experience an increasing cancer burden, cancer research must include diverse Latino communities if we are to reduce the burden of cancer for all Americans. In addition, many cervical cancer survivors—in particular, Latina Americans who are monolingual Spanish speakers—lack adequate information about the overall HRQOL impact of the illness as well as knowledge of resources and relational communication strategies to help them improve their overall well-being after the cancer diagnosis and treatment. Many women may fall through the care net because we have not addressed the risk factors for poor HRQOL and inadequate psychological care among ethnic-minority and underserved cervical cancer survivors. The present study provides preliminary evidence that a culturally infused, problem-solving, solution-focused intervention, administered over the telephone in a culturally sensitive format, is successful in improving physical and functional well-being and overall HRQOL in low-income Latina and European American cervical cancer survivors. Future efforts are needed to test the effectiveness of translating this type of intervention into community-based practices. A community-based approach may be a cost-effective and efficacious strategy for addressing the burden of cancer among cultural and linguistic minority groups.

ACKNOWLEDGMENT

This research was supported by a grant (#RGST-06-136-01-CPPB) from the American Cancer Society.

REFERENCES

Allison, P. J., Edgar, L., Nicolau, B., Archer, J., Black, M., & Hier, M. (2004). Results of a feasibility study for a psycho-educational intervention in head and neck cancer. *Psychooncology, 13*, 482–485.

American Cancer Society. (2007). *Cancer facts and figures 2008*. Atlanta, GA: Author.

American Cancer Society. (2009a). *Cancer facts & figures for African Americans 2009–2010*. Atlanta, GA: Author.

American Cancer Society. (2009b). *Cancer facts and figures 2009*. Atlanta, GA: Author.

Andersen, B., Woods, X., & Copeland, L. (1997). Sexual self-schema and sexual morbidity among gynecologic cancer survivors. *Journal of Consulting & Clinical Psychology, 65*(2), 221–229.

Andersen, B. L., & van Der Does, J. (1994). Surviving gynecologic cancer and coping with sexual morbidity: An international problem. *International Journal of Gynecologic Cancer, 4*(4), 225–240.

Anderson, B. (1985). Sexual functioning morbidity among cancer survivors. Current status and future research directions. *Cancer, 55,* 1835–1842.

Anderson, B. (1993). Predicting sexual and psychologic morbidity and improving the quality of life for women with gynecologic cancer. *Cancer, 71,* 1678–1690.

Anderson, B. (1994). Surviving cancer. *Cancer, 74,* 1484–1495.

Anderson, B., Anderson, B., & deProsse, C. (1989). Controlled, prospective longitudinal study of women with cancer: Psychological outcomes. *Journal of Consulting & Clinical Psychology, 57,* 692–697.

Angen, M. J., MacRae, J. H., Simpson, J. S., & Hundleby, M. (2002). Tapestry: A retreat program of support for persons living with cancer. *Cancer Practice, 10*(6), 297–304.

Ashing-Giwa, K. (1999). The recruitment and retention of African American women into cancer control studies. *Journal of the National Medical Association, 91,* 255–260.

Ashing-Giwa, K. (2000). Quality of life and psychological outcomes in long-term breast cancer survivors: A study of African American women. *Psychosocial Oncology, 17*(3/4), 47–62.

Ashing-Giwa, K. (2005a). Can a culturally responsive model for research design bring us closer to addressing participation disparities? *Ethnicity & Disease, 15*(1), 130–137.

Ashing-Giwa, K. (2005b). The Contextual Model of HRQOL: A paradigm for expanding the HRQOL framework. *Quality of Life Research, 14*(2), 297–307.

Ashing-Giwa, K. (2008). Enhancing physical well-being and overall quality of life among underserved Latina-American cervical cancer survivors: Feasibility study. *Journal of Cancer Survivorship, 2*(3), 215–223.

Ashing-Giwa, K., & Ganz, P. A. (1997). Understanding the psychological and quality of life impacts of breast cancer in African-American survivors. *Psychosocial Oncology, 15,* 19–35.

Ashing-Giwa, K., Gonzalez, P., Lim, J. W., Chung, C., Paz, B., Somlo, G., & Wakabayashi, M. (2010). Diagnostic and therapeutic delays among multiethnic sample of breast and cervical cancer survivors. *Cancer, 116*(13), 3195–3204.

Ashing-Giwa, K., Kagawa-Singer, M., Padilla, G. V., Tejero, J. S., Hsiao, E., Chhabra, R., . . . Tucker, M. B. (2004). The impact of cervical cancer and dysplasia: A qualitative, multiethnic study. *Psychooncology, 13*(10), 675–753.

Ashing-Giwa, K., Kim, J., & Tejero, J. S. (2008). Measuring quality of life among cervical cancer survivors: Preliminary assessment of instrumentation validity in a cross-cultural study. *Quality of Life Research, 17,* 147–157.

Ashing-Giwa, K., Padilla, G., Bohorquez, D. E., Tejero, J. S., Garcia, M., & Meyers, E. A. (2006). Survivorship: A qualitative investigation of Latinas diagnosed with cervical cancer. *Journal of Psychosocial Oncology, 24*(4), 53–88.

Ashing-Giwa, K., Tejero, J. S., Kim, J., Padilla, G. V., Kagawa-Singer, M., Tucker, M. B., & Lim, J. W. (2009). Cervical cancer survivorship in a population based sample. *Gynecologic Oncology, 112,* 358–364.

Auchincloss, S. (1995). After treatment. Psychosocial issues in gynecologic cancer survivorship. *Cancer, 76,* 2117–2124.

Aziz, N., & Rowland, J. (2002). Cancer survivorship research among ethnic minority and medically underserved groups. *Oncology Nursing Forum, 29*(5), 789–801.

Basen-Engquist, K., Paskett, E. D., Buzaglo, J., Miller, S. M., Schover, L., Wenzel, L. B., & Bodurka, D. C. (2003). Cervical cancer: Behavioral factors related to screening, diagnosis, and survivors' quality of life. *Cancer, 98*(9 Suppl.), 2009–2014.

Cella, D., Tulsky, D., Gray, G., Sarafian, B., Linn, E., Bonomi, A., . . . Brannon, J. (1993). The Functional Assessment of Cancer Therapy scale: Development and validation of the general measure. *Journal of Clinical Oncology, 11*(3), 570–579.

Chakraborty, H., & Gu, H. (2009). *A mixed model approach for intent-to-treat analysis in longitudinal clinical trials with missing values.* Research Triangle Park, NC: RIT International.

Chow, E., Taso, M. N., & Harth, T. (2004). Does psychosocial intervention improve survival in cancer? A meta-analysis. *Palliative Medicine, 18*, 25–31.

Corney, R., Everett, H., Howells, A., & Crowther, M., E. (1992). Psychosocial adjustment following major gynecological surgery for carcinoma of the cervix and vulva. *Journal of Psychosomatic Research, 36*(6), 561–568.

Cull, A., Cowie, V.J., Farquharson, D. I., Livingstone, J. R., Smart, G. E., & Elton, R. A. (1993). Early stage cervical cancer: Psychosocial and sexual outcomes of treatment. *British Journal of Cancer, 68*(6), 1216–1220.

Eisemann, M., & Lalos, A. (1999). Psycholosocial determinants of well-being in gynecology cancer patients. *Cancer Nursing, 22*(4), 303–306.

Falagas, M. E., Zarkadoulia, E. A., Ioannidou, E. N., Peppas, G., Christodoulou, C., & Rafailidis, P. I. (2007). The effect of psychosocial factors on breast cancer outcome: A systematic review. *Breast Cancer Research, 9*(R44), 1–23.

Fisher, L. D., & Dixon, D. O. (1990). *Intention-to-treat in clinical trials.* New York, NY: Marcel Dekker.

Frumovitz, M., Sun, C. C., Schover, L. R., Munsell, M. F., Jhingran, A., Wharton, J. T., . . . Bodurka, D. C. (2005). Quality of life and sexual functioning in cervical cancer survivors. *Journal of Clinical Oncology, 23*(30), 7428–7436.

Goodwin, P., Leszcz, M., & Ennis, M. (2001). The effect in group psychosocial support on survival in metastatic breast cancer. *New England Journal of Medicine, 345*, 1719–1726.

Greimel, E., Thiel, I., Peintinger, F., Cegnar, I., & Pongratz, E. (2002). Prospective assessment of quality of life of female cancer patients. *Gynecologic Oncology, 85*, 140–147.

Heiney, S., McWayne, J., Hurley, T., Lamb, L., Bryant, L., Butler, W., & Godder, K. (2003). Efficacy of therapeutic group by telephone for women with breast cancer. *Cancer Nursing, 26*, 439–447.

Hollis, S. (1999). What is meant by intention to treat analysis? Survey of published randomized controlled trials. *BMJ, 319*, 670–674.

Institute of Medicine. (1999). *The unequal burden of cancer: An assessment of NIH research and programs for ethnic minorities and the medically underserved.* Washington, DC: National Academies Press.

Institute of Medicine. (2008). *Cancer care for the whole patient: Meeting psychosocial health needs.* Washington, DC: National Academies Press.

Klee, M., Thranov, I., & Machin, D. (2000). The patients' perspective on physical symptoms after radiotherapy for cervical and vaginal cancer. *Gynecology Oncology, 76*(1), 14–23.

Krieger, N., Quesenberry, C., Peng, T., Horn-Ross, P., Stewart, S., Brown, S., . . . Ward, F. (1999). Social class, race/ethnicity, and incidence of breast, cervix, colon, lung, and prostate cancer among Asian, Black, Hispanic and White residents of the San Francisco Bay Area, 1988–92 (United States). *Cancer Causes & Control, 10*(6), 525–537.

Krumm, S., & Lamberti, J. (1993). Changes in sexual behavior following radiation therapy for cervical cancer. *Journal of Psychosomatic Obstetrics & Gynecology, 14,* 51–63.

Lachin, J. M. (2000). Statistical considerations in the Intent-to-Treat principle. *Controlled Clinical Trials, 21*(3), 167–189.

Lamb, M. (1995). Effects of cancer on the sexuality and fertility of women. *Seminars in Oncology Nursing, 11*(2), 120–127.

Lutgendorf, S., Anderson, B., Rothrock, N., Buller, R. E., Sood, A. K., & Sorosky, J. I. (2000). Quality of life and mood in women receiving extensive chemotherapy for gynecologic cancer. *Cancer, 89,* 1402–1411.

Meyer, T., & Mark, M. (1995). Effects of psychosocial interventions with adults cancer patients: A meta-analysis of randomized experiments. *Health Psychology, 14*(2), 101–108.

Meyerowitz, B., Formenti, S., Ell, K., & Leedham, B. (2000). Depression among Latina cervical cancer patients. *Journal of Social and Clinical Psychology, 19*(3), 352–371.

Meyerowitz, B., Richardson, J., Hudson, S., & Leedham, B. (1998). Ethnicity and cancer outcomes: Behavioral and psychosocial considerations. *Psychological Bulletin, 123*(1), 47–70.

Nelson, E. L., Wenzel, L., Osann, K., Dogan-Ates, A., Chantana, N., Reina-Patton, A., . . . Monk, B. J. (2008). Stress, immunity, and cervical cancer: Biobehavioral outcomes of a randomized clinical trail. *Clinical Cancer Research, 14*(7), 2111–2118.

Office of Minority Health. (2001). Office of Minority Health publishes final standards for cultural and linguistic competence. In *Closing the gap* (pp. 1–2, 10). Washington, DC: Office of Minority Health, DHHS.

Paavonen, J. (1999). Sexual dysfunction associated with treatment of cervical cancer. *Sexually Transmitted Infections, 75,* 375–376.

Rehse, B., & Pukrop, R. (2003). Effects of psychosocial interventions on quality of life in adult cancer patients: Meta analysis of 37 published controlled outcome studies. *Patient Education and Counseling, 50,* 179–186.

Ross, L., Boesen, E. H., Dalton, S. O., & Johansen, C. (2002). Mind and cancer: Does psychosocial intervention improve survival and psychological well-being? *European Journal of Cancer, 38,* 1447–1457.

Schover, L., Fife, M., & Gershenson, D. (1989). Sexual dysfunction and treatment for early stage cervical cancer. *Cancer, 63*(1), 204–212.

SEER. (2004). SEER*Stat Databases: Incidence—SEER 11 Regs +AK Public Use, Nov. 2003 Sub for Expanded Races (1997–2001) and Incidence—SEER 11 Regs Public Use, Nov. 2003 Sub for Hispanics (1997–2001).

Sheard, T., & Maguire, P. (1999). The effect of psychological interventions on anxiety and depression in cancer patients: Results of two meta analysis. *British Journal of Cancer, 80,* 170–180.

Smedslund, G., & Ringdal, G. I. (2004). Meta-analysis of the effects of psychosocial interventions on survival time in cancer patients. *Journal of Psychosomatic Research, 57,* 123–131.

Spiegel, D. (2001). Mind matters—Group therapy and survival in breast cancer. *New England Journal of Medicine, 345,* 1767–1768.

State Health Access Data Assistance Center. (2009). *SHADAC-Enhanced current population survey health insurance coverage estimates: A summary of historical adjustments.* Minneapolis, MN: University of Minnesota.

Steginga, S. K., & Dunn, J. (1997). Women's experiences following treatment for gynecological cancer. *Oncology Nursing Forum, 28,* 1403–1408.

U.S. Census Bureau. (2009). *Current population survey, 2009 annual social and economic supplement.* Washington, DC: Author.

Wenzel, L., DeAlba, I., Habbal, R., Kluhsman, B., Fairclough, D., Krebs, L., . . . Aziz, N. (2005). Quality of life in long-term cervical cancer survivors. *Gynecologic Oncology, 97,* 310–317.

Wenzel, L., Dogan-Ates, A., & Habbal, R. (2005). Reproductive concerns and quality of life in female cancer survivors. *Journal of the National Cancer Institute Monographs,* (34), 94–98.

Wenzel, L., Dogan-Ates, A., Habbal, R., Berkowitz, R., Goldstein, D. P., Bernstein, M., . . . Cella, D. (2005). Defining and measuring reproductive concerns of female cancer survivors. *Journal of the National Cancer Institute Monographs,* (34), 94–98.

Wenzel, L., Robinson, R., & Blake, D. (1995). The effects of problem-focused group counseling early stage gynecologic cancer. *Journal of Mental Health Counseling, 17,* 81–93.

Whelan, T. J., Mohide, E. A., Willan, A. R., Arnold, A., Tew, M., Sellick, S., . . . Levine, M. N. (1997). The supportive care needs of newly diagnosed cancer patients attending a regional cancer center. *Cancer, 80,* 1518–1524.

Zacharias, D., Gilg, C., & Foxall, M. (1994). Quality of life and coping in patients with gynecologic cancer and their spouses. *Oncology Nursing Forum, 21,* 1699–1706.

21

Sexual Minority Women With a History of Breast Cancer: Moving Toward Interventions

Ulrike Boehmer and Deborah Bowen

Sexual minority women (SMW)—that is, lesbian- or bisexual-identified women and women who report a preference for a woman partner—are an underserved population in the United States. The American Cancer Society (ACS) and other cancer agencies recognize sexual orientation as one factor linked to disparities in the cancer burden (American Cancer Society, 2011). Interventions are a powerful tool to address the needs of disparity populations and to alleviate differences in the cancer burden. However, for SMW with breast cancer, evidence about their concerns and needs is mostly lacking, which prevents us from immediately implementing interventions for SMW that are grounded in the literature. Within this chapter, we identify research issues that need to be clarified before we are in a position to conduct evidence-based interventions. Because SMW are a unique population group, this chapter will outline a path toward intervention development for others to replicate. We draw heavily on our ACS-funded study that represents our effort to move closer toward the future goal of implementation of interventions with SMW with breast cancer.

WHY ARE SMW UNLIKE OTHER GROUPS?

One fundamental difference between SMW and other population groups is the absence of surveillance. Sexual orientation is not routinely ascertained in health-related government-sponsored surveys, and if at all, inconsistently recorded in medical records, which results in a lack of information about SMW health. Cancer registries are our premier tool of identifying differences in incidence, treatment, and mortality, but at the present time, data on sexual orientation are absent from registries (Bowen & Boehmer, 2007). Therefore, it is unknown how many of the estimated 12 million cancer survivors currently living in the United States are SMW. In contradistinction, cancer registry data allow for the annual monitoring of changes in cancer incidence by other characteristics, such as age, sex, geographic location, race, ethnicity, or country of birth. The hypothesis of SMW's higher incidence of breast cancer has been confirmed by an ecological study (Boehmer, Ozonoff, & Timm, 2011), but only surveillance data can unequivocally identify SMW as an overrepresented group due to their higher levels of breast cancer risk factors. There is a dearth of information about the quality of life and the functioning of SMW who are breast cancer survivors. SMW may fare worse compared to heterosexual women in some areas and other aspects of SMW survivorship may be similar to heterosexual women's functioning. Such areas of difference or similarity in survivorship have yet to be identified. These data are essential for the development of interventions, programs, and policies that target SMW, thereby responding to these women's needs and reducing detriments in SMW survivorship.

WHAT IS KNOWN TO DATE ABOUT SURVIVORSHIP OF SMW?

SMW are an under-researched group in the context of cancer generally. Knowledge about the survivorship experience of SMW is even less readily available compared to SMW primary and secondary cancer prevention (Brown & Tracy, 2008). Most survivorship studies rely on small samples, use qualitative methods, and some are without a comparison sample of heterosexual women. A recent population-based study of California cancer survivors concluded that lesbian and bisexual cancer survivors report significantly worse health-related quality of life compared to heterosexual cancer survivors (Boehmer, Miao, & Ozonoff, 2011). Other studies inform us that SMW's coping with a cancer diagnosis differs from heterosexual women, in that SMW have less fighting spirit, yet have better coping in that they are more likely to report expression of anger, use less fatalism, and less cognitive avoidance coping (Boehmer, Linde, & Freund, 2005; Fobair et al., 2001). The information about the availability of social support resources for SMW is inconsistent, in that some concluded that SMW have the same level of support and others indicated that they have less support than heterosexual women dealing with a cancer diagnosis (Arena et al., 2006; Fobair et al., 2001). Studies also identified unique concerns of SMW in that SMW reported experiencing additional anxiety relating to their decision on disclosing their sexual orientation to medical providers, and poor communication with health care providers about their sexual orientation (Boehmer & Case, 2004, 2006; Boehmer, Freund, & Linde, 2005; Matthews, Peterman, Delaney, Menard, & Brandenburg, 2002). Some limited data are available on sexual functioning of SMW survivors. Studies find similarities and differences between SMW and heterosexual cancer survivors, identifying areas of strength for SMW, including better body image, and areas of vulnerabilities, such as problems obtaining information and support from medical professionals with respect to sexual functioning (Boehmer, Potter, & Bowen, 2009). A recent review of clinical trials conducted in the United States indicates that gay and lesbian individuals are systematically excluded from trials that have sexual function as the endpoint (Egleston, Dunbrack, & Hall, 2010). So far, while the available studies point to some aspects of SMW's survivorship experience, only thorough and systematic research that recruits a methodologically sound sample will be able to provide the necessary background to guide intervention and program development for SMW survivors.

HOW TO OBTAIN A POPULATION-BASED SAMPLE

When survivors are recruited from the community or through oncologists, selection biases may arise that call into question the generalizability of the findings. Because convenience samples are not well positioned to confidently assess disparities in survivorship due to sexual orientation, we have struggled with the question of how to design a population-based study. Our study (Boehmer et al., 2010) made use of the best source for cancer surveillance data, a statewide cancer registry, to recruit female breast cancer survivors of different sexual orientations. However, because the proportion of SMW among cancer survivors is unknown and is assumed to be a small subgroup, we were concerned about the resources needed to recruit this small subset of cancer survivors. To address this concern, we pulled information from the Census 2000. While the Census does not collect data on sexual orientation directly, it enumerates same-sex–partnered households. We and others have previously used this measure as a proxy for sexual orientation, inferring that women who report living with their same-sex partner would, when given the opportunity, report a sexual minority identity. An advantage of the Census data is that they provide information on where to find SMW, meaning the geographic locations where greater concentrations of female same-sex–partnered households have been recorded by the Census. Using the available geographic information, we restricted the statewide cancer registry data to geographic areas that had the highest concentration of SMW, as measured by female same-sex–partnered households. Because cancer registries do not collect data on sexual orientation, our recruitment necessitated contacting each breast cancer survivor who resided in the specified region to ascertain her sexual orientation. This was done in a screening call, during which also other eligibility criteria were assessed. This screening resulted in a representative sample of eligible breast cancer survivors who either identified to us as heterosexual or SMW. Our study had the goal of recruiting a representative sample of healthy breast cancer survivors, defined as women with a primary diagnosis of breast cancer without a recurrence or a diagnosis of metastatic cancer. The rigorous recruitment resulted in the identification of 6.3% of SMW in the population of breast cancer survivors (Boehmer et al., 2010). All specific details of our recruitment are discussed elsewhere, including a critical analysis of alternatives for finding breast cancer survivors of different sexual orientations (Boehmer et al.). For example, others propose using respondent-driven sampling to obtain a representative sample of hard-to-reach populations of unknown size (Heckathorn, 2002; Salganik & Heckathorn, 2004). However, as has been stated, this sampling methodology is greatly dependent on the connectedness of the population under study (Abdul-Quader, Heckathorn, Sabin, & Saidel, 2006; Meyer & Wilson, 2009; Simic et al., 2006). Our data on breast cancer survivors suggest that they are not highly connected, in the sense of knowing other SMW with whom they share a diagnosis of breast cancer. This suggests that respondent-driven sampling methods are unlikely to be successful. In addition, we also critically examined our registry-based sample by comparing it to a sample we recruited from the community, using the means of convenience sampling (Boehmer, Clark, Timm, Sullivan, & Glickman, 2011). We believe this comparison is of relevance for others who are struggling with the task of obtaining a sample of SMW. Although we readily agree that using a cancer registry is resource intense, the major advantage of registry-based recruitment is the yield of a population-based sample of breast cancer survivors of all sexual orientations. To address the issue of disparities in cancer survivorship due to sexual orientation, we need population-based data.

WHICH DATA ARE NEEDED TO ADEQUATELY ASSESS SURVIVORSHIP OF SMW?

Deciding on outcome measures to include, so that relevant information about disparities in survivorship due to sexual orientation is comprehensively collected, is another process step. Survivorship research, focused on the general population, has identified the profound impact that cancer has on a person's life. There are various ways of partitioning the domains of survivorship. Some point to the multidimensional concept of quality of life (Dow, Ferrell, Haberman, & Eaton, 1999) and the more than 200 cancer-related quality of life instruments available, which include more than 30 dimensions of quality of life (Zebrack, 2000). Others highlight five domains of survivorship, consisting of: (1) ongoing medical follow-up and health planning; (2) the persistent physical effects of cancer and its treatment; (3) altered social and interpersonal relationships; (4) residual psychological and spiritual effects of illness; and (5) the practical implications of having had cancer on such issues as employment and insurance (Alfano & Rowland, 2008).

As one study will not be able to address all domains of SMW survivorship, we decided in this study to be as comprehensive as possible, while being selective to prevent overburdening respondents. Our selection process was driven by two considerations: one was to include aspects of survivorship that were assumed to differ between the general population and SMW; a second one was to focus on domains for which existing programs and interventions are available, which have been shown to improve the outcomes in the population of survivors.

ON WHICH SURVIVORSHIP ASPECTS ARE SMW EXPECTED TO DIFFER?

Relying on evidence from studies that focused on the general noncancer population, we know that disparities due to sexual orientation exist with respect to a number of health behaviors. Studies of the general population have concluded that sexual minority women tend to have poorer health behaviors compared to heterosexual women. For example, population-based data show that both lesbians and bisexual women are more likely to smoke compared to heterosexual women (Tang et al., 2004). There is a well-known weight disparity in noncancer populations, with data indicating that lesbian women are heavier compared to heterosexual women in the general population (Boehmer & Bowen, 2009; Boehmer, Bowen, & Bauer, 2007; Case et al., 2004; Cochran et al., 2001; Valanis et al., 2000). Other aspects on which SMW are known to differ from heterosexual women are SMW's reduced access to health care, lower screening rates, greater alcohol consumption, and so on. A healthy lifestyle among cancer survivors is an important goal to increase the survival and quality of life of cancer survivors. Cancer survivors who do not engage in these behaviors are at risk, in that smoking has been linked to second cancers and cancer recurrence (Do et al., 2004; Khuri et al., 2001) and obesity after breast cancer has been linked to higher breast cancer mortality (Whiteman et al., 2005).

In this study, we selected to focus on body weight among cancer survivors because of the established link between obesity and the risk of developing distant metastases and death as a result of breast cancer or other causes (Ewertz et al., 2011). Specifically, we hypothesized that sexual minority women with breast cancer are more likely overweight and obese compared to heterosexual women with breast cancer, given the existence of such a disparity in the noncancer population (Aaron et al., 2001; Boehmer & Bowen, 2009; Boehmer et al., 2007; Case et al., 2004; Cochran et al., 2001; Dibble, Roberts, Robertson, & Paul, 2002; Valanis et al., 2000). If we can establish that a sexual orientation disparity in body mass index exists among breast cancer survivors, we will have provided the evidence for interventions that target SMW to reduce their weight in an effort to lower their risk for poorer prognosis and mortality.

To date, we have examined this hypothesis using data on 69 SMW and 257 heterosexual survivors of breast cancer whom we asked to self-report weight and height, to derive body mass index (BMI), which we then categorized into healthy or normal weight versus overweight or obese (Boehmer, Mertz et al., 2011). When we compared these two groups of women, bivariate analyses found no significant differences in the prevalence of overweight and obesity by sexual orientation, with more than 50% in each group being overweight or obese. After adjusting for differences in other demographic and clinical factors, including the extent to which these breast cancer survivors were using weight-increasing medications, our final models indicated that, against our expectation, SMW were similar to heterosexual breast cancer survivors with respect to being overweight or greater. This unanticipated similarity between SMW and heterosexual breast cancer survivors raises important questions about the reasons for this similarity. As we have discussed elsewhere (Boehmer, Mertz et al., 2011), one possibility is selection bias, in that our eligibility criteria may have biased our selection toward a particularly lean sample of SMW, because we excluded women with recurrent and metastatic breast cancer, both outcomes associated with greater BMI. Another consideration is that our findings reflect a geographic pattern, as our sample reflected only one state, Massachusetts, which ranks as the state with the second-lowest obesity rates (21.2%) in the nation (Trust for America's Health, 2009). From additional comparisons, we know this does not apply, as SMW recruited from the Massachusetts Cancer Registry do not significantly differ in BMI from the convenience sample of SMW recruited from other U.S. states (Boehmer, Clark, et al., 2011). In conclusion, we suggest it is feasible that we could not establish BMI disparities due to sexual orientation in survivors because SMW respond differently to a breast cancer diagnosis than heterosexual women. It is feasible that SMW are more motivated to engage in healthier lifestyle practices than heterosexual women, which then would explain their similarity in BMI. We hope that future research will test this hypothesis by comparing the weight-related health behaviors of SMW with breast cancer to heterosexual breast cancer survivors. A second method of testing this hypothesis is to compare SMW with breast cancer to a control group of SMW without cancer. Ideally, pre-diagnosis data on SMW with breast cancer provides another opportunity for identifying if SMW are more likely to respond with a change in their health behaviors compared to heterosexual women. For now, these results with respect to BMI do not lead us down a path toward interventions that target specifically SMW with breast cancer; rather, these unexpected findings call for additional assessment studies that help with the understanding of this similarity.

To move toward the identification of differences in survivorship experiences by sexual orientation, which can be addressed with existing programs and interventions, we focused on survivors' psychological adaptation. So far, research in the general population has established differences in SMW's mental health compared to that of heterosexual women (Cochran et al., 2003). This prompted us to examine the psychological adaptation and the well-being of cancer survivors, with the expectation of finding that SMW with breast cancer have worse outcomes.

WHICH MECHANISMS ARE LIKELY TO ACCOUNT FOR THE ASSUMED DIFFERENCES IN PSYCHOLOGICAL ADAPTATION?

A strong need exists for a thorough examination of factors likely to contribute to survivors' psychological outcomes, so that we will then be able to use these data for the adaptation of an intervention that has been effective in improving the quality of life of heterosexual survivors.

Our study draws on an established framework of quality of life and its determinants to guide the selection of factors for inclusion in the assessment (Holland & Gooen-Piels, 2000; Rowland, 1989, 1994). This framework has established three factors that have an impact on survivors' quality of life: (1) society-derived, (2) patient-derived, and (3) cancer-derived factors. However, to understand fully the potential differences in outcomes for SMW, our study added a fourth group of factors, which we called minority-derived factors, as these apply only to the SMW in the proposed study. Society-derived factors capture the general attitudes and beliefs about cancer held in society that impact the patient. As we conducted our study with the intention of resulting in an intervention that focuses on the individual, we omitted collecting data on society-derived factors. Instead, we focused on patient-derived factors, which refer to beliefs and attributes that the individual brings to the illness. We further distinguished patient-derived factors into: (1) intrapersonal factors, which capture the developmental stage of the individual at the time of diagnosis and an individual's coping ability; (2) interpersonal factors, which refers to the available social support; and (3) the socioeconomic status of the individual. The intrapersonal data that we collected include survivors' age, employment status, and marital and relationship status, as well as measures of coping strategies to determine how a survivor manages the stress of being inflicted with cancer. The interpersonal characteristics of survivors were collected using measures of social support to determine the availability of this resource for survivors. Cancer-derived factors include the clinical realities to which the patient has to adapt. In our study, we collected data on cancer stage, the treatments that a survivor endured, the presence of side effects, and survivors' perception of the physician–patient relationship. Finally, to adequately capture the unique situation of SMW cancer survivors, we added a cluster of variables to assess the sexual minority status of the individual, by measuring minority-derived factors. These minority factors include experiences of discrimination, measures of disclosure of sexual orientation to others, which capture the person groups, such as family, friends, coworkers, and neighbors, to which a survivor is "out." We also collected data on the number of years survivors' had identified as lesbian or bisexual, their connectedness to the lesbian, gay, and bisexual community, and their level of comfort with their sexual minority identity. Ultimately, these three factors—patient-derived, cancer-derived, and the minority factors—which we collected data on, are analyzed to identify the mechanisms that explain survivors' psychological outcomes and potential disparities between heterosexual and SMW survivors.

HOW CAN WE DEEPEN OUR UNDERSTANDING OF SMW'S SURVIVORSHIP?

Collecting quantitative survey data from a carefully recruited population-based sample of breast cancer survivors as described above is a necessary step to identify disparities by sexual orientation and the mechanisms that contribute to these disparities. However, large-scale survey studies such as ours are limited in providing a rich understanding of SMW's appraisal of how they perceive their own adjustment. To fully understand SMW experiences and perceptions of their adjustment, we also collected qualitative data from SMW. Specifically, consistent with our prioritization of psychological adjustment, we conducted individual interviews with contrasting groups of SMW, those who adjusted well and those who adjusted poorly. These contrasting accounts from SMW at opposite sides of the spectrum contribute to an in-depth understanding of this population's positive and negative responses, which will further inform the development of an intervention designed to improve this population's quality of life. Because the interviews are open-ended, but semistructured, they complement the data derived from the survey questionnaire. The interview questions are developed after the quantitative data have been analyzed. This allows for selection of topics that appear to be most salient, as identified by the quantitative analysis. The interview guide is designed to elicit extended narratives of SMW's experiences with breast cancer and the subsequent process of adaptation after they completed their treatment. Particular attention is given to eliciting SMW's ways of characterizing their well-being, including negative as well as positive changes due to breast cancer. In these interviews, we also inquire about SMW perceptions of whether their experiences are related to their sexual minority status. Other pieces of information that are particularly valuable for intervention development and design are their preferences for interventions, because SMW may differ on their perceived need for an intervention, their preferences of intervention elements, such as peer support from another SMW with breast cancer, or having a professional conduct the intervention, without concern for the professional's sexual orientation.

To derive this information from the qualitative interviews with SMW, we follow the principles of qualitative research methods. The interviews are audio recorded, and the audiotapes are transcribed verbatim for analysis as word processing text files that may be manipulated by a qualitative software program. The analytic procedures follow the general procedures of grounded theory methodology (Strauss & Corbin, 1990). The objectives of the analysis of the interview data are to understand the experiences of SMW and the process that ensues, leading to adaptation. Other aspects of the analysis focus on determining intervention-specific preferences.

HOW TO CREATE INTERVENTIONS FOR SMW SURVIVORS?

Once the findings from the above research are known, we will then begin to design and test interventions to improve the survivorship experiences of SMW. We plan either to use an established framework for creating an intervention that targets the specific needs of SMW, or to adapt an existing intervention that has been found efficacious in heterosexual samples. Bartholomew's planning framework, with its six steps, is one such framework for creating an intervention. The six steps move from formative data collection, through identification of the objectives and behavioral goals, to feasibility testing in controlled settings (Bartholomew, Parcel, Kok, & Gottlieb, 2006). In detail, Step 1 consists of needs assessment, often of the qualitative and quantitative types mentioned above. Step 2 involves identifying change objectives for each of the areas identified in the formative research. Step 3 involves selecting available theory-informed intervention methods and practical strategies. Step 4 is focused on producing program components and materials, whether through adaptation or new development of such components. Step 5 is the step for planning program adoption, implementation, and sustainability; and Step 6 involves planning the evaluation (Bartholomew et al., 2006). These steps have been used in other settings to target minority populations with interventions to improve health behaviors and health outcomes (Fernandez, Gonzales, Tortolero-Luna, Partida, & Bartholomew, 2005). We will use this method of identifying an intervention if the outcomes of interest (those that show the greatest disparities) have never been tested in other settings. If the data call for creation of an intervention, the quantitative survey data provide the overall framework, such as determining the endpoint of the intervention and the mechanism to be targeted, whereas the qualitative data will bear on the program-specific components, including program components and materials.

We will use the second option, adaptation of an existing intervention, if interventions that target the outcomes of interest are available and tested, but the populations have been different in the published studies. Adapting an intervention is best accomplished through a series of steps, outlined in *Using What Works*, a system of adaptation (National Cancer Institute, 2006). The three steps articulated in this document include identifying of what can and cannot be changed in the intervention, identifying the specific changes in content and format that need to be made, and testing the feasibility of the new intervention plan in an appropriate population. Although lengthy, these procedures will help to ensure that the new intervention will carry the same effect on outcomes as the previously tested one, while being appropriate and culturally relevant for the new target group and setting.

In the case of design or adaptation, the specific components of the intervention will be tightly tied to the data we have collected on predictors of quality of life and on disparities in quality of life and other functional outcomes for SMW. Therefore, it is premature to describe the specific intervention components. However, we provide examples here to illustrate how we will use the data to motivate specific intervention components. For example, one of the hypotheses that we will test is the role of minority-derived factors in predicting SMW's quality of life. If we find that minority-derived factors contribute to the variance in SMW quality of life, over and above the patient- and cancer-derived factors, then we will design specific intervention components to help SMW cope with these minority-derived factors.

One of the minority-derived factors is the experiences of discrimination remembered and understood by SMW as part of daily life. These experiences are likely to affect interactions with heterosexual individuals, including co-workers, friends, family, and providers. To the extent that a SMW has experienced discrimination and that discrimination does affect her interactions with heterosexual others, these effects may inhibit the SMW under study from obtaining support from her provider team in the same positive ways as would a heterosexual woman. The experiences of discrimination do not need to be current; they can be historical and relevant to other heterosexual individuals, not the ones in an ongoing relationship. However, historical experiences such as discrimination do alter interaction patterns, and these learned behaviors could be interfering with an SMW's ability to elicit support in times of need, such as during a cancer treatment period. Therefore, the SMW is left feeling unsupported and her quality of life decreases. These are empirical questions and, once they are answered, we can design intervention components around the specific findings that will improve the quality of life and functioning of SMW.

One issue that we will have to consider even before we see the results of the previously described data collection of this study is the intervention delivery format. Much research has been conducted in which the intervention is delivered to survivors in small groups, often offered at the clinical setting, such as a hospital setting. For SMW, this will not be possible, due to the disparate treatment settings in which SMW receive their treatment and care. Even in an urban setting, SMW patients and survivors are scattered at all clinical settings and treatment facilities, making the formation of group-based interventions for testing not practical. Therefore, we will need to rely on more innovative forms of intervention delivery. Delivering an intervention by telephone is a possibility, as is delivery via the Internet. Both have been used with success as intervention delivery formats for survivorship research. One example of a telephone-delivered intervention is the recently evaluated intervention for survivors of early stage breast cancer, to improve quality of life (Marcus et al., 2009). The CHESS program, led by Gustavson and others (Han et al., 2008), provides clear evidence that breast cancer survivors can benefit from an Internet-delivered intervention to improve quality of life. These examples of successful interventions, delivered using innovative electronic means, provide hope that an intervention for SMW can be created and tested successfully.

WHICH INTERVENTIONS EXIST FOR SMW IN COMMUNITY SETTINGS?

One indicator of the need for interventions that target SMW and their issues is the plethora of existing programs for SMW that have been created and supported by grassroots groups and individuals. Lesbian cancer projects, such as the Mautner Project in Washington, DC (www.mautnerproject.org), were created as grassroots organizations as a result of the cancer diagnosis of a prominent SMW in the local community. They provide a range of services, such as support groups in the community, that are specifically for SMW. These programs are not based on evidence of specific psychosocial issues, nor have they been carefully designed according to the steps we have outlined here. In addition, none of these programs have been evaluated to date and published. However, they do indicate that the perceived need for SMW-specific and -friendly services is great and they can help us in the design of culturally appropriate interventions in the future. Working with community groups to design relevant interventions will help us to improve our ability to reach all SMW with interventions.

Using the principles of community-based participatory research (CBPR) would be a potentially powerful way to design and evaluate these community-based—and, indeed, all—interventions in SMW samples. CBPR involves engagement of community partners in all aspects of research projects, including identification and design, conduct, and analysis. This type of research methodology has been used in intervention design and evaluation for other disparities-defined groups, and could be applied here to improve the design and relevance of the intervention activities for SMW survivors. Bridging the gaps between the academy and community leaders and members is time-consuming and sometimes difficult, but often worth it in terms of community acceptance and impact.

WHAT SHALL WE CONCLUDE AFTER HAVING LAID OUT THESE DEVELOPMENT STEPS?

Our description of these intervention development steps covers a broader range than commonly seen when reviewing intervention studies. As there are multiple gaps in knowledge with respect to SMW, which do not necessarily exist for other disparity populations, this chapter had to describe the means of assessing and identifying disparities due to sexual orientation prior to being able to focus on the intervention that addresses the disparities. This broad spectrum covers a research process that stretches over a number of years and necessitates a team of researchers who collectively possess a variety of expertise and skills to adequately execute the process steps, from assessment to intervention. Further, throughout this process have we stressed that we had to make choices during the development phases. Because so little is known about SMW survivorship, we had to choose domains and aspects of survivorship to be dealt with in the context of one study. In addition, we wish to stress that from the beginning we selected SMW as the target population for intervention. This means that our process covered only one level of intervention. To fully address the disparities of SMW survivorship, other levels of interventions have to be considered. For example, it is possible for others to develop similar process steps to move from assessing disparities in SMW survivorship to educational interventions with physicians who treat these women, or to interventions that target systemic changes of the health care organizations, where these women are treated. Selecting a process that culminates in a patient-level intervention was another decision point, while we are aware that other levels of interventions, with physicians or health care systems or both, may also provide valuable solutions to disparities in SMW survivors worthy of testing and evaluation. We hope that this chapter will provide health care professionals and other researchers with the tools needed to finally develop and test interventions in the population of SMW survivors. In addition, we wish to clarify that we have laid out one process, and that there is ample room for other process steps that lead to other interventions, while pursuing the same goal of reducing disparities for SMW survivors.

REFERENCES

Aaron, D., Markovic, N., Danielson, M., Honnold, J., Janosky, J., & Schmidt, N. (2001). Behavioral risk factors for disease and preventive health practices among lesbians. *American Journal of Public Health, 91*(6), 972–975.

Abdul-Quader, A. S., Heckathorn, D. D., Sabin, K., & Saidel, T. (2006). Implementation and analysis of respondent driven sampling: Lessons learned from the field. *Journal of Urban Health, 83*(Suppl. 1), 1–5.

Alfano, C. M., & Rowland, J. H. (2008). The experience of survival for patients: Psychosocial adjustment. In S. Miller, D. Bowen, R. Croyle,& J. Rowland (Eds.), *Handbook of behavioral science and cancer* (pp. 413–430). Washington, DC: American Psychological Association.

American Cancer Society. (2011). *Cancer facts and figures 2011* (webversion ed.). Atlanta, GA: Author. Retrieved from http://www.cancer.org/Research/CancerFactsFigures/CancerFactsFigures/cancer-facts-figures-2011

Arena, P. L., Carver, C. S., Antoni, M. H., Weiss, S., Ironson, G., & Durán, R. E. (2006). Psychosocial responses to treatment for breast cancer among lesbian and heterosexual women. *Women & Health, 44*(2), 81–102.

Bartholomew, L., Parcel, G., Kok, G., & Gottlieb, N. (2006). *Planning health promotion programs: An intervention mapping approach* (2nd ed.). San Francisco, CA: Jossey-Bass (John Wiley & Sons).

Boehmer, U., & Bowen, D. J. (2009). Examining factors linked to overweight and obesity in women of different sexual orientations. *Preventive Medicine, 48*(4), 357–361.

Boehmer, U., Bowen, D. J., & Bauer, G. R. (2007). Overweight and obesity in sexual minority women: Evidence from population-based data. *American Journal of Public Health, 97*(6), 1134–1140.

Boehmer, U., & Case, P. (2004). Physicians don't ask, some patients tell: Disclosure of sexual orientation among women with breast cancer. *Cancer, 101*(8), 1882–1889.

Boehmer, U., & Case, P. (2006). Sexual minority women's interactions with breast cancer providers. *Women and Health, 44*(2), 41–58.

Boehmer, U., Clark, M., Glickman, M., Timm, A., Sullivan, M., Bradford, J., & Bowen, D. J. (2010). Using cancer registry data for recruitment of sexual minority women: successes and limitations. *Journal of Women's Health, 19*(7), 1289–1297.

Boehmer, U., Clark, M. A., Timm, A., Sullivan, M., & Glickman, M. (2011). Comparing cancer survivors recruited through a cancer registry to convenience methods of recruitment *Women's Health Issues*. DOI: 10.1016/j.whi.2011.03.003

Boehmer, U., Freund, K. M., & Linde, R. (2005). Support providers of sexual minority women with breast cancer: Who they are and how they impact the breast cancer experience. *Journal of Psychosomatic Research, 59*(5), 307–314.

Boehmer, U., Linde, R., & Freund, K. M. (2005). Sexual minority women's coping and psychological adjustment after a diagnosis of breast cancer. *Journal of Women's Health, 14*(3), 214–224.

Boehmer, U., Mertz, M., Timm, A., Glickman, M., Sullivan, M., & Potter, J. (2011). Overweight and obesity in long-term breast cancer survivors: How does sexual orientation impact BMI? *Cancer Investigation, 29*(3), 220–228.

Boehmer, U., Miao, X., & Ozonoff, A. (2011). Cancer survivorship and sexual orientation. *Cancer.* DOI:10.1002/cncr.25950.

Boehmer, U., Ozonoff, A., & Timm, A. (2011). County-level association of sexual minority density with breast cancer incidence: Results from an ecological study. *Sexuality Research and Social Policy, 8*(2), 139–145.

Boehmer, U., Potter, J., & Bowen, D. J. (2009). Sexual functioning after cancer in sexual minority women. [Review]. *The Cancer Journal, 15*(1), 65–69.

Bowen, D. J., & Boehmer, U. (2007). The lack of cancer surveillance data on sexual minorities and strategies for change. *Cancer Causes and Control, 18*(4), 343–349.

Brown, J. P., & Tracy, J. K. (2008). Lesbians and cancer: An overlooked health disparity. *Cancer Causes and Control, 19*(10), 1009–1020.

Case, P., Bryn Austin, S., Hunter, D. J., Manson, J. E., Malspeis, S., Willett, W. C., & Spiegelman, D. (2004). Sexual orientation, health risk factors, and physical functioning in the Nurses' Health Study II. *Journal of Women's Health, 13*(9), 1033–1047.

Cochran, S. D., Mays, V. M., Bowen, D., Gage, S., Bybee, D., Roberts, S. J., . . . White, J. (2001). Cancer-related risk indicators and preventive screening behaviors among lesbians and bisexual women. *American Journal of Public Health, 91*(4), 591–597.

Cochran, S. D., Mays, V. M., & Sullivan, J. G. (2003). Prevalence of mental disorders, psychological distress, and mental health services use among lesbian, gay, and bisexual adults in the United States. *Journal of Consulting and Clinical Psychology, 71*(1), 53–61.

Dibble, S. L., Roberts, S. A., Robertson, P. A., & Paul, S. M. (2002). Risk factors for ovarian cancer: Lesbian and heterosexual women. *Oncology Nursing Forum, 29*(1), E1–E7.

Do, K. A., Johnson, M. M., Lee, J. J., Wu, X. F., Dong, Q., Hong, W. K., . . . Spitz, M. R. (2004). Longitudinal study of smoking patterns in relation to the development of smoking-related secondary primary tumors in patients with upper aerodigestive tract malignancies. *Cancer, 101*(12), 2837–2842.

Dow, K. H., Ferrell, B. R., Haberman, M. R., & Eaton, L. (1999). The meaning of quality of life in cancer survivorship. *Oncology Nursing Forum, 26*(3), 519–528.

Egleston, B. L., Dunbrack, R. L., Jr., & Hall, M. J. (2010). Clinical trials that explicitly exclude gay and lesbian patients. *New England Journal of Medicine, 362*(11), 1054–1055.

Ewertz, M., Jensen, M. B., Gunnarsdottir, K. A., Hojris, I., Jakobsen, E. H., Nielsen, D., . . . Cold, S. (2011). Effect of obesity on prognosis after early-stage breast cancer. *Journal of Clinical Oncology, 29*(1), 25–31.

Fernandez, M. E., Gonzales, A., Tortolero-Luna, G., Partida, S., & Bartholomew, L. K. (2005). Using intervention mapping to develop a breast and cervical cancer screening program for Hispanic farmworkers: *Cultivando La Salud. Health Promotion Practice, 6*(4), 394–404.

Fobair, P., O'Hanlan, K., Koopman, C., Classen, C., Dimiceli, S., Drooker, N., . . . Spiegel, D. (2001). Comparison of lesbian and heterosexual women's response to newly diagnosed breast cancer. *Psychooncology, 10*(1), 40–51.

Han, J. Y., Shaw, B. R., Hawkins, R. P., Pingree, S., McTavish, F., & Gustafson, D. H. (2008). Expressing positive emotions within online support groups by women with breast cancer. *Journal of Health Psychology, 13*(8), 1002–1007.

Heckathorn, D. D. (2002). Respondent-driven sampling II: Deriving valid population estimates from chain-referral samples of hidden populations. *Social Problems, 49*(1), 11–34.

Holland, J. C., & Gooen-Piels, J. (2000). Principles of psycho-oncology. In R. C. Bast, Jr., D. W. Kufe, R. E. Pollock, R. R. Weichselbaum, J. F. Holland,& E. Frei, III (Eds.), *Cancer medicine* (5th ed., pp. 943–958). Hamilton, Ontario: B. C. Decker, Inc.

Khuri, F. R., Kim, E. S., Lee, J. J., Winn, R. J., Benner, S. E., Lippman, S. M., ... Hong, W. K. (2001). The impact of smoking status, disease stage, and index tumor site on second primary tumor incidence and tumor recurrence in the head and neck retinoid chemoprevention trial. *Cancer Epidemiology, Biomarkers & Prevention, 10*(8), 823–829.

Marcus, A. C., Garrett, K. M., Cella, D., Wenzel, L., Brady, M. J., Fairclough, D., ... Flynn, P. J. (2009). Can telephone counseling post-treatment improve psychosocial outcomes among early stage breast cancer survivors? *Psychooncology.*

Matthews, A. K., Peterman, A., Delaney, P., Menard, L., & Brandenburg, D. (2002). A qualitative exploration of the experiences of lesbian and heterosexual patients with breast cancer. *Oncology Nursing Forum, 29*(10), 1455–1462.

Meyer, I. H., & Wilson, P. A. (2009). Sampling lesbian, gay, and bisexual populations. *Journal of Counseling Psychology, 56*(1), 23–31.

National Cancer Institute. (2006) *Using what works: Adapting evidence-based programs to fit your needs.* Retrieved October 9, 2006, from http://cancercontrol.cancer.gov/use_what_works/start.htm

Rowland, J. (1989). Intrapersonal resources: Coping. In J. Rowland (Ed.), *Handbook of psychooncology: Psychological care of the patient with cancer* (pp. 44–57). New York, NY: Oxford University Press.

Rowland, J. H. (1994). Psycho-oncology and breast cancer: A paradigm for research and intervention. *Breast Cancer Research and Treatment, 31*(2–3), 315–324.

Salganik, M. J., & Heckathorn, D. D. (2004). Sampling and estimation in hidden populations using respondent-driven sampling. *Sociological Methodology, 34*, 193–239.

Simic, M., Johnston, L. G., Platt, L., Baros, S., Andjelkovic, V., Novotny, T., & Rhodes, T. (2006). Exploring barriers to "respondent driven sampling" in sex worker and drug-injecting sex worker populations in Eastern Europe. *Journal of Urban Health, 83*(6 Suppl.), i6–i15.

Strauss, A., & Corbin, J. (1990). *Basics of qualitative research: Grounded theory procedures and techniques.* Newbury Park, CA: Sage.

Tang, H., Greenwood, G. L., Cowling, D. W., Lloyd, J. C., Roeseler, A. G., & Bal, D. G. (2004). Cigarette smoking among lesbians, gays, and bisexuals: How serious a problem? (United States). *Cancer Causes and Control, 15*(8), 797–803.

Trust for America's Health. (2009). *F as in fat: How obesity policies are failing in America.* Washington, DC: Robert Wood Johnson Foundation.

Valanis, B. G., Bowen, D. J., Bassford, T., Whitlock, E., Charney, P., & Carter, R. A. (2000). Sexual orientation and health: Comparisons in the women's health initiative sample. *Archives of Family Medicine, 9*(9), 843–853.

Whiteman, M. K., Hillis, S. D., Curtis, K. M., McDonald, J. A., Wingo, P. A., & Marchbanks, P. A. (2005). Body mass and mortality after breast cancer diagnosis. *Cancer Epidemiol, Biomarkers & Prevention, 14*(8), 2009–2014.

Zebrack, B. (2000). Cancer survivors and quality of life: A critical review of the literature. *Oncology Nursing Forum, 27*(9), 1395–1401.

III

LESSONS FOR THE FUTURE

22

Paths for the Future: Using What We've Learned to Eliminate Cancer Disparities

Bruce D. Rapkin

Eliminating cancer health disparities and ensuring the best possible outcomes for anyone affected by cancer are preeminent challenges facing the cancer research community now and in the foreseeable future. As this book amply demonstrates, cancer disparities are largely a product of inequitable distribution of health care, exposures to risk factors, and provisions for a healthy lifestyle. Although biologic factors contribute to some of these disparities, the implications of biologic differences are greatly compounded by environmental, social, and behavioral factors. Eliminating cancer disparities will necessarily entail a social justice agenda that emphasizes universal access to a continuum of high-quality care and infrastructure to promote and support healthy lifestyles.

This chapter will consider the ways in which psychosocial and behavioral research can contribute to the ultimate elimination of cancer disparities. (1) First, it is necessary to examine how trends in the composition of our population, likely advances in technology, and pending changes in health care delivery may each impact cancer health disparities. (2) Based on this analysis, suggestions are made for a number of fundamental solutions to cancer health disparities that are urgently needed now, and that will continue to be imperative in the foreseeable future. (3) Next are lessons learned from the studies summarized in this volume. Beyond their immediate research questions, these studies embody critical perspectives and innovative methods necessary to meet the challenges of the future. (4) These studies provide the basis for future research to empower consumers, strengthen communities, and promote social justice in health care. Aligning our science with the need for social justice will require us to build upon the many innovations embodied in the American Cancer Society's current research portfolio, including community participation in research, empowerment of individuals and families, greater accountability and better communication between providers and consumers, highly adaptive and comprehensive behavioral interventions, and sophisticated use of health information resources to guide and shape policy.

SOCIETAL TRENDS WITH IMPLICATIONS FOR THE FUTURE OF CANCER HEALTH DISPARITIES

If there is one takeaway message that emerges from the in-depth reviews and scholarly research presented in this volume, it is that the future of cancer prevention, early detection, support, and care is already upon us (Albano et al., 2007; Institute of Medicine, 2006; Jemal, Siegel, Xu, & Ward, 2010). Although there have been notable gains in closing some gaps related to cancer screening and health risks, the excess burden of many diseases continues to fall disproportionately on ethnic and racial minorities (Byers, 2010; Shariff-Marco, Klassen, & Bowie, 2010; Stockdale et al., 2007). These groups are subject to greater risk and inadequate access or worse cancer outcomes, associated with specific environmental, cultural, and lifestyle differences (DeLancey, Thun, Jemal, & Ward, 2008; McAlearney et al., 2008). Chapters in this volume touch on demographic trends, technological changes, and health policies that will influence inequities in care and other sources of health disparities. Note that these societal trends interact with the overarching political, social, and economic climate. For over 30 years, the United States has experienced unprecedented imbalances in the distribution of wealth among upper-, middle-, and lower-income citizens and families (Adler et al., 2007; Brunner & Marmot, 2006; Paradies, 2006). It will be worthwhile to consider how historical shifts in demographics, technology, and policy may affect people with different levels of resources.

A Growing, Aging Population, in Poorer Health Than Its Predecessors

As the baby boomers start to retire, an increasing portion of the population of the United States will enter the years when they are at greater risk for cancer. The sheer number of older adults will represent a challenge to the health care system, as more and more individuals require cancer screening and care (Avendano, Glymour, Banks, & Mackenbach, 2009; Smith, 2005). Not only is our population aging, but it is aging with more and more chronic health problems, due to obesity, poor nutrition, and inactivity. The implications of these trends for cancer-related health disparities are many and profound. For example:

- Do we have the health care person-power to meet the growing demand for treatment and care across the cancer continuum? Individuals with lower incomes or living in communities with fewer resources may be subject to greater disparities, if demand for these services outstrips supply.

- Are cancer therapies that have been developed and tested in highly selected samples adequate to meet the needs of populations with comorbid diabetes, cardiovascular disease, and other diagnoses? Lower-income and ethnic-minority groups are more likely to be diagnosed with chronic diseases in addition to cancer, are less likely to be represented in research, and so may experience worse treatment outcomes (Kim, Kumanyika, Shive, Igweatu, & Kim, 2010; Reynolds, Hanson, Henderson, & Steinhauser, 2008).
- How do we serve the growing population of cancer survivors and their family support systems, particularly in light of significant disabilities related to cancer and to their other health needs? In addition to difficulties in affording support and care, lower-income families are more likely to face less job flexibility, inadequate housing and transportation, and multiple members with chronic health needs, all of which can seriously compound the well-being of cancer survivors.

Increasing Diversity of Patients and Families

The recently released results of the 2010 census provide further evidence that the U.S. population is becoming more ethnically and linguistically diverse (U.S. Census Bureau, 2011). Immigrants to the United States are especially affected by barriers associated with language, culture, and stigma, as well as uncertain legal status and intentional impediments to care (Lamont & Small, 2008). These trends suggest that our health care system will have to become increasingly adept at responding to differences in cultural identity (Like, 2008; Smith, Bonomi, Packer, & Wisnivesky, 2010). Unfortunately, minority status will continue to put people at risk for difficulties in cancer treatment:

- Will minority patients continue to encounter pervasive implicit racial bias, with deleterious effects on quality of care? The growth in the number of ethnic-minority health professionals has not kept pace with changes in the population, particularly among African American, Latino, and Native American populations (Alegría, 2009; Terry, 2006; Cargill, 2009).
- How will we respond to the heterogeneity within racial and ethnic categories? As Chen, Gee, Spencer, Danziger, and Takeuchi (2009) point out, Asian, South Asian, and Latino immigrant groups reflect many different nationalities, subcultures, and immigration experiences. Individuals and families relate to health care in many and varied ways, so it is not likely that one-size-fits-all approaches will work, even for members of a single ethnic group.

- In addition to ethnicity and race, how will we accommodate increasing heterogeneity in terms of factors such as family composition? For example, culturally based differences in health behavior and preferences for health care may vary substantially across generations within a given family (Patel, Peacock, McKinley, Clark Carter, & Watson, 2009; Peterson, Dwyer, Mulvaney, Dietrich, & Rothman, 2007). The health care system must be able to accommodate nontraditional families, same-sex marriages, and civil unions. Accommodation not only requires greater awareness and sensitivity on the part of medical professionals, but also changes in everything from medical record keeping through education materials to the attitudes and skills of administrators and staff (Hasnain-Wynia et al., 2007).

Emerging Health Technologies

Ideally, continued advances in cancer detection and treatment will lead to improved health of all members of the population (Cullum, Alder, & Hoodless, 2011; Goldsmith, Dietrich, Du, & Morrison, 2008; Ostroff et al., 2010; Singal & Marrero, 2010). However, as cancer detection and treatment becomes increasingly sophisticated, individuals able to access advanced technology will be the most likely to benefit. For example, for certain surgical procedures, outcomes are associated with access to high-volume cancer specialty centers. Similarly, determining optimal treatment depends on the ability to provide increasingly detailed characterization of tumor genetics and other characteristics:

- Will advances in technologies constrain the number of places where patients are able to receive state-of-the-art care? There is already incredibly wide variation in cancer treatment across settings (Elk et al., chapter 4). Economically disadvantaged patients, as well as those living in communities without academic cancer centers, are least likely to have access to settings where the latest technologies are available (MacDonald, Blazer, & Weitzel, 2010; Price, 2010).
- Similarly, will increasingly complicated choices present greater challenges in terms of health decision making and provider–patient communication? Oncologists may avoid offering certain treatments if they expect patients to have difficulty in understanding choices or providing informed consent.
- Will patients face increasing challenges with adherence as self-administered oral treatment for cancers become more widely available? As we have seen with complex oral regimens for treatment of HIV, adherence is often more problematic for patients facing challenging physical, emotional, or socioeconomic circumstances, contributing to poorer outcomes of care.

Health Care Reform

At this writing, the outcome of federal health care reform efforts is far from certain. In principle, improving individuals' access to health care insurance ought to reduce health disparities (Errickson et al., 2011). However, even if current legislation is successful, increased coverage in and of itself does not assure access to good-quality care (Fiscella, 2011). Initiatives to promote greater accountability and coordination of care hold much promise, but top-down regulatory and structural systems alone are unlikely to overcome cancer health disparities (Burgess, 2010). Pressures to maximize corporate profits combined with challenges in defining, measuring, and regulating quality of care will continue to affect cancer disparities. Several additional factors may contribute to even greater cancer-related health disparities. For example:

- Do providers and systems have the training and tools they need to address the changes in patient populations? Health care reform is intended to expand access for patients who have previously been closed out of health care (Epstein, Fiscella, Lesser, & Stange, 2010). This will increase the numbers and proportions of patients that providers see who have previously been under-served. Clearing this bottleneck means more patients with lower levels of adherence to screening and health behavioral guidelines, higher levels of medical and psychiatric comorbidities, and more complex psychosocial needs (Boyer & Lutfey, 2010). Without special steps to absorb these patients into the current health delivery system, already overtaxed providers and systems in low health resource and low-income communities may be overwhelmed, contributing to greater disparities (Paredes, 2008; Varkey et al., 2009).
- How will increased access impact transitions in care and communications across systems? Already, fragmentation in care accounts for outcomes for cancer patients due to delays in adjuvant chemotherapy or radiation treatment after surgery. Similarly, communications between oncology and primary care systems are often inadequate to address the special needs of cancer survivors. Increasing numbers of complex patients, limited re-sources, and greater requirements for documentation and accountability may further impede communications across systems. Even with the as-sistance of patient navigators and the like, outcomes will be worse for in-dividuals who are not able to participate fully in the management of their own cancer care.

IMPERATIVES FOR ELIMINATING CANCER DISPARITIES

This brief discussion of societal trends in population composition and health, distribution of cancer treatment and screening technologies, and pressures on health service delivery systems leads to an uncomfortable conclusion: Without significant, widespread efforts to offset these trends, disparities in cancer are likely to continue and even expand. Of course, the best way to eliminate cancer disparities would be to eliminate cancer. However, we cannot defeat cancer in the same way that our predecessors in medicine and public health defeated polio. There is no single technological innovation on the horizon that will eradicate any one of the major cancer killers, let alone all cancer. Instead, our best hope in defeating cancer requires engaging people in prevention, detecting disease early, and ensuring universal access to state-of-the-art treatment and supportive care (Epstein et al., 2010). In short, reducing disparities and making headway against cancer will require continued mobilization and expansion of public health resources and infrastructure. Although not exhaustive, it is possible to outline a number of steps that are necessary to counter the forces that drive cancer disparities. These are labeled as "imperatives" because elimination of cancer health disparities will require efforts at the following levels:

1. *Effective health behavioral interventions must become the standard of care.* Research presented in this volume highlights the ways in which effective strategies can be developed and implemented to improve diet and physical activity, reduce smoking, improve access to screening and care, and achieve adherence to recommended treatment. As discussed below, these studies demonstrate considerable sophistication and depth of understanding in their approaches to complicated decision making and behavior change, particularly for people in challenging life circumstances. Outcomes of cancer and associated disparities are fundamentally related to these health behaviors and lifestyle choices, as reflected in national health goals and plans (U.S. Department of Health and Human Services, 2011). Unfortunately, these interventions are not at all the norm in public health. For example, national efforts to promote breast and cervical screening provide coverage for tests but very few resources for education and outreach, and no incentives to incorporate (or develop) evidence-based interventions. Recent efforts to encourage providers to use smoking cessation guidelines emphasize the use of specific steps to promote cessation (Ask, Advise, Assist, Assess, and Arrange), but there is no standard of care available to ensure that these different steps are carried out effectively (cf. Dixon et al., 2009). The lack of awareness of techniques available to encourage these behaviors and the wide variation in quality of care is a travesty. To make progress against disparities in cancer and other chronic diseases, we must help communities use evidence-based methods to establish continua of public health care that will provide effective education and ensure access to necessary behavioral and preventive health care. This would be a substantial undertaking,

involving the mass media, community organizations, employers, education systems, and, of course, health and mental health providers. Recent advances in dissemination and implementation research offer strategies for promoting sustainable transfer of effective behavioral and psychosocial interventions into widespread practice (cf. Brownson et al., 2007).

2. *All primary care and frontline providers must have the time, information, communication skills, and support staff needed to support patients' behavioral change and ability to participate in their own health decisions.* This imperative is acknowledged in recent health policy. For example, development of the patient-centered medical home concept includes steps to promote greater opportunities to support patients (Goode, Haywood, Wells, & Rhee, 2009; McMillen & Stewart, 2009). However, there is no incentive for incorporation of evidence-based interventions to improve patients' health literacy, lose weight, or accomplish behavioral change. More generally, overcoming disparities means reimagining what we can and cannot expect from primary care. Time constraints such as the proverbial "15 minute" primary care visits are frequently invoked by physicians, policy makers, and researchers as the reason why certain interventions cannot be incorporated into primary care (Bodenheimer & Laing, 2007). However, the "15 minute" visit is not an inviolable law of nature. We need to determine how much time physicians and their support staff need to spend with patients to accomplish different goals. Although evidence-based stepped interventions should be employed to ensure the greatest cost-efficiency, we must insist that sufficient care be provided to accomplish behavioral outcomes.

3. *Hospitals and oncology care providers must provide the highest standard of care for the cancers that they treat.* The wide variation in oncology care available to cancer patients in communities is unacceptable. All oncologists must have access to technology needed to provide the agreed standard of care to all of the patients that they treat (Myers & Teel, 2008). Patients must have access to all available treatment options and assistance to consider the alternatives. Providers have the responsibility to be aware of advances in care of patients that they treat, and they must be held accountable if treatment moves beyond their areas of competence or the technology at their disposal. This may drive more oncologists into collaborative practices, or require them to affiliate with high-volume centers that can offer advanced surgical care, pathology, and clinical trials as needed. Patients rely upon their doctors to provide the best possible care for their condition. To eliminate cancer disparities, we have to make sure that this trust is well founded.

4. *Systems must be in place to ensure that appropriate transitions in care occur in a well-coordinated and timely fashion.* No matter how well each

component of the health care system performs its particular function, patient outcomes are adversely affected by problems in coordination of care and transitions across systems (Feldstein & Glasgow, 2008; Hong, Wright, Gagliardi, & Paszat, 2010). A variety of strategies have been implemented to foster better coordination of cancer care, including multidisciplinary care teams, integrated medical records, and regional health information systems (Lamb et al., 2011). Shared care and colocated care models have been proposed, to ensure integration of necessary oncology follow-up with routine primary care for cancer survivors (Gilbert et al., 2011; Thorne & Truant, 2010). Over the past several years, there has been wide dissemination of patient navigation models to facilitate transitions (Shelton et al., 2011; Yosha et al., 2011). Although patient navigation may provide vital assistance to individuals on a case-by-case basis, navigation may not be the ideal long-term solution to facilitating transitions and coordination of care (Robie, Alexandru, & Bota, 2011; Thorne & Truant, 2010). Rather, it is vital to examine the health system, community, and financial barriers that create the need for navigation in the first place. Navigation programs may serve as stopgap measures until procedures are put into place to reduce fragmentation and poor coordination, and to make it easier for patients to make routine transitions without additional assistance (Nguyen, Tran, Kagawa-Singer, & Foo, 2011; Phillips et al., 2011). This would allow navigation programs to focus on patients experiencing more complex needs or with greater likelihood of getting lost in the system (Guadagnolo et al., 2010; Jean-Pierre et al., 2011; Schapira & Schutt, 2010).

5. *Effective treatment for mental health issues, family functioning, spiritual support, and palliative care should be universally available to all patients.* Mental health is the linchpin of physical health, and we will not succeed in eliminating disparities in access and outcomes along the cancer continuum if we ignore this aspect of health (Kadan-Lottick, Vanderwerker, Block, Zhang, & Prigerson, 2005; Neighbors et al., 2007; Siegel, Hayes, Vanderwerker, Loseth, & Prigerson, 2008). Individuals with untreated psychiatric, substance abuse, and social problems have markedly worse health behaviors, utilization of screening services, and health outcomes. Although evidence-based interventions have been developed to address the emotional and psychosocial needs of cancer patients, these programs are not universally available, particularly in low-income communities and areas that lack major academic centers (Hughes, 2005; Weng et al., 2009). Lack of access to palliative care in minority and low-income communities has also been widely documented (Anderson, Green, & Payne, 2009; Barnato, Anthony, Skinner, Gallagher, & Fisher, 2009; Fitzsimons et al., 2007; Johnson, 2009; O'Mahony et al., 2008). As several of the

authors in this volume argue, eliminating cancer disparities means eliminating undue pain and distress and promoting optimal quality of life (Ashing-Giwa, Lim, & Serrano, Chapter 20).

It is worthwhile to reflect on these imperatives. Although expressed with some urgency, the ideas offered here are hardly radical. After all, why shouldn't all patients benefit from access to well-coordinated systems offering the best available medical, behavioral, and mental health care? From a technical point of view, these solutions are well within our reach. Indeed, if anything, readily available information technology would make it easier to take on these challenges than ever before. Patients anywhere can benefit from the tele-presence of top surgical specialists (Stewart & Switzer, 2011). Expert systems, such as IBM's "Watson," are becoming sophisticated to the point that providers can pose questions about diagnostic and treatment quandaries in natural language. Electronic medical records are being designed to support coordination of care. Patients are gaining the ability to exchange information with providers and obtain information and support from telephone and online resources. Thanks to these emerging technologies, it is possible to imagine more and more ways in which we can increase the availability of state-of-the-art cancer resources to isolated communities and disadvantaged patients (Stewart & Switzer, 2011). On the other hand, even with these technological advantages, doing what we know we must do to eliminate cancer health disparities will take enormous political will and a major investment of money. Many of these solutions would involve changing the clinical practices and business models of health providers and hospitals, insurance companies, and government agencies. We continue to have cancer health disparities because the steps that we must take to truly eliminate them will cut into corporate profits and place additional strain on public resources.

This is the point in discussions of health inequities at which most social and behavioral scientists sign off. Although most of us who conduct research with medically underserved and vulnerable groups are highly concerned about equity and social justice, these issues involve economic and policy decisions that are beyond the scope of our research. It is not even clear if those issues are at all amenable to methods of social science and public health. Despite our best and most creative efforts, the root causes of cancer health disparities often seem intractable and necessary solutions out of reach.

This brings us to the crux of the argument. *Rather than being irrelevant, I contend that the social and behavioral sciences have a fundamental role in making these imperative solutions happen.* Indeed, the scholarship presented in this volume embodies many of the strategies that will be needed. *However, to truly eliminate cancer disparities, it will be necessary to reframe and expand our research to look beyond individual health behavior and access to care, to consider our societal and cultural responses to cancer health disparities and inequitable health care.* If we want to overcome disparities, we must ultimately be concerned about public support for necessary solutions (Small, Harding & Lamont, 2010). There must be a sufficiently broad consensus that elimination of cancer health disparities is a priority for funding, and an issue that will affect consumers' purchases and voters' decisions (Reichlin, 2011).

The concept of using social science to promote social justice may seem quite foreign to many. Yet there is a long-standing tradition in social sciences concerned with fostering the empowerment of underserved communities in the face of political oppression, social disenfranchisement, and economic stress. Consider that in the 1970s and 1980s, many people in the field of community psychology—my field—were concerned with overcoming policies that "blamed the victims" of poverty programs that fostered dependence and made it more difficult for individuals to act on their own behalves. Rappaport (1981) discussed the inherent tensions between a top-down and paternalistic prevention agenda versus an empowerment agenda that provided individuals with resources to discover and organize community solutions to problems that plagued them. Helping disparate groups of stakeholders develop a shared sense of community to foster collective action to improve local conditions was an important theme. Community psychology, and sister disciplines such as action-oriented anthropology, were involved in fostering and supporting social movements in areas such as mental health care, juvenile justice, education, and housing (Schensul & Trickett, 2009).

Although strands of this work are still under way, research in public health has generally distanced itself from community empowerment and advocacy, in favor of individual-level solutions. Over the past 25 years, the emphasis in many areas of public health has been on the development of individual behavioral interventions. The reasons for this shift are many: A cultural backlash against the civil rights and poverty programs of the 1960s and 1970s; the growing reliance on medical-model solutions to psychological, social, and behavioral health problems; the dissolution of the Alcohol, Drug Abuse, and Mental Health Administration, and the incorporation of all federally sponsored social and psychological research under the umbrella of the National Institutes of Health; and the emphasis on top-down randomized trials as the best, if not the only acceptable, approach for identifying solutions to public health problems. To be sure, research on community work in public health has continued and grown to encompass behavioral health promotion and disease prevention, but the emphasis has largely been on discovering how to promote individual-level behavioral change in a wider variety of settings. Changing the underlying conditions of inequity and social injustice that contribute to health disparities has largely been off the table.

LESSONS FROM THE AMERICAN CANCER SOCIETY DISPARITIES RESEARCH PORTFOLIO: STRATEGIES TO MOBILIZE COMMUNITY ACTION

Clearly, the research summarized in this volume offers very important approaches for changing individual health behavior, supporting better decisions, enhancing quality of care, and promoting quality of life. These are the kinds of strategies that must we must bring to scale. However, taking these interventions to scale is largely dependent on the availability of resources and, hence, the political will that our health care system must be rededicated and redesigned to eliminate cancer disparities.

As such, the most important lessons we can draw from these examples involve ways to raise public awareness and build a national consensus for broad-based social policies to eliminate disparities. The studies in this volume demonstrate the kinds of strategies necessary to mobilize and guide a nationwide grassroots campaign to address cancer health disparities in a way that is comprehensive and sustainable. Reading through this volume study after study, it becomes apparent that researchers have arrived at powerful new techniques for activating communities and transforming delivery systems. What remained in writing this closing chapter was simply to recognize and label this potential. The lessons learned fall into eight distinct areas, outlined below:

Lesson 1: Acknowledging individuals' multiple identities, and addressing stigma and discrimination, is empowering. Perhaps the most fundamental cause of health disparities in our society is that we view access to care and healthy living conditions as a privilege rather than as a human right. Public acceptance of inequitable access to health care is tied into politically motivated images and stereotypes that serve to justify disenfranchisement and inequitable treatment (Ryan, 1976). The prevailing social construction of ethnic, sexual, or religious minority groups often includes explanation and justification for why they are to blame for their poor health, unwilling to take care of themselves, or otherwise unworthy of society's benefits. *These stigmatizing attitudes and beliefs are amenable to change by promoting greater familiarity and providing countervailing examples.*

Several studies in this volume help bring to the fore the concerns and the potential of groups that are often ignored or demeaned. For example, Christopher and colleagues (Chapter 12) discuss the history of their work in partnership with the Apsáalooke community. Research of this sort would be impossible without validation of the communities' concerns and ownership of the research process. However, many underserved communities are not geographically centered or as highly organized as the Apsáalooke. Levels of stigma and disorganization can impede evaluation of needs and tailoring of programs. Boehmer and Bowen (Chapter 21) discuss how sexual minority women's social networks and relationships can influence their health behavior. This work offers a rich and nuanced perspective of a social group that has often been subject to stigma and ignorance in the health care system and beyond. These examples show how social science research can help to organize segments of the community, and help give voice and legitimacy to their concerns.

No group in this country suffers from worse health disparities than African American men. However, it is overly simplistic to presume that one-size-fits-all solutions are appropriate for these men. For instance, Griffith and colleagues (Chapter 8) discuss efforts to tailor interventions according to men's multiple identities, to determine competing priorities that interfere with health behavior as well as potential avenues for change. It is noteworthy that settings that may be suitable for reaching some segments of the community (such as workplaces or fraternal organizations) would entirely omit other segments.

Regardless of the specific health behavioral targets or intervention strategies, studies such as these emphasize the efforts of marginalized groups to pursue better health and quality of life. They also highlight some of the historical and social factors that have impeded success. Individual projects such as these serve to express the particular struggles and challenges faced by each group. Taken together, these studies help to put a human face on cancer health disparities statistics. Examples such as these must be communicated to the broader public, to contribute to a greater sense of commonality with disenfranchised groups. It becomes much harder to deny access to health and quality of life to people who are seen as "us" rather than "them."

Lesson 2: Raising public awareness of disparities is a vital tool for mobilizing community support. The introductory chapters of this volume present overwhelming evidence concerning the extent, nature, and consequences of cancer health disparities. These data are absolutely vital for analyzing the extent and nature of disparities. However, what is not clear is whether and to what extent individuals who are subject to these disparities are aware that they exist. Although there have been decades-long campaigns focused on health risk behaviors, there is virtually no widespread or sustained attempt to raise consumer awareness of disparities in cancer care. *The next generation of research to reduce cancer health disparities must include efforts to build public awareness of health disparities, including risk for receiving inaccurate information and substandard care.*

Of course, there have been arguments against releasing information grading physician or hospital outcomes to the general public. The concern is that ratings do not take into account the variation of cases across providers and settings, and that the public is not sophisticated enough to understand this information. As several studies in this volume demonstrate, these problems may be readily addressed. For example, Latini and colleagues (Chapter 17) show how attention to health literacy helped men to understand choices related to prostate cancer, while Makoul and colleagues (Chapter 13) discuss approaches to communicating information about colonoscopy. We have the tools that we need to help many patients understand quantitative concepts such as relative risk and likelihood of benefit. These same concepts can be applied to helping consumers evaluate information about their local health care system. Providing consumers with question lists and other tools can also help them to determine whether that they know what to ask their providers and that they are getting more complete information. *Research related to health literacy must be broadened to help individuals and families become more effective and better informed health care consumers.*

In addition to supporting health literacy interventions to inform consumers, lay health advisors (LHAs) and community health advocates could be trained to help patients understand their choices in care. In the work of Erwin and colleagues (Chapter 15), LHAs employed to encourage individual behavior change are in a great position to also help consumers obtain and interpret information about the treatment facilities and providers available in their communities. Just as we train LHAs to access and provide accurate information about cancer treatment, screening, nutrition, and other topics, we can ensure that they provide appropriate information about local health choices. *We need to develop support systems in communities that can provide guidance and support for active health care consumers.*

Community organizers and change agents for social justice would necessarily share many of the same characteristics that we look for in community LHAs. People in this role must have the skills to share their own stories and elicit these stories from others. They must understand the tacit concerns and assumptions that members of their communities would bring to discussions of health inequities, to anticipate and address these issues. They must be able to establish the trust necessary to encourage community members to take action at the individual level (e.g., insisting on appropriate time and attention from providers) or at the collective level (e.g., participating in meetings to share information about disparities that they have experienced).

Lesson 3: Health care delivery and research must join together to create learning systems. Patient navigation also provides a powerful tool for addressing system sources of health disparities. In programs such as the one described by Hendren and colleagues (Chapter 14), navigators do more than address individual motivation and lack of knowledge. Through their work, navigators necessarily encounter problems in health systems that impede access to screening and care. Information from navigation could be used to determine where to employ quality improvement strategies to reduce disparities, and to evaluate the efficacy of these systemic strategies. Ideally, navigation should not only link individuals to services one at a time; it should contribute to systemic solutions that make navigation less necessary. *Future studies of patient navigation must be conducted in conjunction with systems-level interventions to reduce health disparities.*

The interventions in this volume are already providing a safety net for cancer patients who may be subject to fragmented or poorly coordinated care. It is noteworthy that the Sisters Informing Sisters[SM] intervention by Sheppard and colleagues (Chapter 16) is helping to ensure that women receive adjuvant treatment that ought to be the standard of care. Although it is necessary to assist these women, it is also important to address the reasons why they are falling through the cracks. Data from projects like Sisters Informing Sisters[TM] shed light on systemic problems, and can contribute to systemic solutions by identifying the reasons for gaps in care. Individual-level interventions to ensure that patients receive a widely accepted standard of care are only necessary because the health delivery system is failing to do its job. *Future individual-level interventions to foster access to care must also include systems research to identify and close gaps in care.*

Adams and Chien's (Chapter 11) discussion of the use of linked datasets to examine the impact of policy demonstrates another important lesson. Datasets must be available to track the impact of policy changes on health disparities. What is perhaps most remarkable about Adams' work is the lengths that she needed to go to link datasets so that she could examine the impact of major changes in public health policy on system uptake and performance. For purposes of accountability, stakeholders and researchers should be involved in the implementation of all major policies that affect public health and health disparities. Plans to ensure the rigorous evaluation of performance should be in place before programs are implemented. Involvement of health services researchers in the planning process should help to ensure that data are captured in ways that facilitate implications of programs for health disparities. *Evaluation of public health policy should be a priority from the outset, with mechanisms to gather the necessary information and link databases designed into implementation plans from the outset.*

Lesson 4: Determine points of contact with communities where interventions can be introduced. The intervention studies described in this volume were each successful in finding natural and acceptable ways to intersect with people's lives. For instance, reaching young adolescents through Boy Scout programs (Chapter 7) is a very important example. Clearly, offering these young men incentives and encouragement to engage in healthy behavior is a natural. It is possible to consider taking this to another level in several ways. Scouts and other youth leaders can be empowered to serve as champions for preventive health advocates in their communities.[1]

---

[1] For the sake of full disclosure, the author of this chapter participated in a Boy Scouts Explorer Program for medical careers in his junior year of high school.

Very valuable information about community-specific cancer statistics and the quality of local health care can also be provided in venues such as beauty salons (Linnan et al., Chapter 9) or on line (Anderson et al., Chapter 18). Again, interventions in these settings must be designed to ensure that individuals receive accurate information about health disparities and local choices in care. These settings can also facilitate consumers sharing information with one another about their experiences in care. In fact, it is highly likely that consumers in these settings already exchange information about the quality of doctors, hospitals, screening programs, and the like. Our interventions can support this process by ensuring that information is complete, accurate, and understood in the proper context. *The next generation of research must foster the exchange of information about available health care choices, to help people make decisions about where to go for care.*

Lesson 5: Communities should experience immediate benefits from involvement in research. In addition to specific strategies to promote informed decision making, motivate change, and build necessary skills and supports, many of the interventions in this volume have incorporated "nonspecific" components that are important to the success of health behavioral interventions. These same nonspecific factors are also important to the efforts to promote community support and involvement for social justice efforts. It is necessary to carry out interventions in ways that help people to build their social networks, learn something of value, receive recognition for their accomplishments, or simply have a good time—strategies employed by many of the interventions in this volume. As with any other community interventions, grassroots efforts to eliminate disparities must provide a positive, meaningful experience for participants.

In addition, participants in our interventions may be interested in health careers, including public health research. Our research programs should be involved in facilitating health careers by linking to training programs such as the NCIs CURE opportunities (National Cancer Institute [NCI], 2011). Programs that employ LHAs and other community health workers have also provided entrée to health careers for people in underserved communities. *Future community-based research efforts should be linked to existing and new training opportunities, to broaden health career participation for people in low-income and underrepresented minority communities.*

Lesson 6: Efforts to eliminate cancer disparities must engage the family. Several of the interventions described in this volume have included spouses, partners, and other family members of "target" populations. Focus on the family is intrinsically more complicated and challenging than working with individuals, particularly in underserved communities. At a minimum, involving family members entails logistical challenges, particularly in light of partners' or family caregivers' multiple roles. Family members may also face their own unaddressed health issues. A family history of conflict or communication problems adds even more challenges. In addition, delivery and financing of health services is often organized around individuals rather than families, and providers and settings may not be trained to engage families in care. Nonetheless, the advantages of working with families make it necessary to find ways to overcome these challenges, such as described in the work of Ayala and colleagues (Chapter 10). More generally, implementing health promotion in ways that engage families is more consistent with the kinds of lifestyle changes that people must make in key areas such as diet, physical activity, sexual risks, and tobacco and substance use. Similarly, health decisions are often made in the family context. Empowering consumers means assisting families in making use of information about health care. *The role of the family in reducing cancer health disparities should be a major focus of research across the cancer continuum.*

Lesson 7: Eliminating disparities means enhancing quality of life. The research by both Ashing-Giwa and colleagues (Chapter 20) and Moadel and colleagues (Chapter 19) offers an interesting and important twist on the question of health disparities by focusing on diminished quality-of-life outcomes. This is a critical focus, especially if we are concerned about consumer empowerment. Recent research in the area of quality-of-life appraisal and response shift (Rapkin & Schwartz, 2004) suggests that people vary widely in the personal criteria and standards of comparison that they use to evaluate their own quality of life. Consumer empowerment means ensuring that people are evaluating their health and well-being and the quality of care available to them using appropriately high standards and expectations. In fact, helping to raise people's standards and expectations for their own health or the quality of care that they receive may lead to expressions of dissatisfaction and reduced ratings of quality of life. This brings the discussion of our future research agenda full circle. Making people aware of disparities and inequities in their lives is a necessary part of the empowerment process, and such awareness may contribute to a diminished level of quality of life, increased medical mistrust, and a reduced sense of control. From an ethical point of view, it seems more acceptable to make people aware of the disparities that they face than to skirt the issue or encourage them to access care that we know is substandard. Nonetheless, pursuing a consumer empowerment agenda means that interventions must strive to ensure that people have ways to act on their own behalf to improve their access to quality. For example, in some communities, there may simply be no good options for quality cancer care for anyone, or for people with the wrong type of health insurance. Raising awareness of this fact makes it possible for health consumers and their families to take action on their own behalf. *Research on empowerment-oriented interventions must be concerned with raising individuals' standards for quality of life, and ensuring that avenues to take action on their own behalf are available.*

Lesson 8: Theoretical constructs and frameworks that guide health behavioral and decision-making interventions are highly relevant to community mobilization and organizing. Several authors in this volume have discussed the importance of theory in designing interventions. Theoretical aspects included intrapersonal, interpersonal, and social contextual factors that could impact health behavior. Very similar theoretical constructs can be brought to bear to understand factors that would help raise individual awareness of the health disparities that affect them, their families, and their communities. For example, the PEN-3 framework (Sheppard et al., Chapter 16; Erwin et al., Chapter 15) includes constructs to identify factors that affect desired behaviors. Individuals necessarily hold positive, existential, and negative perceptions about the forces that affect the quality of health care available in their communities, and their ability to take actions. Enabling factors might include providing them with evidence about the comparative quality of care, or strategies that have been implemented in other communities to reduce disparities. Community organizing to promote awareness of others with similar concerns and a shared sense of struggle may help to nurture and sustain grassroots action.

Another important concept is the notion of intervention tailoring. Several of the interventions discussed in this volume build in procedures to assess the needs and priorities of individuals at the point of intervention delivery, to ensure that approaches are most responsive to individual circumstances. Tailoring is also relevant to community organizing. Determining and addressing individuals' sources of greatest concern, or the most daunting barriers to involvement, must be a critical component to efforts to empower communities. It is certainly possible to imagine community organizers using a motivational interviewing approach to better understand how to engage individuals in taking action at a variety of levels. A number of the interventions described in this volume have incorporated multiple components, to support individuals through a progression of changes. A similar logic can be applied to community-organizing efforts.

As Griffith and colleagues (Chapter 8) discuss, tailoring must address both surface and deep-level realities and concerns. As with behavioral interventions, initiatives to expand social justice in health care must be appealing, accessible, and practical in order to encourage community participation. At a deeper level, interventions must take into account communities' narratives of political struggle, transitions, and efforts to achieve quality of life. Interventions may need to elicit these narratives to guide change or to help communities develop alternatives to narratives of hopelessness and inevitable defeat. This can be an advantage of rooting interventions in geographically defined settings (Landrine et al., Chapter 6). Clearly, in many communities, spirituality and religious identity may be an important part of these narratives, just as they are in other struggles for civil rights and social justice.

TRANSFORMING CANCER HEALTH DISPARITIES RESEARCH TO PLACE SOCIAL JUSTICE AT THE CORE

As the lessons gleaned from the studies in this volume amply demonstrate, concepts and techniques that have been used successfully to bring people together for interventions and motivate behavioral change can be readily applied to efforts to empower health care consumers, build local capacity for delivering and adapting effective programs and services, and hold the health care system accountable for effective prevention and outcomes of cancer care. Nonetheless, it is a very different thing to conduct a study to help people quit smoking, or get a mammogram compared to a study to help people hold their local doctors and hospitals accountable for high-quality care. We have come to accept the aims of research to promote health behavior as legitimate, scientific questions. Is the same true for research to promote equitable treatment in health care and social justice, or is this tantamount to hijacking science for a political agenda? Should scarce research resources be spent on organizing communities and building self-advocacy skills to demand better health care in poor and underserved communities, rather than continuing to incrementally find ways to help individuals modify behaviors that we know lead to cancer?

Of course, in some ways this is a false dichotomy. For example, efforts to promote screening or smoking cessation could serve as an entrée to broader consumer education and empowerment. *Even so, it is important to address a key ethical question.* The justification for encouraging individuals to take a particular test or eat particular foods is that scientific research has shown that it is good for them. We do not have this same sort of justification when it comes to social justice. We cannot say that providing consumers with information about the poor quality of cancer care available in their community will be helpful. Even though we may have ample evidence that individuals in some communities are at high risk for receiving substandard care, we do not (yet) know whether there is any direct benefit if we raise awareness and help them to act on this information. Indeed, such information might be construed as harmful if it scares people away from necessary treatment.

However, there is another ethical dimension to this discussion. Much of our research is predicated on findings that strongly link cancer disparities to conditions of poverty and inequitable distribution of health resources. Is it ethical to withhold (or fail to actively communicate) this information? No matter how effective our efforts to promote health behavior, improve patient–provider communication or even enhance conditions in specific neighborhoods or communities, we researchers know that the findings of all of the individual research projects sponsored by the American Cancer Society (ACS), the NCI, and other major funders are highly unlikely to alter cancer disparities without major investment to get these programs into practice. Shouldn't research participants also be made aware of this, as part of providing informed consent? Should the lack of social justice in health care be part of the risk–benefits equation in research participation (Powell, Rapkin, & Weiss, 2009)? More generally, even without guarantee of benefit, shouldn't individuals have the right to know about the quality of health care available to them, to make informed choices in care? As Rappaport (1981) argued 30 years ago, this discussion reflects the tension between medical paternalism and patient empowerment, between a system driven by attention to caring for patient needs versus helping them to exercise and attain their human rights.

It is no coincidence that this portfolio of ACS-supported studies on health disparities uses methods and concepts that are so consonant with the social justice agenda. We have arrived at a point in the development of our understanding of science and public health at which we can no longer rest with the assumption that "normal science," predicated on a needs-based, individual-level, medical-model approach to overcoming health disparities, is viable. Rather, we are in the midst of a paradigm shift that involves a rethinking of the ways in which research can contribute to the elimination of cancer health disparities and other pervasive inequities in health care. *Rather than being anti-scientific, the social justice agenda must propel this paradigm shift.*

Recently, the NCI and other agencies have called upon the research community to consider a new generation of research designs and methods, to foster dissemination of evidence-based interventions. For example, the NCI has produced recommendations based on an ongoing series of "Dialogues on Dissemination" (NCI, 2010). Specific suggestions include support for community organizations involved in dissemination, incorporation of surveillance systems to monitor intervention implementation, and uptake of evidence-based practices. Key strategies include the need to involve representative stakeholders from all who might potentially benefit from dissemination (Barton-Villagrana, Bedney, & Miller, 2002; Miller & Shinn, 2005; Yoshikawa et al., 2003), to establish lasting partnerships between investigators and community collaborators (Altman, 1994; Lamb, Greenlick, & McCarty, 1998), to encourage a culture of evidence-based practice with community organizations (Foster-Fishman, Berkowitz, Lounsbury, Jacobsen, & Allen, 2001; Guerra & Knox, 2008), to create models of collaboration based on mutual self-interest (Wandersman, 2003; Stokols et al., 2005), and to make it easier for communities to institutionalize evidence-based strategies

(Goodman, McLeroy, Steckler, & Holye, 1993;Goodman & Steckler, 1989). Recommended areas of study for dissemination research include factors that affect adoptions of innovation in practice, studies of motivational factors that affect implementation and uptake at multiple levels, research on the effective use of change agents, and contextual factors that influence and support implementation. The NCI has emphasized that research designs must move beyond exclusively individual outcomes to also address systems- and population-level changes, with priority given to targeted dissemination efforts able to reach middle-to-late adopters of evidence-based practices (Von Eschenbach, 2003).

There is great potential for dissemination research to foster social justice in the service of eliminating health disparities. To realize this potential, dissemination research must eschew the traditional medical-model view of dissemination, which places a premium on direct replication of behavioral interventions with high fidelity to core elements. There is a very strong scientific and ethical rationale for moving away from top-down technology transfer (Bull, Gillette, Glasgow, & Estabrooks, 2003; Glasgow, 2003; Glasgow, Goldstein, Ockene, & Pronk, 2004; Kerner, 2002). Due to an almost complete lack of attention to external validity in research, we cannot claim with any certainty that an intervention found to be effective in one setting will be equally efficacious in another setting (Bonfill Cosp, Marzo Castillejo, Pladevall Vila, Marti, & Emparanza, 2001; Green, 2001; Green & Glasgow, 2006; Greenhalgh, Robert, Macfarlane, Bate, & Kyriakadou, 2004). Thus, it is generally not warranted to offer behavioral interventions to communities as well-established solutions or best practices. Rather, the most rigorous way to gain any clarity on the question of "what to disseminate" is to try out different interventions in different places (Brownson et al., 2007; Green & Ottoson, 2004). This would allow us to gain an understanding of "program-context interaction" through what Green and Glasgow (2006) refer to as practice-based evidence. Green and Ottoson (2004) discuss dissemination as a joint process of problem-solving, involving key stakeholders in making decisions about proper approaches to implement in different contexts. Similarly, Sandler (2007) argues that it is necessary to engage communities in critical thinking and reflection about what programs they need and how they are working.

The key is that we cannot expect to overcome disparities by applying any particular solution in a given community. Rather, research must foster a shared process of critical reflection and problem-solving over time, using scientific methods to progressively arrive at optimal solutions for specific settings. We need to stop funding research designed to be "definitive trials," intended to establish universal "intervention effects." Rather, *the science that we need to overcome disparities will be advanced by garnering a deep understanding of how to use behavioral science principles, methods, and interventions to support community problem-solving.*

In addition to being scientifically and ethically superior, community-engaged approaches to dissemination of evidence-based practice provide a strong platform for advancing social justice. There is no better way to foster this scientific direction than to expand the criteria that reviewers consider in evaluating research proposals and journal articles. Lessons learned from the portfolio of ACS-supported research presented in this volume point to criteria that will serve to ensure that the next generation of cancer health disparities interventions advances social justice. Consider how emphasis on the following review criteria would start to transform the science of cancer health disparities:

1. Does the research foster community ownership of research methods as a problem-solving strategy to stimulate ongoing community dialogue about disparities and health promotion based on research?
2. Are intervention outcomes understood in terms of improvement in indicators of overall performance, including reach, efficiency, sustainability, and fit with the local service ecology, not merely efficacy?
3. Do interventions designs incorporate quality improvement and tailoring strategies to maximize intervention performance in the local community?
4. Does research empower health consumers by increasing the communities' understanding of local cancer health disparities and by providing action steps to address those disparities?
5. Does the research project increase the accountability of local providers and make it possible for providers to earn the greater trust of the community through effective communications and improved services?
6. Does the research provide information needed by policy makers to guide allocation of resources?
7. Does the research project offer opportunities for leadership, skill development, and access to health careers for local community members?
8. Does the intervention make provisions to include people experiencing multiple physical, psychological, and/or social problems that may interfere with intervention outcomes?
9. Does the research champion the value of diversity, and enhance the social identities of groups that are subject to marginalization, disenfranchisement, and stigma?
10. Does the intervention strive to affect all relevant outcomes, including noncancer-specific outcomes such as better access to primary care and improved overall quality of life?

11. Does the research contribute to a transparent, ongoing relationship between care providers, community stakeholders, and academic researchers that extends beyond the life of any one study?
12. Will planned analyses place findings in context, to permit comparison with other studies and to determine the external validity of results?

Each of these criteria may be operationally defined and evaluated in the context of grant review, and in the evaluation of studies for inclusion in meta-analysis and the like. Of course, there is considerable need to determine standards for how research projects can incorporate these criteria. Nonetheless, thinking of quality research in these dimensions (as opposed to applying the randomized control trial as the single standard of excellence) would go a long way in fostering research to address the sources of social injustice that underlie cancer health disparities.

REFERENCES

Adler, N., Stewart, J., Cohen, S., Cullen, M., Diez Roux, A., Dow, W., . . . Williams, D. (2007). *Reaching for a healthier life: Facts on socioeconomic status and health in the United States.* San Francisco, CA: The John D. and Catherine T. MacArthur Foundation Research Network on Socioeconomic Status and Health.

Albano, J.D., Ward, E., Jemal, A., Anderson, R., Cokkinides, V.E., Murray, T., . . . Thun, M. J. (2007). Cancer mortality in the United States by education level and race. *Journal of the National Cancer Institute, 99,* 1384–1394.

Alegría, M. (2009). Training for research in mental health and HIV/AIDS among racial and ethnic minority populations: Meeting the needs of new investigators. *American Journal of Public Health, 99*(Suppl. 1), S26–S30.

Altman, D. (1994). *Power and community: Organizational and cultural responses to AIDS.* Bristol, PA: Taylor & Francis.

Anderson, K. O., Green, C. R., & Payne, R. (2009). Racial and ethnic differences in preferences for end-of-life treatment. *Journal of Pain, 10,* 1187–1204.

Avendano, M., Glymour, M. M., Banks, J., & Mackenbach, J. P. (2009). Health disadvantage in U.S. adults aged 50 to 74 years: A comparison of the health of rich and poor Americans with that of Europeans. *American Journal of Public Health, 99,* 540–548.

Barnato, A. E., Anthony, D. L., Skinner, J., Gallagher, P. M., & Fisher, E. S. (2009). Racial and ethnic differences in preferences for end-of-life treatment. *Journal of General Internal Medicine, 24,* 695–701.

Barton-Villagrana, H., Bedney, B. J., & Miller, R. L. (2002). Peer relationships among community-based organizations providing HIV prevention services. *Journal of Primary Prevention, 23,* 217–236.

Bodenheimer, T., & Laing, B. Y. (2007). The teamlet model of primary care. *Annals of Family Medicine, 5* (5), 457–461.

Bonfill Cosp, X., Marzo Castillejo, M., Pladevall Vila, M., Marti, J., & Emparanza, J. I. (2001). Strategies for increasing the participation of women in community breast cancer screening. *Cochrane Database of Systematic Reviews* (1), CD002943.

Boyer, C. A., & Lutfey, K. E. (2010). Examining critical health policy issues within and beyond the clinical encounter: Patient–provider relationships and help-seeking behaviors. *Journal of Health and Social Behavior, 51*(Suppl.), S80–S93.

Brownson, R. C., Ballew, P., Dieffenderfer, B., Haire-Joshu, D., Heath, G. W., Kreuter, M. W., . . . Myers, B. A. (2007). Evidence-based interventions to promote physical activity: What contributes to dissemination by state health departments? *American Journal of Preventive Medicine, 33*(Suppl.1), S66–S73.

Brunner, E., & Marmot, M. (2006). Social organization, stress and health. In M. Marmot & R. G. Wilkinson (Eds.), *Social determinants of health* (2nd ed., pp. 6–30). Oxford, UK: Oxford University Press.

Bull, S. S., Gillette, C., Glasgow, R. E., & Estabrooks, P. (2003). Worksite health promotion research: To what extent can we generalize the results and what is needed to translate research to practice? *Health Education and Behavior, 30*, 537–549.

Burgess, D.J. (2010). Are providers more likely to contribute to healthcare disparities under high levels of cognitive load? How features of the healthcare setting may lead to biases in medical decision making. *Medical Decision Making, 30*, 246–257.

Byers, T. (2010). Two decades of declining cancer mortality: Progress with disparity. *Annual Review Public Health, 31*, 121–132.

Cargill, V. A. (2009). Recruiting, retaining, and maintaining racial and ethnic minority investigators: Why we should bother, why we should care. *American Journal of Public Health, 99*, S5–S7.

Chen, J., Gee, G. C., Spencer, M. S., Danziger, S. H., & Takeuchi, D. T. (2009). Perceived social standing among Asian immigrants in the US: Do reasons for immigration matter? *Social Science Research, 38*(4), 858–869.

Cullum, R., Alder, O., & Hoodless, P. A. (2011). The next generation: Using new sequencing technologies to analyse gene regulation. *Respirology, 16*, 210–222.

DeLancey, J., Thun, M., Jemal, A., & Ward, E. (2008). Recent Black–White disparities in cancer mortality. *Cancer Epidemiology, Biomarkers & Prevention,17*, 2908–2912.

Dixon, L. B., Medoff, D., Goldberg, R., Lucksted, A., Kreyenbuhl, J., DiClemente, C., . . . Afful, J. (2009). Is implementation of the 5 A's of smoking cessation at community mental health centers effective for reduction of smoking by patients with serious mental illness? *American Journal of Addiction, 18*(5), 386–392.

Epstein, R. M., Fiscella, K., Lesser, C. S., & Stange, K. C. (2010). Why the nation needs a policy push on patient-centered health care. *Health Affairs (Millwood), 29*, 1489–1495.

Errickson, S. P., Alvarez, M., Forquera, R., Whitehead, T. L., Fleg, A., Hawkins, T., . . . Schoenbach, V. J. (2011). What will health-care reform mean for minority health disparities? *Public Health Reports, 126*, 170–175.

Feldstein, A. C., Glasgow, R. E. (2008). A Practical, Robust Implementation and Sustainability Model (PRISM) for integrating research findings into practice. *Joint Commission Journal on Quality and Patient Safety, 34*(4), 228–243.

Fiscella, K. (2011). Health care reform and equity: Promise, pitfalls, and prescriptions. *Annals of Family Medicine, 9*, 78–84.

Fitzsimons, D., Mullan, D., Wilson, J. S., Conway, B., Corcoran, B., Dempster, M., . . . Fogarty, D. (2007). The challenge of patients' unmet palliative care needs in the final stages of chronic illness. *Palliative Medicine, 21*, 313–322.

Foster-Fishman, P. G., Berkowitz, S. L., Lounsbury, D. W., Jacobsen, S., & Allen, N. A. (2001). Building collaborative capacity in community coalitions: A review and integrative framework. *American Journal of Community Psychology, 29,* 241–261.

Gilbert, J. E., Green, E., Lankshear, S., Hughes, E., Burkoski, V., & Sawka, C. (2011). Nurses as patient navigators in cancer diagnosis: Review, consultation and model design. *European Journal of Cancer Care, 20,* 228–236.

Glasgow, R. E. (2003). Translating research to practice: Lessons learned areas for improvement, and future directions. *Diabetes Care, 26,* 2451–2456.

Glasgow, R. E., Goldstein, M. G., Ockene, J., & Pronk, N. P. (2004). Translating what we have learned into practice: Principles and hypotheses for addressing multiple behaviors in primary care. *American Journal of Preventive Medicine, 27,* 88–101.

Goldsmith, B., Dietrich, J., Du, Q., & Morrison, R. S. (2008). Variability in access to hospital palliative care in the United States. *Journal of Palliative Medicine, 11,* 1094–1102.

Goode, T. D., Haywood, S. H., Wells, N., & Rhee, K. (2009). Family-centered, culturally, and linguistically competent care: Essential components of the medical home. *PediatricAnnals, 38,* 505–512.

Goodman, R. M., & Steckler, A. (1989). A model for the institutionalization of health promotion programs. *Family and Community Health, 11*(4), 63–78.

Goodman, R. M., McLeroy, K. R., Steckler, A., & Hoyle, R. H. (1993). Development of level of institutionalization (LoIn) scales for health promotion programs. *Health Education Quarterly, 20*(2), 161–178.

Green, L.W. (2001). From research to "best practices" in other settings and populations. *American Journal of Health Behavior, 25,* 165–178.

Green, L. W., & Glasgow, R. E. (2006). Evaluating the relevance, generalization, and applicability of research: Issues in external validity and translation methodology. *Evaluation & Health Professions, 29,* 126–153.

Green, L. W., & Ottoson, J. M. (2004). *From efficacy to effectiveness to community and back: Evidence-based practice vs. practice-based evidence.* Paper presented at "From Clinical Trials to Community: The Science of Translating Diabetes and Obesity Research," Bethesda, MD.

Greenhalgh, T., Robert, G., Macfarlane, F., Bate, P., & Kyriakadou, O. (2004). Diffusion of innovations in service organizations: Systematic review and recommendations. *The Milbank Quarterly, 82*(4), 581–629.

Guadagnolo, B. A., Boylan, A., Sargent, M., Koop, D., Brunette, D., Kanekar, S., . . . Petereit, D. G.(2010). Patient navigation for American Indians undergoing cancer treatment: Utilization and impact on care delivery in a regional healthcare center. *Cancer* Retrieved April 1, 2001 from http://onlinelibrary.wiley.com/doi/10.1002/cncr.25823/pdf

Guerra, N. G., Knox, L. (2008). How culture impacts the dissemination and implementation of innovation: A case study of the Families and Schools Together program (FAST) for preventing violence with immigrant Latino youth. *American Journal of Community Psychology, 41*(3–4), 304–313.

Hasnain-Wynia, R., Baker, D. W., Nerenz, D., Feinglass, J., Beal, A. C., Landrum, M. B., . . . Weissman, J. S. (2007). Disparities in health care are driven by where minority patients seek care: Examination of the hospital quality alliance measures. *Archive of Internal Medicine, 167,* 1233–1239.

Hong, N. J., Wright, F. C., Gagliardi, A. R., & Paszat, L. F. (2010). Examining the potential relationship between multidisciplinary cancer care and patient survival: An international literature review. *Journal of Surgical Oncology, 102,* 125–134.

Hughes, A. (2005). Racial and ethnic disparities in pain: Causes and consequences of unequal care. *International Journal of Palliative Nursing, 11,* 6–13.

Institute of Medicine. (2006). *Examining the health disparities research plan of the National Institutes of Health: Unfinished business.* Washington, DC: National Research Council, Institute of Medicine National Academies Press.

Jean-Pierre, P., Fiscella, K., Freund, K. M., Clark, J., Darnell, J., Holden, A., . . . Patient Navigation Program Group. (2011). Structural and reliability analysis of a patient satisfaction with cancer-related care measure: A multisite patient navigation research program study. *Cancer, 117,* 854–861.

Jemal, A., Siegel, R., Xu, J., & Ward, E. (2010). Cancer statistics, 2010. *CA: A Cancer Journal for Clinicans, 60,* 277–300.

Johnson, M. R. D. (2009). End of life care in ethnic minorities. *British Medical Journal, 338,* a2989.

Kadan-Lottick, N. S., Vanderwerker, L. C., Block, S. D., Zhang, B., & Prigerson, H. G. (2005). Psychiatric disorders and mental health service use in patients with advanced cancer. A report from the coping with cancer study. *Cancer, 104,* 2872–2881.

Kerner, J. F. (2002). *Closing the gap between discovery and delivery.* Washington, DC: National Cancer Institute.

Kim, A. E., Kumanyika, S., Shive, D., Igweatu, U., & Kim, S. H. (2010). Coverage and framing of racial and ethnic health disparities in US newspapers, 1996–2005. *American Journal of Public Health, 1,* S224–S231.

Lamb, B.W., Brown, K.F., Nagpal, K., Vincent, C., Green, J. S., & Sevdalis, N. (2011). Quality of care management decisions by multidisciplinary cancer teams: A systematic review. *Annals of Surgical Oncology, 18*(8), 2116–2125.

Lamb, S., Greenlick, M. R., & McCarty, D. (1998). *Bridging the gap between practice and research: Forging partnerships with community-based drug and alcohol treatment.* Washington, DC: National Academies Press.

Lamont, M., & Small, M. L. (2008). How culture matters: Enriching our understanding of poverty. In Linn, A. C., & Harris, D. R. (Eds.), *The colors of poverty* (pp. 76–102). New York: Russell Sage Foundation.

Like, R. C. (2008). Culturally competent medicine: An American perspective. *Diversity in Health & Social Care, 5*(2), 83– 86.

MacDonald, D. J., Blazer, K. R., & Weitzel, J. N. (2010). Extending comprehensive cancer center expertise in clinical cancer genetics and genomics to diverse communities: The power of partnership. *Journal ofthe NationalComprehensive Cancer Network, 8,* 615–624.

McAlearney, A. S., Reeves, K. W., Dickinson, S. L., Kelly, K. M., Tatum, C., Katz, M. L., & Paskett, E. D. (2008). Racial differences in colorectal cancer screening practices and knowledge within a low-income population. *Cancer, 112,* 391–398.

McMillen, M., & Stewart, E. (2009). The patient-centered medical home: 12 tips to help you lead the way. *Family Practice Management, 16,* 15–18.

Miller, R. L., & Shinn, M. (2005). Learning from communities: Overcoming difficulties in dissemination of prevention and promotion effort. *American Journal of Community Psychology, 35*(3–4), 169–183.

Myers, J. S., & Teel, C. (2008). Oncology nurses' awareness of cognitive impairment secondary to chemotherapy. *Clinical Journal of Oncology Nursing, 12,* 725–729.

National Cancer Institute (2010). *Dialogue on dissemination: Facilitating dissemination research and implementation of evidence-based cancer prevention, early detection, and treatment practices.* Retrieved from http://cancercontrol.cancer.gov/d4d/info_dod.html

National Cancer Institute (2011). *Continuing Umbrella of Research Experiences (CURE).* Retrieved from http://crchd.cancer.gov/diversity/cure-overview.html

Neighbors, H. W., Caldwell, C., Williams, D.R., Nesse, R., Taylor, R. J., Bullard, K. M., . . . Jackson, J. S. (2007). Race, ethnicity, and the use of services for mental disorders. *Archive of General Psychiatry, 64,* 485–494.

Nguyen, T. U., Tran, J. H., Kagawa-Singer, M., & Foo, M. A. (2011). A qualitative assessment of community-based breast health navigation services for Southeast Asian women in Southern California: Recommendations for developing a navigator training curriculum. *American Journal of Public Health, 101,* 87–93.

O'Mahony, S., McHenry, J., Snow, D., Cassin, C., Schumacher, D., & Selwyn, P. A. (2008). A review of barriers to utilization of the Medicare hospice benefits in urban populations and strategies for enhanced access. *Journal of Urban Health, 85,* 281–290.

Ostroff, R. M., Bigbee, W. L., Franklin, W, Gold, L., Mehan, M., Miller, Y. E., . . . Brody, E. N. (2010). Unlocking biomarker discovery: Large scale application of aptamer proteomic technology for early detection of lung cancer. *PLoS One,5*(12), e15003.

Paradies, Y. (2006). A systematic review of empirical research on self-reported racism and health. *InternationalJournal of Epidemiology, 35,* 888–901.

Paredes, M. J. (2008). Quality of health care. *Issue Brief Health Policy Track Service, 7,* 1–21.

Patel, S., Peacock, S. M., McKinley, R. K., Clark Carter, D., & Watson, P. J. (2009). GPs' experience of managing chronic pain in a South Asian community: A qualitative study of the consultation process. *Journal of Health Psychology, 14*(7), 909–918.

Peterson, N. B., Dwyer, K. A., Mulvaney, S. A., Dietrich, M. S., & Rothman, R. L. (2007). The influence of health literacy on colorectal cancer screening knowledge, beliefs and behavior. *Journal of the National Medicine Association, 99,* 1105–1112.

Phillips, C. E., Rothstein, J. D., Beaver, K., Sherman, B. J., Freund, K. M., & Battaglia, T. A. (2011). Patient navigation to increase mammography screening among inner city women. *Journal of General Internal Medicine, 26,*123–129.

Powell, T., Rapkin, B. D., & Weiss, E. S. (2009). Participating in biomedical research. *Journal of the American Medical Association, 302* (20), 2201.

Price, R.A. (2010). Association between physician specialty and uptake of new medical technologies: HPV tests in Florida Medicaid. *Journal of General Internal Medicine, 25,* 1178–1185.

Rapkin, B. D., & Schwartz, C. E. (2004). Toward a theoretical model of quality-of-life appraisal: Implications of findings from studies of response shift. *Health and Quality of Life Outcomes, 2,* 14. Retrieved from http://www.hqlo.com/content/2/1/14

Rappaport, J. (1981). In praise of paradox. A social policy of empowerment over prevention. *American Journal of Community Psychology, 9*(1), 1–25.

Reichlin, M. (2011). The role of solidarity in social responsibility for health. *Medicine Health Care &* Philosophy, 27, 179–195.

Reynolds, K. S., Hanson, L.C., Henderson, M., & Steinhauser, K. E. (2008). End-of-life care in nursing home settings: Do race or age matter? *Palliative & Supportive Care, 6*, 21–27.

Robie, L., Alexandru, D., & Bota, D. A. (2011). The use of patient navigators to improve cancer care for Hispanic patients. *Clinical Medical Insights: Oncology, 2*, 1–7.

Ryan, W. (1976). *Blaming the victim*. New York: Vintage Books.

Sandler, J. (2007). Community-based practices. Integrating dissemination theory with critical theories of power and justice. *American Journal of Community Psychology, 40*, 272–289.

Schapira, L., & Schutt, R. (2010). Training community health workers about cancer clinical trials. *Journal of Immigrant & Minority Health*. DOI: 10.1007/s10903-010-9432-7.

Schensul, J. J., & Trickett, E. (2009). Introduction to multi-level community based culturally situated interventions. *American Journal of Community Psychology, 43* (3–4), 232–240.

Shariff-Marco, S., Klassen, A., & Bowie, J. V. (2010). Racial/ethnic differences in self-reported racism and its association with cancer-related health behaviors. *American Journal of Public Health, 100*, 364–374.

Shelton, R. C., Thompson, H. S., Jandorf, L., Varela, A., Oliveri, B., Villagra, C., . . . Redd, W. H.(2011). Training experiences of lay and professional patient navigators for colorectal cancer screening. *Journal of Cancer Education, 26*(2), 277–284.

Siegel, M. D., Hayes, E., Vanderwerker, L. C., Loseth, D. B., & Prigerson, H. G. (2008). Psychiatric illness in the next of kin of patients who die in the intensive care unit. *CriticalCare Medicine, 36*, 1722–1728.

Singal, A. G., & Marrero, J. A. (2010). Recent advances in the treatment of hepatocellular carcinoma. *Current Opinion in Gastroenterology, 26*, 189–195.

Small, M. L., Harding, D., & Lamont, M. (2010). Reconsidering culture and poverty. *Annals of the American Academy of Political and Social Science, 629*, 6–27.

Smith, J. (2005). Unraveling the SES–health connection. In Waite, L. (Ed.), *Aging, health, and public policy: Demographic and economic perspectives*. New York, NY: Population Council.

Smith, C. B., Bonomi, M., Packer, S., Wisnivesky, J. P. (2011) Disparities in lung cancer stage, treatment and survival among American Indians and Alaskan Natives. *Lung Cancer, 72*(2), 160–164.

Stewart, S. F., & Switzer, J. A. (2011). Perspectives on telemedicine to improve stroke treatment. *Drugs Today, 47*, 157–167.

Stockdale, S., Wells, K.B., Tang, L., Belin, T. R., Zhang, L., & Sherbourne, C. D. (2007). The importance of social context: Neighborhood stressors, stress-buffering mechanisms, and alcohol, drug, and mental health disorders. *Social Science & Medicine 65*, 1867–1881.

Stokols, D., Harvey, R., Gress, J., Fuqua, J., & Phillips, K. (2005). In vivo studies of transdisciplinary scientific collaboration: Lessons learned and implications for active living research. *American Journal of Preventive Medicine, 28*(2S2), 202–213.

Terry, F. (2006). *Diversity in the physician workforce* Retrieved March 31, 2011 from http://www.aamc.org/diversity/start.htm

Thorne, S., & Truant, T. (2010). Will designated patient navigators fix the problem? Oncology nursing in transition. *Cancer Oncology & Nursing Journal, 20*, 116–128.

U.S. Census Bureau. (2011). Retrieved March 31, 2011, from http://www.census.gov

U.S. Department of Health and Human Services. (2011). *Healthy people 2020*. Retrieved April 1, 2011, from http://www.healthypeople.gov

Varkey, A. B., Manwell, B., Williams, E.S., Ibrahim, S. A., Brown, R. L., Bobula, J. A., . . . MEMO Investigators. (2009). Separate and unequal: Clinics where minority and nonminority patients receive primary care. *Archives of Internal Medicine, 169,* 243–250.

Von Eschenbach, A. (2003). NCI sets goal of eliminating suffering and death due to cancer by 2015. *Journal of the National Medical Association, 95,* 637–639.

Wandersman, A. (2003). Community science: Bridging the gap between science and practice with community-centered models. *American Journal of Community Psychology, 31,* 227–242.

Weng, L. C., Huang, H. L., Wilkie, D. J., Hoenig, N. A., Suarez, M. L., Marschke, M., & Durham, J. (2009). Predicting survival with the Palliative Performance Scale in a minority-serving hospice and palliative care program. *Journal of Pain & Symptom Management, 37,* 642–648.

Yosha, A. M., Carroll, J. K., Hendren, S., Salamone, C. M., Sanders, M., Fiscella, K., & Epstein, R. M. (2011). Patient navigation from the paired perspectives of cancer patients and navigators: A qualitative analysis. *Patient Education and Counseling, 82,* 396–401.

Yoshikawa, H., Wilson, P. A., Hsueh, J., Rosman, E. A., Chin, J., & Kim, J. H. (2003). What front-line CBO staff can tell us about culturally anchored theories of behavior change in HIV prevention for Asian/Paci?c Islanders American. *Journal of Community Psychology, 32,* 143–158.

Index